Inherited Metabolic Epilepsies

Inherited Metabolic Epilepsies

Phillip L. Pearl, MD
Division Chief, Child Neurology
Children's National Medical Center
Professor of Neurology, Pediatrics, and Music
The George Washington University School of Medicine and
Columbian College of Arts and Sciences
Washington, DC

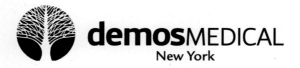

demosMEDICAL
New York

Visit our website at www.demosmedpub.com

ISBN: 9781936287253
e-book ISBN: 9781617050565

Acquisitions Editor: Beth Barry
Compositor: Techset composition

Medicine is an ever-changing science. Research and clinical experience are continually expanding our knowledge, in particular our understanding of proper treatment and drug therapy. The authors, editors, and publisher have made every effort to ensure that all information in this book is in accordance with the state of knowledge at the time of production of the book. Nevertheless, the authors, editors, and publisher are not responsible for errors or omissions or for any consequences from application of the information in this book and make no warranty, express or implied, with respect to the contents of the publication. Every reader should examine carefully the package inserts accompanying each drug and should carefully check whether the dosage schedules mentioned therein or the contraindications stated by the manufacturer differ from the statements made in this book. Such examination is particularly important with drugs that are either rarely used or have been newly released on the market.

Library of Congress Cataloging-in-Publication Data

Inherited metabolic epilepsies / [edited by] Phillip L. Pearl.
    p. ; cm.
 Includes bibliographical references and index
 ISBN 978-1-936287-25-3 - - ISBN 978-1-61705-056-5 (e-book)
 I. Pearl, Phillip L.
 [DNLM: 1. Brain Diseases, Metabolic, Inborn - - complications. 2. Epilepsy - - etiology. 3. Brain Diseases, Metabolic, Inborn - - diagnosis. 4. Brain Diseases, Metabolic, Inborn - - therapy. 5. Epilepsy - - diagnosis. 6. Epilepsy - - therapy. WL 385]
   616.85'3–dc23- -dc23

2012023320

Special discounts on bulk quantities of Demos Medical Publishing books are available to corporations, professional associations, pharmaceutical companies, health care organizations, and other qualifying groups. For details, please contact:

Special Sales Department
Demos Medical Publishing, LLC
11 West 42nd Street, 15th Floor
New York, NY 10036
Phone: 800-532-8663 or 212-683-0072
Fax: 212-941-7842
E-mail: rsantana@demosmedpub.com

Printed in the United States of America by Strategic Content Imaging.
15 16 17/9 8 7 6 5

*This book is dedicated to my wife, Maria Tartaglia Pearl, MD,
whose sacrifices for my work are fortunately outmatched
by our mutual love for medicine.*

Contents

Contributors

Nicholas S. Abend, MD   Assistant Professor of Neurology and Pediatrics, Division of Neurology, Children's Hospital of Philadelphia, Department of Neurology, Perelman School of Medicine, University of Pennsylvania School of Medicine, Attending Physician, Department of Pediatrics (Neurology), Children's Hospital of Philadelphia, Philadelphia, Pennsylvania

Mona S. Al-Dulaligan, MD   Division of Clinical Neurophysiology, Children's National Medical Center, Washington, DC, Department of Pediatric Neurology, Ministry of Health, Riyadh, Saudi Arabia

Frances Ashcroft, PhD   Professor, OXION Initiative, Henry Wellcome Centre for Gene Function, and Department of Physiology, Anatomy and Genetics and OXION, University of Oxford, Oxford, UK

Kristin W. Barañano, MD, PhD   Clinical Associate, Pediatric Neurology, Department of Neurology, Johns Hopkins Hospital, Instructor of Neurology, Johns Hopkins School of Medicine, Baltimore, Maryland

Nenad Blau, PhD   Professor of Clinical Biochemistry, Division of Inborn Metabolic Diseases, University Children's Hospital, Department of General Pediatrics, Heidelberg, Germany, Division of Metabolism and Division of Clinical Chemistry and Biochemistry, University Children's Hospital, Zürich, Switzerland

Andrew Breeden, BA   Center for Functional and Molecular Imaging, Department of Neurology, Georgetown University, Washington, DC

Kimberly A. Chapman, MD, PhD   Assistant Professor, George Washington University, Genetics and Metabolism, Children's National Medical Center, Washington, DC

Dimitar Gavrilov, MD, PhD   Assistant Professor of Laboratory Medicine & Pathology, Co-Director, Biochemical Genetics Laboratory, Departments of Laboratory Medicine & Pathology, and Medical Genetics, Mayo Clinic College of Medicine, Rochester, Minnesota

K. Michael Gibson, PhD   Department of Biological Sciences, Michigan Technological University, Houghton, Michigan

Sidney M. Gospe, Jr, MD, PhD   Herman and Faye Sarkowsky Endowed Chair, Professor and Head, Division of Pediatric Neurology, Departments of Neurology and Pediatrics, The Center on Human Development and Disability, University of Washington, Division of Neurology, Seattle Children's Hospital, and Seattle Children's Research Institute, Seattle, Washington

Ton de Grauw, MD, PhD   Professor and Chief, Pediatric Neurology, Emory University School of Medicine, Atlanta, Georgia

Andrea L. Gropman, MD   Department of Neurology, Children's National Medical Center, George Washington University of the Health Sciences, Washington, DC

Julia B. Hennermann, MD   Charité Universitätsmedizin Berlin, Department of Pediatrics, Metabolic Unit, Berlin, Germany

Cornelis Jakobs, PhD   Metabolic Laboratory, Departments of Pediatrics and Clinical Chemistry, Vrje University Medical Center, Amsterdam

Parastoo Jangouk, MD   Research Fellow, Department of Neurology, Kennedy Krieger Institute, Johns Hopkins School of Medicine, Baltimore, Maryland, Research Fellow, Department of Neurogenetics, Kennedy Krieger Institute, Baltimore, Maryland

Hyder A. Jinnah, MD, PhD   Professor, Departments of Neurology, Human Genetics, and Pediatrics, Atlanta, Georgia

Andrea Kelly, MD, MSCE   Assistant Professor of Pediatrics, Division of Endocrinology & Diabetes, Children's Hospital of Philadelphia, Department of Pediatrics, Perelman School of Medicine, University of Pennsylvania School of Medicine, Children's Hospital of Philadelphia, Attending Physician, Department of Endocrinology & Diabetes, Children's Hospital of Philadelphia, Philadelphia, Pennsylvania

Zarir P. Khademian, MD, PhD   Assitant Professor of Radiology and Pediatrics, Staff Neurologist, Division of Diagnostic Imaging and Radiology, Children's National Medical Center, Washington, DC

Tom J. de Koning, MD, PhD   Pediatrician for Inborn Errors of Metabolism, Department of Genetics, University Medical Center Groningen, RB Groningen, The Netherlands, Former address: Department of Metabolic Diseases, University Medical Centre Utrecht, AB Utrecht, The Netherlands

Eric H. W. Kossoff, MD   Associate Professor, Department of Neurology and Pediatrics, The John M. Freeman Pediatric Epilepsy Center, The Johns Hopkins Hospital, Baltimore, Maryland

Carolina Lahmann, BSc   OXION Initiative, Henry Wellcome Centre for Gene Function, and Department of Physiology, Anatomy and Genetics and OXION, University of Oxford, Oxford, UK

Brendan Lanpher, MD   Assistant Professor of Pediatrics, George Washington University, Division of Genetics and Metabolism, Children's National Medical Center, Washington, DC

Beth Leeman, MD, MA, MMSc   Assistant Professor, Department of Neurology, Emory University, Director, Emory University Epilepsy Monitoring Unit, and Atlanta VA Epilepsy Unit, Atlanta, Georgia, Physician, Department of Neurology, Atlanta VA Medical Center, Decatur, Georgia

Dietrich Matern, MD   Professor of Laboratory Medicine & Pathology, Medical Genetics, and Pediatrics, Biochemical Genetics Laboratory, Mayo Clinic College of Medicine, Rochester, Minnesota

William M. McClintock, MD   Children's National Medical Center, Associate Professor of Neurology and Pediatrics, The George Washington University School of Medicine, Washington, DC

Thomas Opladen, MD   Division of Inborn Metabolic Diseases, Department of General Pediatrics, University Children's Hospital, Heidelberg, Germany

Sumit Parikh, MD   Division of Neurology, Section on Neurogenetics and Metabolism, Cleveland Clinic, Cleveland, Ohio

Phillip L. Pearl, MD   Division Chief, Child Neurology, Children's National Medical Center, Professor of Neurology, Pediatrics, and Music, George Washington University School of Medicine, and Columbian College of Arts and Sciences, Washington, DC, Clinical Epilepsy Branch, National Institute of Neurological Disorders and Stroke, National Institutes of Health, Bethesda, Maryland

Barbara Plecko-Startinig, Dr. med. univ.   Abteilung Neurologie, Universitäts-Kinderspital Zürich, Zürich, Switzerland

Anna Lecticia Pinto, MD   Fellow in Neurogenetics, Boston Children's Hospital, Boston, Massachusetts

Amanda Wai-Yun Pong, MD, MSc   Assistant Professor in Pediatric Epilepsy, Neurological Institute of New York, Columbia University Medical Center, New York, New York

Morgan Prust, BS Department of Neurology, Children's National Medical Center, Washington, DC, Harvard Medical School, Boston, Massachusetts

Gerald V. Raymond, MD Director of Neurogenetics, Department of Neurogenetics, Kennedy Krieger Institute, Professor of Neurology, Johns Hopkins School of Medicine, Baltimore, Maryland

Debra S. Regier, MD, PhD Department of Pediatrics, Children's National Medical Center, Washington, DC

Jörn Oliver Sass, Dr. rer. nat. Professor, Labor für Klinische Biochemie und Stoffwechsel, Zentrum für Kinder- und Jugendmedizin, Universitätsklinikum Freiburg, Freiburg, Germany

Fernando Scaglia, MD, FACMG Associate Professor, Department of Molecular and Human Genetics, Baylor College of Medicine, Houston, Texas

Susan Sparks, MD, PhD Clinical Geneticist, Department of Pediatrics/Clinical Genetics, Levine Children's Hospital at Carolinas Medical Center, Adjunct Clinical Assistant Professor, Pediatrics, University of North Carolina at Chapel Hill, Chapel Hill, North Carolina

Marshall L. Summar, MD Chief, Division of Genetics, Children's National Medical Center, Washington, DC

Pranoot Tanpaiboon, MD Assistant Professor of Pediatrics, Division of Genetics and Metabolism, The George Washington University School of Medicine and Health Sciences, Children's National Medical Center, Washington, DC

Davide Tonduti, MD Fellow in Child Neurology, Department of Child Neurology and Psychiatry, IRCCS C. Mondino Institute of Neurology Foundation, Pavia, Italy

Adeline Vanderver, MD Assistant Professor of Neurology, Pediatrics and Integrated Systems Biology, Children's National Medical Center, Washington, DC

Jodie Martin Vento, MGC, CGC Certified Genetic Counselor, Department of Neurology, Children's National Medical Center, Clinical Instructor in Pediatrics, George Washington University School of Medicine and Health Sciences, Washington, DC, Division of Child Neurology, Children's Hospital of Pittsburgh of UPMC, Pittsburgh, Pennsylvania

Darryl C. De Vivo, MD Sidney Carter Professor of Neurology, Professor of Pediatrics, Associate Chairman (Neurology) for Pediatric Neurosciences, Director, Pediatric Neurology, Emeritus, Director, Colleen Giblin Research Laboratories, Director, Pediatric Neuromuscular Disease Center, Co-Director, Center for Motor Neuron Biology and Disease, Columbia University Medical Center, The Neurological Institute, New York, New York

Lynne Wolfe, MS, CRNP, BC Undiagnosed Disorders Program, National Human Genome Research Institute, National Institutes of Health, Bethesda, Maryland

Robert A. Zimmerman, MD Department of Radiology, Children's Hospital of Philadelphia, Philadelphia, Pennsylvania

Preface

The inherited metabolic epilepsies represent a group of disorders that are rare individually but in aggregate represent a substantial clinical burden as well as vexing area for physicians, investigators, and students to master. The sheer amount and complexity of information are overwhelming and require the physician to synthesize key concepts in neurology, genetics, and epilepsy. As a pediatric epileptologist and medical educator, I have found this area among the most challenging and rewarding in practice and research. This monograph is an attempt to bring expertise in the various inherited metabolic epilepsies under one roof with a sense of clarity and purpose that will enable other clinicians and investigators to appreciate the same confluence of neurogenetics and epilepsy that I have attempted to bring to my work.

This monograph was borne following the organization of the Pediatric State-of-the-Art Symposium on Treatable Metabolic Epilepsies presented at the annual meeting of the American Epilepsy Society in Boston in 2009. At the time of proposing the topic a year earlier, I had emerged from the fall meeting of the Society for the Study of Inborn Errors of Metabolism (SSIEM) in Lisbon awestruck with both the significance of disorders being discussed and the chiasmic gap in communication between the remarkable experts in genetic–metabolic medicine and my other equally remarkable community of epileptologists. For example, a storybook series of investigations elucidated not only the surprising antiquitin defect in pyridoxine-dependent epilepsy but also the highly charged requirement that physicians consider a pivotal role for folinic acid and pyridoxal-5-phosphate in patients with virtually the same clinical presentation. I also perceived a relative lack of awareness of disorders such as glucose transporter 1 deficiency, serine synthetic defects, DEND, and HI–HA, among others, that had very specific therapeutic implications with potential for dramatically improving outcome but with an even greater likelihood that they were escaping diagnosis.

There are multiple ways to organize these disorders. Conceptually, the traditional inborn errors of metabolism may be viewed as abnormalities of synthesis, metabolism, and transport. Others have come to be recognized as channelopathies or receptor defects. Others may be viewed principally as defects in cofactors including vitamins. Alternatively, one could have organized this work based on the epilepsy, for example, using a scheme such as idiopathic, cryptogenic, or symptomatic. Neurologists may begin an organizational scheme based on the clinical course, that is, static versus progressive encephalopathies, and then organize the latter by principal site of involvement, whether by anatomy (leukodystrophy, poliodystrophy, basal ganglionopathy), systems approach (cortical projections, cerebellar pathways, basal ganglia projections, brainstem mediated, multisystem), or maximal organelle of involvement (eg, mitochondria, peroxisome, etc).

Ultimately, this book was divided into four sections: General Principles, Small Molecule Diseases, Large Molecule Diseases, and Conclusions. This appeared to be the most logical structure and sequence to present this material in a digestible format for physicians and researchers with an interest in this field. The part on General Principles begins with a "high impact" presentation of particularly treatable metabolic epilepsies in which early diagnosis and targeted intervention may afford a profound alteration in prognosis in what otherwise typically lends to a much worse if not catastrophic outcome, and ends with attention to the special role of the ketogenic diet, itself a metabolic intervention, in the metabolic epilepsies. The other chapters provide overviews with many specific examples of the vital roles of neuroradiology, electroencephalography, and genetic counseling in the evaluation and management of patients with inherited metabolic epilepsies.

From the viewpoint of the neurologist and epileptologist, it was thought that the grouping of these seemingly disparate disorders into the metabolic specialist's view of small versus large molecules may be instructive. The part on Small Molecule Diseases brings expertise together in disorders of amino acids, organic acids, urea cycle, neurotransmitters, transporters, cofactors, purines, and mitochondria. Owing to their special importance in the metabolic epilepsies, there is specific disease related coverage in several of these areas, such as glycine encephalopathy, Lesch–Nyhan disease, sulfite oxidase/molybdenum cofactor deficiency, cerebral folate deficiencies, and homocysteinemias including MTHFR (methylenetetrahydrofolate reductase) deficiency. Other specific epileptic encephalopathies, for example, neuronal ceroid lipofuscinoses, are covered in the existing chapters, for example, large molecules chapter on lysosomal storage diseases. A grouping of the "glucose regulation defects": glucose transporter 1 deficiency, DEND (developmental delay, epilepsy, neonatal diabetes), and HI–HA (hyperinsulinism–hyperammonemia) was purposefully chosen in the sequencing of the chapters. Although their pathophysiologic mechanisms are quite different, the clinician will recognize the logic of organizing defects in glucose metabolism as a subsection within the small molecule disorders. The part on Large Molecule

Diseases covers defects of glycosylation, lysosomal and peroxisomal function, and leukodystrophies.

The final Conclusion part provides an algorithm designed to be a resource for the physician in search of direction while considering an inherited metabolic disorder as the explanation for a patient with epilepsy. Hence, what began as a quest to increase awareness of treatable metabolic epilepsies became a multiauthored monograph to feature not only the fundamentals of the metabolic epilepsies, a subspecialty that crosses over between epilepsy and neurogenetics, but also a collection of thoughtful writings on the role and pathomechanisms of seizures within these disorders.

Each author was charged with addressing an audience of physicians caring for patients with metabolic epilepsies who are not necessarily experts in metabolic disease, highlighting the relation between the metabolic error(s) and epilepsy, and providing insight into Future Directions and "Clinical Pearls" to serve as take-home messages. I carefully edited each chapter to provide a uniform voice and continuity, and failings in this regard are my own. Certainly one could argue that certain diseases deserved more, or perhaps less, representation. In addition, at some point the scope of the book had to be limited, so that the burgeoning area of genetic epilepsies that would not be particularly viewed as inborn errors of metabolism per se (there are many examples, from the phakomatoses to sodium channelopathies, among others) were not given specific attention; these entities and their relation to epilepsy are time honored and covered well in many other sources. It is truly hoped that this book will educate if not enlighten physicians, particularly specialists and trainees in pediatric and adult neurology, neurodevelopmental disabilities, epilepsy, and genetics, while caring for patients with inherited metabolic epilepsies, as well as spur further research into basic mechanisms and clinical trials in this group of maladies.

Phillip L. Pearl, MD

Acknowledgments

This book was suggested to me by Beth Barry from Demos Medical Publishers following my organization of the Pediatric State-of-the-Art Symposium on Treatable Metabolic Epilepsies presented at the American Epilepsy Society 2009 meeting, and I remain indebted to Beth and her colleagues at Demos for their persistence and dedication to this project. My education in child neurology and epilepsy is grounded in great mentors, including Ralph D. Feigin, MD in pediatrics and Marvin A. Fishman, MD in pediatric neurology at Baylor College of Medicine in Houston, and Gregory L. Holmes, MD in epilepsy and clinical neurophysiology, then at Children's Hospital, Harvard Medical School in Boston. I wish to take this opportunity to acknowledge these teachers of mine.

My foray into metabolic disorders has been made possible by the always helpful, brilliant, and steadfast work of Mike Gibson, PhD, whose collaboration in the area of GABA (gamma-amino butyric acid) disorders, specifically SSADH (succinic semialdehyde dehydrogenase) deficiency, has been a constant source of intellectual nourishment and encouragement. My clinical and departmental work at Children's National Medical Center has sustained my professional development, and there are a multitude of people to whom I am grateful. At the risk of omitting so many of them from this all too brief section of acknowledgments, I wish to thank William D. Gaillard, MD, my co-chief who handles matters large and small in clinical neurophysiology, epilepsy, and critical care neurology at Children's National, Roger J. Packer, MD, executive vice president of neuroscience who has guided the careers of many junior and mid-career faculty including my own, and William H. Theodore, MD, Chief of the Clinical Epilepsy Section at the NINDS, who has served as my mentor in our ongoing investigative work on metabolic epilepsies at the NIH.

I thank each of the contributors to this book for receiving and re-receiving my pleas, deadlines, and edits to accomplish this task. Many will be recognized as world-class authorities, if not the initial investigators, in their particular topic. I am humbled by their contributions to the book. Others may have less eponymic fame but are equally impressive and progressing rapidly along their academic trajectories. I am grateful for the time they too have taken to share their knowledge and insights. Danniele Provost, research assistant and neurology education coordinator, and Colleen McGavin, post-baccalaureate student who has now matriculated into medical school, meticulously helped me with the massive organizational and editing effort that went into this project. As a group, I thank the many patients and families, as well as students, residents, and fellows, who inspire our work. I thank my own family who, as with all of us, make the most in personal sacrifices and provide the most inspiration.

Phillip L. Pearl, MD

Inherited Metabolic Epilepsies

1

Inherited Metabolic Epilepsies: The Top 10 Diagnoses You Cannot Afford to Miss

Phillip L. Pearl

INTRODUCTION

This topic, which served as the stimulus for the Pediatric State-of-the-Art Symposium during the 2009 annual meeting of the American Epilepsy Society and subsequently countless other presentations, became the impetus for this book. The imperative of the clinician is to identify treatable conditions, and this mandate has become increasingly prominent with the rapid discoveries in neurogenetics and metabolic diseases. The theme of this presentation is to identify those conditions that meet three criteria: each is eminently treatable, epilepsy may be prominent in the clinical presentation, and the prognosis is linked to early diagnosis and introduction of therapy (Table 1.1). Case presentations are used to introduce the diseases, which are either the author's personal cases or, when indicated, published cases. While one could certainly consider and include other conditions not covered here, the writer challenges fellow clinicians and investigators

TABLE 1.1   Criteria for the Top 10 Inherited Treatable Metabolic Epilepsies

- Eminently treatable
- Epilepsy prominent in presentation
- Prognosis linked to early Dx and Rx

to modify the list, adding one entity at the expense of another, to come up with one's own, "Top Ten!"

CASE PRESENTATIONS

NUMBER 10: PARKINSONISM, LEARNING DISABILITIES, AND SEIZURES

A 7-year-old girl from Guatemala presented with a history of recurrent weakness and rash over 1–2 years duration. Her past medical history indicated that she had an abnormal newborn screen for phenylketonuria (PKU) and she was placed on a restricted diet until 4 years of age. Her family immigrated to the United States then and compliance with the diet was reduced and eventually lost without apparent ill effects. Over the prior 1–2 years she developed fluctuated weakness and gait impairment during which she was described as having stiff legs. She complained of knee pain and had recurrent unexplained erythematous skin rash. A neurologist described a normal neurological examination and obtained brain MRI and MR angiography studies which returned as unremarkable. She was referred to a rheumatologist, who diagnosed seronegative juvenile rheumatoid arthritis and prescribed prednisone for a number of months. This was ineffective, and her treatment was converted to methotrexate.

Within a week her abnormalities worsened dramatically and she became bedridden, unable to ambulate or speak, although her mentation was preserved. She was hospitalized and serum phenylalanine was elevated at 163 mg/dL. Urine pterin showed decreased biopterin of 3.7% (control range 18%–70%). She was diagnosed with a biopterin synthesis defect, which on specific enzyme assay testing was confirmed as the most common in this group, PTPS (pyruvoyltetrahydropterin synthase) deficiency. She improved with L-DOPA, 5-hydroxytryptophan, and biopterin supplementation. She continues to have mild gait stiffness and has intermittent generalized seizures, treated with levetiracetam and clonazepam.

This represents the disorders of synthesis or recycling of tetrahydrobiopterin (BH4). These disorders are usually identified by hyperphenylalanine on newborn screening, although blood phenylalanine levels may be normal and some of these conditions are associated with a normal blood phenylalanine (Table 1.2). Thus, evaluation for a disorder in the BH4 pathway should be done in infants with unexplained neurological disease. BH4 is essential in the synthesis of the monoamine neurotransmitters, that is, dopamine, norepinephrine, epinephrine, as well as serotonin (Figure 1.1). There is an ongoing cycle where BH4 is converted from BH2 (dihydrobiopterin) via dihydropterin reductase (DHPR) (Figure 1.2). Urine biopterin is helpful in distinguishing between various disorders in this pathway. In the biopterin synthesis defects, as in the present case, levels are very low, whereas urine biopterin is normal in classic PKU and elevated in DHPR deficiency. There is a salvage pathway from sepiapterin to BH4 using dihydrofolate reductase (DHFR).

The major phenotype of the BH4 disorders includes intellectual disability, epilepsy (typically myoclonic seizures, as is the case with metabolic encephalopathies), and extrapyramidal manifestations (Table 1.3). Of interest, neuroimaging may show basal ganglia calcifications, especially in DHPR deficiency. The treatment of BH4 disorders include compounds aimed to replenish the diminished supply of the monoamine neurotransmitters using L-DOPA and monoamine oxidase or catechol-O-methyltransferase (COMT) inhibitors, biopterin supplementation, and 5-hydroxytryptophan as a precursor to 5-hydroxytryptamine, that is, serotonin. In DHPR deficiency, the basal ganglia calcifications may be reversible with folinic acid supplementation (1). The case analysis in the present patient is that she decompensated with the methotrexate intervention, prescribed for the misdiagnosis of juvenile rheumatoid arthritis. The folate antagonist methotrexate interfered with her salvage pathway and she lost this vital source of BH4, leading to collapse of biopterin, and hence catecholamine neurotransmitter production. The biopterin synthesis defects are covered in more detail in Chapter 12 by Drs Nenad Blau and Thomas Opladen.

Diagnosis: PTPS deficiency (biopterin synthesis defect)

NUMBER 9: IRRITABILITY, CRANIAL DECELERATION, AND SEIZURES IN INFANCY

A 2-year-old infant presented with generalized tonic–clonic seizures at 5 months of age, and was treated with phenobarbital without recurrence until 12 months of age. EEG and MRI studies were normal, and the clinical impression was that of mild developmental delay (2). The child was then hospitalized at

TABLE 1.2 Defects of Biopterin Metabolism Based on Whether Hyperphenylalaninemia Is Present

	BH$_4$ Metabolism
• + ↑ [PHE] – arGTPCH[1] – PTPS deficiency[2] – PCD deficiency[3] – DHPR deficiency[4] – Defects	• Normal [PHE] – adGTPCH[1] – SR deficiency[5] – [1]GTP cyclohydrolase – [2]Pyruvoyl-4H-pterin synthase – [3]Pterin-carbinolamine reductase – [4]Dihydropteridine reductase – [5]Sepiapterin reductase

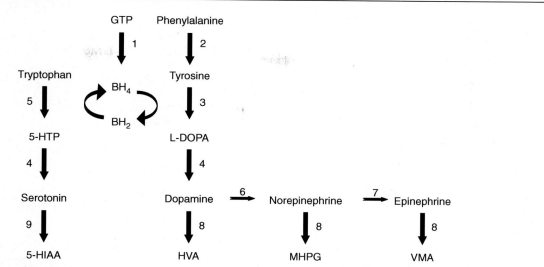

FIGURE 1.1 Monoamine and serotonin synthesis pathway. 5-HTP, 5-hydroxytryptophan; 5-HIAA, 5-hydroxyindoleacetic acid; GTP, guanosine triphosphate; BH4, tetrahydrobiopterin; BH2, quinonoid dihydrobiopterin; L-DOPA, levodopa; HVA, homovanillic acid; MHPG, 3-methoxy-4-hydroxyphenylglycol; VMA, vanillylmandelic acid. **1,** GTP-cyclohydroxylase I; **2,** phenylalanine hydroxylase; **3,** tyrosine hydroxylase; **4,** aromatic-L-amino acid decarboxylase; **5,** tryptophan hydroxylase; **6,** dopamine β-hydroxylase; **7,** phenylethanolamine-*N*-methyltransferase; **8,** monoamine oxidase, aldehyde dehydrogenase, catechol-*O*-methyltransferase; **9,** monoamine oxidase.

17 months of age with serial generalized tonic–clonic seizures and lapsed into a coma of 5 days duration. EEG showed high-voltage slowing and irregular periods of voltage attenuation. MRI was normal. The child emerged as profoundly impaired. Extensive laboratory testing ultimately revealed low 5-methyltetrahydrofolate in CSF of 28 nmol/L (normal range 40–187) and subsequently was positive for antifolate receptor antibodies. The diagnosis was cerebral folate deficiency. This child was treated with folinic acid 1 mg/kg/d without significant improvement, but other published cases have had improvement in seizures, mental status, and involuntary movements (3).

Cerebral folate deficiency has been associated both with auto-antibodies and gene mutations of the folate FR1 receptor (4). While folate is stored in erythrocytes, FR1-mediated endocytosis is required to transport folate across the blood–brain barrier, from which it is transported into the neuron. The manifestations of cerebral folate deficiency are infantile onset irritability, cranial growth deceleration, and seizures, along with pyramidal and extrapyramidal tract deficits (Table 1.4). Both optic atrophy and cortical visual loss are observed after 3 years of age. This disorder is covered in more detail in Chapter 22 by Dr Fernando Scaglia.

Diagnosis: Cerebral Folate Deficiency

NUMBER 8: SEIZURES, HYPOTONIA, OPTIC ATROPHY, AND RASH

The phenotypic components of this disorder are developmental delay, hypotonia, seizures, ataxia, and rash (Table 1.5). This combination is manifest in biotinidase deficiency, an organic acidopathy that can also present with intermittent metabolic acidosis and an organic acid profile of lactic and propionic acidemia. The fundamental defect is an inability to cleave biocytin (Figure 1.3). This leads to impaired ability to form free biotin and to catalyze holocarboxylase synthetase, causing a biochemical scenario of multiple carboxylase deficiency (which itself can be caused by holocarboxylase synthetase deficiency). There are variants with partial deficiency and variable penetrance. Newborn screening has yielded a frequency estimate of one in 60,000 births, and screening is still not yet mandatory in all 50 states plus may not occur in international births.

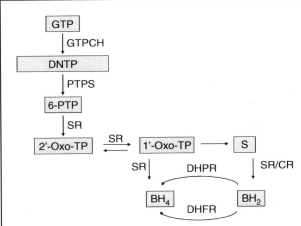

FIGURE 1.2   Biopterin metabolism. GTP, guanine triphosphate; GTPCH, GTP cyclohydrolase I; DNTP, dihydroneopterin triphosphate; PTPS, 6-pyruvoyl-tetrahydropterin synthase; 6-PTP, 6-pyruvoyl-tetrahydropterin; SR, sepiapterin reductase; 2′-Oxo-TP, 1′-hydroxy-2′-oxo-tetrahydropterin; 1′-Oxo-TP, 1′-oxo-2′-hydroxy tetrahydropterin; S, sepiapterin; BH$_4$, tetrahydrobiopterin; DHPR, dihydropterin reductase; DHFR, dihydrofolate reductase; BH$_2$, 7,8-dihydrobiopterin; CR, carbonyl reductase.

The treatment is 10 mg/d of biotin and the outcome is gratifying, although if sensorineural hearing loss and optic atrophy with vision loss occur, they tend to persist. There are pitfalls and traps in particular for even an experienced clinician pertaining to biotinidase deficiency. Cases of biotinidase deficiency have been misdiagnosed as "atypical" or "childhood" multiple sclerosis. Patients have presented in adolescence with spastic paraparesis. The dermatologic manifestations have been misdiagnosed as acrodermatitis

TABLE 1.3   Major Phenotype of BH$_4$ Disorders

- Intellectual disability
- Myoclonic seizures
- Muscular rigidity
- Dystonia
- Drooling
- Microcephaly
- Neuroimaging:
    - Cerebral atrophy, lucency of the white matter, basal ganglia calcifications

TABLE 1.4   Manifestations of Cerebral Folate Deficiency

- Infantile onset (4–6 months)
    - Irritability
    - Decelerating head growth
    - Seizures
    - Psychomotor retardation
    - Cerebellar ataxia
    - Pyramidal tract signs
    - Ballismus, choreoathetosis
- After 3 years of age:
    - Optic atrophy
    - Cortical blindness

enteropathica or anhidrotic ectodermal dysplasia. Furthermore, seizures (generalized, myoclonic, and infantile spasms) occur in the majority of patients and may be the *only obvious symptom*. Thus, testing for biotinidase deficiency is warranted in any patient with unexplained seizures.

Diagnosis: Biotinidase deficiency

NUMBER 7: CONGENITAL MICROCEPHALY AND PSYCHOMOTOR RETARDATION

The phenotype of congenital microcephaly and psychomotor retardation is nonspecific and the pediatric practitioner is likely to suspect in utero processes such as TORCH or perinatal, static difficulties. Yet a treatable metabolic disorder would be important indeed to consider. While rare, there are disorders of serine biosynthesis in which greatly improved outcomes have been reported, including prenatal treatment, using supplemental serine (400–600 mg/kg/d)

TABLE 1.5   Biotinidase Deficiency: Clinical Phenotype

- Developmental delay
- Hypotonia
- Seizures
- Ataxia
- Alopecia, perioral rash
- Episodic metabolic acidosis
- Hearing loss
- Vision loss, optic atrophy
- Lactic and propionic acidemia

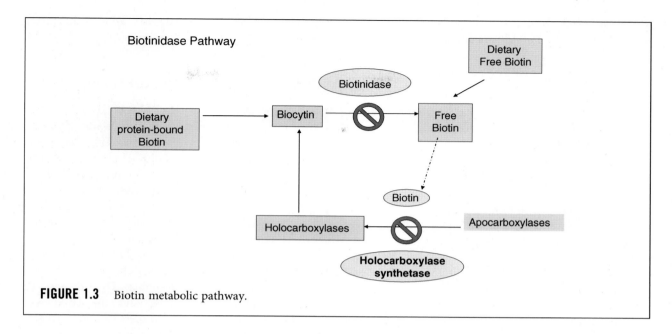

FIGURE 1.3   Biotin metabolic pathway.

and glycine (200–300 mg/kg/d) (5). The serine biosynthesis and catabolism pathway (Figure 1.4) involves interconversion with glycine and includes folate and methylation transfer as shown. Enzymatic deficiency of either the dehydrogenase or phosphatase may occur. The diagnosis can be screened using amino acid analysis of plasma or CSF for low serine levels. The prognosis is poor except when the specific dietary supplementation is implemented. This disorder is covered in more detail in Chapter 18 by Dr De Koning.

Diagnosis: Serine synthesis defect

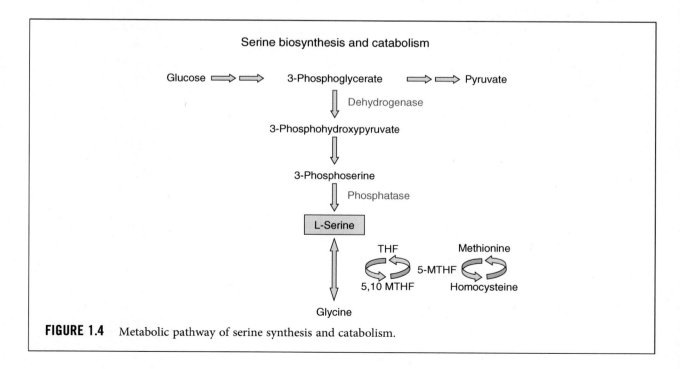

FIGURE 1.4   Metabolic pathway of serine synthesis and catabolism.

NUMBER 6: FEBRILE SEIZURES TO STATUS EPILEPTICUS; INFANTILE SEIZURES TO CHILDHOOD EPILEPSY WITH LANGUAGE DELAY

A 4-year-old Honduran girl of nonconsanguinous parents presented with a history of seizures and language delay. Seizures began at $3\frac{1}{2}$ years of age with fever and she developed mixed generalized seizures including atypical absences, myoclonias, and drops. Her language was characterized by only single or two-word utterances. Findings on examination included increased appendicular tone, truncal hypotonia, and right upper extremity dystonia noted with gait. EEG showed mild diffuse background slowing and generalized and multifocal spike discharges. Extensive laboratory testing was unremarkable for various causes of myoclonic epilepsy. MR spectroscopy using single voxel technique over the basal ganglia was obtained and showed a decreased ratio of creatine to choline (Figure 1.5). A creatinine-to-creatine ratio was determined in serum as mildly increased; serum GAA level was normal. Fibroblasts were sent for mutational analysis and revealed a missense mutation of SLC6A8, the creatine transporter gene, located at Xq28. The diagnosis of creatine transporter deficiency was established, which has an epileptic spectrum of recurrent febrile seizures to status epilepticus (6).

Metabolic disorders of creatine were first described in 1994 with the discovery of GAMT deficiency (7). The creatine synthesis and transport pathway involves two enzymatic reactions starting from arginine with GAA being the intermediate (Figure 1.6). The GAA level will be elevated in GAMT deficiency, decreased in AGAT (arginine:glycine aminidotransferase) deficiency, and normal in creatine transporter deficiency. The phenotype of this group of disorders includes failure to thrive and early developmental delay, neurologic regression, intellectual disability, autistic behavior, hypotonia, epilepsy, movement disorders, and abnormal pallidal signal on MRI. The disorders cannot be reliably distinguished by clinical criteria and require laboratory identification. The treatment is creatine supplementation in GAMT and AGAT deficiency, as well as arginine restriction and ornithine supplementation in GAMT deficiency. On the contrary, creatine transporter deficiency is at best partially amenable to pharmacologic therapy, with improvement reported in peripheral but not central nervous system (CNS) manifestations (8). This group of disorders is covered in more detail in Chapter 21 by Dr Ton de Grauw.

Diagnosis: Creatine synthesis and transporter deficiencies

CASE 5: STIFF NEWBORN WITH EXCESSIVE STARTLE

A full-term newborn was described as having seizures within minutes from birth with fisting and rhythmic movements of the extremities and eyes. There was possible improvement following administration of phenobarbital and pyridoxine. EEG monitoring showed no epileptiform correlates and a background largely obscured due to widespread myogenic artifact. The child's tone was increased since birth and experienced severe choking and apnea during laryngoscopy.

The helpful bedside test was the nose tap, using the finger to tap the nose in search of a prominent and, in reality, dramatic startle response. The diagnosis of hyperekplexia was established, and the child was treated with clonazepam with progressive improvement.

Hyperekplexia, or stiff baby syndrome, appears to have a major form with significant hypertonia and symptoms of infantile falling, shaking, hyperreflexia, and unsteady gait. There also appears to be a more common minor form with isolated but excessive startle reactions. Both forms may involve frequent difficulty with swallowing and choking, which appears to be responsible for the known unfortunate complication of sudden death.

The disorder is due to impairment in glycine-mediated inhibition at the brainstem and spinal cord level. Whereas GABA is the major inhibitory neurotransmitter of the brain, glycine is the major inhibitory transmitter of the brainstem and cord. Mutations may be identified in the glycine inhibitory receptor GLRA1 or glycine transporters. Attacks have been described as preventable by sudden flexion of the head and limbs, and clonazepam is recommended (9). The patient described in this vignette gradually improved on this therapy and by 15 months of age was alert, interactive, cruising, standing 5–10 seconds duration, and had recently begun clapping and babbling. The tone was just mildly increased. By 4 y of age, the clonazepam was discontinued with no further deficits noted on exam. While this condition would be considered an epilepsy mimic, the notion that sudden death could be prevented with an inexpensive benzodiazepine in a condition that may be misdiagnosed as epilepsy is compelling.

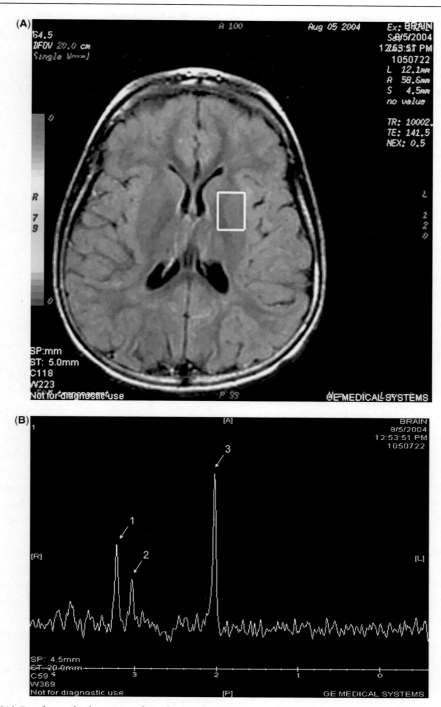

FIGURE 1.5   (A) Basal ganglia location of single voxel MR spectroscopy on T-1 weighted MRI. (B) Elevated choline (1) to creatine (2) ratio noted in 4-year-old girl with creatine transporter deficiency. The *N*-acetylasparate level (3) was normal.

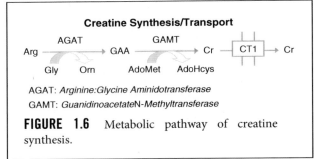

Creatine Synthesis/Transport

AGAT   GAMT

Arg → GAA → Cr — CT1 → Cr

Gly Orn   AdoMet AdoHcys

AGAT: *Arginine:Glycine Aminidotransferase*
GAMT: *Guanidinoacetate*N-*Methyltransferase*

FIGURE 1.6 Metabolic pathway of creatine synthesis.

Diagnosis: Hyperekplexia (Congenital startle disorder or stiff baby syndrome)

CASE 4: NEONATAL EPILEPSY WITH DIABETES

A syndrome has been recently elucidated that combines the problems of Developmental Delay, Epilepsy, and Neonatal Diabetes acronymized as DEND. This involves a mutation in a potassium channel that is gated by ATP concentrations. These channels normally close with hyperglycemia, associated with an elevated ATP/ADP ratio, promoting depolarization and physiologic insulin release. Sulfonylurea binds to these receptors, promoting closure and augmenting insulin release which could treat this disorder due to channel mutations and hence impaired channel closure in the face of hypoglycemia. This therapy was reported as effective in a child diagnosed with the condition at $3\frac{1}{2}$ years of age who otherwise had a profound encephalopathy (10). Thus, DEND bears highlighted awareness of a neonatal epileptic channelopathy with diabetes where insulin administration may correct systemic hyperglycemia but have no effect on the otherwise poorly understood CNS effects of the disorder. This disorder is covered in more detail in Chapter 15 by Frances Ashcroft and Carolina Lahmann from Oxford University.

Diagnosis: DEND

CASE 3: EPILEPSY ASSOCIATED WITH HYPOGLYCEMIA AND LEARNING DISABILITIES

A 13-year-old boy is followed with generalized tonic–clonic seizures, typical absence seizures (associated with 3 Hz spike-and-wave EEG discharges), and moderate learning disabilities) (Figure 1.7). He presented with focal right-sided neonatal seizures and had a left

Case: 13 yr old boy with GTCS & absence, learning disabilities, generalized spike-wave

- Neonatal seizures
- Hypoglycemia
- Frontal lobe hemorrhagic infarction
- Dx "noccidioblastosis"
- Pancreatectomy refused (wisely)
- Worsened pre-prandially and post-protein meals
- Doing well with protein restriction & diazoxide

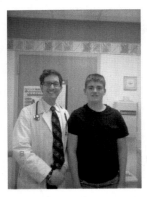

FIGURE 1.7 A 13-year-old boy with HI–HA syndrome pictured by the author, with permission from the patient and the family.

frontal-lobe hemorrhagic infarction on CT. He had persistent hypoglycemia and was diagnosed with suspected noccidioblastosis based on hyperinsulinism. A pancreatectomy was recommended but the parents refused. Over time the child stabilized but was observed to worsen in seizure control, behavior, and mood both preprandially and postprandially. He was later identified as having hyperammonemia and was diagnosed with a syndrome known as hyperinsulinism–hyperammonemia, or HI–HA.

HI–HA is a syndrome of congenital hyperinsulinism and hyperammonemia that has been related to activating mutations of glutamate dehydrogenase (GLUD1). This enzyme serves to promote the formation of alpha-ketoglutarate from glutamate, which ultimately leads to an increase in the ATP:ADP ratio in pancreatic beta cells. This serves to inhibit the ATP-sensitive potassium channel resulting in channel closure, membrane depolarization, calcium influx, and insulin release. Patients develop recurrent symptomatic hypoglycemia with fasting or following a high protein meal. The constellation of (generalized) epilepsy, learning disorders, and behavior problems is characteristic. The condition is manageable with a combination of protein restriction, antiepileptic medications, and diazoxide, a KATP channel agonist which inhibits insulin release (11). This disorder is covered in more detail in Chapter 16 by Drs Andrea Kelly and Nicholas Abend, endocrinologist and neurologist, respectively, from the Children's Hospital of Philadelphia.

Diagnosis: HI–HA

CASE 2: FROM NEONATAL SEIZURES TO A CONTINUING WIDENING SPECTRUM RELATED TO GLUCOSE

The presence of seizures and developmental delay associated with hypoglycorrhacia was reported by DeVivo and colleagues in 1991, and a breathtaking array of neurologic phenotypes has been associated with this problem of glucose entry into the brain. The diagnosis is glucose transporter I deficiency, and has emerged as the leading metabolic indication for the ketogenic diet, a previously established dietary therapy to restrict glucose so that the CNS reverted to the ketone bodies, predominantly acetoacetate and beta-hydroxybutyrate, as alternative fuels. The clinical spectrum appears to include early onset absence seizures with postprandial improvement as well as cases of isolated adult onset ataxia. This disorder is covered in more detail in Chapter 14 by Drs Darryl C. De Vivo and Amanda Pong from Columbia University.

Diagnosis: Glucose transporter 1 deficiency

CASE 1: ". . . THE PROTOTYPE OF THE SEVERE BUT EMINENTLY TREATABLE CONDITIONS THAT NO CLINICIAN WANTS TO MISS" (12)

Pyridoxine-dependent epilepsy was reported as a single case from Hunt et al in *Pediatrics* 1954 (13). The description of the third pregnancy to a mother who lost a prior conceptus due to neonatal seizures revealed severe hyperemesis gravidarum that responded to a multivitamin preparation. The newborn had severe seizures that were refractory to standard medical therapy and for which a series of vitamins were tried, simulating the compound's contents that were ameliorative during the gestation. After much empirical trial and error therapy, it was discovered that low dose (2 mg) pyridoxine stopped the seizures and improved the EEG. While the supplement was discontinued and renewed to prove the point, it became recognized over the ensuing decades that this therapy should be given continuously if effective and over a prolonged period, with confirmation based on an accompanying EEG showing a response with concomitant administration of intravenous pyridoxine at usually a 100-mg dose.

Subsequently considerable research showed that the traditional thinking that pyridoxine augmented GABA synthesis in its role as a cofactor to glutamic acid decarboxylase did not serve as a pathophysiology explanation, as there was no consistent demonstration of impaired GABA synthesis. Genetic linkage and the finding of a precipitate involving pipecolic acid ultimately led to the discovery of a mutation in antiquitin, involved in the lysine degradation pathway (Figure 1.8). There is accumulation of a carboxylate, as shown in the figure, which sequesters pyridoxal-5-phosphate, the biologically active form of pyridoxine which is integral to over 100 enzymatic reactions in the brain (Table 1.6).

The condition of pyridoxine dependency was further extended, based largely on serendipity, to cases that appeared instead to respond to folinic acid, either together with pyridoxine or, in the initial reports, to folinic acid alone. Folinic acid-dependent seizures were subsequently found to be allelic to pyridoxine dependency (14). In addition, atypical cases with long asymptomatic periods without pyridoxine supplementation, and cases diagnosed later in infancy after apparently being ruled out in the neonatorum, have been described.

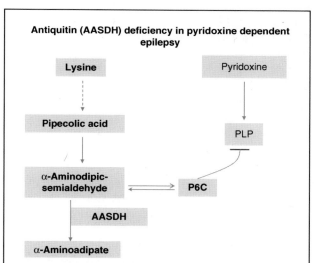

FIGURE 1.8 Antiquitin (AASDH) pathway. When antiquitin activity is deficient, pipecolic acid and P6C both accumulate, sequestering intracellular PLP. AASDH, alpha-aminodipic-semialdehyde dehydrogenase *(antiquitin)*; P6C, delta-piperideine-6-carboxylate; PNPO = pyridox(am)ine oxidase; PLP, pyridoxal-5-phosphate.

TABLE 1.6   Selected PLP-Dependent Enzymes and Their Respective Functions

AADC	DA, 5-HT Synthesis
2-Oxoglutarate NH_3-transferase	Glutamate synthesis
GABA transaminase	GABA catabolism
GAD	GABA synthesis
Glycine cleavage system	Glycine catabolism
Kynureninase	Quinolinic acid synthesis
Kynurenine NH_3-transferase	Kynurenic acid synthesis
L-serine racemase	D-serine synthesis

AADC, aromatic aminoacid decarboxylase; DA, dopamine; GABA, gamma-amino butyric acid; GAD, glutamic acid decarboxylase; NH_3, ammonia.

The pyridoxine-dependent epilepsies, long a source of fascination to neurologists interested in vitamin-dependent neurologic disorders (15), developed yet another twist, as documented in this case report:

A full-term 3220-g male newborn presented with abnormal eye movements and grunting 12 hours following birth. EEG showed bilateral sharp discharges and episodic background suppression. MRI was unremarkable. Following trials of phenobarbital and levetiracetam, the patient became seizure-free for 6 weeks on pyridoxine. Breakthrough tonic seizures then occurred, followed by myoclonic and tonic–clonic seizures, unresponsive to topiramate and prednisolone. The seizures stopped upon the first dose of PLP but breakthrough events occurred as a dose became due. CSF PLP level was 23 nmol/L (normal range of 23–64 nmol/L). CSF amino acids showed a slight increase in threonine. Neurotransmitter metabolites were normal and there was no indication of biomarkers for pyridoxine responsive seizures, although an unidentified peak was detected. Subsequent PNPO gene sequencing identified a homozygous mutation in a highly conserved area in exon 3: c.352G > A p.G118R. Parental testing confirmed heterozygosity for this mutation in both parents.

The biologically active form of pyridoxine is pyridoxal-5-phosphate, which is derived from dietary pyridoxine (the main source being vegetables), pyridoxamine (from meat), and pyridoxal through kinases (Figure 1.9). The phosphorylated pyridoxine-P

and pyridoxamine-P are then oxidized to pyridoxal-5-phosphate through the enzyme PNPO, that is, pyridox(am)ine phosphate oxidase. The pyridoxal-P is able to cross the blood–brain barrier through membrane-associated phosphatases, and then become rephosphorylated in the neuron to function as intracellular pyridoxal-5-phosphate.

In the case of our patient, the cerebrospinal fluid (CSF) pyridoxal phosphate level was just below the reference range, indicating this mutation led to a partially functioning protein. The elevated CSF threonine is compatible with PLP-dependency of threonine dehydratase. The unexplained peak has been seen consistently in patients with PNPO deficiency receiving exogenous pyridoxine (K. Hyland, personal communication), which was the case in our patient. Clinical observations indicate that initial temporary pyridoxine responsiveness may be seen in partial PNPO deficiency. Partial pyridoxine responsiveness is an indication for possible PNPO deficiency and trial of pyridoxal-5-phosphate.

The spectrum of the phenotype, along with an update on diagnosis and treatment, is covered in Chapter 11 by Dr S. Gospe.

Diagnosis: Pyridoxine-related responsive seizures

AN ELEVENTH CASE . . .

Similar to a baker's dozen, there is always room for an extra case. A full-term 3-day-old male newborn presented with poor feeding, dyspnea, and lethargy. He had been discharged home from his newborn admission the prior day. The perinatal circumstances were normal. On examination, suprasternal retractions, flattened anterior fontanelle, and hepatomegaly were noted. The evaluation demonstrated cerebral edema on CT imaging, mild respiratory alkalosis on arterial blood gas analysis, normal serum glucose and anion gap, but markedly elevated plasma ammonia of 770 micrograms/deciliter (mcg/dL). EEG showed intermittent multifocal ictal seizure discharges. The child was treated with phenobarbital, sodium phenylacetate, and hemodialysis. The metabolic laboratory studies showed low citrulline and elevated glutamine and alanine. The diagnosis was confirmed as ornithine transcarbamylase (OTC) deficiency.

The urea cycle disorders require rapid recognition and therapy and can present with encephalopathy

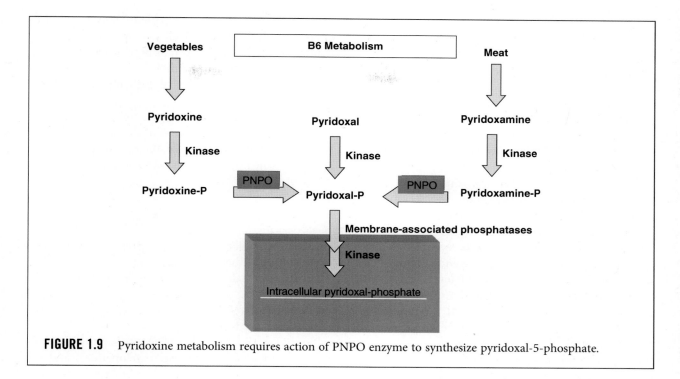

FIGURE 1.9 Pyridoxine metabolism requires action of PNPO enzyme to synthesize pyridoxal-5-phosphate.

including seizures and hypotonia, particularly associated with poor feeding after protein intake. The neonatal presentation is consistent with complete enzyme deficiency. There are six urea cycle enzymes, all of which are inherited as autosomal recessive except for the X-linked OTC. While elevated ammonia levels are the hallmark, this may be normal in arginase deficiency. The survival rate for acute neonatal hyperammonemia due to urea cycle defects is about 75%, compared to a better prognosis with later presentation. Poor factors for survival are coma at admission and peak ammonia levels greater than 1,000 mcg/dL. The most common is OTC deficiency, with an incidence of 1:14,000, with half of all cases being of neonatal onset. Males typically present as neonates and have higher morbidity and mortality. Female heterozygotes can become symptomatic, with the severity and timing dependent on the extent of hepatic lionization. While orthotopic liver transplant may be curative, this will not reverse neurologic injury, emphasizing the need for rapid recognition of diagnosis and initiation of therapy. This group of disorders is covered in more detail in Chapter 9 by Drs D. Regier, B. Lanpher, and M. Summar.

Diagnosis: OTC deficiency (Urea cycle disorders)

CONCLUSION

A selected group of eminently treatable but otherwise catastrophic inherited epilepsies were described. These disorders represent a vexing clinical challenge because a sufficiently low diagnostic threshold must be maintained for rare and esoteric diseases (Table 1.7).

TABLE 1.7 **The Top 10 Inherited Treatable Metabolic Epilepsies**

- 10. Biopterin synthesis disorders
- 9. Cerebral folate deficiency
- 8. Biotinidase deficiency
- 7. Serine biosynthesis defects
- 6. Creatine synthesis disorders
- 5. Hyperekplexia
- 4. DEND (Dev Delay, Epilepsy, Neonatal Diabetes)
- 3. HI/HA (Hyperinsulinism/ammonemia)
- 2. Glucose transporter I deficiency
- 1. B6/PLP/folinic acid dependencies

See text for explanation and eleventh case.

Newborn screening may lead to a misdiagnosis of PKU whereas an infant presenting with seizures may have a *biopterin-responsive hyperphenylalaninemia*. Dihydropteridine reductase deficiency additionally requires folinic acid which may result in resolution of basal ganglia calcifications. *Cerebral folate deficiency*, also treatable with folinic acid, is associated with decreased CSF 5-methyltetrahydrofolate with normal peripheral folate levels. Seizures (including infantile spasms or myoclonic) may be the sole feature in *biotinidase deficiency*, which is not universally covered in newborn screening. *Serine biosynthesis disorders* are treatable with combined L-serine and glycine but otherwise result in microcephaly and epilepsy. *Creatine synthesis disorders* feature intellectual disability and epilepsy, may be diagnosed with abnormal guanidinoacetic acid (GAA) levels in urine or plasma (or MR spectroscopy), and respond to creatine and ornithine supplementation and arginine restriction. Benzodiazepines appear to have an ameliorative role in *hyperekplexia*, an epilepsy mimicker due to mutations in the glycine inhibitory receptor or transport system associated with sudden death. A neonate presenting with seizures and diabetes may have a potassium-regulated ATP channelopathy of pancreas and brain, *DEND*, whereas the hyperglycemia is corrected by insulin but a profound encephalopathy may be preventable with utilization of a sulfonylurea. In contrast, congenital hyperinsulinism with hyperammonemia (*HI–HA*), a mutation of glutamate dehydrogenase, is associated with generalized epilepsy and learning disabilities, and is treated with diazoxide and protein restriction. *Glucose transporter 1 deficiency* has an enlarging phenotype, requires CSF analysis for hypoglycorrhachia, and is treatable with the ketogenic diet, offering an alternative metabolic fuel to glucose.

Pyridoxine (vitamin B6) dependency is the prototype and recently identified as antiquitin deficiency involving lysine degradation. Urine or plasma pipecolic acid is a valuable laboratory aid in addition to the standard concomitant administration of 100 mg IV pyridoxine during EEG. There are alternative approaches to making this diagnosis with trials of enteral therapy. Empirical discontinuation of therapy as a diagnostic maneuver is inadvisable, and the diagnosis must be resuspected even in initial treatment failures. The enigmatic folinic acid dependency is allelic to pyridoxine dependency, and patients may respond to either or both therapies. Pyridoxal-5-phosphate dependency is a newly recognized variant which is due to pyridox(am)ine oxidase deficiency and requires supplementation with the biologically active form of pyridoxine.

An 11th case was added, the urea cycle disorder OTC deficiency, in recognition of the quest to identify other important examples of the treatable metabolic epilepsies which no clinician wants to miss!

CLINICAL PEARLS

- Hyperphenylalaninemia may represent a disorder of biopterin synthesis or recycling instead of PKU. Intracranial calcifications may be reversible with folinic acid.
- Cerebral folate deficiency requires assay of CSF methyltetrahydrofolate.
- Biotinidase deficiency has been misdiagnosed as atypical demyelinating disease, myelopathies, and GI and cutaneous conditions. Seizures may the only obvious symptom in biotinidase deficiency and includes infantile spasms. International patients may not have been screened at birth.
- Treatable serine synthesis defects can present with congenital microcephaly, developmental disorder, or epilepsy.
- Treatable creatine synthesis defects have a wide and often nonspecific phenotype.
- Hyperekplexia is an epilepsy mimic with a risk of sudden death that can be mitigated with an oral benzodiazepine.
- Neonatal epilepsy with diabetes may represent a potassium channelopathy responsive to oral hypoglycemic agents but not insulin.
- Hypoglycemia with hyperinsulinism may be associated with hyperammonemia and respond to limited protein intake as well as diazoxide rescue when needed.
- Glucose transporter defect has a widening spectrum and is treated with the ketogenic diet as an alternative cerebral fuel to glucose.
- Pyridoxine and folinic acid dependency are allelic. Some patients require the biological form of pyridoxine, pyridoxal-5-phosphate, is a separate but related disorder of an oxidase deficiency.

REFERENCES

1. Blau N, Thöny B, Cotton RGH, et al. Disorders of tetrahydrobiopterin and related biogenic amines. In: CR Scriver, AL Beaudet, WS Sly, et al. eds. *The Metabolic & Molecular Bases of Inherited Disease*. New York: McGraw-Hill; 2001:1725–1776.
2. Bonkowsky JL, Ramaekers VT, Quadros EV, et al. Progressive encephalopathy in a child with cerebral folate deficiency syndrome. *J Child Neurol*. 2008;23(12):1460–1463.
3. Ramaekers VT, Häusler M, Opladen T, et al. Psychomotor retardation, spastic paraplegia, cerebellar ataxia and dyskinesia associated with low 5-methyltetrahydrofolate in cerebrospinal fluid: a novel neurometabolic condition responding to folinic acid substitution. *Neuropediatrics*, 2002;33(6):301–308.
4. Raemakers VT, Blau N. Cerebral folate deficiency. *Dev Med Child Neurol*. 2004;46:843–851.
5. de Koning TJ, Klomp LW, Van Oppen AC, et al. Prenatal and early postnatal treatment in 3-phosphoglycerate-dehydrogenase deficiency. *Lancet*. 2004;364(9452):2221–2222.
6. Fons C, Sempere A, Sanmarti FX, et al. Epilepsy spectrum in cerebral creatine transporter deficiency. *Epilepsia*. 2009;50(9):2168–2170.
7. Stöckler S, Holzbach U, Hanefeld F, et al. Creatine deficiency in the brain: a new, treatable inborn error of metabolism. *Pediatr Res*. 1994;36(3):409–413.
8. Valayannopoulos V, Boddaert N, Chabli A, et al. Treatment by oral creatine, L-arginine and L-glycine in six severely affected patients with creatine transporter defect. *J Inherit Metab Dis*. 2011;35:151–157.
9. Mineyko A, Whiting S, Graham GE. Hyperekplexia: treatment of a severe phenotype review of the literature. *Can J Neurol Sci*. 2011;38:411–416.
10. Shimomura K, Hörster F, de Wet H, et al. A novel mutation causing DEND syndrome: a treatable channelopathy of pancreas and brain. *Neurology*. 2007;69(13):1342–1349.
11. Palladino AA, Stanley CA. The hyperinsulinism/hyperammonemia syndrome. *Rev Endocr Metab Disord*. 2010;11(3):171–178.
12. Pearl PL, Gopse SM. Pyridoxal phosphate dependency, a newly recognized treatable catastrophic epileptic encephalopathy. *J Inherit Metab Dis*. 2007;30(1):2–4.
13. Hunt AD, Stokes J, McCrory WW, et al. Pyridoxine dependency: report of a case of intractable convulsions in an infant controlled by pyridoxine. *Pediatrics*. 1954;13(2):140–145.
14. Gallagher RC, Van Hove JL, Scharer G, et al. Folinic acid-responsive seizures are identical to pyridoxine-dependent epilepsy. *Ann Neurol*. 2009;65(5):550–556.
15. Baxter P. Pyridoxine dependent pyridoxine responsive seizures. In: P Baxter ed. *Vitamin Responsive Conditions in Paediatric Neurology*. London: Mac Keith Press, 2001:109–165.

2

Neuroimaging in the Metabolic Epilepsies

Robert A. Zimmerman and Zarir P. Khademian

INTRODUCTION

MRI IMAGING

Structural brain imaging including computed tomography (CT), MRI, and magnetic resonance spectroscopy (MRS) are part of the diagnostic work-up for the patient presenting with seizures, and can assist with identifying underlying inborn errors of metabolism (1). Imaging studies are used to supplement the routine development of a differential diagnosis based on the patient's clinical and family history, physical examination, and subsequent laboratory evaluation. The goal of neuroimaging is to arrive at an imaging phenotype that matches the clinical and genetic phenotype of the metabolic abnormality, thus giving some specificity to the diagnosis. Common imaging features of inborn errors of metabolism are atrophy of brain tissue over time, symmetry of involvement of brain structures such as the basal ganglia, abnormalities in myelination of the brain, and, less frequently,

abnormalities of contrast enhancement and malformation of structure (Table 2.1). Proton MRS adds a second dimension to MRI, demonstrating the presence of metabolites that are not normally detected, such as galactitol in galactosemia and ketones in diabetic ketoacidosis. Additionally, proton MRS reveals abnormalities in the concentrations of normal metabolites that may be increased, as in Canavan's disease, or decreased, as in creatine deficiency. One of the most useful metabolites for diagnosing a neurometabolic disease is lactate, as the presence of lactate in increased amounts within the brain tissue results from defects in enzymatic pathways of energy metabolism. The purpose of this chapter is to focus on the MRI and MRS features that need to be considered when evaluating a patient with epilepsy and a suspected metabolic disorder.

CT IMAGING

While CT of the brain is not considered to be as useful as MRI and MRS, the CT findings should not be ignored, as they are potentially useful or even disease-specific. Acute hypodensity of the basal ganglia may be seen in many decompensating processes of energy metabolism such as Leigh's disease, glutaric aciduria, methylmalonic aciduria, and propionic aciduria. Hypodensity may also be seen in disorders involving more extensive regions such as the cortex as in MELAS (mitochondrial myopathy, encephalopathy, lactic acidosis, and stroke) and ornithine transcarbamylase deficiency (OTC) (Figure 2.1). White matter

TABLE 2.1   MR Features of Metabolic Disease

1. Atrophy—common
2. Symmetry—common (eg, basal ganglia)
3. Myelination abnormalities
4. Enhancement—infrequent
5. Malformation—dysmorphic (mainly in lysosomal and peroxisomal diseases)

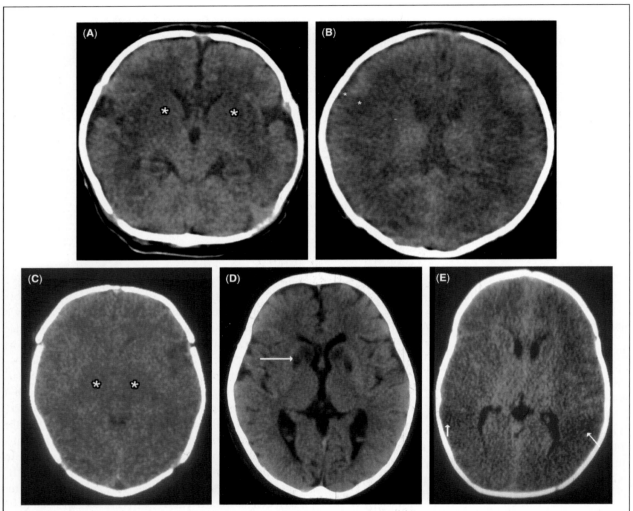

FIGURE 2.1   Computed tomography: Hypodensity due to metabolic edema and/or injury. (A) and (B) Ornithine transcarboxylase deficiency (OTC). A 2-week-old infant with abnormal hypodensity of (A) basal ganglia (*'s) and (B) cortical areas (*'s). (C) MSUD. A 8-day-old male infant with hypodensity of thalami (*'s). (D) Leigh's disease, chronic stage of insult to basal ganglia with tissue loss (arrow). (E) Molybdenum cofactor deficiency. Cortical and subcortical white matter hypodensity due to brain edema involving both cerebral hemispheres (arrows). Courtesy of Elsevier.

hypodensity on CT may be more difficult to appreciate in the newborn and infant than in the older child, but can be highly significant in maple syrup urine disease (MSUD), galactosemia, metachromatic leukodystrophy (MLD), and Pelizaeus–Merzbacher disease (PMD), among others. Hyperdensity in central gray matter on CT, for example, the basal ganglia, may be an important clue in mitochondrial disease and Aicardi–Goutières syndrome, while thalamic hyperdensity can be a clue to Krabbe disease and Sandhoff syndrome

(Figure 2.2). Any of these CT findings in a patient with or without seizures should indicate the need for MRI and MRS.

DISCUSSION

Some metabolic diseases have relatively specific MRI imaging features (Table 2.2), while other diseases have findings that are more suggestive than specific

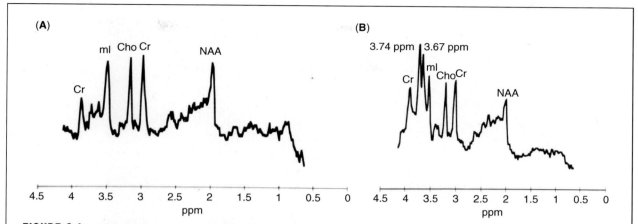

FIGURE 2.4 Normal short echo TE and short echo TE at 1.5 T of galactosemic with galactitol, relative to normal control. (A) A 7-day-old infant with single voxel through the basal ganglia shows normal spectra. (B) Abnormal spectra in a galactosemic patient with elevation of galactitol at 3.67 and 3.74 ppm. Courtesy of Elsevier.

(Figure 2.9C), Pelizaeus–Merzbacher more generalized and diffuse (Figure 2.9D), and L2-hydroxyglutaric aciduria more peripheral (Figure 2.9E).

Alexander's disease also shows evidence of contrast enhancement in the basal ganglia and brainstem (Figure 2.10C) that are not seen in Canavan's, where

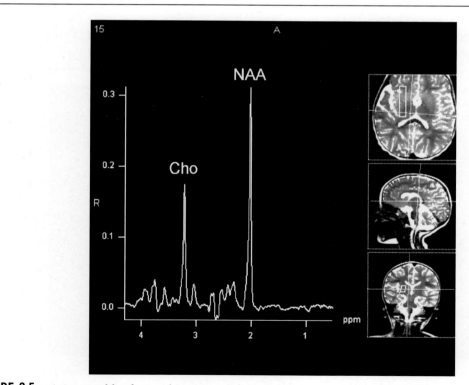

FIGURE 2.5 A 2-year-old infant with creatine deficiency. Proton spectra (long TE 270 msec at 3 T) shows absent creatine peak. Normal NAA and choline (Cho). Courtesy of Elsevier.

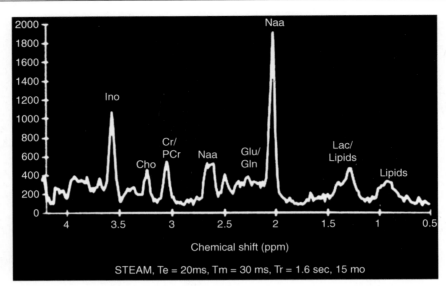

FIGURE 2.6   Canavan's disease. Proton spectra (short TE at 1.5 T) show marked elevation of *N*-acetyl aspartate, decreased choline, and elevation of myoinositol. Courtesy of Elsevier.

there is no gadolinium enhancement. ALD, shown in Figures 2.9B and 2.11A, presents as a white matter abnormality in the splenium of the corpus callosum and shows elevation of choline at the site (Figure 2.11B) as its initial presentation (8, 9). The advancing demyelinating margins in ALD show gadolinium

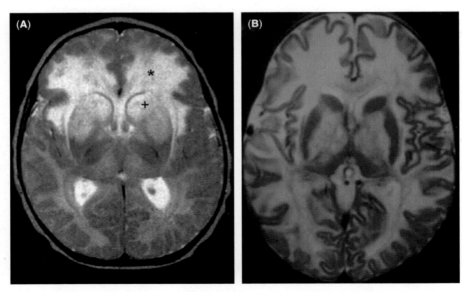

FIGURE 2.7   Macrocephaly. (A) Axial T2-weighted image in a macrocephalic infant with Alexander's disease shows frontal predominance in white matter (*) and basal ganglia involvement (+). (B) Axial T2-weighted image shows diffuse white matter involvement in infant with Canavan's disease. Courtesy of Elsevier.

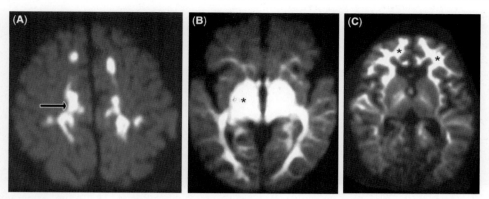

FIGURE 2.8 Diffusion positive imaging and its reversibility. (A) Axial diffusion-weighted image in patient with Leigh's disease showing irreversible white matter damage (arrow). (B) Axial diffusion image in patient with MSUD showing white matter abnormality that was reversible (*). (C) Axial diffusion-weighted image in patient with Canavan's disease showing stable vacuolar diffusion restriction (*'s). Courtesy of Elsevier.

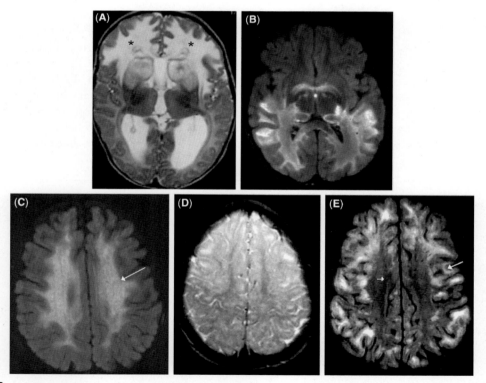

FIGURE 2.9 Differential patterns of white matter involvement on T2 and FLAIR imaging. (A) Frontal white matter involvement in Alexander's disease on axial T2 (*'s). (B) Posterior white matter involvement in ALD on axial FLAIR (*). (C) Diffuse central white matter involvement (arrow) with spared subcortical u-fibers in metachromatic leukodystrophy. (D) Diffuse white matter involvement and hypomyelination involving subcortical u-fibers in Pelizaeus–Merzbacher disease. (E) Axial T2 with peripheral white matter hyperintensity (large arrow) sparing central white matter in L2-hydroxyglutaric aciduria (small arrow). Courtesy of Elsevier.

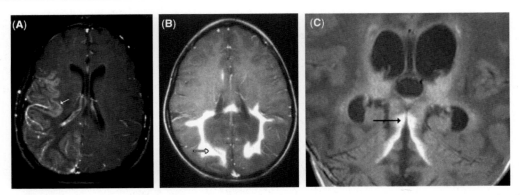

FIGURE 2.10   Abnormal gadolinium enhancement in neurometabolic disease. (A) Axial T1-weighted image post-gadolinium injection in patient with MELAS, showing cortical contrast enhancement at sites of infarction (arrow). (B) Axial post-gadolinium T1-weighted image in ALD showing contrast enhancement of the advancing edge of demyelination (arrow). (C) Coronal T1-weighted gadolinium-enhanced image showing enhancement in the brainstem as a result of Alexander's disease (arrow). Courtesy of Elsevier.

enhancement (Figure 2.10B) in a posterior distribution of white matter (Figure 2.9B), which helps to characterize the disease from an imaging standpoint (10). Gadolinium enhancement occurs not only in ALD and Alexander's, but also in cases of MELAS where there has been infarction (Figure 2.10A).

MRIs performed during acute decompensation on neurometabolic patients presenting with seizures

should be evaluated with attention paid to the gray matter in the cerebral cortex (Figure 2.12), including the hippocampi (Figure 2.13). Acute swelling can be seen on the FLAIR and T2-weighted images, and restricted motion of water due to cytotoxic edema can be seen on diffusion imaging, as shown in Figure 2.14B with OTC deficiency (11, 12). The subsequent evolution of such injuries is frequently loss

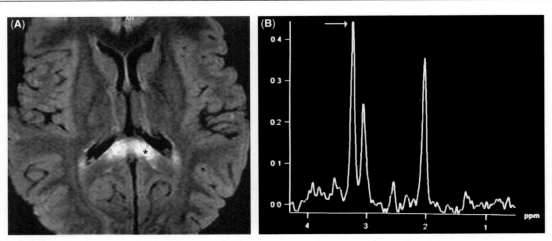

FIGURE 2.11   A 10-y-old male individual with ALD, x-linked. (A) Axial FLAIR shows abnormal increased signal intensity in the splenium of the corpus callosum (*). (B) Proton spectra (long TE, 135 msec) shows elevated choline in a single voxel taken from the splenium of the corpus callosum (arrow). Courtesy of Elsevier.

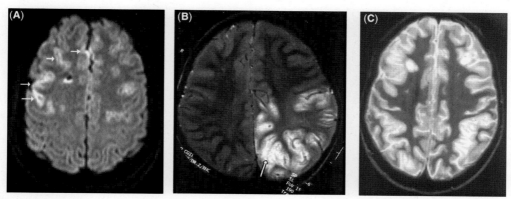

FIGURE 2.12   Acute cortical T2/FLAIR cortical hyperintensity. (A) Hypoglycemic brain injury. Axial FLAIR shows cortical increased signal intensity involving the frontal lobes (arrows). (B) MELAS with cortical hyperintensity seen on axial T2 involving the left parietal lobe (arrow). (C) Diffuse increased T2 cortical signal intensity in acute metabolic decompensation of OTC deficiency. Courtesy of Elsevier.

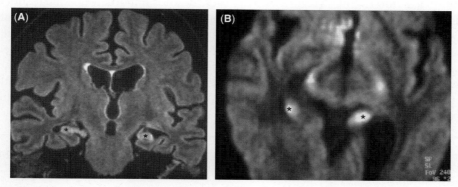

FIGURE 2.13   Acute hippocampal injury. Mitochondrial disease in a 16-y-old male adolescent. (A) Coronal FLAIR image shows increased signal intensity in bilateral hippocampi (*'s). (B) Axial diffusion-weighted image shows restricted motion of water in the bilateral hippocampi (*'s). Courtesy of Elsevier.

of tissue, eventually seen as cortical atrophy (Figure 2.15C). Cortical atrophy also accompanies neurodegenerative processes of neurometabolic origin, as shown in Figure 2.15A with neural ceroid lipofuscinosis (13), and following metabolic injury, as in Kearns–Sayre syndrome (Figure 2.15B). The gray matter in the basal ganglia and portions of the brainstem is also vulnerable to acute metabolic injury, as seen in Leigh's disease on T2 and FLAIR images (Figure 2.16A,B). In acute situations, these changes can also be seen on diffusion imaging as restricted motion of water (Figure 2.14C), including in Leigh's and glutaric aciduria

type 1 (14, 15). With permanent injury, the structures involved undergo atrophy, but continue to have abnormally increased signal intensity on T2 and FLAIR. Restricted motion of water on diffusion imaging is not always a sign of irreversibility. As mentioned earlier, in contrast with Leigh's disease (Figure 2.8A), this may be reversible in MSUD (Figures 2.14A and 2.8B) when appropriate dietary measures are applied (16).

Patterns of white matter involvement are often important clues to the nature of the underlying neurometabolic disease (17). Central white matter involvement with sparing of subcortical u-fibers is seen

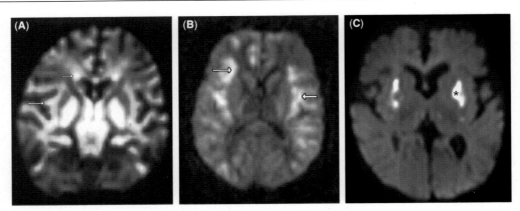

FIGURE 2.14   Acute metabolic decompensation with swelling of cortex, white matter, or basal ganglia on diffusion imaging. (A) Axial diffusion of MSUD showing acute swelling of the myelinated white matter (arrows). (B) Acute metabolic decompensation in OTC deficiency with cortical cytotoxic edema (arrows). (C) Acute basal ganglionic cytotoxic edema in a case of Leigh's disease (asterisk). Courtesy of Elsevier.

in metachromatic leukodystrophy (Figure 2.9C) (18). With Pelizaeus–Merzbacher disease, there is diffuse hypomyelination of all of the involved white matter supratentorially (Figure 2.9D). However, in L2-hydroxyglutaric aciduria, the peripheral white matter is involved and the central white matter is spared, except in the internal capsule (Figure 2.9E)

(19, 20). It is important to evaluate not only the supratentorial white matter, but also the infratentorial region as well. High signal intensity abnormalities on T2 and FLAIR involving the dentate nucleus region are seen in L2-hydroxyglutaric aciduria (Figure 2.17), Leigh's disease, cerebrotendinous xanthomatosis, and Wilson's disease (14, 19, 20–22). Malformation of the

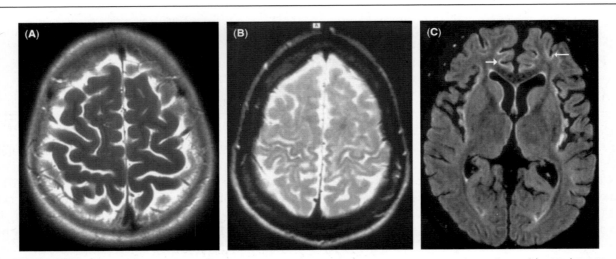

FIGURE 2.15   Thinning of the cortex as a result of neurometabolic injury seen as cortical atrophy and/or T2/FLAIR hyperintensity. (A) Axial T2 shows thin cortex secondary to neuronal ceroid lipofuscinosis. Note the prominent sulci. (B) T2 axial shows cortical atrophy as a result of Kearns–Sayre disease. Note the prominent sulci. (C) Focal thinning of the cortex with FLAIR hyperintensity post injury in OTC deficiency (arrows). Courtesy of Elsevier.

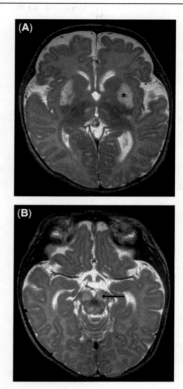

FIGURE 2.16 A 3-month-old infant with Leigh's disease. (A) Basal ganglia hyperintensity seen on T2 and FLAIR (*). (B) Brainstem hyperintensity seen on T2 and FLAIR (arrow). Courtesy of Elsevier.

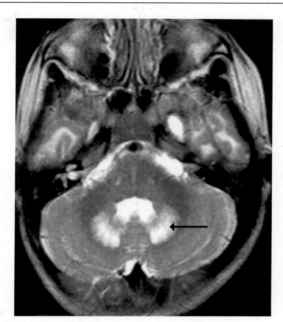

FIGURE 2.17 Dentate T2/FLAIR high signal intensity abnormality. L2-hydroxyglutaric aciduria with high signal in the dentate nuclei on axial T2 (arrow). Courtesy of Elsevier.

brain depends on metabolic effects altering the brain structure in utero. Examples of this are seen in glycine encephalopathy and pyruvate dehydrogenase

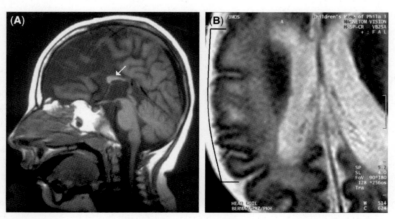

FIGURE 2.18 Cerebral malformation. (A) Sagittal T1 of a 4-year-old patient with pyruvate dehydrogenase deficiency and severe hypoplasia of the corpus callosum (arrow). (B) Axial T2 of a infant with polymicrogyria in Zellweger syndrome. A portion of involved cortex is indicated. Courtesy of Elsevier.

deficiency, producing degrees of corpus callosal agenesis (Figure 2.18A), and in Zellweger's syndrome, with polymicrogyria (Figure 2.18B) (23, 24).

CONCLUSION

MRI and MRS contribute to the diagnostic evaluation of patients with neurometabolic diseases. Careful evaluation of structures by T2, FLAIR, and diffusion imaging reveals patterns of findings that, to a greater or lesser degree, may indicate an etiology. Further correlation between imaging, clinical, and genetic evaluation should further enhance our diagnostic ability regarding phenotypic expression.

KEY POINTS

- Imaging phenotypes may be relatively specific for metabolic diseases.
- Acute hypodensity of basal ganglia on CT may indicate decompensating processes.
- Hyperdensity in central gray matter on CT may indicate mitochondrial disease or Aicardi Goutieres syndrome. Thalamic hyperdensity on CT may suggest Krabbe or Sandhoff disease.
- On MRI, diffusion restriction may be a sign of irreversible and progressive (Leigh disease) or reversible pathology (MSUD), or remain stable (Canavan's disease).
- Anatomic white matter involvement is more anterior in Alexander's, posterior in ALD, central in MLD, diffuse in Pelizaeus-Merzbacher, and peripheral in L2-OH-glutaric aciduria.
- Cortical atrophy accompanies neurodegenerative processes (eg, NCL) or metabolic injury (eg, Kearns-Sayre syndrome).
- Malformations of brain development may result from in utero effects of metabolic diseases (eg, corpus callosal agenesis in glycine encephalopathy and pyruvate dehydrogenase deficiency) or polymicrogyria in Zellweger's syndrome.

Chapter adapted from: Zimmerman RA. Neuroimaging of inherited metabolic disorders producing seizures. *Brain Dev.* 2011;33(9):734–744. All tables are published and all figures have been modified and published with permission from Elsevier.

REFERENCES

1. Wang ZH, Zimmerman RA. The value of proton MR spectroscopy in pediatric metabolic brain disease. *Am J Neuroradiol.* 1997;18:1872–1879.
2. Berry GT, Hunter JV, Wang Z, et al. In vivo evidence of brain galactitol accumulation in an infant with galactosemia and encephalopathy. *J Pediatr.* 2001;138:260–262.
3. Wang ZJ, Berry GT, Dreha SF, et al. Proton magnetic resonance spectroscopy of brain metabolites in galactosemia. *Ann Neurol.* 2001;50:266–269.
4. Stockler S, Holzbach U, Hanefeld F, et al. Creatine deficiency in the brain: A new, treatable inborn error of metabolism. *Pediatr. Res.* 1994;36:409–413.
5. Marks HG, Caro PA, Wang Z, et al. Use of computed tomography, magnetic resonance imaging, and localized 1H magnetic resonance spectroscopy in Canavan disease: A case report. *Ann Neurol.* 1991;30:106–110.
6. Brismar J, Brismar G, Gascon G, et al. Canavan disease: CT and MR imaging of the brain. *Am J Neuroradiol.* 1990;11:805–810.
7. van der Knaap MS, Naidu S, Breiter SN, et al. Alexander disease: Diagnosis with MR imaging. *Am J Neuroradiol.* 2001;22:541–552.
8. Moser HW, Loes DJ, Melhem ER, et al. X-linked adrenoleukodystrophy: Overview and prognosis as a function of age and brain magnetic resonance imaging abnormality. A study involving 372 patients. *Neuropediatrics.* 2000;31:227–239.
9. Confort-Gouny S, Vion-dury J, Chabrol B, et al. Localised proton magnetic resonance spectroscopy in x-linked adrenoleukodystrophy. *Neuroradiology.* 1995;37:568–575.
10. Melhem ER, Loes DJ, Georgiades CS, et al. X-linked adrenoleukodystrophy: The role of contrast-enhanced MR imaging in predicting disease progression. *Am J Neuroradiol.* 2000;21:839–844.
11. de Grauw TJ, Smit LM, Brockstedt M, et al. Acute hemiparesis as the presenting sign in a heterozygote for ornithine transcarbamylase deficiency. *Neuropediatrics.* 1990;21:133–135.
12. Takanashi J-I, Barkovich AJ, Cheng SF, et al. Brain MR imaging in acute hyperammonemic encephalopathy arising from late-onset ornithine transcarbamylase deficiency. *Am J Neuroradiol.* 2003;24:390–393.
13. Santavuori P, Vanhanen SL, Autti T. Clinical and neuroradiological diagnostic aspects of neuronal ceroid lipofuscinoses disorders. *Eur J Paediatr Neurol.* 2001;5(Suppl A):157–161.
14. Detre JA, Wang Z, Bogdan AR, et al. Regional variation in brain lactate in Leigh syndrome by localized 1H magnetic resonance spectroscopy. *Ann Neurol.* 1991;29:218–221.
15. Bismar J, Ozand PT. CT and MR of the brain in glutaric aciduria type I: A review of 59 published cases and a report of 5 new patients. *Am J Neuroradiol.* 1995;16:675–683.
16. Jan W, Zimmerman RA, Wang ZJ, et al. MR diffusion imaging and MR spectroscopy of maple syrup urine disease during acute metabolic decompensation. *Neuroradiology.* 2003;45:393–399.
17. Schiffmann R, van der Knaap MS. An MRI-based approach to the diagnosis of white matter disorders. *Neurology.* 2009;72:750–759.
18. Faerber EN, Melvin JJ, Smergel EM. MRI appearances of metachromatic leukodystrophy. *Pediatr Radiol.* 1999;29:669–672.

19. Nezu A, Kimura S, Takeshita S, et al. An MRI and MRS study of Pelizaeus–Merzbacher disease. *Pediatr Neurol.* 1998;18: 334–347.

20. D'Incerti L, Farina L, Moroni I, et al. L-2-Hydroxyglutaric aciduria: MRI in seven cases. *Neuroradiology.* 1998;40:727–733.

21. DeStefano N, Dotti MT, Mortilla M, et al. Magnetic resonance imaging and spectroscopic changes in brains of patients with cerebrotendinous xanthomatosis. *Brain.* 2001;124:121–131.

22. DeHaan J, Grossman RI, Civitello L, et al. High field MRI of Wilson's disease. *CT: J Comput Tomogr.* 1987;11:132–135.

23. Shevell MI, Matthews PM, Scriver CR, et al. Cerebral dysgenesis and lactic academia: an MRI/MRS phenotype associated with pyruvate dehydrogenase deficiency. *Pediatr Neurol.* 1994;11: 224–249.

24. Barkovich AJ, Peck WW. MR of Zellweger syndrome. *Am J Neuroradiol.* 1997;18:1163–1170.

3

Advances in MR Spectroscopy for Inherited Epilepsies

Andrew Breeden, Morgan J. Prust, and Andrea L. Gropman

INTRODUCTION

Magnetic resonance spectroscopy (MRS) is a powerful clinical tool that has gained increased attention as new diagnostic applications become more widespread, such as early disease detection, therapy monitoring, and biochemical profiling. The most common MRS scan, ^{1}H spectroscopy, can be conducted on a standard MRI hardware setup at 1.5 T field strength and above, with conventional sequences taking 3–10 min. The technique is FDA approved and can be ordered by physicians. Most major MRI manufacturers now include relatively automated sequences for acquiring and processing MRS data. Unlike traditional MRI scans, however, MRS does not output an image. Instead, it produces a spectrum of peaks that contain information about biochemical concentrations in a region of interest (typically 1–10 cm^3) within the brain.

A correct reading of MR spectra can reveal information about brain metabolite concentrations relevant to a variety of neurological conditions including brain tumors, neonatal injury, white matter disorders, metabolic disorders, and epilepsy (1). Researchers and clinicians have used the technique in epilepsy to identify regions of neuronal injury, lateralize seizure foci, predict surgical outcomes, and elucidate the mechanisms of bio-energetic failure. In these instances it provides information that is not revealed by a standard MRI T1/T2 brain image.

It is important to note that spectra do not contain absolute quantification of biochemicals per se, and as such, a correct reading of spectra relies on examining resonance ratios between metabolites or absolute quantitation. There are also a variety of sequences and techniques available, with some reporting higher reliability and spectral quality than others. Thus it is important to understand not only how MRS data is clinically relevant in epilepsy, but some basic concepts regarding spectroscopy, its acquisition, processing, and interpretation.

CONCEPTS: THE BASIS FOR MR SPECTROSCOPY

MRS relies on concepts that chemists and physicists have used for decades in chemical analysis. Physicists determined in the 1920s that protons spin due to thermal energy and can spin only at certain frequencies, as predicted by quantum mechanics. It was later discovered that because of this, protons can absorb electromagnetic energy if it matches the frequency at which the proton is spinning. The absorption of this energy changes the energy state of the spin. This forms the basis of the concept of magnetic resonance, and the frequency at which energy is absorbed is known as the resonant frequency. The resonant frequencies of protons depend on the static magnetic field applied to them—with the resonance frequency of hydrogen being around 63 MHz at 1.5 T, and 126 MHz at 3 T.

To understand how the concept of magnetic resonance allows for the creation of images or spectra, one needs to examine the behavior of nuclei in the presence of an applied static magnetic field. Because of its prevalence in biological tissue, hydrogen is the most commonly imaged nucleus in MRI and MRS. Note, however, that substances with unfilled molecular orbitals (ie, an odd number of protons or neutrons, including ^1H, ^{13}C, and ^{31}P) create magnetic moments and are detectable with MR. Each nucleus has its own resonant frequency. These nuclei act like tiny magnets that, when in the presence of a static magnetic field, change their orientation and rotate at their resonant frequency in a motion known as precession, akin to a spinning top. The vast majority of nuclei enters a lower-energy stable state and begins to spin parallel to the magnetic field. In a normal environment, the earth's magnetic field is too weak and thus the direction of spinning is essentially random and the net magnetization of a group of protons is almost negligible. In high field strength such as in an MRI scanner, however, the majority of proton spins begin to align and create a net magnetic moment parallel to the static field (2). Thus, in a strong magnetic field, a group of protons goes from random alignment to a cumulative magnetic force that becomes visible in an MRI. The large amount of hydrogen in the human body allows us to examine tissue contrast in MRI, or certain hydrogen containing metabolites in MRS.

Aligning protons in a magnetic field is not, in itself, enough for detection of signal from the protons. We must also utilize the principles of magnetic resonance and electromagnetic absorption described above. To generate a signal, the protons are bombarded with electromagnetic waves in the radiofrequency (RF) range, known as an RF excitation pulse that oscillates at the resonant frequency of hydrogen. This excites the protons and their spins absorb energy and enter a transitory high-energy state, changing their net magnetization to become perpendicular to the static field. The spins then reemit electromagnetic energy that can be measured by a RF coil tuned to the resonant frequency (3). In summary, MR functions by using a large magnetic field to align the spins of protons, and then transmit a pulse of RF energy so these spins can be measured. This measurement is mathematically transformed to create images or spectra.

While these principles of generating a signal, and the hardware required to do so, are the same in standard MRI and MRS, they differ in some important ways. Structural MR images are created by applying magnetic gradients that change the magnetic field slightly with space. Excited protons then emit energy at different frequencies in different spatial locations. This information is used in a mathematical technique called Fast Fourier Transform (FFT) to deconstruct the signal (predominately from hydrogen in water molecules) into units of space called voxels, which renders a brain image. In MRS, however, one does not localize water signal to examine tissue contrast. Instead, the goal is to examine metabolites that are 10,000 times less prevalent than the concentration of brain water. In order to visualize metabolites of interest, a pulse known as water suppression is first applied to disperse the water signal. The MR signal within a region of interest (a voxel) is then read out, and a Fourier Transform creates a plot of resonances at different frequencies. This is the MR spectrum. Why, however, do protons resonate with different frequencies in MRS?

Unlike MRI, the answer to this question hinges not on controlled magnetic gradients, but on variations in the local magnetic environment in different metabolites due to their chemical structure. Chemical bonds within metabolites distribute their electron clouds differently, based on bonding structure and chemical confirmation of neighboring nuclei, which slightly changes the magnetic field experienced by protons. Thus, protons appear in different locations on an MR spectrum based on their chemical environment. Even protons in different bonding locations in the same molecule show up differently on spectra. Each proton in the molecule gives an MR detectable signal and chemically equivalent protons will resonate at the same place on the spectrum with additive signal. The frequency of absorption of a metabolite in reference to a molecular standard is known as chemical shift. In neurospectroscopy the standard is a large peak around 2.0 parts per million (ppm), corresponding to the peptide *N*-acetylaspartate (NAA), a neuronal marker.

By having prior knowledge of metabolite chemical structure, and based on previous experimental information, one can construct an expected chemical fingerprint of how and where a brain metabolite will resonate in the spectrum. Specialized software can be used to analyze spectral data, incorporating a priori information acquired from an in vitro basis set with known concentrations, and model the spectrum as a linear combination of individual chemicals. This information is used to assign resonances to specific metabolites and the software finds the area under these peaks, which gives a value proportional to the concentration of the metabolite (4). Software also carries out important processing steps such as filtering remaining water signal, correcting for electrical current distortions caused by localization gradients known as eddy current distortion, correction for phase shifts due to hardware settings, and correcting for baseline distortions. Some MR facilities have automated processing software. Other common software packages for processing and fitting MRS data include LCModel, QUEST, and AMARES (1). Various software use different mathematical approaches to spectral interpretation, but a detailed description of these is beyond the scope of this chapter. Using software packages, one can detect the concentration of metabolites that are present. At lower field strength there is a lower signal-to-noise ratio (SNR) making it more difficult to resolve metabolites with similar, overlapping resonances into distinct peaks on the spectrum. Higher field strengths tend to produce spectra with better resolution.

Unfortunately, not all hydrogen-containing compounds are visible on the MR time scale. In general, small, mobile molecules with concentrations above approximately 0.5 μmol/g tissue are detectable. To get signal robust enough to examine these metabolites, voxels are typically big (1–10 cm^3). Some measurable metabolites include some amino acids, carbohydrates, and fatty acids. In total there are roughly 35 metabolites measurable in the human brain (5). Some of these include unexpected chemicals such as ethanol. In practice, not all of these metabolites will be in sufficient concentration, or there will not be sufficient signal to resolve their peaks. Because many of these resolvable biochemicals are part of well-regulated pathways, there is an extensive literature on normal metabolite concentration ratios in gray and white matter. By looking at aberrations in the concentration of these metabolites one can glean information that is clinically relevant to a particular disease process. A more extensive treatment of common biochemical alterations revealed in patients with epilepsy is discussed later in this chapter.

Acquisition Techniques

^{1}H MRS scans may be acquired as a single spectrum from one area of the brain (single voxel scans—SVS) or as many spectra from different locations simultaneously (chemical shift imaging—CSI). Each provides different benefits to the study of epilepsy.

^{1}H MRS localizes signal acquisition by acquiring data from the intersection of three excited orthogonal planes that defines an ROI. There are two main types of acquisitions in SVS—Simulated Echo Acquisition Mode (STEAM) and Point-Resolved Spectroscopy (PRESS)—known as pulse sequences because they send excitation pulses of RF energy and apply magnetic gradients in a sequence designed to acquire the desired signal in the desired location. STEAM provides a well-delineated voxel, and good water suppression, but less signal than PRESS (3). When using either technique, the time that signal is read out after excitation (TE) can be varied to examine metabolites differently. Long TE (135 ms or greater) scans can separate NAA, creatine (Cr), and choline (Cho) very well, and short TE (35 ms or less) scans resolve more metabolites such as glutamate (Glu), glutamine (Gln), and myoinositol, and have better signal (6). Single voxel scans (SVS) usually acquire many spectra over time from the same voxel location and average them to achieve sufficient signal. Optimal results from SVS are achieved when the area of measurement is placed in a homogeneous gray or white matter location. Standard clinical voxel placements for examination of nonfocal disorders are in occipital gray matter to assess neuronal health, and in a posterior white matter voxel to assess axonal condition (1).

While MRS focused on one location is of high clinical utility to examine specific areas of neuronal damage, or to describe metabolite changes in gray or white matter when there are global disease abnormalities, studies of human epilepsy often benefit from looking at a large number of locations to localize pathology and metabolic abnormalities (7). Multivoxel MRS, or CSI, achieves this aim by simultaneously acquiring multiple spectra in voxels across a region of space called a brain slice. Regions of interest within the slice can also be selected even after the scan has already been acquired through a post-processing step called voxel shifting. Multivoxel scans are not without drawbacks, however. Acquisitions are more time intensive than SVS—up to 30–40 min. Additionally, the spectra acquired tend to be lower resolution and susceptible to artifacts, especially in regions adjacent to the paranasal sinuses.

In addition to ^{1}H MRS, ^{31}P and ^{13}C MRS are available. These require specialized receiver head-coils that are tuned to the resonant frequency of the desired nuclei. They can also be time consuming, and ^{13}C may require oral administration or intravenous infusion of compounds such as $(1-^{13}C)$ glucose (8).

Reading a Spectrum

MRS spectra are displayed on an x-axis with units of parts per million (ppm), and values increase right to left (somewhat counter-intuitively). The first step when reading a spectrum is to determine if it meets a quality threshold acceptable for use in a clinical work-up. Signs of poor spectral quality include peaks not appearing in the correct expected location (discussed below), peaks overlapping extensively when not expected, or the baseline sloping dramatically across the spectrum (6). If a spectrum is acceptable, metabolite concentrations can then be used to describe brain biochemistry in that region. A spectrum will reveal these biochemically relevant metabolites: lactate, NAA, glutamine–glutamate, creatine, choline metabolites, and myoinositol (Figure 3.1). Visual inspection of the spectrum can reveal disease processes

as evidenced by abnormal metabolite peak heights. A more rigorous approach utilizes software packages to provide calculated area under resonance peaks to determine concentration.

Because concentrations are proportional, they are sometimes expressed in ratio to a reference metabolite—often creatine (Cr) (eg, NAA/Cr ratio). This is premised on the assumption that Cr is relatively constant, even in diseased brains. Sometimes, however, this assumption does not hold. Other techniques to standardize concentration values have emerged, such as expressing concentrations after applying a mathematical correction for the proportion of gray matter, white matter, and CSF present in a voxel. This is done by segmenting an anatomical MRI scan and determining tissue proportions where the MRS voxel was acquired.

Each metabolite present in sufficient concentration to be commonly examined in clinical MRS provides different information. *N*-Acetylaspartate (present at 2.02 ppm) is an amino acid derivative synthesized in neurons, transported down axons, and broken down

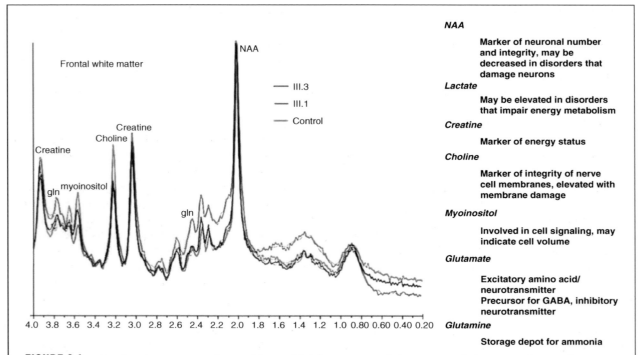

FIGURE 3.1   Overlapping spectrum from subjects with inborn errors of nitrogen metabolism is used as an illustration of the location of metabolite peaks and variations that reflect stage of disease.

in oligodendrocytes. While its role in vivo is not well understood, studies have shown that it is present almost entirely in neurons and axons (9), and thus correlates with the number of intact neurons in gray matter and density of intact neurons in white matter (1). This property makes NAA a very powerful diagnostic marker. It is present in consistent levels in normal populations, with some heterogeneity. Decreased NAA can indicate neuronal damage, focal disorders, and tumors, with the level of reduction commonly used as a proxy for the extent of neuronal or axonal loss. In epilepsy, decreased NAA may be indicative of neuronal metabolic dysfunction. For reasons discussed later, low NAA can also localize seizure onset location. Clinicians working with pediatric populations should note that NAA levels are lower in the developing brain and typically peak at age 10 to 15 years (10). "Normal" NAA levels in younger individuals should therefore be assessed on the basis of age.

Glutamate and glutamine (combined referred to as Glx) resonances overlap in spectra acquired in scanners below 7 T. These closely related amino acids are involved in neurotransmission and have peaks at 2.12 to 2.35 ppm (representing the beta and gamma protons) and another peak at 3.74 to 3.75 ppm (representing the alpha proton) (1). Glutamate is mainly present in neurons. Increased glutamate levels can lead to neuronal damage due to overexcitation. Glutamine is present in higher levels in astrocytes, and is thus said to be an astrocyte marker (6). Increased glutamine can be found in Reyes syndrome, hypoxic–ischemic events, and hyperammonemia (11, 12).

A peak present at 3.22 is sometimes deemed choline (Cho), but is better referred to as "choline containing compounds," or total Choline (tCho) because it is comprised of several compounds, mainly phosphorylcholine, phosphorylated cholines, and glycerophosphorylcholine. These are membrane and myelin markers, and can increase with pathological changes to membrane turnover (13). Fluctuations in tCho compounds can indicate malignant tumors, multiple sclerosis, or diffuse axonal injury (14).

The major resonance of creatine (Cr) is present at 3.00 ppm and, in a healthy brain, is comprised of equal proportions of free creatine and phosphocreatine (PCr), with Cr and PCr in constant enzymatic exchange. PCr is a bioenergetic marker because of its large role in the synthesis of ATP (1). Cr is sometimes assumed to be constant and is used to scale other metabolites. Cr is transported to the brain from the liver, however, so some systemic diseases can change cerebral Cr levels. This needs to be taken into consideration when using Cr in metabolite ratios. Additionally, Cr levels are normally low in the newborn brain (6).

Lactate can be seen at 1.33 ppm but is not at a high enough concentration in healthy tissue to yield a visible signal. In general, the presence of a lactate peak is indicative of gliotic injury in which the normal processes of oxidative metabolism are disrupted (1).

Gamma-aminobutyric acid (GABA) is the major inhibitory neurotransmitter in the central nervous system and plays a large role in epilepsy. GABA levels may be of great interest in epilepsy. Its resonances, however, overlap with other metabolites such as Glu, NAA, and Cr, making it difficult or impossible to resolve on a traditional spectrum. Pulse sequences typically employed at high field (3 T or greater), and known as editing sequences, have been designed to resolve the one or more GABA signals. A common editing sequence called MEGA-PRESS uses editing pulses to cancel the Cr signal and enable a more clear resolution of GABA (15).

MRS AND EPILEPSY

Over the past two decades, MRS has been extensively used to probe the neurometabolic underpinnings of epileptiform illness. Findings from MRS studies in epilepsy have given rise to a disease model in which bioenergetic failure in neuronal mitochondria disrupts the clearance of excitatory neurotransmitters, principally glutamate, increasing neuronal excitability and, ultimately, risk for epileptiform discharges. This seizure activity, in turn, exerts oxidative stress on neuronal mitochondria, perpetuating bioenergetic failure and hypometabolism, and ultimately compromising the active transport-mediated maintenance of ionic gradients. Loss of effective neuronal repolarization in epileptogenic zones disrupts the coordinated activity of neuronal assemblies, increasing the risk for further seizure activity.

The overwhelming majority of MRS investigations of epilepsy have been conducted in patients with medial temporal-lobe epilepsy (MTLE). We will describe the relevant findings in MTLE as a model with which to explore other more rare epilepsies, such as seen in inborn errors of metabolism and West syndrome. We describe 1H, 31P, and 13C MRS as individual components of this investigative model.

THE GLIAL-NEURONAL UNIT, BIOENERGETIC FAILURE AND HYPEREXCITABILITY IN EPILEPSY

In order to understand how metabolic failure increases the risk of seizure activity, one must appreciate the pathways through which excitatory neurotransmitters are cycled through the neuron, synapse, and glia. Pan et al (16) have proposed the glial-neuronal unit (GNU) as a model to illustrate how astrocytes, sensitive to increases in neurotransmission, couple synaptic activity with metabolic flux (Figure 3.2). It has been demonstrated that when glutamate (Glu), the brain's primary excitatory neurotransmitter, is released into the synapse, it is cleared via Na+-dependent transport by the GNU into the astrocyte (17). This process triggers the astrocytic uptake of glucose, which is subsequently metabolized to provide the cellular energy necessary to drive the metabolic flux of Glu and the activity of neuronal Na+/K+ ATP-ase pumps, which further drive the synaptic Na+ gradient and maintain neuronal polarization. When Glu enters the astrocyte, a molecular cascade stimulates the glycolytic production of 2 ATP molecules and lactate. Glu is converted by glutamine synthetase into glutamine (Gln), a metabolic conversion that consumes one of the glycolytic ATP molecules. Gln is then transported back into the neuron, where it is converted back into Glu by glutaminase, a process which consumes the other ATP. Lactate is shuttled from the astrocyte to the neuron, where, under normal conditions, it undergoes oxidative phosphorylation to produce an additional 17 ATP molecules, which fuel the activity of the Na+/K+ ATP-ase pump (17).

The flow of GABA, the brain's primary inhibitory neurotransmitter, through the GNU also stems from the Glu cycle. Glu is converted into GABA in the neuron by glutamic acid decarboxylase (GAD). Once released into the synapse, GABA is either repackaged into neurotransmitter vesicles following reuptake, or transported into the astrocyte where GABA-transaminase (GABA-T) converts it into succinate, which ultimately enters the TCA cycle. Roughly 20% of Glu flux is devoted to GABA cycling (16). Neurons and glia are thus inherently interdependent with respect to neurotransmission and metabolism, which are susceptible to disturbances in the GNU.

1H MRS

Beginning in the mid-1990s, numerous 1H MRS studies on MTLE identified local reductions in *N*-acetyl aspartate (NAA) as markers of seizure foci (18–21). NAA is synthesized exclusively in neuronal mitochondria and its concentration in brain tissue is closely correlated with oxidative phosphorylation (22), making it a useful index of local bioenergetic activity in the brain. NAA levels derived from MRS spectra are often reported as a ratio of NAA to creatine and/or choline. Reductions in NAA have consistently been shown to localize to epileptogenic zones (18, 23) as opposed to normal NAA levels in epilepsy patients with well-controlled seizures (24). Hippocampal NAA reduction is correlated with severity of hippocampal sclerosis, duration of illness, and early onset in MTLE (25). Decreases in hippocampal NAA correlate robustly with the frequency of epileptiform discharges (26).

Given that NAA synthesis occurs exclusively in neuronal mitochondria, it was initially thought that reduced NAA signal on MRS reflected neuronal loss (27). Several studies, however, have demonstrated that in patients who have undergone surgical resection of the seizure focus, NAA signals may resolve postoperatively in the contralateral hippocampus and throughout the broader network of affected structures (16, 18, 28, 29). Furthermore, in patients whose seizures localize to malformations of cortical development, NAA signal reductions are seen in seizure foci in the absence of neuronal loss (24). Additionally, it has been shown that NAA reductions in the hippocampi of MTLE patients do not correlate with the ratio of hippocampal glia to hippocampal neurons in resected ex vivo tissue (30). Given the reversibility of aberrant NAA signals in contralateral hippocampi, and its association with electron transport in neuronal mitochondria (22), in the context of epilepsy, NAA reductions appear to reflect metabolic dysfunction that originates in a seizure focus and affects an array of downstream structures.

Thus, NAA signal on 1H MRS reflects neuronal metabolic state, and reduced NAA is associated

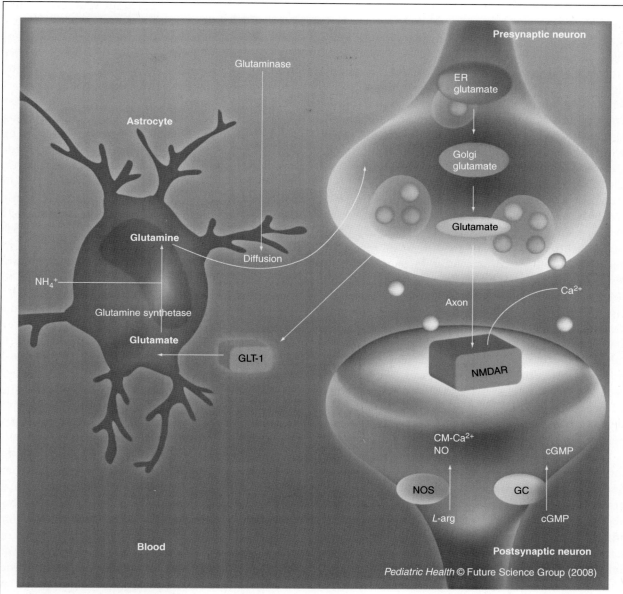

FIGURE 3.2 Glutamate–glutamine neuronal unit. The glial-neuronal unit (GNU), comprised of pre- and postsynaptic neurons and the adjacent astrocyte. Glutamate (Glu) is synthesized in the presynaptic axon terminal and packaged into vesicles for neurotransmission. Following release, excess Glu enters the adjacent astrocyte, where glutamine synthetase converts it into glutamine (Gln) through the addition of an amine group. Gln diffuses back into the presynaptic neuron and is deaminated by glutaminase to reform Glu, allowing the cycle of neurotransmission and metabolic conversion to repeat. Refer to text for details. Reproduced from *Pediatric Health.* 2008;2(6):701–713 with permission of Future Medicine Ltd.

with regional hypometabolism and epileptogenic foci. If NAA reduction is a marker of hypometabolism, what are its consequences? How is neuronal hypometabolism linked to hyperexcitability and ictal discharges? The answer lies in the neurotransmission and metabolic cycling of Glu through the neuron, synapse and astrocyte. As described above, the metabolic flux that regulates Glu cycling, and buffers against increases in synaptic Glu under conditions of high neurotransmission, is an energy-expensive process that depends on oxidative metabolism of one glucose for each Glu that enters the astrocyte. When this process is compromised by injury to the mitochondria, neuronal polarization and synaptic $Na+$ gradients cannot be optimally maintained, disrupting the astrocytic uptake of Glu through excitatory amino acid transporters. This disruption causes synaptic levels of Glu to rise, ultimately leading to increased postsynaptic excitation and risk for epileptiform discharges. MRS evidence suggests that, beyond the local environment of the epileptic focus, the effects of metabolic dysfunction of neuronal excitability are distributed through a network of connected structures, presumably as a result of oxidative stress experienced by the downstream neuronal targets of epileptiform discharges (16). NAA reductions are seen in both ipsilateral and contralateral hippocampi as well as bilateral thalami and putamena (31). Localizing a seizure focus is a clinical challenge for cases in which inter-hemispheric distribution of epilepsy signals is present. 1H MRS has been shown to more accurately predict the location of seizure foci in MTLE than PET (32) and EEG (33), suggesting that it is a powerful complement to neuroimaging work-ups in epilepsy patients.

Finally, 1H MRS has also been used to characterize the neuropsychological and phenomenological manifestations of seizure-induced injury in the epileptic brain. Post-ictal elevations in lactate have been observed within seizure foci, with lactate elevations and NAA reductions correlating with measures of seizure severity (34). Additionally, in patients with left hemisphere seizure foci, NAA reductions predict lower performance on tests of medial temporal-lobe-mediated neuropsychological performance (35) and verbal working memory (36).

31P MRS

31P MRS is another spectroscopic imaging modality that allows clinicians and researchers to index the relative concentrations of phosphate-containing compounds in the brain, principally ATP, phosphocreatine (PCr), and inorganic phosphate. Although the need for RF coils equipped to process both 1H and 31P MRS signals has limited the widespread clinical use of 31P MRS in diagnostic imaging of epilepsy patients, 31P MRS has provided further corroboration of the bioenergetic model of epilepsy through studies examining the concentrations of inorganic phosphate, PCr, ATP, and the PCr/ATP ratio within nervous tissue (16, 27). Creatine serves as an intracellular storage buffer for high-energy phosphates, binding phosphates during energetic excess and transferring them to ADP when cellular energetic demand exceeds production in order to maintain normal energy levels within the cell. Under hypermetabolic conditions, in which the mitochondria fail to meet cellular energetic demands through oxidative ATP production, neurons are forced to draw on their reserves of PCr to meet cellular energy demands, causing PCr concentrations to fall and Cr concentrations to rise as phosphates are transferred from ADP to form ATP. The ability to measure the PCr/ATP ratio makes 31P MRS a very useful measure of neuronal bioenergetics. Epileptogenic regions have been shown to have lower PCr/ATP ratios relative to controls (37). Additionally, it has been demonstrated that, just as NAA signal reductions show recovery in contralateral hippocampi following surgical resection of the seizure focus, the PCr/ATP signal derived from 31P MRS spectra also shows recovery following successful seizure management with the ketogenic diet (38).

Beyond allowing researchers and clinicians to identify seizure foci in epilepsy patients, MRS has been used in concert with other measures of neuronal function to elucidate not only the presence of bioenergetic failure in epilepsy, but also its consequences for the regulation of cerebral electric currents. Analysis of pre-operative PCr/ATP and the recovery rate of membrane potentials in resected epileptogenic tissue has shown a robust positive correlation between neurometabolism and neuronal firing patterns (37). Neurons resected from regions of low PCr/ATP on preoperative MRS show markedly reduced recovery rates following suprathreshold stimulation in ex vivo neuron cultures. Thus, compromised bioenergetics appears to diminish the ability of neurons to restore ionic gradients following a pre-synaptic stimulus. This in turn may disrupt the metabolic cycling of Glu and GABA, tipping the balance of synaptic neurotransmitters in favor of increased post-synaptic excitation and increasing the epileptogenic potential of affected regions.

13C MRS

The 13C isotope is present in only 1% of naturally occurring compounds, but may be used as a source of MRS contrast when exogenous 13C-labeled glucose is administered to patients prior to MRS scanning. As the labeled glucose is metabolized in the brain, it is converted into glutamate, glutamine and GABA, allowing investigators to image glucose metabolism and glutamate–glutamine cycling between neurons and glia (39). Ex vivo analysis with 13C MRS of resected human epileptic hippocampus reveals significantly reduced glutamate–glutamine cycling in patients with hippocampal sclerosis, resulting in increased extracellular glutamate and decreased glutamine concentrations (40). To date, however, 13C MRS has yet to be broadly applied clinically, and further work is needed to fully characterize 13C MRS phenotypes in human epilepsy and to determine its utility in clinical diagnosis and disease management.

CLINICAL APPLICATIONS OF MRS TO EPILEPSY BEYOND MTLE

Now that we have a model with which to interpret MRS findings in epilepsy, rarer inherited metabolic epilepsies present fertile territory for the study and clinical management of epileptic manifestations in these disorders. A host of inherited metabolic diseases, such as urea cycle disorders, mitochondrial disorders, infantile spasms and epileptiform channelopathies are characterized by debilitating seizures. To date, however, MRS has not been rigorously applied to the study of the epileptic components of these disorders. MRS studies using sequences, such as CSI, that can be applied throughout the brain are needed to characterize the location and distribution of epileptic zones, the degree of metabolic impairment in widespread regions, and the response of relevant 1H, 31P, and 13C MRS signals to pharmacologic and neurosurgical treatments. While neuroradiologists currently employ MRS studies to determine the presence or absence of lactate peaks in structural brain lesions, the potential of MRS to detect nonlesional, that is, MRI-negative, epileptogenic zones and to more thoroughly characterize the metabolic dysfunction in those zones demands further exploration.

FUTURE DIRECTIONS

MRS has the potential to demonstrate how alterations in relative levels of excitatory and inhibitory neurotransmitters contribute to epilepsy. MRS measurements will reflect not only neurotransmitter pools, but also overall brain levels of related measurable compounds such as GABA and creatine. 1H MRS results will reflect brain metabolism as well as synaptic activity.

KEY POINTS

- 1H MRS localizes signal acquisition by acquiring data from the intersection of three excited orthogonal planes that defines an ROI (region of interest).
- MRS spectra are displayed on an x-axis with units of parts per million (ppm), and values increase from right to left.
- Glutamate and glutamine (combined as a single "Glx" peak) resonances overlap in spectra acquired in scanners below 7 T. These closely related amino acids are involved in neurotransmission and have peaks at 2.12 to 2.35 ppm (representing the beta and gamma protons) and another peak at 3.74 to 3.75 ppm (representing the alpha protons).
- Glutamate is mainly present in neurons. Increased levels can lead to neuronal damage due to overexcitation. Glutamine is present in higher levels in astrocytes, and is said to be an astrocyte marker.
- Increased glutamine can be found in hypoxic–ischemic events, hyperammonemia, and Reye syndrome.
- Neuronal hypometabolism is linked to hyperexcitability and epileptic discharges in the neurotransmission and metabolic cycling of glutamate through the neuron, synapse, and astrocyte.

REFERENCES

1. Mountford CE, Stanwell P, Lin A, et al. Neurospectroscopy: The past, present and future. Chem Rev. 2010;110(5):3060–3086.
2. Huettel S, Song A, McCarthy G. Functional Magnetic Resonance Imaging. UK, Sunderland: Sinauer Associates, Inc; 2004.
3. Brown M, Semelka R. MRI Basic Principles and Applications. 3rd ed. Hoboken: John Wiley and Sons, Inc.; 2003.
4. Poullet JB, Sima DM, Van Huffel S. MRS signal quantitation: a review of time- and frequency-domain methods. J Magn Reson. 2008;195(2):134–144.

5. Govindaraju V, Young K, Maudsley AA. Proton NMR chemical shifts and coupling constants for brain metabolites. *NMR Biomed*. 2000;13(3):129–153.

6. Panigrahy A, Nelson MD, Blüml S. Magnetic resonance spectroscopy in pediatric neuroradiology: clinical and research applications. *Pediatr Radiol*. 2010;40(1):3–30.

7. Hetherington HP, Kim JH, Pan, et al. 1H and 31P spectroscopic imaging of epilepsy: spectroscopic and histologic correlations. *Epilepsia*. 2004;45(4):17–23.

8. Ross B, Lin A, Harris K, et al. Clinical experience with 13C MRS in vivo. *NMR Biomed*. 2003;16(6–7):358–369.

9. Moffett JR, Namboodiri MA, Neale JH. Enhanced carbodiimide fixation for immunohistochemistry: application to the comparative distributions of N-acetylaspartylglutamate and N-acetylaspartate immunoreactivities in rat brain. *J Histochem Cytochem*. 1993;41:559.

10. Kreis R, Ernst T, Ross B. Development of the human brain: in vivo quantification of metabolite and water content with proton magnetic resonance spectroscopy. *Magn Reson Med: Off J Soc Magn Reson Med/Soc Magn Reson Med*. 1993;30(4): 424–437.

11. Mardini H, Smith FE, Record CO, et al. Magnetic resonance quantification of water and metabolites in the brain of cirrhotics following induced hyperammonaemia. *J Hepatol*. 2011; 54(6):1154–1160.

12. Ross BD. Biochemical considerations in 1H spectroscopy. Glutamate and glutamine; myo-inositol and related metabolites. *NMR Biomed*. 1991;4(2):59–63.

13. Blüml S, Seymour KJ, Ross BD. Developmental changes in choline- and ethanolamine-containing compounds measured with proton-decoupled (31) P MRS in in vivo human brain. *Magn Reson Med: Off J Soc Magn Reson Med/Soc Magn Reson Med*. 1999;42(4):643–654.

14. Xu V, Chan H, Lin AP, et al. MR spectroscopy in diagnosis and neurological decision-making. *Sem Neurol*. 2008;28(4):407–422.

15. Bogner W, Gruber S, Doelken M, et al. In vivo quantification of intracerebral GABA by single-voxel (1)H-MRS-How reproducible are the results? *Eur J Radiol*. 2010;73(3):526–531.

16. Pan JW, Williamson A, Cavus I, et al. Neurometabolism in human epilepsy. *Epilepsia*. 2008;49(Suppl 3):31–41.

17. Magistretti PJ, Pellerin L. Cellular mechanisms of brain energy metabolism and their relevance to functional brain imaging. *Philos Trans R Soc Lond B Biol Sci*. 1999;354(1387):1155–1163.

18. Cendes F, Andermann F, Preul MC, et al. Lateralization of temporal lobe epilepsy based on regional metabolic abnormalities in proton magnetic resonance spectroscopic images. *Ann Neurol*. 1994;35(2):211–216.

19. Connelly A, Jackson GD, Duncan JS, et al. Magnetic resonance spectroscopy in temporal lobe epilepsy. *Neurology*. 1994;44(8): 1411–1417.

20. Hetherington H, Kuzniecky R, Pan J, et al. Proton nuclear magnetic resonance spectroscopic imaging of human temporal lobe epilepsy at 4.1 T. *Ann Neurol*. 1995;38(3):396–404.

21. Vainio P, Usenius JP, Vapalahti M, et al. Reduced N-acetylaspartate concentration in temporal lobe epilepsy by quantitative 1H MRS in vivo. *Neuroreport*. 1994;5(14):1733–1736.

22. Goldstein FB. The enzymatic synthesis of N-acetyl-L-aspartic acid by subcellular preparations of rat brain. *J Biol Chem*. 1969;244(15):4257–4260.

23. Shih JJ, Weisend MP, Lewine J, et al. Areas of interictal spiking are associated with metabolic dysfunction in MRI-negative temporal lobe epilepsy. *Epilepsia*. 2004;45(3):223–229.

24. Kuzniecky R, Hetherington H, Pan J, et al. Proton spectroscopic imaging at 4.1 tesla in patients with malformations of cortical development and epilepsy. *Neurology*. 1997;48(4):1018–1024.

25. Duc CO, Trabesinger AH, Weber OM, et al. Quantitative 1H MRS in the evaluation of mesial temporal lobe epilepsy in vivo. *Magn Reson Imaging*. 1998;16(8):969–979.

26. Hammen T, Schwarz M, Doelken M, et al. 1H-MR spectroscopy indicates severity markers in temporal lobe epilepsy: correlations between metabolic alterations, seizures, and epileptic discharges in EEG. *Epilepsia*. 2007;48(2):263–269.

27. Garcia PA, Laxer KD, Ng T. Application of spectroscopic imaging in epilepsy. *Magn Reson Imaging*. 1995;13(8):1181–1185.

28. Hugg JW, Kuzniecky RI, Gilliam FG, et al. Normalization of contralateral metabolic function following temporal lobectomy demonstrated by 1H magnetic resonance spectroscopic imaging. *Ann Neurol*. 1996;40(2):236–239.

29. Vermathen P, Ende G, Laxer KD, et al. Temporal lobectomy for epilepsy: Recovery of the contralateral hippocampus measured by (1)H MRS. *Neurology*. 2002;59(4):633–636.

30. Kuzniecky R, Palmer C, Hugg J, et al. Magnetic resonance spectroscopic imaging in temporal lobe epilepsy: Neuronal dysfunction or cell loss? *Arch Neurol*. 2001;58(12):2048–2053.

31. Hetherington HP, Kuzniecky RI, Vives K, et al. A subcortical network of dysfunction in TLE measured by magnetic resonance spectroscopy. *Neurology*. 2007;69(24):2256–2265.

32. Park SW, Chang KH, Kim HD, et al. Lateralizing ability of single-voxel proton mr spectroscopy in hippocampal sclerosis: comparison with mr imaging and positron emission tomography. *AJNR Am J Neuroradiol*. 2001;22(4):625–631.

33. Maton B, Gilliam F, Sawrie S, et al. Correlation of scalp EEG and 1H-MRS metabolic abnormalities in temporal lobe epilepsy. *Epilepsia*. 2001;42(3):417–422.

34. Najm IM, Wang Y, Shedid D, et al. MRS metabolic markers of seizures and seizure-induced neuronal damage. *Epilepsia* 1998;39(3):244–250.

35. Kikuchi S, Kubota F, Hattori S, et al. A study of the relationship between metabolism using 1H-MRS and function using several neuropsychological tests in temporal lobe epilepsy. *Seizure*. 2001;10(3):188–193.

36. Sawrie SM, Martin RC, Knowlton R, et al. Relationships among hippocampal volumetry, proton magnetic resonance spectroscopy, and verbal memory in temporal lobe epilepsy. *Epilepsia*. 2001;42(11):1403–1407.

37. Williamson A, Patrylo PR, Pan J, et al. Correlations between granule cell physiology and bioenergetics in human temporal lobe epilepsy. *Brain*. 2005;128(Pt 5):1199–1208.

38. Pan JW, Bebin EM, Chu WJ, et al. Ketosis and epilepsy: 31P spectroscopic imaging at 4.1 T. *Epilepsia*. 1999;40(6):703–707.

39. Sibson NR, Mason GF, Shen J, et al. In vivo (13) C NMR measurement of neurotransmitter glutamate cycling, anaplerosis and TCA cycle flux in rat brain during. *J Neurochem*. 2001;76(4):975–989.

40. Petroff OA, Errante LD, Rothman DL, et al. Glutamate–glutamine cycling in the epileptic human hippocampus. *Epilepsia*. 2002;43(7):703–710.

4

Electroencephalography in the Metabolic Epilepsies

Mona S. Alduligan and Phillip L. Pearl

Seizures are a common symptom in a great number of metabolic disorders, occurring mainly in infancy and childhood. In some, seizures may occur only until adequate treatment is initiated or as a consequence of acute metabolic decompensation. Epilepsy in inborn errors of metabolism can be classified in different ways. One useful way utilizes possible pathogenetic mechanisms. Seizures can arise from lack of energy, intoxication, impaired neuronal function in storage disorders, disturbances of neurotransmitter systems with excess of excitation or lack of inhibition, or associated malformations of the brain (Table 4.1). Other approaches take into account the clinical presentation, with emphasis on seizure semiology, epilepsy syndrome, and associated EEG findings (Table 4.2) or the age of manifestation (Table 4.3) (1).

Metabolic disorders may result from an absence or abnormality of an enzyme or its cofactor, leading to either accumulation or deficiency of a specific metabolite. Patients with inborn errors may present at birth or in early infancy with seizures or severe hypotonia (2). Although inborn errors of metabolism are a rare cause of seizures in children, seizures may occur in virtually all inborn errors of metabolism. Seizures may be the only manifestation of pyridoxine-dependent seizures or folinic acid responsive seizures (3).

ELECTROENCEPHALOGRAPHIC FEATURES THAT SUGGEST INBORN ERRORS OF METABOLISM

Epileptic encephalopathies presenting in early life present a diagnostic and therapeutic challenge. These disorders often present with multiple seizure types that are treatment resistant and associated with

TABLE 4.1 Classification of Epilepsies of Metabolic Origin According to Their Pathogenesis

Energy deficiency	Hypoglycemia, GLUT1-deficiency, respiratory chain deficiency, creatine deficiency
Toxic effect	Amino acidopathies, organic acidurias, urea cycle defects
Impaired neuronal function	Storage disorders
Disturbance of neurotransmitter systems	Nonketotic hyperglycinemia, GABA transaminase deficiency, succinic semialdehyde dehydrogenase deficiency
Associated brain malformations	Peroxisomal disorders (Zellweger), O-glycosylation defects
Vitamin/Co-factor dependency	Biotinidase deficiency, pyridoxine-dependent and pyridoxal phosphate dependent epilepsy, folinic acid-responsive seizures, Menkes' disease
Miscellaneous	Congenital disorders of glycosylation, serine biosynthesis deficiency and inborn errors of brain excitability (ion channel disorders)

TABLE 4.2 Classification of Epilepsies of Metabolic Origin According to Age at Onset

Neonatal period	Hypoglycemia, pyridoxine-dependency, PNPO deficiency, nonketotic hyperglycinemia, organic acidurias, urea cycle defects, neonatal adrenoleukodystrophy, Zellweger syndrome, folinic acid-responsive seizures, holocarboxylase synthase deficiency, molybdenum cofactor deficiency, sulfite oxidase deficiency
Infancy	Hypoglycemia, GLUT1-deficiency, creatine deficiency, biotinidase deficiency, amino acidopathies, organic acidurias, congenital disorders of glycosylation, pyridoxine dependency, infantile form of neuronal ceroid lipofuscinosis (NCL1)
Toddlers	Late infantile form of neuronal ceroid lipofuscinosis (NCL2), mitochondrial disorders including Alpers' disease, lysosomal storage disorders
School age	Mitochondrial disorders, juvenile form of neuronal ceroid lipofuscinosis (NCL3), progressive myoclonus epilepsies

significant abnormalities on electroencephalographic (EEG) studies (4). Classification systems using simple descriptions of ictal behaviors can be reliably applied and may aid in the recognition of these disorders. Myoclonic seizures in infancy in particular suggest an inborn error of metabolism. In addition, certain epileptic syndromes are known to be associated with metabolic disorders, including some forms of neonatal seizures, West syndrome, early myoclonic encephalopathy, and early infantile epileptic encephalopathy. There is limited literature regarding specific EEG features in infants with inborn errors of metabolism. In some circumstances distinctive EEG findings have been identified which point to a limited list of etiologies (Table 4.4).

CLASSIFICATION OF EPILEPSIES OF METABOLIC ORIGIN ACCORDING TO AGE OF ONSET

METABOLIC DISORDERS IN THE NEWBORN

Neonatal seizures are most commonly the marker of acute brain injury rather than of epilepsy. Seizures often attenuate within days of onset. In neonates whose seizures do not spontaneously remit, inborn errors of metabolism must be suspected (5).

Nonketotic Hyperglycinemia (Glycine Encephalopathy)

Nonketotic hyperglycinemia, preferentially called glycine encephalopathy to avoid confusion with the nonketotic hyperglycemia in the diabetic, represents a set of defects

TABLE 4.3 Classification of Epilepsies of Metabolic Origin According to the Type of Presenting Seizures or Epilepsy Syndrome

Infantile spasms	Biotinidase deficiency, Menkes' disease, mitochondrial disorders, organic acidurias, amino acidopathies
Epilepsy with myoclonic seizures	Nonketotic hyperglycinemia, mitochondrial disorders, GLUT1-deficiency, storage disorders
Progressive myoclonic epilepsies	Lafora disease, MERRF, MELAS, Unverricht-Lundborg disease, sialidosis
Epilepsy with generalized tonic–clonic seizures	GLUT1-deficiency, NCL2, NCL3, other storage disorders, mitochondrial disorders
Epilepsy with myoclonic–astatic seizures	GLUT1-deficiency, NCL2
Epilepsy with (multi-)focal seizures	NCL3, GLUT1-deficiency, and others
Epilepsia partialis continua	Alpers' disease, other mitochondrial disorders

TABLE 4.4 Electroencephalogram Patterns and Associated Disorders

Pattern	Disorder
Comb-like rhythm	Maple syrup urine disease, propionic acidemia
Fast central spikes	Tay–Sachs disease, biotinidase deficiency
Rhythmic vertex-positive spikes	Sialidosis (type I)
Vanishing electroencephalogram	Infantile NCL (early infantile/type I/Haltia-Santavouri, locus 1p32, mutation in the palmitoyl-protein thioesterase gene)
High-amplitude (16–24 Hz) activity	Infantile neuroaxonal dystrophy
Giant SSEPs	Progressive myoclonic epilepsy
Marked photosensitivity	Progressive myoclonic epilepsy (Lafora) and NCL, particularly late infantile (type II/Bielschowsky, CLN2)
Burst suppression	Adrenoleukodystrophy (neonatal), citrullinemia, D-glyceric acidemia, holo-carboxylase synthetase deficiency, Leigh disease, Mb cofactor deficiency, Menkes, MTHFR deficiency, NKH, PDH/PC deficiency, propionic acidemia, sulfite oxidase deficiency
Hypsarrhythmia	Adrenoleukodystrophy (neonatal), CDG (type III), HHH, Menkes, neuroaxonal dystrophy, NKH, PDH, PEHO, phenylketonuria, Zellweger
Low-amplitude slowing	Urea cycle defects (carbamylphosphate synthetase, OTC, argininosuccinate synthetase)

CDG, congenital disorders of glycosylation; CLN2, ceroid lipofuscinoses 2; HHH, hyperornithinemia, hyperammonemia, homocitrullinuria; MTHFR, methylene tetrahydrofolate reductase; NCL, neuronal ceroid lipofuscinoses; NKH, nonketotic hyperglycinemia; OTC, ornithine transcarbamylase; PEHO, progressive encephalopathy with edema and hypsarrhythmia; PDH/PC, pyruvate dehydrogenase/pyruvate carboxylase.

in the multienzyme complex for glycine cleavage and has been identified as one of the most important metabolic disorders responsible for Ohtahara syndrome (6).

The most prominent seizure type is myoclonic, particularly fragmentary or erratic. Erratic focal seizures and massive myoclonus are the seizure types most suggestive of this disorder. Tonic spasms nearly always develop long after the initial seizures, usually around 3 to 4 months of age.

EEG findings are characterized by suppression-burst patterns which consist of bursts lasting 1 to 5 sec alternating with almost flat periods lasting 3 to 10 sec (Figures 4.1 and 4.2). The pattern may be enhanced in sleep. The discontinuous EEG may be replaced by atypical hypsarrhythmia or a multifocal epileptiform pattern.

Peroxisomal Disorders

The peroxisomal disorders represent a group of inherited metabolic disorders that derive from defects of peroxisomal biogenesis or from dysfunction of single or multiple peroxisomal enzymes (7). These have been divided into three categories: disorders of peroxisome biogenesis (Zellweger's syndrome, neonatal adrenoleukodystrophy [ALD], infantile Refsum's disease); disorders of a single peroxisomal enzyme (x-linked ALD, acyl-CoA oxidase deficiency); disorders with deficiencies of multiple peroxisomal enzymes [rhizomelic chondrodysplasia punctata (RCPD)].

Zellweger Syndrome: (Cerebro–Hepato–Renal Syndrome)

First described as a familial syndrome of multiple congenital defects in 1964, Zellweger syndrome is the most frequent peroxisomal disorder in early infancy. The syndrome is characterized by the presence of dysmorphism and multiple congenital malformations, severe failure to thrive and usually early death (8).

Seizures occur in 80% of patients, including partial, generalized tonic–clonic (rare), myoclonic, and atypical flexor spasms. The partial motor seizures originating in the arms, legs, or face typically do not culminate into generalized seizures and are responsive to antiepileptic drugs.

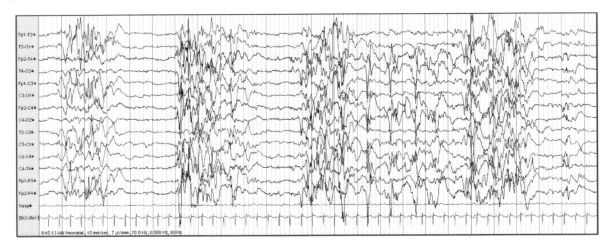

FIGURE 4.1   Ohtahara syndrome: Term infant (38 weeks). On DOL 2, noted to have left eye twitching, bilateral arm extension, and oxygen desaturation. EEG shows minimal background organization with excessive asynchrony.

Interictal EEG shows infrequent bilateral independent multifocal spikes, predominantly in the frontal motor cortex and the surrounding regions (9) (Figure 4.3). Less frequently hypsarrhythmia is observed.

Neonatal Adrenoleukodystrophy

This is an autosomal recessive disorder with onset of disability in the neonatal period, involvement of adrenal cortex and cerebral white matter, and increased very long-chain fatty acids in plasma, cultured skin fibroblasts, brain, and adrenal gland (10). Frequent intractable seizures occur that may include tonic, clonic, myoclonic, or epileptic spasms (11).

No characteristic EEG pattern has been defined, but descriptions include high-voltage slowing, polymorphic delta activity, multifocal paroxysmal discharges, burst-suppression, and hypsarrhythmia (11). The abnormality is almost continuous. This aspect gives an impression of chaotic disorganization that is

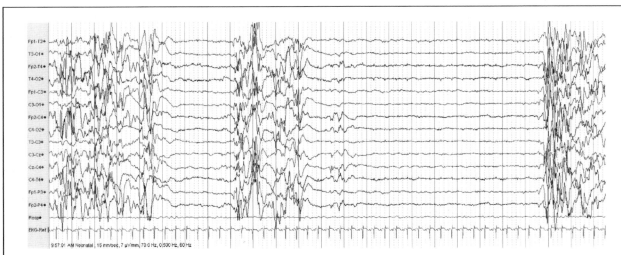

FIGURE 4.2   The same patient in Figure 4.1, background with burst suppression and multifocal epileptiform discharges. Periods of generalized burst suppression lasting between 3 and 8 sec, followed by bursts of high-voltage (>50 μV) activity, intermingled with abnormal sharp waves in the temporal and occipital lobes bilaterally.

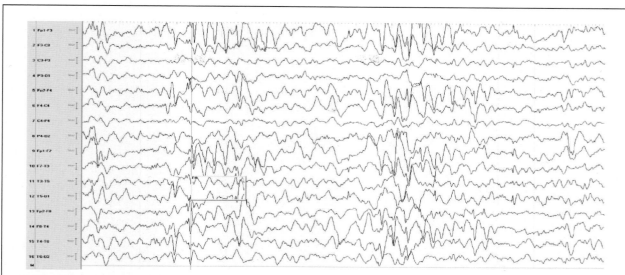

FIGURE 4.3 Zellweger syndrome: EEG shows multifocal independent epileptiform discharges predominantly seen over the frontal regions. Sensitivity 10 μV/mm, TC 0.1 s, HF 70 Hz.

continuous in the awake state (Figures 4.4 and 4.5). During sleep, there is an increase in spike and polyspike activity, with increased synchronization, and some fragmentation of hypsarrhythmic activity (Figure 4.6) (12).

Spasms are usually grouped in clusters of 20 to 40 occasionally up to 100, occurring 5 to 30 seconds apart.

The EEG during the spasm demonstrates a medium- to high-voltage, positive slow-wave maximal

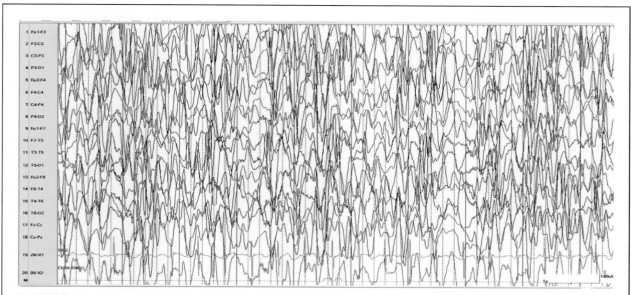

FIGURE 4.4 Infant with neonatal adrenoleukodystrophy: 4-month-old baby girl with history of one to two clusters per day of 4 to 5 seizures characterized by arching and eye fluttering. EEG shows hypsarrhythmia. Sensitivity 20 μV/mm, TC 0.1 s, HF 70 Hz.

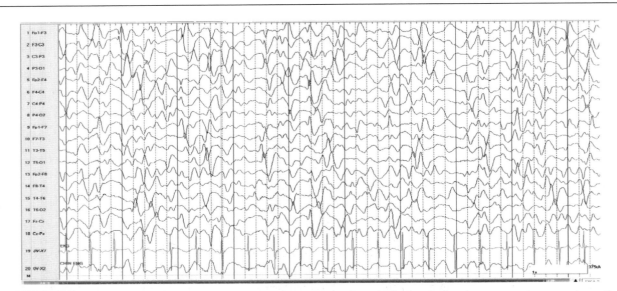

FIGURE 4.5 The same patient in Figure 4.4 with neonatal adrenoleukodystrophy during a quieter portion of the interictal recording vis-à-vis epileptiform activity (note very high-voltage background given sensitivity of 75 μV/mm). Sensitivity 75 μV/mm, TC 0.1 s, HF 70 Hz.

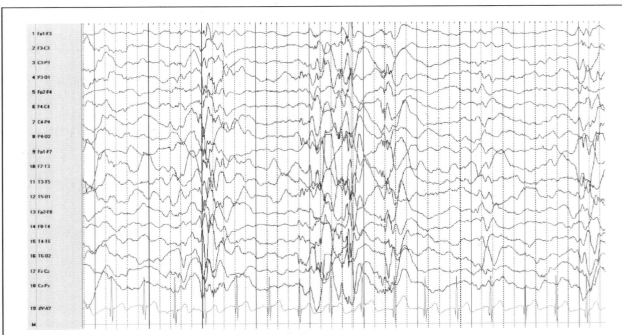

FIGURE 4.6 The same patient in Figure 4.4 during sleep: discontinuous with bursts of irregular high-amplitude sharp activity followed by periods of attenuation. Normal sleep architecture was not seen. Sensitivity 75 μV, TC 0.1 s, HF 70 Hz.

at the central and vertex regions. Very-low-voltage fast activity is often superimposed (13). In most cases generalized low-amplitude fast activity or a high amplitude, frontally dominant, generalized slow-wave transient occurs, followed by diffuse voltage attenuation (electrodecremental event) (14) (Figure 4.7).

Acyl-CoA Oxidase Deficiency

This is a disorder of a single peroxisomal enzyme characterized by the absence of dysmorphic features, elevation of very long-chain fatty acids, and onset of seizures shortly after birth. The interictal EEG may show continuous, diffuse, high-voltage theta activity (9).

Pyridoxine Dependency

Pyridoxine dependency typically manifests as refractory seizures within the first several days after birth. The phenomenon of pyridoxine-dependent epilepsy has been known since 1954 (15). Pyridoxine-dependent epilepsy is classified into a typical, early-onset group presenting within the first few days of life, and may appear in utero from the 5th month of pregnancy.

Atypical, later-onset groups presenting thereafter and up to 3 years of age have been reported (16).

Multiple seizure types start within the first few days and may be combined in the same infant, including spasms, myoclonic seizures, partial clonic, and secondary generalized seizures, generally evolving into status resistant to conventional antiepileptic drugs. EEG findings can be very heterogeneous, with abnormal background activity, no sleep organization, discontinuous EEG with suppression burst-like pattern and spike and polyspike discharges with bilateral high-voltage delta slow-wave activity (17).

Treatment with high doses of pyridoxine can result in cession of seizures, conversion of the EEG to a burst-suppression pattern, and later normalization of the EEG (18).

Pyridoxal Phosphate Responsive Seizures [Pyridox (Am)Ine-5′-Phosphate Oxidase (Pnpo) Deficiency]

Neonates with deficiency of the PNPO enzyme are unresponsive to treatment with pyridoxine but respond to pyridoxal 5′-phosphate (PLP), the biologically active form (19).

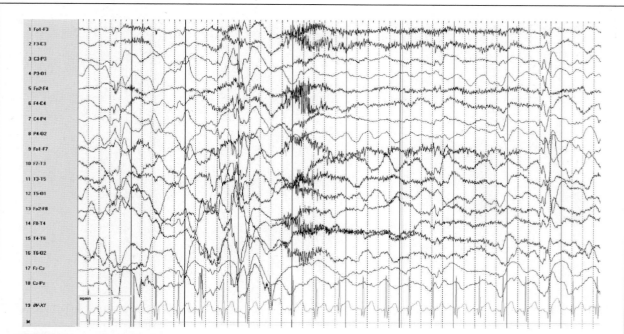

FIGURE 4.7 Infantile spasm in child with neonatal ALD. The patient has clusters of extensor spasms consisting of an initial myoclonic jerk followed by a tonic spasm. EEG during the spasms showed high-voltage diffuse slowing followed by 3 to 4 sec of background voltage attenuation (electrodecremental response). Sensitivity 75 μV, TC 0.1 s, HF 70 Hz.

Neonates with this condition are often premature and have lactic acidosis and hypoglycemia at presentation. Seizure types include tonic, generalized tonic–clonic, complex partial, spasms, and myoclonus. The EEG commonly shows a burst-suppression pattern, multifocal sharp waves, or spike and slow-wave discharges (20, 21) (Figures 4.8).

associated with abnormal mitochondrial metabolism. Progressive neurological symptoms may include developmental delay, intermittent ataxia, poor muscle tone, lactic acidosis, and seizures in the form of myoclonic seizures and infantile spasms (22). The EEG shows multifocal slow spike-and-wave discharges (Figures 4.9 and 4.10).

Pyruvate Dehydrogenase Complex Deficiency

Pyruvate dehydrogenase complex deficiency is one of the most common neurodegenerative disorders

Pyruvate Carboxylase Deficiency

Deficiency of pyruvate carboxylase is an autosomal recessive disease. Based on the severity of the clinical

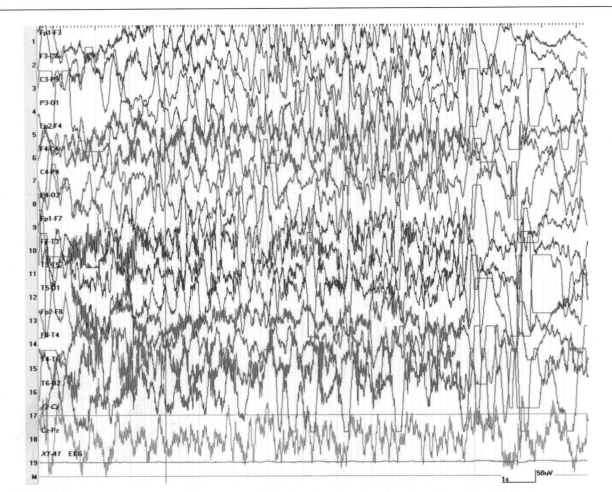

FIGURE 4.8   EEG of a 5-month-old with PNPO deficiency (pyridoxal-5-phosphate dependency), showing paroxysms of diffuse spike-wave discharges accompanied by thrashing movements. These were separated by periods of relative background suppression, accompanied by an initial tonic spasm and then quieting until the next paroxysm. This sequence persisted 25 minutes until intravenous lorazepam administration led to temporary resolution. Settings: 20 sec epoch, Sensitivity 10 μV/mm, TC 0.1 s, HF 70 Hz.

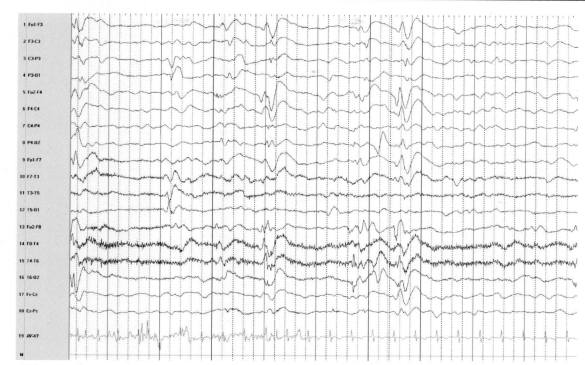

FIGURE 4.9   A 4-month-old girl with PDH deficiency presents in the neonatal period with hypotonia, somnolence and high lactic acidosis. During the awake state the EEG showed poorly formed background with frequent multifocal independent epileptiform foci. Sensitivity 7 μV/mm, TC 0.1 s, HF 70 Hz.

presentation and the biochemical disturbances, two clinical forms have been described representing the extremes of a spectrum of clinical variation (23). The neonatal type manifests with severe lactic acidosis and death in the first few months of life. The juvenile presentation begins in the first 6 months of life, with moderate lactic acidosis, global developmental delay with intellectual deficiency, and seizures. In milder forms, diffuse 1.5- to 3-Hz slowing have been noted on EEG (24).

Leigh Syndrome

Also known as subacute necrotizing encephalomyelopathy, Leigh syndrome may be caused by mutations in mitochondrial DNA (25). A variety of different seizures including partial and generalized seizures have been described. Infantile spasms with hypsarrhythmia have been reported. In addition, there have been several cases of epilepsia partialis continuans (26).

EEG features do not appear to be specific. Focal or multifocal EEG epileptiform activity prominent during sleep may be seen. During partial seizures, the ictal EEG has been reported to show posterior or hemispheric background attenuation or ictal fast activity (27).

Molybdenum Cofactor Deficiency and Sulfite Oxidase Deficiency

This condition is associated with deficiency of the molybdenum-containing cofactor and presents shortly after birth with progressive encephalopathy, feeding difficulties, hypotonia, and refractory partial, myoclonic, or generalized seizures (28). EEG is characterized by multifocal paroxysms and a burst-suppression pattern (29).

Urea Cycle Disorders

There are six enzymes in the urea cycle that convert ammonia into urea; deficiency of five are associated

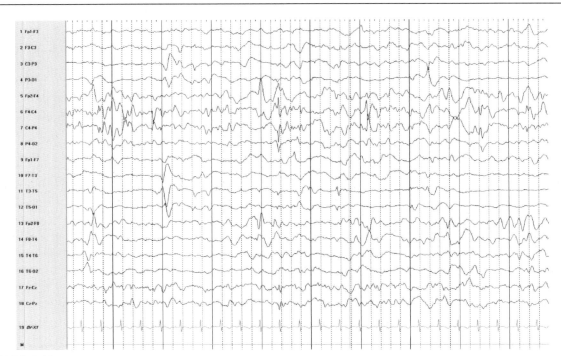

FIGURE 4.10   The same patient in Figure 4.9 with PDH deficiency, sleep EEG with poor sleep architecture and frequent multifocal independent epileptiform foci. Sensitivity 7 μV/mm, TC 0.1 s, HF 70 Hz.

with neonatal seizures: ornithine transcarbamylase (OTC), argininosuccinic acid synthetase (ASD), arginase (AG), arginosuccinase lyase (ALD), carbamyl phosphate synthetase (CPS). *N*-acetylglutamate synthetase (NAGS) will typically manifest later in infancy.

Affected newborns present with convulsions 1 to 5 days after birth. The EEG may show a low-voltage pattern with diffuse slowing and multifocal epileptiform discharges (30) or monorhythmic theta activity (31). Burst-suppression has been described in patients with citrullinemia (32) (Figures 4.11 and 4.12).

Maple Syrup Urine Disease

Maple syrup urine disease is an aminoacidopathy secondary to an enzyme defect in the catabolic pathway of the branched-chain amino acids: leucine, isoleucine, and valine, as first reported by Menkes and colleagues in 1954 (33). Patients present in the first to second weeks of life with myoclonic, partial, and generalized seizures. The EEG shows diffuse slowing and loss of

reactivity to auditory stimuli. A unique EEG pattern, the "comb-like rhythm," has described in neonatal (classic) maple syrup urine disease. This pattern consists of bursts and runs of 5 to 7 Hz primarily monophasic surface negative mu-like activity in the central and parasagittal regions. This pattern seems peculiar to maple syrup urine disease (34), appears during the first 2 weeks of life, and tends to resolve after the initiation of dietary therapy (35).

Organic Acidurias

Several organic acidurias may lead to seizures during the time of initial presentation or episodic acute decompensation. The more common entities are methylmalonicacidemia and propionic acidemia. Progressive neurocognitive deterioration is almost invariably present in propionic and methylmalonic acidurias (36). Isovaleric acidemia may present in the neonatal period with an acute episode of severe metabolic acidosis, ketosis, seizures, and vomiting and may lead to coma

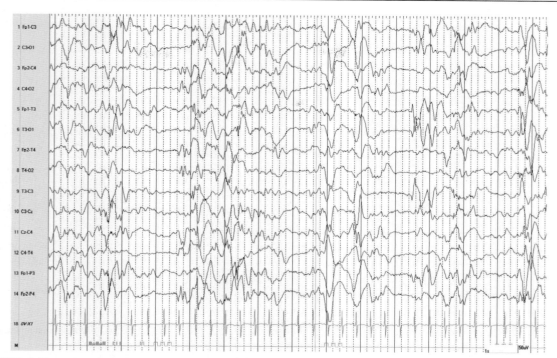

FIGURE 4.11   A 2-month-old boy with citrullinemia, presenting with 1 to 2 min episode of cyanosis and unresponsiveness and poor feeding. Awake EEG shows multifocal epileptiform discharges with discontinuous background. Sensitivity 7 μV/mm, TC 0.1 s, HF 70 Hz.

and death in the first 2 months of life. Seizures are most often partial motor or generalized tonic. EEG shows dysmature features during sleep.

Propionic acidemia also appears during neonatal period, with 20% of affected newborns having partial or generalized seizures as the first symptoms. EEG shows background disorganization with marked frontotemporal and occipital slow-wave activity (24). In 40% of children, myoclonic seizures develop in later infancy, and older children may have atypical absence seizures.

In methylmalonic acidemia, seizures are a major feature. Diffuse tonic seizures and partial seizures with secondary generalization are the most frequent types. Seizures may be characterized by eyelid myoclonus with simultaneous upward ocular deviation. EEG shows multifocal epileptiform discharges, depressed background activity, and lack of sleep spindles (24) (Figures 4.13 and 4.14). Myoclonus and hypsarrhythmic EEG patterns have been reported (37).

DISORDERS OF VITAMIN METABOLISM

Early-Onset Multiple Carboxylase Deficiency (Holocarboxylase Synthetase Deficiency)

Holocarboxylasesynthetase (HCS) is an essential enzyme for the biotinylation of several mammalian carboxylases. Deficiency is accountable for early onset biotin-responsive multiple carboxylase deficiency (38). This is an enzyme that catalyzes biotin incorporation into carboxylases and histones (39). This condition presents in the first week of life with varied presentations, with dermatological signs (dermatitis and alopecia), neurological abnormalities (seizures, hypotonia, and ataxia), and recurrent infections (40).

Seizures occur in 25% to 50% of cases, characterized by generalized tonic seizures, partial motor seizures, and multifocal myoclonic seizures (1). EEG shows multifocal spikes or a burst-suppression pattern.

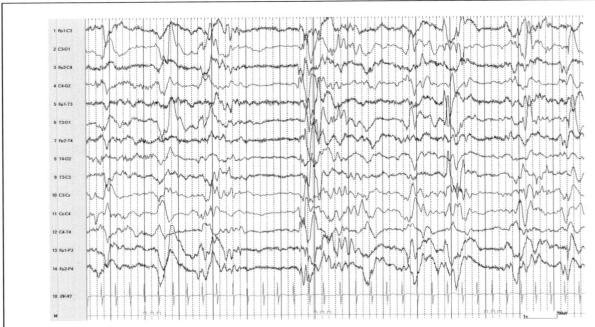

FIGURE 4.12   Same patient in Figure 4.11 (dx citrullinemia), sleep state. The background activity demonstrates burst suppression pattern. Sensitivity 7 μV/mm, TC 0.1 s, HF 70 Hz.

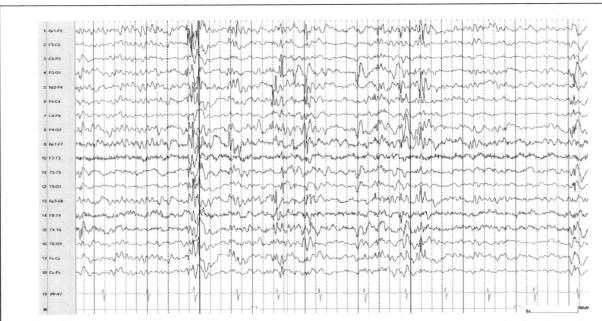

FIGURE 4.13   A 5-year-old girl with methylmalonic acidemia. EEG shows multifocal spike and polyspike-and-wave discharges. Sensitivity 7 μV/mm, TC 0.1 s, HF 70 Hz.

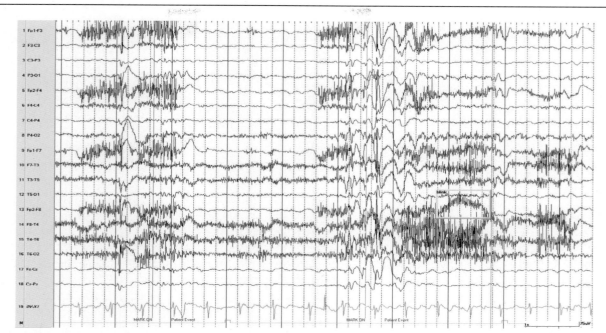

FIGURE 4.14 The same child in Figure 4.13 with methylmalonic acidemia, presenting with frequent eyelid myoclonias. EEG showed generalized irregular 3 Hz spike and wave complexes, maximal in bifrontal regions intermixed with EMG. Sensitivity 7 µV/mm, TC 0.1 s, HF 70 Hz.

METABOLIC DISORDERS OF EARLY INFANCY

Lysosomal Storage Disorders

Tay-Sachs Disease and Sandhoff Disease

GM2 gangliosidosis is a lysosomal disorder that invariably includes seizures as a prominent feature. The infantile forms of GM2 gangliosidosis include Tay-Sachs disease, caused by a deficiency in hexosaminidase A, and Sandhoff disease, caused by deficiency in hexosaminidase A and B (41).

Epileptic seizures are rare and generally appear later, although spasms sometimes appear around 6 months. By the age of 1 to 2 years, seizures become prominent, with frequent partial motor, complex partial, and atypical absence seizures. Myoclonic seizures are frequent and are often triggered by an exaggerated startle response to noise.

The EEG is normal early in the course of the disease. Gradually background activity slows, with bursts of high-voltage delta waves and very fast central spikes (Figure 4.15) (42).

As the disease progresses, EEG voltage declines, and background activity becomes undifferentiated.

Krabbe Disease

Also known as globoid cell leukodystrophy, Krabbe disease can be divided according to the age of onset into four main forms: infantile, late infantile, juvenile, and adult.

Early infantile Krabbe disease is a progressive neurodegenerative disease caused by deficiency of lysosomal enzyme galactocerebroside beta-galactosidase, with onset before the age of 6 months. Partial or generalized seizures, as well as infantile spasms, are reported (43–45).

EEG characteristics include a hypsarrhythmia-like pattern with irregular slow activity and multifocal discharges of low voltage. A prominent beta pattern independently occurring in the posterior temporal regions and vertex superimposed over slow high-amplitude waves has been recorded in long runs without any apparent clinical manifestation (46). In the terminal stages, little electrical activity is detected. Excess of irregular slow activity, polyphasic spikes, and very large amplitude discharges in response to slow rates of photic stimulation have been reported (47).

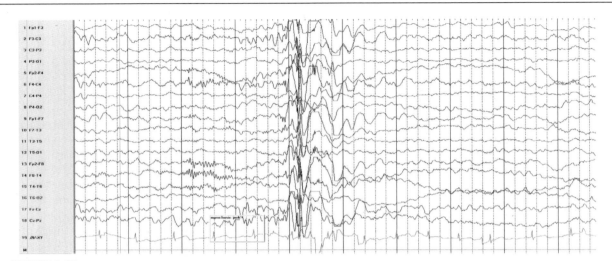

FIGURE 4.15   Diagnosis of GM2. A 4-year-old boy with developmental delay and history of myoclonic seizures. EEG shows high-amplitude generalized spike and wave discharge. Sensitivity 7 μV/mm, TC 0.1 s, HF 70 Hz.

GM1 Gangliosidosis

GM1-gangliosidosis is caused by a genetic deficiency of lysosomal acid beta-galactosidase (beta-gal). The disease manifests itself either as an infantile, juvenile, or adult form and is primarily a neurological disorder with progressive brain dysfunction (48).

Infantile GM1 gangliosidosis (type 1) is the most common and severe form, with clinical features of hypotonia, failure to thrive in the neonatal period, and clonic–tonic seizure activity The late infantile or juvenile form (type 2) begins with progressive mental and motor retardation between 1 and 5 years of age. Seizures are common (49). In both types, a progressive deterioration of the EEG with irregular background slowing evolves as the disease progresses.

Paroxysmal features are not necessarily prominent, despite the occurrence of seizures (50). Type 2 patients may show fluctuating 4 to 5 Hz rhythmic activity especially prominent in the temporal regions (51).

Disorders of Vitamin Metabolism

Late-Onset Multiple Carboxylase Deficiency: Biotinidase Deficiency

Biotinidase deficiency is the primary defect in most individuals with late-onset multiple carboxylase deficiency (52). It is characterized clinically by skin rash, alopecia, seizures, ataxia, and developmental delay.

Seizures are a prominent feature of late-onset multiple carboxylase deficiency, occurring in 50% to 75% of patients. Generalized clonic or tonic–clonic, partial, and myoclonic seizures, as well as infantile spasms, are the presenting feature in nearly half of patients. EEG may include a burst-suppression pattern, absence of physiological sleep patterns, poorly organized and slow background activity, and frequent spike and spike-and-slow-wave discharges (Figure 4.16) (53).

Methylene Tetrahydrofolate Reductase Deficiency

Methylene tetrahydrofolate reductase deficiency is the most common inborn error of folate metabolism. Most patients present in early life. The main clinical findings are neurologic signs such as severe developmental delay, marked hypotonia, acquired microcephaly, apnea, and seizures characterized by intractable infantile spasms, partial, atonic and myoclonic seizures. EEG findings vary from diffuse background slowing to continuous spike-and-wave complexes or multifocal discharges (Figure 4.17).

Disorders of Creatine Metabolism

Disorders of creatine metabolism comprise three different defects: impaired creatine transport into the brain in the x-linked creatine transporter defect (54), and impaired creatine synthesis in GAMT

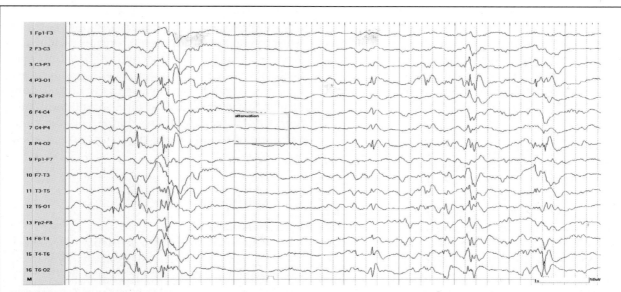

FIGURE 4.16   Biotinidase deficiency: EEG showed poorly organized and slow background activity, poorly formed sleep architecture, and independent bilateral epileptiform discharges. Sensitivity 7 μV/mm, TC 0.1 s, HF 70 Hz.

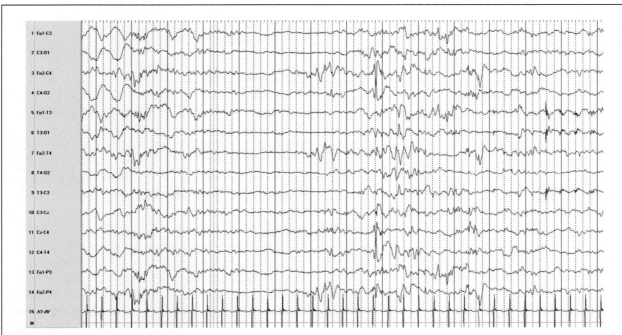

FIGURE 4.17   MTHFR deficiency: A 2-month-old girl presented with lethargy, irritability, and poor feeding. CT brain showed ventriculomegaly. EEG shows a multifocal discontinuous pattern. Sensitivity 7 μV/mm, TC 0.1 s, HF 70 Hz.

(guanidinoacetate methyltransferase) and AGAT (arginine–glycine amidinotransferase) deficiencies.

Seizures present in the first months of life, and include infantile spasms, atypical absences, astatic, myoclonic, and ultimately generalized tonic–clonic. Multifocal epileptiform discharges have been reported on the electroencephalogram (55).

Glucose Transporter Type 1 Deficiency Syndrome

Glucose transporter type 1 deficiency syndrome was initially described in 1991 by De Vivo et al (56). The condition results from a loss of functional glucose transporters, encoded by GLUT-1, that mediate glucose transport across the blood–brain barrier. Clinical features include infantile seizures, developmental delay, acquired microcephaly, spasticity, ataxia, and hypoglycorrhachia (57). Seizures are often the first identified feature of this syndrome. Seizure types include generalized tonic or clonic, myoclonic, atypical absence, atonic, and unclassified. Multifocal spike-wave discharges are seen, although a normal interictal electroencephalogram is well described. Seizures became more synchronized with brain maturation and are associated with generalized 2.5- to 4-Hz spike-wave discharges (58).

Hyperinsulinism/Hyperammonemia Syndrome

The hyperinsulinism/hyperammonemia (HI/HA) syndrome is a form of congenital hyperinsulinism in which affected children have recurrent symptomatic hypoglycemia together with asymptomatic, persistent elevations in plasma ammonia levels. The disorder is caused by dominant mutations of the mitochondrial enzyme, glutamate dehydrogenase (59). The main clinical feature in children is recurrent episodes of symptomatic hypoglycemia. These may occur during fasting or following high-protein intake. Neurological disorders consist of cognitive impairment and typically generalized seizures (in contrast with focal or multifocal seizures as in patients with epilepsy secondary to hypoglycemic insults). Seizures may be related to hypoglycemia in the early phase of the disease or may occur later in childhood without a known hypoglycemic event (60). Myoclonic absence seizures with photosensitivity have been reported with photosensitive generalized and irregular spike-wave discharges and runs of multiple spikes (61).

Organic Acidurias

Convulsive seizures or infantile spasms may be the presenting symptoms in several organic acidurias of infancy, including 3-methylcrotonyl-CoA carboxylase deficiency, 3-methylglutaconic aciduria, glutaric aciduria, and isovaleric acidemia. EEG findings reported include background slowing, focal or multifocal epileptiform discharges (including during episodic clinical deterioration), and intermittent background attenuation (24).

Amino Acid Disorders

Phenylketonuria

Phenylketonuria, caused by a deficiency of the enzyme phenylalanine hydroxylase, is associated with hyperphenylalaninemia. Seizures are present in 25% of the affected children. The vast majority of affected children (>80%) are found to have abnormalities on the electroencephalogram. Young children present with infantile spasms and hypsarrhythmia, while the older child will present with myoclonic or tonic–clonic seizures (62, 63). The EEG pattern includes diffuse background slowing, focal sharp waves, and irregular generalized spike-and-slow-wave discharges (55, 64) (Figure 4.18). An increase in delta activity has been seen with increasing phenylalanine levels (65).

Tyrosinemia Type III

Tyrosinemia III, an autosomal recessive disorder caused by deficiency in 4-hydroxyphenylpyruvate dioxygenase activity, has a wide phenotypic spectrum. It has been reported in intractable neonatal seizures as well as infantile spasms (66). EEG has been described as low-voltage, with spike and polyspike discharges in the parietal–occipital regions.

Menkes Disease

Menkes disease, also known as kinky hair disease, is an x-linked neurodegenerative disease of impaired copper transport. Children usually present at 2 to 3 months of age with loss of developmental milestones, twisted hair, and spasticity (67). Based on seizures type and EEG findings, three stages have been classified (68):

(a) an early stage (median age 3 months), characterized by focal clonic status epilepticus with ictal runs of

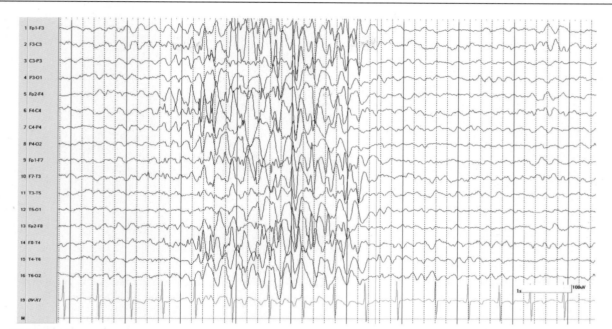

FIGURE 4.18 A 4-year-old boy with phenylketonuria presents with staring spells and periods of confusion. EEG showed bursts of high-amplitude diffuse irregular spike and slow-wave activity of 3 to 4 Hz with bifrontal predominance maximally involving the right frontal region. Sensitivity 20 μV/mm, TC 0.1 s, HF 70 Hz.

slow spike wave and slow waves in the posterior regions, and interictal multifocal and polymorphic slow waves, or mixed slow spike-and-wave; (b) an intermediate stage (median age 10 months) with intractable infantile spasms and interictal modified hypsarrhythmia (Figure 4.19) or diffuse irregular slow waves and spike waves; (c) a late stage (median age 25 months) with multifocal seizures, tonic spasms, and myoclonus, with electrographic multifocal high-amplitude activity mixed with irregular slow waves (69).

Progressive Encephalopathy With Edema, Hypsarrhythmia, and Optic Atrophy (PEHO)

PEHO syndrome is a rare neurodegenerative syndrome first reported in 1991 (70) with profound psychomotor retardation, hypotonia, edema, and loss of visual contact. The patients have characteristic facial features. Seizures generally begin as infantile spasms with associated hypsarrhythmia on EEG. Later other seizure types may be seen, including tonic, tonic–clonic, and absence seizures. The EEG may evolve to a slow spike-and-wave pattern, and otherwise is nonspecific (71).

METABOLIC DISORDERS OF LATE INFANCY

Metachromatic Leukodystrophy

This progressive white matter disease is caused by deficiency in the lysosomal enzyme sulfatide sulfatase, otherwise known as arylsulfatase. Recurrent seizures are common and may occur at any stage of the disease, particularly in patients with juvenile onset. Generalized seizures are more frequent in patients with late infantile-onset, whereas partial seizures develop over time in 25% of patients with the late infantile form and in 50% to 60% of patients with the juvenile-onset form (72, 73). EEG early in the course may be normal or show mild background slowing and paroxysmal electrographic discharges usually appear during the later stages (74).

Schindler Disease

Schindler disease is a recognized infantile neuroaxonal dystrophy resulting from deficient activity of the lysosomal hydrolase, alpha-*N*-acetylgalactosaminidase (75). Seizures with generalized tonic–clonic and

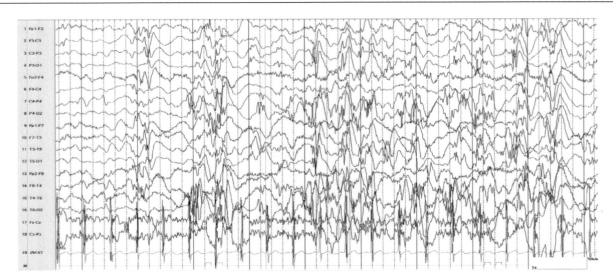

FIGURE 4.19   A 10-month-old infant with Menkes disease. Interictal EEG: Multifocal high-amplitude and polymorphic activity, mixed with irregular slow waves (modified hypsarrhythmia). Sensitivity 20 μV/mm, TC 0.1 s, HF 70 Hz.

myoclonic activity are common. EEG shows multifocal spikes and spike-wave complexes.

Mucopolysaccharidoses

The mucopolysaccharidoses are genetic disorders of glycosaminoglycan metabolism, and are characterized by excessive intralysosomal accumulation of partially degraded mucopolysaccharides. The clinical consequences of such storage range from skeletal abnormalities to cardiovascular problems, and to developmental motor and cognitive impairment (76). The most common mucopolysaccharidosis is Sanfilippo disease (MPS type III).

Generalized seizures develop in about 40% of patients with Sanfilippo syndrome. EEG changes include lack of normal sleep staging, absence of vertex waves and sleep spindles, and low-amplitude fast (12–15 Hz) activity with generalized delta frequencies (77). Epileptiform paroxysms are seen in patients with or without histories of clinical seizures (78).

Neuronal Ceroid Lipofuscinoses

The neuronal ceroid lipofuscinoses (NCL) are severe neurodegenerative lysosomal storage disorders characterized by accumulation of autofluorescent ceroid lipopigment in most cells. NCLs are caused by mutations in at least 10 recessively inherited human genes, eight of which have been characterized (79).

In the infantile form (NCL1), seizures start at the end of the first year of life, with myoclonus and atonic and tonic–clonic seizures. The EEG shows early attenuation and progressive loss of background (Figure 4.20).

In the late-infantile form (NCL2), onset is usually after the second year of life. The seizures include generalized tonic–clonic, atonic, astatic, and myoclonic (Figures 4.21 and 4.22). The clinical picture may resemble myoclonic–astatic epilepsy. The EEG shows spike and slow-wave activity and photoparoxysmal responses (1).

Alpers' Syndrome (Progressive Infantile Poliodystrophy)

Alpers' disease represents a group of disorders characterized by a rapidly progressive encephalopathy with intractable seizures and diffuse neuronal degeneration.

Intractable seizures are characteristic and include generalized tonic–clonic, focal, myoclonic, epilepsia partialis continuans, and convulsive status epilepticus. Status epilepticus may be the presenting symptom (80).

EEG findings show a pattern of continuous, anterior, high-voltage l- to 3-Hz spike-and-wave activity

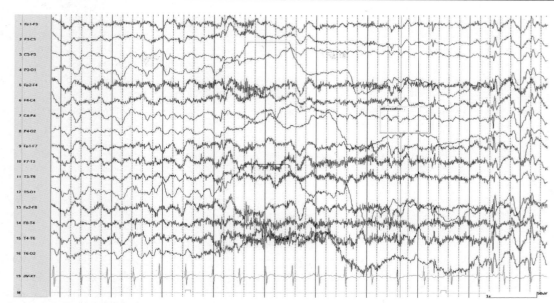

FIGURE 4.20   A 3-year-old patient with NCL1 presented with myoclonic seizures and drop attacks. Awake EEG shows slow background with ictal attenuation. Sensitivity 7 μV/mm, TC 0.1 s, HF 70 Hz.

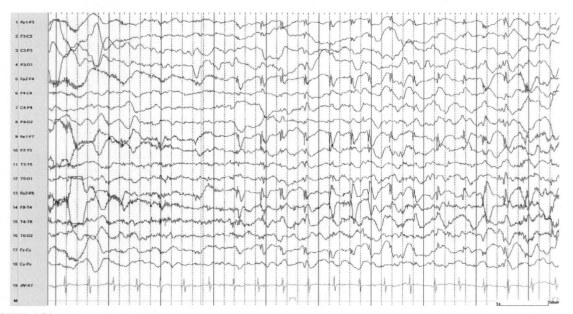

FIGURE 4.21   A 4-year-old girl with NCL2 presents with progressive regression of developmental skills, myoclonic seizures and drop attacks. Awake EEG showed slow background and anterior dominant slow spike-and-wave activity of 2.5 Hz/sec. Sensitivity 7 μV/mm, TC 0.1 s, HF 70 Hz.

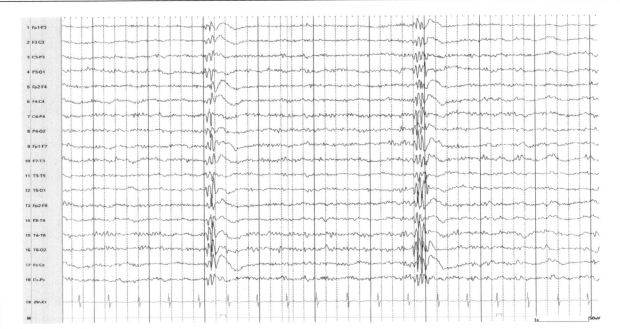

FIGURE 4.22   NCL2 (same patient as Figure 4.21, during sleep state). EEG showed generalized bilaterally synchronous polyspike and wave discharges. Sensitivity 7 μV/mm, TC 0.1 s, HF 70 Hz.

that persists despite intermittent focal seizures. There is furthermore progressive slowing of the background with disease progression (81) (Figure 4.23).

Congenital Disorders of Glycosylation

This group refers to a complex group of hereditary defects in glycoprotein metabolism involving organelle dysfunction of the endoplasmic reticulum and Golgi body. Predominant symptoms are cognitive deficiency, epilepsy, cerebellar ataxia, polyneuropathy, strabismus, and retinitis pigmentosa. Systemic symptoms include growth impairment, hepatic steatosis, pericardial effusion, hypothyroidism, and dysmorphism including wide-spaced nipples and excessive subcutaneous fat pads. Interictal EEG shows hypsarrhythmia or epileptiform discharges (82).

METABOLIC DISORDERS OF CHILDHOOD AND ADOLESCENCE

Homocystinuria

This disorder of transsulfuration is caused by deficiency in cystathionine beta-synthase.

Symptoms include psychomotor delay, ectopic lenses, and osteoporosis (83). Generalized seizures occur in about 20% of patients with pyridoxine-nonresponsive homocystinuria and in approximately 15% of patients with the pyridoxine-responsive form. EEG features are nonspecific with slowing and focal interictal epileptiform discharges (84).

Adrenoleukodystrophy

X-linked adrenoleukodystrophy (ALD) is a rare metabolic disorder caused by peroxisomal enzyme failure. It is characterized by the accumulation of very long-chain fatty acids in the brain and adrenal tissues. The cerebral form presents between 4 and 8 years of age (85). Seizures, including versive, focal motor, and secondarily generalized, appear between 2 and 4 years after the clinical onset (74).

Status epilepticus, including epilepsia partialis continuans, has been reported early in the course. Initial EEGs may be normal or minimally abnormal, with diffuse slowing of posterior rhythms (corresponding to the localization of pathology as seen on MRI) (74). As the disease progresses, slow-wave abnormalities

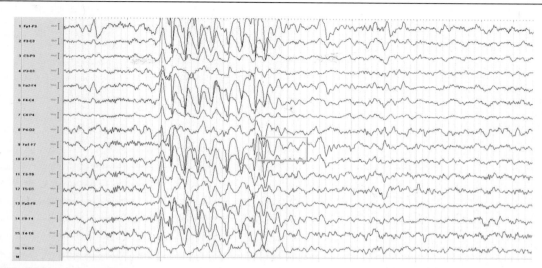

FIGURE 4.23 A 7-year-old boy diagnosed with Alpers syndrome presented with encephalopathy, tonic–clonic seizures and myoclonic seizures. EEG shows high-amplitude anterior poorly formed 2 to 3 Hz sharp and slow activity.

became progressively widespread, together with paroxysmal discharges and loss of faster frequencies over the posterior regions (74, 86).

Lysosomal Disorders

Sialidosis Type I (Cherry-Red Spot Myoclonus Syndrome)

Sialidosis I is a slowly progressive syndrome that combines action-sensitive and stimulus-sensitive myoclonus with a cherry-red spot at the macula and optic atrophy (87). Electrophysiological findings include low-voltage fast EEG background activity and paroxysmal bursts of bilateral 10 to 20 Hz positive spikes over the vertex which increase in frequency during sleep and are time locked to the myoclonus (88, 89).

Sialidosis Type II/Galactosialidosis

This is a rare neuronal storage disease that begins in childhood with cognitive impairment, skeletal abnormalities, progressive myoclonus and a cherry-red spot in the macula (90). This diagnosis has mainly been reported in Japanese patients. Electrophysiological studies show paroxysmal moderate-voltage generalized 4 to 6 Hz spike-wave. Intention myoclonus in this disorder is consistent with "cortical reflex" myoclonus (Figure 4.24) (91).

Gaucher Disease Type III

Gaucher Disease type III, glucocerebrosidase deficiency, has a variable age of onset, from childhood to early adulthood. The first symptoms are often impairment of saccadic horizontal eye movements and supranuclear gaze palsy with strabismus (92). Myoclonic and tonic–clonic seizures are present, and EEG shows a normal to slow background with bursts of multifocal or predominantly posterior polyspike waves (Figure 4.25), rhythmical trains of rapid (6–10 Hz) spikes or sharp waves, and photosensitivity (93).

Neuroaxonal Dystrophies

The neuroaxonal dystrophies constitute a group of neurodegenerative disorders characterized by a common axonal lesion. These disorders include infantile (Seitelberger disease), late-infantile, and juvenile forms as well as neuroaxonal leukodystrophy and neuro-ferritinopathy associated with pantothenate kinase deficiency (formerly known eponymically as Hallervorden–Spatz syndrome, with this attribution erased due to unethical behavior during the Nazi atrocities). Seizures occur in one-third of patients, with onset of convulsions after 3 years of age. Myoclonic and tonic seizures are the presenting and predominant clinical feature in infantile neuroaxonal dystrophy (94–96).

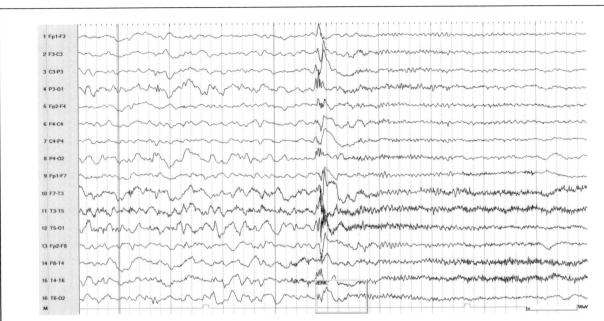

FIGURE 4.24   Sialidosis type 2: 15-month-old girl with global developmental delay, myoclonic seizures, and cherry-red spot of the macula. Ictal event shown; interictal EEG showed paroxysmal moderate voltage, generalized 4 to 5 Hz spike-wave activity. Sensitivity 10 µV/mm, TC 0.1 s, HF 70 Hz.

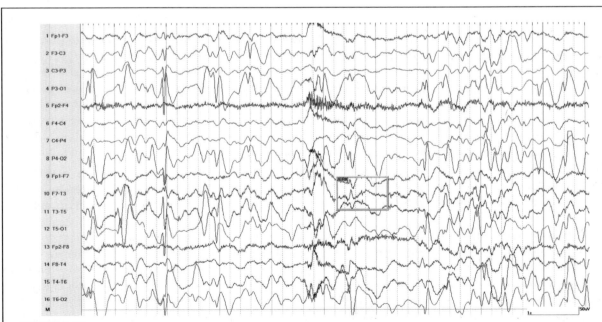

FIGURE 4.25   Patient with Gaucher disease type III showing a myoclonic seizure. EEG background showed slowing and runs of predominantly posterior spike and wave. Sensitivity 7 µV/mm, TC 0.1 s, HF 70 Hz.

The characteristic EEG pattern is high-voltage, fast (16–24 Hz) rhythmic activity and absence of reactivity on eye-opening or closure or during intermittent photic stimulation. During sleep, the fast activity persists as the dominant feature, with absence of central sleep transients or K-complexes (97). A series of symmetrical tonic spasms of both upper extremities with a corresponding electrographic diffuse irregular high-voltage sharp and slow-wave transient followed by desynchronization has been described (96).

Neuronal Ceroid Lipofuscinosis Type III (Batten Disease)

Batten disease (juvenile onset neuronal ceroid lipofuscinosis, sometimes called Spielmeyer–Vogt) has symptom onset between ages 5 and 10 years, with gradual onset of vision problems and myoclonic seizures. Tonic–clonic and sometimes atypical absence seizures begin 1 to 4 years after onset. Segmental myoclonias occur, and myoclonus is aggravated by passive movements. Massive myoclonias can proceed to clonic seizures, and clonic status is common at the terminal stages (98–99). EEG changes are nonspecific.

Progressive Myoclonus Epilepsies

The progressive myoclonus epilepsies are a collection of rare disorders presenting with the triad of myoclonus (typically cortical), tonic–clonic seizures, and neurological deterioration.

Onset generally begins in late childhood and adolescence (100). The differential diagnosis includes Lafora disease, Unverricht Lundborg, and MERRF, which are described below.

Lafora Disease

Seizures are the initial symptom, which include partial visual seizures and generalized tonic–clonic events. The visual phenomena are simple or more complex hallucinations or scotomata (101). Severe resting and action myoclonus ensue. At onset, generalized bursts of irregular spike and polyspike discharges superimposed upon a normal background and a photoparoxysmal response are seen on EEG (Figure 4.26). As the disease progresses, the EEG background becomes disorganized and slow, with focal spikes particularly over the occipital regions as well as loss of normal sleep architecture (Figure 4.27) (102).

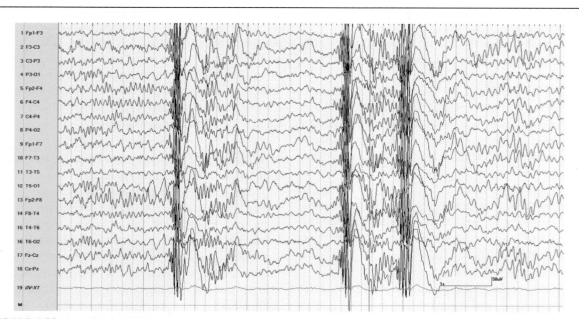

FIGURE 4.26 A 15-year-old boy with Lafora body disease presents with increased generalized seizures. Sleep EEG shows significant activation of epileptiform activity in sleep characterized by generalized polyspike and wave activity (as shown) and fragmentary spike discharges. Sensitivity 7 µV/mm, TC 0.1 s, HF 70 Hz.

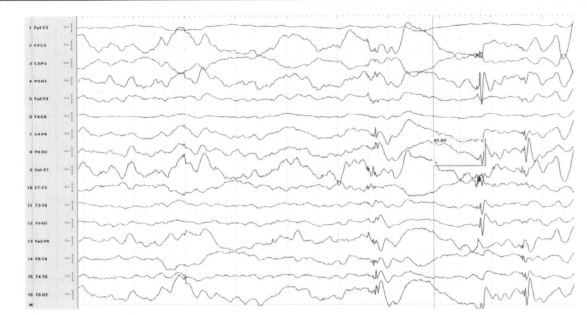

FIGURE 4.27   Patient with advanced Lafora body disease, showing disorganized background activity with focal spikes over the occipital regions. Sensitivity 7 μV/mm, TC 0.1 s, HF 70 Hz.

Unverricht Lundborg Disease

More commonly reported in Scandinavian countries, this disorder has onset between the ages 6 and 15 years. The characteristic feature is stimulus-sensitive myoclonus (103). Either myoclonic or tonic–clonic seizures may be the presenting sign (104). The myoclonias may be provoked by light, physical exertion, noise, stress, and awakening. They occur predominantly in proximal muscles and are asynchronous; they may be focal or multifocal and may generalize to a series of myoclonic seizures or even status myoclonicus (105).

EEG may be normal or mildly slow at the beginning, followed by progressive slowing with generalized 3- to 5-per-second frontally dominant spike-wave bursts. Photic stimulation elicits generalized spike and polyspike discharges (104, 106).

Myoclonic Epilepsy and Ragged Red Fibers (MERRF)

Myoclonic epilepsy and ragged-red fibers (MERRF) is a multisystem mitochondrial cytopathy characterized by myoclonic seizures, tonic–clonic seizures, and progressive neurologic dysfunction (ataxia and myopathy) with the presence of ragged-red fibers on skeletal muscle biopsy. It is associated with a mitochondrial tRNA gene point mutation (107).

EEG findings include background slowing, focal epileptiform discharges, and atypical spike or sharp and slow-wave complexes that have a variable association with the myoclonic activity. Sporadic occipital spikes and sharp waves as well as photosensitivity may be seen, suppression of these discharges during sleep is characteristic (108).

Mitochondrial Encephalomyopathy, Lactic Acidosis, and Stroke-Like Episodes (MELAS)

Mitochondrial encephalomyopathy, lactic acidosis, and stroke like episodes, or MELAS, is characterized by seizures with focal clonic and myoclonic activity, severe headaches resembling migraines, and sudden onset of stroke-like episodes (109). Epilepsia partialis continuans occurs in MELAS, and seizures often evolve into partial or generalized status epilepticus (Figures 4.28–4.30) (110).

Ictal EEG shows focal high-voltage delta slow waves with polyspikes (Figures 4.28–4.30). Frequent focal spikes or sharp waves and 14- and 6-Hz positive bursts are also noted (111).

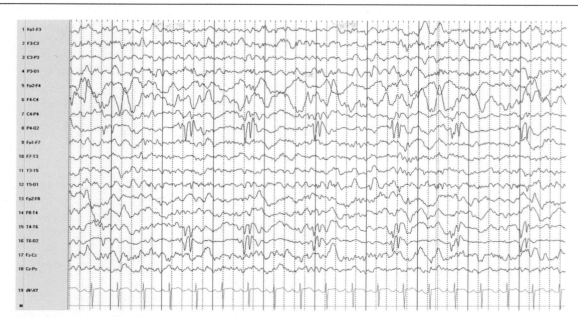

FIGURE 4.28 A 14-year-old girl with a history of MELAS presents with epilepsia partialis continuans manifest by clonic activity of the left fingers, wrist and arm. EEG is most notable for right hemispheric polymorphic slowing and PLEDS maximally involving the right occipital lobe. Sensitivity 7 μV/mm, TC 0.1 s, HF 70 Hz.

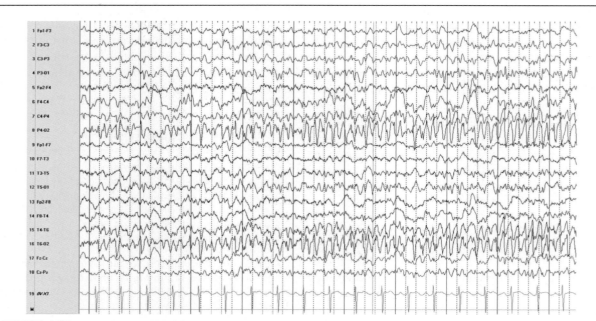

FIGURE 4.29 Same patient with MELAS as in Figure 4.27. EEG shows seizure discharge of right occipital origin. Sensitivity 7 μV/mm, TC 0.1 s, HF 70 Hz.

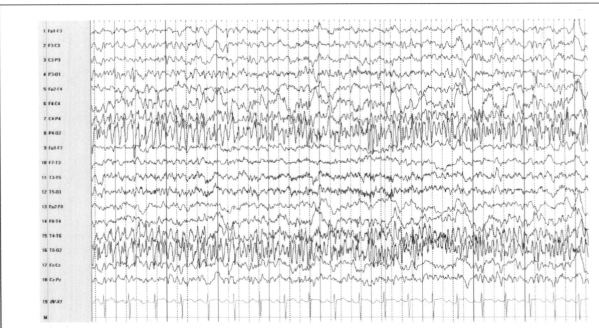

FIGURE 4.30   Same patient in Figure 4.28 with MELAS; EEG shows ongoing seizure activity with propagation over the right hemisphere. Sensitivity 7 μV/mm, TC 0.1 s, HF 70 Hz.

Dentatorubral-Pallidoluysian Atrophy

Dentatorubral-pallidoluysian atrophy (DRPLA) is a rare neurodegenerative disease first described in 1958, and subsequently associated with a CAG trinucleotide repeat sequence on chromosome 12p (112). DRPLA is most prevalent in Japan. Symptoms begin in infancy to early childhood with myoclonus, ataxia, dementia, opsoclonus, or seizures that can be generalized tonic–clonic, atypical absence, or atonic.

EEG is characterized by bursts of slowing, irregular spike-and-wave, and multifocal paroxysmal discharges (113). Photoparoxysmal responses are characteristic, and myoclonic seizures are often triggered by photic stimulation.

CLINICAL PEARLS

Metabolic epilepsies present with myoclonic seizures and infantile spasms, as well as partial and generalized seizures.

EEGs typically reveal burst-suppression or hypsarrhythmia in early onset metabolic epileptic encephalopathies, although more specific patterns such as the comb like rhythm in maple syrup urine disease have been described.

Serial EEGs in the progressive metabolic epilepsies progress from normal to background slowing and loss of sleep architecture to an increasing burden of generalized spike-and-wave activity and sometimes photoparoxysmal responses.

REFERENCES

1. Nicole I, Wolf TB, Surtees R. Epilepsy in inborn errors of metabolism. *Epileptic Disorder.* 2005;7(2):67–81.
2. Leonard JV. MA, Biochemistry, Endocrinology and Metabolism Unit, Institute of Child Health, London, UK. Diagnosis and early management of inborn errors of metabolism presenting around the time of birth. *Acta Paediatr.* 2006;95(1): 6–14.
3. Torres OA, MV, Buist NM, Hyland K. Folinic acid-responsive neonatal seizures. *J Child Neurol.* 1999;14(8),529–532.
4. Prasad AN, HGCN. Early onset epilepsy and inherited metabolic disorders: Diagnosis and management. *Can J Neurol Sci.* 2010;37(3):350–358.
5. Nordli and DVDC. Classification of infantile seizures: implications for identification and treatment of inborn errors of metabolism. *J Child Neurol.* 2002;17(3) 3S3–3S7.

6. Ohtahara S, OY, Yamatogi Y. Early-infantile epileptic encephalopathy with suppression-bursts: developmental aspect. *Brain Dev.* 1997;9:371–376.

7. Brown FR, III, Voigt PR, Singh AK, et al. Peroxisomal disorders: Neurodevelopmental and biochemical aspects. *Am J Dis Child.* 1993;147(6):617–626.

8. Baumgartner MR, Saudubray JM. Peroxisomal disorders. *Sem Neonatol: SN.* 2002;7(1):85–94.

9. Takahashi Y, SY, KK., et al. Epilepsy in peroxisomal diseases. *Epilepsia.* 1997;38(2):182–188.

10. Benke PJ, Reyes PF, et al. New form of adrenoleukodystrophy. *Human Genetics.* 1981;58(2):204–208.

11. Verma NP, Hart ZH, et al. Electrophysiologic studies in neonatal adrenoleukodystrophy. *Electroencephalography and Clinical Neurophysiology.* 1985;60(1): 7–15.

12. Gastraut H, RJ, Soulayrol R, et al. (1964). Infantile spasms and West syndrome. In J Roger, M Bureau, C Dravet, et al. eds. *Epileptic Syndromes in Infancy, Childhood and Adolescence.* 4th ed. Montrouge, France: John Libbey Eurotext Ltd., 2005:53–72.

13. Lucia Fusco FV. Ictal clinical electroencephalographic findings of spasms in West syndrome. *Epilepsia.* 1993;34(4):671–678.

14. Kellaway P, HR, Frost JD, Jr, Zion T. Precise characterization and quantification of infantile spasms. *Ann Neurol.* 1979; 6(3):214–218.

15. Hunt AD, SJJ, Jr, McCrory WW, Stroud HH. Pyridoxine dependency: report of a case of intractable convulsions in an infant controlled by pyridoxine. *Pediatrics.* 1954;13:140–145.

16. Baxter P. Epidemiology of pyridoxine dependent and pyridoxine responsive seizures in the UK. *Arch Dis Child.* 1999;81:431–433.

17. Nabbout R, Soufflet C, et al. Pyridoxine dependent epilepsy: A suggestive electroclinical pattern. *Archives of Disease in Childhood—Fetal and Neonatal Edition.* 1999;81(2):F125–F129.

18. Lin J, Lin K, et al. Pyridoxine-dependent epilepsy initially responsive to phenobarbital. *Arq Neuropsiquiatr.* 2007; 65(4-A):1026–1029.

19. Mills PB, Surtees RAH, et al. Neonatal epileptic encephalopathy caused by mutations in the PNPO gene encoding pyridox (am)ine 5′-phosphate oxidase. *Hum Mol Genet.* 2005;14(8): 1077–1086.

20. Pearl P, Gospe S. Pyridoxal phosphate dependency, a newly recognized treatable catastrophic epileptic encephalopathy. *J Inherited Metab Dis.* 2007;30(1):2–4.

21. Veerapandiyan A, Winchester SA, et al. Electroencephalographic and seizure manifestations of pyridoxal 5′-phosphate-dependent epilepsy. *Epilepsy Behav.* 2011;20(3):494–501.

22. Brown GK, OL, LeGris M, Brown RM. Pyruvate dehydrogenase deficiency. *J Med Genet.* 1994;31(11):875–879.

23. Robinson BH. Lactic acidemia: disorders of pyruvate carboxylase, pyruvate dehydrogenase. In: CR Scriver, AL Beaudet, WS Sly, et al. eds. *The Metabolic and Molecular Bases of Inherited Disease.* 8th ed. New York: McGraw-Hill; 2001:2275–2295.

24. Stigsby B, YS, Rahbeeni Z, Dabbagh O, et al. Neurophysiologic correlates of organic acidemias: A survey of 107 patients. *Brain Dev.* 1994;16(Suppl):125–144.

25. DiMauro S, Moraes CT. Mitochondrial encephalomyopathies. *Arch Neurol.* 1993;50(11):1197–1208.

26. Elia M, Musumeci SA, et al. Leigh syndrome and partial deficit of cytochrome c oxidase associated with epilepsia partialis continua. *Brain Dev.* 1996;18(3):207–211.

27. Canafoglia L, Franceschetti S, et al. Epileptic phenotypes associated with mitochondrial disorders. *Neurology.* 2001;56(10): 1340–1346.

28. Johnson JL, Waud WR, et al. Inborn errors of molybdenum metabolism: combined deficiencies of sulfite oxidase and xanthine dehydrogenase in a patient lacking the molybdenum cofactor. *Proc Natl Acad Sci.* 1980;77(6):3715–3719.

29. Kurlemann G, SG. EEG in diagnosis of other disease pictures than epilepsy. *Klin Padiatr.* 1994;206(2):100–107.

30. Garcia-Alvarez M, ND, De Vivo DC Inherited metabolic disorders. In J Engel, TA Pedley, eds. *Epilepsy: A Comprehensive Textbook.* Philadelphia: Lippincott-Raven; 1998:2547–2562.

31. Verma NP, HZ, Kooi KA. Electroencephalographic findings in urea-cycle disorders. *Electroencephalogr Clin Neurophysiol.* 1984;57(2):105–112.

32. Rudolf C, Engel NRMB. The EEGs of infants with citrullinemia. *Dev Med Child Neurol.* 1985;27(2):199–206.

33. Peinemann F, Danner DJ. Maple syrup urine disease 1954 to 1993. *J Inherited Metab Dis.* 1994;17(1):3–15.

34. Trottier A, KM, Geoffroy G, Andermann F. A characteristic EEG finding in newborns with maple syrup urine disease (branched-chain keto aciduria). *Electroencephalogr Clin Neurophysiol.* 1975;38:108.

35. Tharp BR. Unique EEG pattern (comb-like rhythm) in neonatal maple syrup urine disease *Pediatr Neurol.* 1992;8(1): 65–68

36. Dionisi-Vici C, Deodato F, et al. "Classical" organic acidurias, propionic aciduria, methylmalonic aciduria and isovaleric aciduria: long-term outcome and effects of expanded newborn screening using tandem mass spectrometry. *J Inherited Metab Dis.* 2006;29(2):383–389.

37. Guevara-Campos J, González-De Guevara L, et al. Methylmalonic aciduria associated with myoclonic convulsions, psychomotor retardation and hypsarrhythmia. *Rev Neurol.* 2003; 36(08):0735–0737.

38. Aoki Y, Suzuki Y, et al. Characterization of mutant holocarboxylase synthetase (HCS): AKm for biotin was not elevated in a patient with HCS deficiency. *Pediatr Res.* 1997;42(6): 849–854.

39. Suzuki Y, Yang X, et al. Mutations in the holocarboxylase synthetase gene HLCS. *Hum Mutat.* 2005;26(4):285–290.

40. Williams ML, Packman S, et al. Alopecia and periorificial dermatitis in biotin-responsive multiple carboxylase deficiency. *J Am Acad Dermatol.* 1983;9(1):97–103.

41. Vellodi A. Lysosomal storage disorders. *Br J Haematol.* 2005;128(4):413–431.

42. Cobb W, MF, Pampiglione G. Cerebral lipidosis: An electroencephalographic study. *Brain.* 1952;75(3):343–357.

43. Zafeiriou DI, Anastasiou AL, et al. Early infantile Krabbe disease: deceptively normal magnetic resonance imaging and serial neurophysiological studies. *Brain Dev.* 1997;19(7): 488–491.

44. Blom S, Hagberg B. EEG findings in late infantile metachromatic and globoid cell leucodystrophy. *Electroencephalogr Clin Neurophysiol.* 1967;22(3):253–259.

45. Hagberg B. Krabbe's disease: clinical presentation of neurological variants. *Neuropediatrics.* 1984;15(S1):11,15.

46. Kliemann FA, HA, Pampiglione G. Some EEG observations in patients with Krabbe's disease. *Dev Med Child Neurol.* 1969;11(4):475–484.

47. Pampiglione G, Harden A. Neurophysiological identification of a late infantile form of "neuronal lipidosis". *J Neurol, Neurosurg Psychiatry.* 1973;36(1):68–74.

48. Brunetti-Pierri N, Scaglia F. GM1 gangliosidosis: review of clinical, molecular, and therapeutic aspects. *Mol Genet Metab.* 2008;94(4):391–396.

49. Chen C, Zimmerman R, et al. Neuroimaging findings in late infantile GM1 gangliosidosis. *AJNR Am J Neuroradiol.* 1998;19(9):1628–1630.

50. Pampiglione G, Harden A. Neurophysiological investigations in GM1 and GM2 gangliosidoses. *Neuropediatrics.* 1984;15(S1): 74,84.

51. Harden A, Martinovic Z, et al. Neurophysiological studies in GM_1, gangliosidosis. *Italian J Neurol Sci.* 1982;3(3): 201–206.

52. Cole H, Wolf B, et al. Localization of serum biotinidase (BTD) to human chromosome 3 in band p25. *Genomics.*1994;22(3): 662–663.

53. Salbert BA, Pellock JM, et al. Characterization of seizures associated with biotinidase deficiency. *Neurology.* 1993;43(7): 1351–1355.

54. Salomons GS, van Dooren SJM, et al. X-Linked creatine-transporter gene (SLC6A8) defect: A new creatine-deficiency syndrome. *Am J Hum Genet.* 2001;68(6):1497–1500.

55. KF S. Aminoacidopathies and organic acidemias resulting from deficiency of enzyme activity and transport abnormalities. In: KF Swaiman, S Ashwal eds. *Pediatric Neurology, Principles and Practice.* 3rd ed. St. Louis: Mosby-year book, Inc.; 1999: 377–410.

56. De Vivo DC, Trifiletti RR, et al. Defective glucose transport across the blood–brain barrier as a cause of persistent hypoglycorrhachia, seizures, and developmental delay. *New Eng J Med.* 1991;325(10):703–709.

57. Wang D, Pascual JM, et al. Glut-1 deficiency syndrome: clinical, genetic, and therapeutic aspects. *Ann Neurol.* 2005;57(1): 111–118.

58. Leary LD, Wang D, et al. Seizure characterization and electroencephalographic features in glut-1 deficiency syndrome. *Epilepsia.* 2003;44(5):701–707.

59. Stanley CA. Hyperinsulinism/hyperammonemia syndrome: insights into the regulatory role of glutamate dehydrogenase in ammonia metabolism. *Mol Genet Metab.* 2004;81(Supp 1): 45–51.

60. Bahi-Buisson N, Roze E, et al. Neurological aspects of hyperinsulinism–hyperammonaemia syndrome. *Devl Med Child Neurol.* 2008;50(12):945–949.

61. Bahi-Buisson N, El Sabbagh S, et al. Myoclonic absence epilepsy with photosensitivity and a gain of function mutation in glutamate dehydrogenase. *Seizure: J Br Epilepsy Assoc.* 2008;17(7):658–664.

62. Low NL, BJ, Armstrong MD. Studies on phenylketonuria. VI. EEG studies in phenylketonuria. *AMA Arch Neurol Psychiatry.* 1957;77(4):359–365.

63. Yanling Y, QG, Zhixiang Z, Chunlan M, et al. A clinical investigation of 228 patients with phenylketonuria in mainland China. *Southeast Asian J Trop Med Public Health.* 1999; 30(Suppl 2):58–60.

64. Pietz J, Schmidt E, et al. EEGs in phenylketonuria I: Follow-up to adulthood; II: Short-term diet-related changes in EEGs and cognitive function. *Dev Med Child Neurol.* 1993;35(1): 54–64.

65. Donker DNJ, Reits D, et al. Computer analysis of the EEG as an aid in the evaluation of dietetic treatment in phenylketonuria. *Electroencephalogr Clin Neurophysiol.* 1979;46(2):205–213.

66. Seshia SS, Perry TL, et al. Tyrosinemia and intractable seizures. *Epilepsia.* 1984;25(4):457–463.

67. Menkes JH. Kinky hair disease. *Pediatrics.* 1972;50(2): 181–183.

68. Bahi-Buisson N, Kaminska A, et al. Epilepsy in Menkes disease: analysis of clinical stages. *Epilepsia.* 2006;47(2): 380–386.

69. Friedman E, Harden A, et al. Menkes' disease: neurophysiological aspects. *J Neurol, Neurosur Psychiatry.* 1978;41(6): 505–510.

70. Salonen R, Somer M, et al. Progressive encephalopathy with edema, hypsarrhythmia, and optic atrophy (PEHO syndrome). *Clin Genet.* 1991;39(4):287–293.

71. Somer M, Sainio K. Epilepsy and the electroencephalogram in progressive encephalopathy with edema, hypsarrhythmia, and optic atrophy (the PEHO syndrome). *Epilepsia.* 1993;34(4): 727–731.

72. Fukumizu M, Matsui K, et al. Partial seizures in two cases of metachromatic leukodystrophy: Electrophysiologic and neuroradiologic findings. *J Child Neurol.* 1992;7(4):381–386.

73. Balslev T, Cortez MA, et al. Recurrent seizures in metachromatic leukodystrophy. *Pediatr Neurol.* 1997;17(2):150–154.

74. Wang P-J, Hwu W-L, et al. Epileptic seizures and electroencephalographic evolution in genetic leukodystrophies. *J Clin Neurophysiol.* 2001;18(1):25–32.

75. Wang AM, Schindler D, et al. Schindler disease: the molecular lesion in the alpha-N-acetylgalactosaminidase gene that causes an infantile neuroaxonal dystrophy. *J Clin Invest.* 1990;86(5): 1752–1756.

76. Cantz M, Gehler J. The mucopolysaccharidoses: inborn errors of glycosaminoglycan catabolism. *Hum Genet.* 1976;32(3): 233–255.

77. Kriel RL, Hauser WA, et al. Neuroanatomical and electroencephalographic correlations in Sanfilippo syndrome, Type A. *Arch Neurol.* 1978;35(12): 838–843.

78. Albuquerque RML, Liberalesso PBN, et al. Aspectos eletrencefalográficos em crianças com mucopolissacaridose. *J Epilepsy Clin Neurophysiol.* 2010;16:162–166.

79. Jalanko A, BT. Neuronal ceroid lipofuscinoses. *Biochim Biophys Acta.* 2009;1793(4):697–709.

80. Wolf NI, Rahman S, et al. Status epilepticus in children with Alpers' disease caused by POLG1 mutations: EEG and MRI features. *Epilepsia.* 2009;50(6):1596–1607.

81. Brick IE, WI, Gomez MR. The electroencephalogram in Alper's disease [abstract]. *Electroencephalogr Clin Neurophysiol.* 1984;58:31.

82. Tayama M, HT, Miyazaki M, Murakawa K, et al. Pathophysiology of carbohydrate-deficient glycoprotein syndrome—

neuroradiological and neurophysiological study. *No To Hattatsu.* 1993;25(6):537–542.

83. Mudd SH, SF, Levy HL, Pettigrew KD, et al. The natural history of homocystinuria due to cystathionine beta-synthase deficiency. *Am J Hum Genet.* 1985;37(1):1–31.

84. Del Giudice E, SS, Andria G. (1983). Electroencephalographic abnormalities in homocystinuria due to cystathionine synthase deficiency. *Clin Neurol Neurosurg.* 85(3):165–168.

85. Igarashi M, Schaumburg HH, et al. Fatty acid abnormality in adrenoleukodystrophy. *J Neurochem.* 1976;26(4):851–860.

86. Mamoli B, Graf M, et al. EEG, pattern-evoked potentials and nerve conduction velocity in a family with adrenoleucodystrophy. *Electroencephalogr Clin Neurophysiol.* 1979;47(4):411–419.

87. Franceschetti S, Uziel G, et al. Cherry-red spot myoclonus syndrome and alpha-neuraminidase deficiency: neurophysiological, pharmacological and biochemical study in an adult. *J Neurol, Neurosurg Psychiatry.* 1980;43(10):934–940.

88. Engel J, Rapin I, et al. Electrophysiological studies in two patients with cherry red spot-myoclonus syndrome. *Epilepsia.* 1977;18(1):73–87.

89. Louboutin JP, Nogues B, et al. Multimodality evoked potentials and EEG in a case of cherry red spot-myoclonus syndrome and alpha-neuraminidase deficiency (sialidosis Type 1). *Eur Neurol.* 1995;35(3):175–177.

90. O'Brien JS, Warner TG. Sialidosis: delineation of subtypes by neuraminidase assay. *Clin Genet.* 1980;17(1):35–38.

91. Tobimatsu S, Fukui R, et al. Electrophysiological studies of myoclonus in sialidosis type 2. *Electroencephalogr Clin Neurophysiol.* 1985;60(1):16–22.

92. Tripp JH, Lake BD, et al. Juvenile Gaucher's disease with horizontal gaze palsy in three siblings. *J Neurol, Neurosurg Psychiatry.* 1977;40(5):470–478.

93. Nishimura R, Omos-Lau N, et al. Electroencephalographic findings in Gaucher disease. *Neurology.* 1980;30(2):152–159.

94. Schindler D, Bishop DF, et al. Neuroaxonal dystrophy due to lysosomal alpha-N-acetylgalactosaminidase deficiency. *New Engl J Med.* 1989;320(26):1735–1740.

95. Butzer JF, Schochet SS, et al. Infantile neuroaxonal dystrophy. *Acta Neuropathol.* 1975;31(1):35–43.

96. Wakai S, Asanuma H, et al. Ictal video-EEG analysis of infantile neuroaxonal dystrophy. *Epilepsia.* 1994;35(4):823–826.

97. Ferriss GS, Happel LT, et al. Cerebral cortical isolation in infantile neuroaxonal dystrophy. *Electroencephalogr Clin Neurophysiol.* 1977;43(2):168–182.

98. Gardiner M, Sandford A, et al. Batten disease (Spielmeyer–Vogt disease, juvenile onset neuronal ceroid-lipofuscinosis) gene (CLN3) maps to human chromosome 16. *Genomics.* 1990;8(2):387–390.

99. Berkovic SF, Andermann F, et al. Progressive myoclonus epilepsies: Specific causes and diagnosis. *New Engl J Med.* 1986;315(5):296–305.

100. Samuel F, Berkovic JC, Eva Andermann FA. Progressive myoclonus epilepsies: Clinical and genetic aspects. *Epilepsia.* 1993;34(Suppl S3):S19–S30.

101. Roger J, PJ, Bureau M, Dravet C, et al. Early diagnosis of Lafora disease. Significance of paroxysmal visual manifestations and contribution of skin biopsy. *Rev Neurol (Paris).* 1983;139(2):115–124.

102. Ponsford S, IFP, Elliot EJ. Posterior paroxysmal discharge: an aid to early diagnosis in Lafora disease. *J Roy Soc Med.* 1993;86(10):597–599.

103. Sinha S, Satishchandra P, et al. Progressive myoclonic epilepsy: a clinical, electrophysiological and pathological study from South India. *J Neurol Sci.* 2007;252(1):16–23.

104. Koskiniemi M, Toivakka E, et al. Progressive myoclonus epilepsy. Electroencephalographical findings. *Acta Neurol Scand.* 1974;50(3):333–359.

105. Kalviainen R, Khyuppenen J, et al. Clinical picture of EPM1-Unverricht–Lundborg disease. *Epilepsia.* 2008;49(4):549–556.

106. Ferlazzo E, MA, Striano P, Vi-Hong N, et al. Long-term evolution of EEG in Unverricht–Lundborg disease. *Epilepsy Res.* 2007;73(3):219–227.

107. Shoffner JM, LM, Lezza AM, Seibel P, et al. Myoclonic epilepsy and ragged-red fiber disease (MERRF) is associated with a mitochondrial DNA tRNA(Lys) mutation. *Cell.* 1990;61(6):931–937.

108. So N, Berkovic S, et al. 1. Myoclonus epilepsy and ragged-red fibres (MERRF). 2. Electrophysiological studies nad comparison with other progressive myoclonus epilepsies. *Brain.* 1989;112(5):1261–1276.

109. Hirano M, Ricci E, et al. MELAS: an original case and clinical criteria for diagnosis. *Neuromusc Disord.* 1992;2(2):125–135.

110. Berkovic SF, AF, Karpati G, et al. The epileptic syndromes associated with mitochondrial disease. *Electroencephalogr Clin Neurophysiol.* 1988;69: 50P.

111. Fujimoto S, Mizuno K, et al. Serial electroencephalographic findings in patients with MELAS. *Pediatr Neurol.* 1999;20(1):43–48.

112. Nagafuchi S, Yanagisawa H, et al. Dentatorubral and pallidoluysian atrophy expansion of an unstable CAG trinucleotide on chromosome 12p. *Nat Genet.* 1994;6(1):14–18.

113. Saitoh S, Momoi MY, et al. Clinical and electroencephalographic findings in juvenile type DRPLA. *Pediatr Neurol.* 1998;18(3):265–268.

5

Genetic Counseling in Metabolic Epilepsies

Jodie M. Vento

It has long been known that genetics plays a role in a large proportion of neurological disorders. Recent advancements in molecular genetics have expanded our understanding of the etiology of many neurological diseases and neurodevelopmental abnormalities. Having a comprehensive understanding of genetics is essential in treating patients with metabolic epilepsies. Many neurology and neurology subspecialty programs have recognized the need for genetic counseling services and decided to employ genetic counselors within their department. Other programs may refer patients out to a genetics clinic for genetic counseling. Providers of genetic counseling services are not limited to genetic counselors, but rather include clinical geneticists, genetic nurses or nurse practitioners, and laboratory geneticists. The unique role of a genetic counselor is important to understand, as genetic counselors play an integral part of the multidisciplinary team that treats and evaluates patients with metabolic epilepsies.

Genetic counselors have specialized graduate degrees and clinical experience in the areas of pediatric, adult, prenatal, and cancer genetics and counseling. Many genetic counselors have a background in a variety of different disciplines, including biology, genetics, clinical research, nursing, psychology, public health, and/or social work. Genetic counselors provide a unique and vital service to patients and families.

Genetic counseling has been defined a process of helping people understand and adapt to the medical, psychological and familial implications of genetic contributions to disease. Some of the components of a genetic counseling interaction include: interpretation of family and medical histories to assess the chance of disease occurrence or recurrence, education about inheritance, testing, management, prevention, resources and research, and counseling to promote informed choices and adaptation to the risk or condition (1). In the pediatric neurology setting, some of the key components of the genetic counseling interaction are summarized in Table 5.1.

TABLE 5.1 Components of the Genetic Counseling Interaction

- Eliciting a detailed medical, developmental, and family history
- Assessing and communicating personal, family, and future reproductive genetic risks
- Reviewing past metabolic and molecular testing to establish/verify diagnoses, determine phenotypic correlation, and guide future testing options
- Communicating potential testing results, risks, and benefits with families to establish informed consent
- Providing information about a condition, prognosis, family and reproductive implications once a diagnosis has been established
- Offering psychosocial counseling support for the powerful emotions that often accompany genetic diagnoses

PATTERNS OF INHERITANCE

FAMILY HISTORY

A detailed, three-generation pedigree is a fundamental tool in the evaluation of an individual with a suspected metabolic epilepsy syndrome. Family history can be utilized as a cost-effective means for genetic diagnosis by aiding in the identification of patterns of inheritance, establishing rapport with the patient and family, distinguishing genetic risk factors from other environmental risk factors, and determining medical surveillance for at-risk relatives (2). While the collection of a comprehensive family history is ideal, the potential time burden may make this impractical. The clinician must determine what level of detail to collect based upon the patient's specific symptoms and circumstances. For many patients with epilepsy, frequent neurology visits allow for the collection of an evolving and dynamic family history over time.

While most genetics clinics utilize the traditional pedigree method, many neurology clinics may choose to use a checklist format to collect and record family health history. Pedigrees are especially useful because they utilize standard symbols and terminology to represent a large amount of information within a single diagram. This diagram format organizes complex information and allows for visualization of traits clustering together and inheritance patterns. Standardized pedigree nomenclature and an example pedigree are demonstrated in Figure 5.1 (3). No matter what method is utilized, the method must be medically accurate, easily updatable, amenable to pattern recognition, and clear to other healthcare professionals. The clinician recording the information should focus on several key elements, shown in Table 5.2.

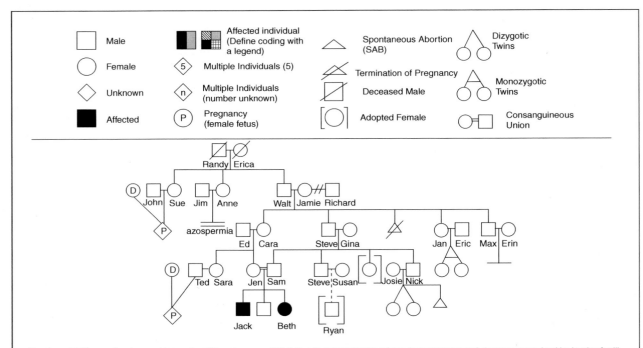

Randy and Erica are the deceased parents of Sue, Anne, and Walt. Sue is pregnant with a fetus (gender unknown) that was conceived by in *vitro* fertilization with John's sperm and a donor egg. Anne and Jim do not have any children secondary to infertility (Jim's a zospermia). Jamie was in a previous relationship with Richard, but now has children withWalt. Jamie and Walt have four children (Cara, Steve, Jan, and Max) and had one termination of pregnancy. Care and Ed have two children, Sara and Jen. Steve and Gina had four biological children, one of which has been given up for adoption. Jan and Eric have monozygotic twin girls. Max and Erin have no children by choice. Ted is Sara's partner and his sperm has been used to inseminate an unrelated woman, who is also carrying the fetus as a surrogate. Jen and Sam are first cousins, and thus in a consanguineous union. Jen and Sam have three children, two of which are affected with a genetic syndrome (which is presumably autosomal recessive). Steve and Susan have no biological children, but have adopted Ryan. Josie and Nick have dizygotic twin girls and had one spontaneous abortion.

FIGURE 5.1 Standardized pedigree symbols and example pedigree.

TABLE 5.2   Key Elements of a Genetic Family History

Family members:

- First-degree relatives (parents, children, siblings)
- Second-degree relatives (half-siblings, grandparents, aunts, uncles, grandchildren)
- Third-degree relatives (cousins)

Conditions:

- Seizures, fits, syncope, black-outs, staring spells
- Mental retardation/intellectual disability
- Learning disability, speech and language disorders
- Psychiatric conditions
- Deafness, blindness
- Neuromuscular issues
- Birth defects, congenital anomalies
- Pregnancy losses
- Sudden or unexpected death

History

- Age of onset
- Age and cause of death
- Ancestral origins
- Consanguinity
- Pregnancy outcomes

The pedigree serves as a useful tool to analyze inheritance patterns and genetic red flags. Some genetic red flags include: family history of multiple affected members with the same or related disorders, earlier age at onset of disease than expected, condition in the less-often-affected sex, disease in the absence of known risk factors, close biological relationship between parents (ie, consanguinity), and/or ethnic predisposition to certain genetic disorders (4).

Inheritance Patterns

While recognition of inheritance patterns can be useful in guiding diagnostic testing, it is also essential for accurate genetic counseling of other family members that may be at risk. To best understand various inheritance patterns, it is helpful to review some basic genetics. Humans should have 46 total chromosomes, 44 of which are autosomes, and the other two are sex chromosomes. All of our chromosomes come in pairs; one inherited from the mother and one from the father. As such, all of our genes (except for sex-linked genes) also come in pairs. The main inheritance patterns are described below and also in Figure 5.2.

Autosomal Dominant Inheritance

Autosomal dominant (AD) conditions are characterized by only requiring one mutant gene (allele) to manifest disease. The mutated gene copy "dominants" the normal gene product. In reviewing family history information, one will often note affected male and female members, multiple affected generations, and male-to-female transmission. For an individual affected by an AD condition, each offspring will either inherit the mutant allele or the normal allele. As such, someone with an AD condition has a 50% recurrence risk. If a child is diagnosed with AD metabolic epilepsy, it is important to analyze family history and offer parental testing to properly counsel about recurrence risk. Two of the sodium channel genes, *SCN1A* and *SCN1B*, are involved with varying AD epilepsy phenotypes. The spectrum of phenotypes associated with the sodium channelopathies include: simple febrile seizures, generalized/genetic epilepsy with febrile seizures plus (GEFS+), and severe myoclonic epilepsy of infancy (SMEI)/Dravet syndrome. Many children with the more severe phenotype of Dravet syndrome have an identifiable *de novo* (new) mutation in *SCN1A*. When a child is identified to have an AD condition and parental testing is negative, it is considered a *de novo* mutation. This differs from children that may present with the milder GEFS+ and an identifiable *SCN1B* mutation. *SCN1B* mutations are also AD, but typically not *de novo*. As such, family history can help to guide appropriate diagnostic testing and recurrence risk counseling.

Autosomal Recessive Inheritance

Autosomal recessive (AR) conditions are characterized by requiring two mutated alleles to manifest disease. Most of the time, carriers (those with only one mutated allele) do not manifest disease, or may only have milder symptoms. Family history will often be unremarkable, unless there is an affected sibling or

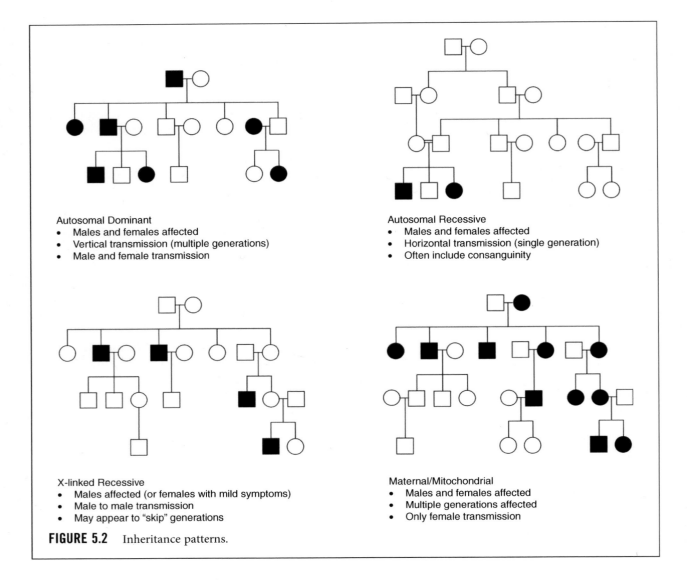

Autosomal Dominant
- Males and females affected
- Vertical transmission (multiple generations)
- Male and female transmission

Autosomal Recessive
- Males and females affected
- Horizontal transmission (single generation)
- Often include consanguinity

X-linked Recessive
- Males affected (or females with mild symptoms)
- Male to male transmission
- May appear to "skip" generations

Maternal/Mitochondrial
- Males and females affected
- Multiple generations affected
- Only female transmission

FIGURE 5.2 Inheritance patterns.

consanguinity present, and there is an equal risk for both male and female members. If a child is diagnosed with an AR condition, it is important to offer targeted testing to parents to confirm carrier status. Two carriers of an AR condition have a 25% chance of having an affected offspring, a 50% chance of having a carrier offspring, and a 25% chance of having an unaffected, noncarrier offspring with each pregnancy. Most metabolic conditions are AR, and seizures may often be complicating symptoms of these conditions. The neuronal ceroid lipofucinoses (NCL) often present with epilepsy, vision loss, and cognitive and motor decline. There are at least 10 different types of NCL, each having a

different causative genetic etiology. While there are varying ages of onset and at least 10 different genes that are responsible, all of the NCL's are inherited in an AR fashion.

X-Linked Recessive Inheritance

Female individuals have two X chromosomes, and male individuals have an X and a Y chromosome. X-linked recessive inheritance is caused by a mutated X chromosome. Female individuals only require one working copy of the X chromosome in each cell in their body, and randomly inactivate the other copy of the X chromosome. This is a protective mechanism in women, and one of the key characteristics of X-linked inheritance is a family history with only men affected (or male individuals affected more severely than female individuals), and no male-to-female transmission. These family histories will often present with disease that appear to "skip" generations. Some X-linked disorders are lethal in male members, and will cause symptoms in female members. These are often referred to as X-linked dominant disorders. One of the urea cycle disorders, ornithine transcarbamylase deficiency (OTC), is caused by alterations in the *OTC* gene located on the X-chromosome. In OTC deficiency, the urea cycle cannot normally process proteins, and nitrogen accumulates in the bloodstream in the form of ammonia. OTC deficiency is typically more severe in males who often rapidly develop hyperammonemic coma in the newborn period. Whereas only approximately 15% of carrier female individuals will develop symptoms ranging from behavioral and learning disabilities to protein intolerance, cyclical vomiting, and hyperammonemic crises during their lifetime (5).

Mitochondrial Inheritance

Mitochondrial diseases are a clinically diverse group of disorders that arise as a result of dysfunction of the mitochondria, which are responsible for making most of a cell's energy in the form of adenosine triphosphate (ATP). Some of the commonly observed symptoms associated with mitochondrial disease can be classified into discrete clinical syndromes. However, most often, the presentation and severity of these conditions may have wide variation, creating challenges in diagnosis and recurrence risk counseling. Mitochondrial disorders can be caused by alterations in nuclear DNA (nDNA) and/or mitochondrial DNA (mtDNA). The mtDNA and nDNA have a symbiotic relationship that is essential for normal functioning of the electron transport chain and mitochondria. As such, this group of disorders may be inherited in different manners. The nDNA alterations are most often AD or recessive. While not always possible, establishing a molecular genetic diagnosis is fundamental in proving accurate recurrence risk counseling. If mutations are identified in a nDNA gene known to be inherited in an AR manner such as, *SURF1* or *DGUOK*, there may not be other family members affected except for one or more siblings. The risk for

future offspring in this case is 25% or $\frac{1}{4}$. Some of the nDNA genes can be inherited in either an AR or dominant fashion (ie, *POLG1*). In this case, it is important to offer parental testing and research genotype/phenotype correlations to accurately discuss recurrence risks. Often, childhood onset mitochondrial diseases are caused by nDNA alterations, while those that present in later childhood or adulthood are more likely to be due to mtDNA abnormalities.

Mitochondrial diseases, caused by alterations in the mtDNA, are always maternally inherited since ova contain mitochondria, whereas any mitochondria in the sperm are either diluted or destroyed. Mitochondrial encephalomyopathy with lactic acidosis and stroke-like episodes (MELAS) most commonly presents with stroke-like episodes, encephalopathy with seizures or dementia, and myopathy during childhood. However, there can be much intra-familial phenotypic variability. Some individuals may only have hearing loss or diabetes mellitus. The difficulty in accurately predicting the clinical consequences and inheritance of mtDNA abnormalities is due to several complicating factors, including: heteroplasmy, the bottleneck effect, and threshold effect. Heteroplasmy describes a mixture of mitochondria within one single cell, with some containing mutant DNA and some containing normal DNA. As technology improves, there is increased ability to detect heteroplasmy levels. Predicating clinical consequences, however, can be challenging. While a mother with mtDNA alterations transmits mutant mtDNA to all of her offspring, the degree of heteroplasmy can vary form egg to egg because of the random bottleneck effect during oogenesis. The threshold effect describes the minimum amount of energy required by a cell, tissue, or organ to function properly. This threshold can vary over the course of development, during times of physiological stress (illness), and from tissue to tissue. Some tissues require more energy (ie, brain and muscle) than others (ie, skin) and therefore have a lower energy threshold and tolerance for mutant mitochondria.

While most mtDNA point mutations are maternally inherited, most mtDNA deletions are *de novo*, occurring either in the mother's oocyte or during embryogenesis. The three overlapping phenotypes associated with mtDNA deletions are Kearns–Sayre syndrome (KSS), Pearson syndrome, and progressive external ophthalmoplegia (PEO). Determining if an mtDNA deletion is maternally inherited or *de novo* is essential for proper genetic counseling.

Factors Affecting Genetic Disease Manifestation

Germline Mosaicism

Once a genetic alteration is identified in a child, it is often appropriate to offer parental testing. If the parents are tested and found to not be carriers of genetic alteration, then it is most typically believed to be a *de novo* alteration. While the risk to the future off-spring of these parents is likely very low, it is important to discuss the risk for germline mosaicism. Individuals with germline mosaicism will not typically suffer from any of the symptoms of the genetic disorder, but may have the mutation(s) present in some or all of their germline cells. This means that there is a theoretical possibility of having normal parental carrier testing, but passing the disorder on to their children. As such, it is important to offer genetic counseling and repro-ductive testing options. Depending on the condition, the risk for germline mosaicism may vary, but is typi-cally very low.

Penetrance

Penetrance describes the possibility that a given gene alteration will manifest itself in an individual in the form of disease and is most often associated with AD inheritance. Complete penetrance is when clinical symptoms are present in all individuals who have the disease-causing genetic alteration, and reduced or incomplete penetrance describes the condition when clinical symptoms are not always present in individuals who have the disease-causing genetic alteration. Incomplete penetrance often creates a pedigree that looks like a generation is "skipped." Sometimes, however, comprehensive molecular and clinical exam-ination reveals minimal signs of a particular syndrome, indicating variable expressivity of the disease symp-toms, rather than incomplete penetrance.

Variable Expressivity

Variable expressivity refers to the variation in severity of disease manifestation in different people with the same genetic condition. Both inter-familial and intra-familial variability has been demonstrated in a number of genetic syndromes. Variations between families can be due to different mutations at the same disease locus, while variation within families is most likely due to other modifier genes, environmental factors, or other stochastic events. For example, inter-familial variability can be noted in hexosaminidase A defi-ciency. The classic, severe form of hexosaminidase A deficiency is a result of homozygous, null (nonsense) mutations in the *HEXA* gene that lead to Tay-Sachs disease. Other mutations in *HEXA* in either the homozygous or compound heterozygous state can produce a milder, adult-onset version of hexosamin-idase A deficiency.

Skewed X-Inactivation

X-inactivation is the phenomenon in female individ-uals by which one X chromosome (either maternally or paternally derived) is randomly inactivated in each somatic cell as a method of dosage compensation. Typi-cally, this is a random pattern with about 50% paternal and 50% maternal X chromosomes inactivated. This becomes important when a carrier female individual of an X-linked recessive condition demonstrates skewed X-inactivation. In cases where this process leads to the skewed inactivation of more X chromo-somes containing the affected gene, there can be a milder phenotype. Transversely, if more of the unaf-fected X chromosome is inactivated, there can be more severe symptoms. This phenomenon explains the clinical variability in female individuals with X-linked diseases. Females with mutations in the X-linked *PDHA* gene associated with pyruvate dehy-drogenase deficiency can have quite a range in the severity of their symptoms, depending on their X-inactivation pattern.

Anticipation

Anticipation describes the tendency, in certain genetic disorders, for individuals in successive generations to present with more severe disease manifestations often at an earlier age of onset than expected. This process is often observed in genetic syndromes that are the result of a trinucleotide repeat mutation, such as myo-tonic dystrophy type 1 and fragile X syndrome. Antici-pation in fragile X syndrome may not happen every generation, as many families transmit premutation alleles for generations with little or no presentation of clinical symptoms until a trinucleotide repeat expan-sion leads to the full mutation, resulting in an affected individual.

GENETIC TESTING

DIAGNOSTIC TESTING

Diagnostic testing is used in the clinical setting to either confirm or rule out a known or suspected genetic syndrome in an individual presenting with consistent symptoms. If the testing comes back positive, then a genetic diagnosis is confirmed. If the testing comes back negative, it could be due to technical limitations of the testing or genetic heterogeneity. Sometimes, genetic variants of uncertain pathogenic significance are identified. Typically this is because the laboratories are not able to classify the variant as either a benign polymorphism or a pathogenic mutation due to limited data. Often, a comprehensive family history and parental genetic testing can help to better elucidate these variants of uncertain significance.

Predictive Testing

Asymptomatic individuals with a family history of a genetic disorder are often offered predictive testing. Predictive testing might reveal that an individual will eventually develop a known disease (eg, presymptomatic testing in an individual with a family history of Huntington disease) or that an individual has an increased risk to develop a disease over time (eg, *BRCA* mutations lead to an increased risk of breast and ovarian cancers). Generally speaking, the predictive testing of an asymptomatic child is discouraged unless medical interventions are available to help ameliorate the effects of disease. Predictive genetic testing can have long-term psychological ramifications; therefore informed consent, counseling, and follow-up are critical.

Carrier Testing

Carrier testing is available to individuals who have family members with a known AR or X-linked recessive genetic condition or individuals of certain ancestry or ethnic background that are known to have a higher carrier rate for a particular genetic conditions. Sometimes carrier testing is offered because of a known genetic diagnosis in an offspring or other family member. In these cases, targeted analysis for the identified genetic alteration is the most appropriate testing. When carrier testing is offered because of known population risks based on an individual's ethnicity or ancestry, targeted testing for one or several known, common disease-causing mutations reveals the large majority (but not all) carriers. Carrier status is important for genetic counseling and reproductive testing options.

Pre-Conceptional and Prenatal Testing

Prenatal diagnostic testing is available to women who are at an increased risk of having a fetus with a genetic condition due to advanced maternal age, family history, ethnicity, or other prenatal screening examinations. A molecular diagnosis in an affected individual needs to be identified before targeted prenatal or preconceptional testing can be offered. When a molecular diagnosis cannot be elucidated in an affected individual, consultation with a genetic counselor is appropriate to discuss risks and screening options (ie, detailed ultrasound, fetal MRI, etc). Preimplantation genetic diagnosis (PGD) is done in conjunction with in vitro fertilization to allow for genetic testing on the early embryo and selective implantation of the unaffected embryo(s). PGD is usually offered to couples with a high risk of having an offspring with a serious disorder. Due to possible errors in PGD, follow-up prenatal diagnostic testing is currently recommended to monitor the pregnancy.

Types of Genetics Testing

Clinical genetic testing typically involves analysis of DNA, chromosomes, or certain metabolites in order to detect alterations related to a known syndrome. This testing can be accomplished by many different technologies, which are outlined in Table 5.3. Genetic testing has some unique considerations that may not apply to other type of laboratory testing:

- Genetic testing is voluntary and patient or guardian informed consent should be obtained prior to testing.
- Medical management and personal decision making may change as a result of genetic testing.
- Genetic technology and knowledge is rapidly evolving; thus, results and testing should be reviewed and updated over time if applicable.
- Genetic testing can be expensive and insurance coverage varies.
- Psychosocial counseling, support, and appropriate follow-up planning should be made available to every patient before testing is initiated.

TABLE 5.3   Types of Genetics Testing

Genetic Testing Strategy	Description of Testing	Limitation(s)	Example
Full gene sequencing	Scans for mutations across the entire gene or genes of interest	• Some deep intronic and promoter mutations may not be identified • Some laboratories will only offer sequencing of select exons • Deletions may not be detected, unless large regions of homozygosity are noted	*SCN1A* sequencing to investigate a clinical suspicion of Severe Myoclonic Epilepsy of Infancy (SMEI)
Targeted mutation analysis or targeted mutation panel	Looks for specific mutation(s) in a gene or genes of interest	• Not all mutations will be detected	*OTC* targeted analysis for a known mutation in a family member of an affected individual
Multiplex ligand-dependent probe amplification (MLPA) or array-based intragenic deletion/duplication analysis	Looks for larger sections of DNA that may be deleted or duplicated; these deletions or duplications may not be detected through gene sequencing. Some array-based technologies may detect smaller intra-genic deletions or duplications.	• Will not identify mutations	MLPA analysis for the detection of deletions in the *MECP2* gene in someone with suspected Rett syndrome
Chromosome, oligo, and SNP array analysis	Examines selected areas of the genome to detect gains or losses of genetic material (ie, microdeletions, duplications and copy number variants)	• Balanced rearrangements such as translocations and inversions will not be identified • Point mutations, small intragenic deletions/duplications, and insertions will not be detected • Low level mosaicism will not be identified • Arrays are only as sensitive as the amount and coverage of their genetic probes; imbalances in regions not covered will not be detected • Copy number variants of uncertain significance will often require parental testing	Chromosome microarray to detect a microdeletion or microduplication associated with epilepsy (ex: 15q13.3 deletion syndrome)
Karyotype (chromosome analysis)	Detects aneuploidy, translocations, inversions, and large deletions or duplications. May identify mosaicism (if enough cells are counted)	• Point mutations, microdeletions, microduplications, and insertions will not be detected	Karyotype reveals an inversion of chromosome 2 associated with epilepsy

(continued)

TABLE 5.3 Types of Genetics Testing (*continued*)

Genetic Testing Strategy	Description of Testing	Limitation(s)	Example
FISH	Analysis of selected chromosome deletions based on a targeted probe	• Coverage is only as sensitive as the pre-designed probe, so small deletions could be missed	FISH probe of the 17p13.3 region detects a large deletion associated with Miller-Dieker syndrome
Methylation analysis	Detects alterations in imprinting	• Does not detect point mutations or other small genetic changes	Abnormal methylation studies of chromosome 15 consistent with Angelman syndrome
Whole exome or whole genome sequencing	Comprehensive analysis of the entire genome	• Data to explain all genetic variations is lacking	Whole exome sequencing as part of a research protocol for a child with an undiagnosed genetic condition

KEY POINTS

- Genetic counseling interactions include detailed histories including drafting of accurate pedigrees, assessment of disease and reproductive risks, and psychosocial support.
- SCN1A mutations are typically de novo in Dravet syndrome in contrast to inherited in GEFS + as well as SCN1B mutations.
- 15% of carrier females of X-linked OTC deficiency will be symptomatic with a wide phenotype including learning and behavior problems, protein intolerance, cyclic vomiting, or hyperammonemic crises.
- Mitochondrial disorders are maternally inherited when involving mitochondrial DNA, but ausotomal dominantly or recessively inherited when involving mutations of nuclear DNA, including either possibility with some nuclear genes, eg, POLG.
- Heteroplasmy, the bottleneck effect, and the threshold effect all contribute to the difficulty in predicting the clinical consequences and inheritance of mtDNA mutations.
- Germline mosaicism is a confounding factor for reproductive counseling when a parent has normal testing results.
- Reduced penetrance, variable expressivity, skewed X inactivation, anticipation, imprinting, and uniparental disomy are all non-Mendelian factors altering phenotype that must be explained by the genetic counselor to patients and families.
- The comprehensive family history and parental genetic testing are used to elucidate laboratory variants of uncertain significance.

REFERENCES

1. Resta R, Biesecker BB, Bennett RL, et al. A new definition of Genetic Counseling: National Society of Genetic Counselors' Task Force report. *J Genet Counsel.* 2006;15(2):77–83.
2. Bennett RL. *The Practical Guide to the Genetic Family History.* 2nd ed. Hoboken, NJ: Wiley-Blackwell; 2010.
3. Bennett RL, French KS, Resta RG, et al. Standardized pedigree nomenclature: update and assessment of the recommendations of the National Society of Genetic Counselors. *J Genet Counsel.* 2008;17(5):424–433.
4. National Coalition for Health Professional Education in Genetics (NCHPEG). Core Principles in Family History. 2008. Available at: http://www.nchpeg.org/ Accessed April 12, 2011.
5. Gyato K, Wray J, Huang ZJ, et al. Metabolic and neuropsychological phenotype in women heterozygous for ornithine transcarbamylase deficiency. *Ann Neurol.* 2004;55:80–86.

Ketogenic Diet in Metabolic Epilepsies

Eric H. Kossoff

INTRODUCTION

One of the earliest treatments on record for epilepsy, the ketogenic diet (KD) has experienced a resurgence of both clinical and research interest in the past few decades (1). This high-fat, low carbohydrate diet is considered "nonpharmacologic" rather than alternative, providing a typically adjunctive option for children and recently adults with difficult-to-control epilepsy. Recent years have seen neurologists taking the use of dietary therapies to new levels; investigations have revealed benefits of less restrictive forms of the KD, uses of this treatment for infants and adults, first-line use for severe, dramatic-onset epilepsies such as infantile spasms and myoclonic–astatic epilepsy, and even most intriguing, indications for conditions other than epilepsy.

What about using the KD for children with metabolic epilepsies? This concept stems back to some of the earliest modern studies of dietary treatment. Specifically, the use of the KD in glucose transporter-1 (GLUT-1) deficiency strongly placed this treatment in the realm of a definitive treatment addressing metabolic disturbances (2). Similarly, pyruvate dehydrogenase (PDH) deficiency is also considered an indication for the KD (3). Recent work has shifted the prevailing concept of mitochondrial disease from a relative contraindication to use of the KD to now an absolute indication. As basic science evidence has indicated that dietary treatment profoundly affects metabolism (in the case of epilepsy, perhaps for the better), researchers have even recently proposed changing the term "dietary treatment" to "metabolism-based therapy."

This chapter will discuss the basics of KD treatment, from its origins to recent research, covering its history, initiation, maintenance, adverse effect profile, and use for conditions other than epilepsy. In the second half of this review, the use of this nonpharmacologic treatment specifically for metabolic epilepsies will be addressed.

THE BASICS OF DIETARY TREATMENT

History of Ketogenic Diets

The KD is a high-fat, adequate protein, low carbohydrate diet that has been in continuous use since Dr. Wilder at the Mayo Clinic in 1921 realized that the centuries' old treatment of fasting could be mimicked indefinitely with a "ketogenic" diet (4). Over the next decade, the KD was a popular therapeutic option, especially in comparison to the currently available phenobarbital and bromides. Both children as well as adults were treated and had remarkable success (5, 6).

With the introduction of new anticonvulsants such as phenytoin, carbamazepine, and diazepam, the field of epilepsy shifted toward pharmacologic treatments and the KD was used sporadically and only as a last resort. This changed in 1993 when a 20-month-old boy from California named Charlie Abrahams was cured of his generalized epilepsy at Johns Hopkins Hospital by the KD after multiple failed medications and epilepsy surgery. His father, a movie producer, created the Charlie Foundation (www.charliefoundation.org) and a movie titled "First Do No Harm" with Meryl Streep in order to raise awareness, funds, and research into the KD.

The result has been dramatic. The KD is now available in nearly 100 countries worldwide (7). Not just one, but four different diets (KD, medium-chain triglyceride, modified Atkins diet, and low glycemic index treatment) are available for adults as well as children. In 1995, the first poster on the KD ever was presented at the annual meeting of the American Epilepsy Society. In 2008, an international symposium gathered over 300 attendees in Phoenix, Arizona for 5 days solely to discuss dietary treatments. This was repeated with greater success in Edinburgh, Scotland 2 years later. The world of the KD has changed.

Overall Outcomes for Seizure Control

In 2000, an article written for Blue Cross Blue Shield insurance company reviewed all studies to date and concluded the KD led to a "significant reduction in seizure frequency" and that "it is unlikely that this degree of benefit can result from a placebo response and/or spontaneous remission" (8). In this meta-analysis, they found that children treated had a 16% likelihood of seizure freedom and overall, 56% improved by more than 50%. Most studies of anticonvulsants in children with intractable seizures will report approximately 30% responder rates, of which 5% become seizure-free in comparison.

Despite this strong evidence for efficacy, until recently one of the largest criticisms of the KD was the lack of randomized and controlled studies. A Cochrane Library meta-analysis in 2003 concluded "there is no reliable evidence from randomized controlled trials to support the use of KDs for people with epilepsy" (9). This became no longer valid in 2008, after publication of a study examining the MCT (medium-chain triglyceride) and LCT (long-chain triglyceride) diets, with a 4-wk waiting period for each arm serving as its own control, was completed at Great Ormond Street Hospital in London (10). Each arm was also then randomized with an additional 12-wk control period of anticonvulsants continued at current doses. These investigators found that the seizure frequency after 4 months was significantly lower in the 54 children on the KD (38% decrease in seizures), compared to the 49 controls (37% *increase* in seizures) ($P < .0001$). No child in the control group had a greater than 90% reduction in seizures, compared to 5 with the KD ($P = .06$). There was also no difference seen in efficacy between the classical and medium chain triglyceride diets.

A randomized, double blind, placebo-controlled trial of 20 patients (60 g daily glucose vs saccharin solution given sequentially as a crossover during an initial fasting period) was completed at the Johns Hopkins Hospital that same year (11). The blind was successful with parents and investigators being unaware of which solution the child was given or their level of ketosis. There was a strong yet not significant trend identified in favor of the saccharin (treatment) group over the glucose (placebo) group, $P = .07$. In addition, there was overall a mean decrease of 34 seizures per day over the 12-d study period ($P = .003$).

The most common usage of the diet in regards to seizure types is for children with symptomatic generalized epilepsies such as Lennox–Gastaut syndrome. Myoclonic–astatic epilepsy (Doose syndrome), Dravet syndrome, tuberous sclerosis complex, Rett syndrome, and mitochondrial disorders also appear to do very well with dietary treatment (12). The two most widely reported conditions for which the KD is indicated include GLUT-1 deficiency and PDH deficiency, which will be discussed later in this chapter.

The KD also appears to be very helpful for intractable infantile spasms (13). In a recent study of 104 infants, 64% had at least a greater than 50% decrease in their spasms within 6 months of treatment, of which 38 (37%) became spasm-free for at least 6 months (13). As a result of this growing evidence for intractable infantile spasms, our center has used the KD in children for new-onset infantile spasms (if the family brings the child in within 2 wk). Approximately half of children treated in this manner have had their spasms resolve within days (14).

Children receiving KD formulas only (eg, infants or those with gastrostomy tubes) may be ideal for KD use in regards to both efficacy and compliance. Several KD formulas exist including Microlipid™, Ross Carbohydrate-Free™, and Polycose™, or as a pre-packaged 4:1 or 3:1 powdered or liquid form (Nutricia KetoCal™ or Solace Nutrition KetoVolve™). In a study from our center of 61 children formula-fed (30 had gastrostomy tubes), 59% had a greater than 90%

seizure reduction at 12 months, which is nearly double that of the overall population treated with the diet (15).

Initiation and Maintenance

The KD has changed little over the past century in terms of its core composition. Calories may be slightly restricted to 90% of the estimated daily requirements, and fluids are also slightly reduced (12). The evidence for both fluid and calorie restriction is scant, however, and most centers no longer strictly do this. The diet "prescription" includes a ratio of fat-to-carbohydrate and protein grams combined, with 4:1 the most common starting ratio, with 3:1 or 2.5:1 used for infants, adolescents, and patients in whom higher protein contents are desired (12). Children are all universally given a multivitamin, mineral, and calcium supplement. Foods given often include butter, heavy whipping cream, oils, mayonnaise, various meats, and green vegetables. A new development in the past decade is the availability of KD formulas which can be given to infants or children with gastrostomy tubes easily, including a 4:1 or 3:1 premixed powder or liquid (15).

In the past decade, many investigators have attempted to change the methods of providing and starting the KD in order to improve tolerability. Although the KD is traditionally implemented in the hospital by a trained dietitian with calories advanced slowly after a 24 to 48 hr fasting period, recent evidence from a randomized trial suggests that both the fast and perhaps the admission may not be universally required, although the seizure control may occur quicker when children are fasted (16, 17). Once started, a dietitian often adjusts the diet at follow-up clinics every few months in order to optimize growth, nutrition, and efficacy (12). An international group of physicians and dietitians, experts in the KD, have published a consensus statement regarding ideal implementation and management (12).

"Alternative" Diets

In 1976, a new dietary treatment was devised by using large quantities of a very ketogenic product, medium-chain triglyceride (MCT) oil, in the foods (18). The "MCT diet" had similar efficacy but allowed more carbohydrates and therefore improved tolerability. Rather than calculations with ketogenic ratios, the MCT diet calculates a set percentage of MCT oil; increasing as tolerated. Side effects do include bloating and diarrhea, but can be ameliorated by using lower MCT percentages. This diet is used primarily in the United Kingdom and Canada today.

The past decade has seen the emergence of two new diets designed to be started as an outpatient, without a fasting period, and without calorie or fluid calculations. The "modified Atkins diet" (MAD) was introduced in 2003 at our institution, following observations by parents that after years on the traditional KD the restrictiveness could be reduced without loss of efficacy (19). The MAD does not limit protein, calories, or fluid; instead, it solely limits carbohydrates to 10 g/d (20 g/d for adults) and encourages high-fat food ad lib. Studies worldwide in over 200 children and adults have shown similar efficacy to the KD. The MAD may be particularly helpful for children in developing countries, adolescents, and adults (20, 21).

The low glycemic index treatment (LGIT) limits carbohydrates to 40–60 g/d, but specifies the use of only low glycemic carbohydrates (glycemic index less than 50) such as berries and whole grains (22). Fat is not encouraged to the extent of the MAD. This diet theoretically works by preventing the wide (but normal) fluctuations in serum glucose on a standard diet, which may be beneficial for epilepsy as well as diabetes. Although fewer studies exist for this treatment, preliminary data is encouraging.

Both the MAD and LGIT may be of particular benefit for metabolic epilepsies in terms of their ability to maintain stable serum glucose, induce ketosis and a metabolic shift, yet perhaps be less extreme and potentially stress inducing for a child with such a condition. In addition, should dietary treatment for metabolic epilepsies be a lifelong proposition, these diets may be more appealing due to their inherent flexibility and improved tolerability. The group in Japan has started to investigate the MAD for GLUT-1 deficiency in this manner (23).

Side Effects

Side effects with the KD are often transient and do not usually require the diet to be stopped. The most common include constipation, acidosis (increased with illness), gastrointestinal upset (typically during the initiation of the diet predominantly), and lack of significant weight gain (occasionally weight loss)

(12). Children who do not receive adequate vitamin and calcium supplementation can have nutritional deficiencies, especially Vitamin D, selenium, and B complex vitamins. Hypoglycemia and acidosis are more common when the KD is started with a fasting approach, and as stated previously, fasting is not required for long-term seizure control (16). For this reason, our center tends to avoid fasting children with metabolic epilepsies due to potential risk for creating a metabolic crisis or stress situation unnecessarily.

Other, late-onset side effects are also possible and need to be closely monitored. Total cholesterol and LDL cholesterol will often rise by 30% on the diet, but then stabilize after 6 months and, after several years on the KD, typically normalize (24). Kidney stones occur in 6% of children placed on the diet, but appear to be nearly completely prevented by treatment with oral alkalinizing agents such as Polycitra K™ especially if given to all children starting the KD automatically (25). Decreased linear growth may occur, especially in young infants, and may be related to the level of ketosis rather than protein content of the KD (26). Less common side effects such as selenium deficiency, cardiomyopathy, pancreatitis, increased infections, bone density decrease, and basal ganglia changes have also been reported. Long-term side effects for children continuously on the KD for over 6 years include predominantly kidney stones, bone fractures, and decreased linear growth (27).

Nonepilepsy Investigational Uses

Today many anticonvulsants are used for conditions other than epilepsy, especially pain and psychiatric disorders. As some basic science evidence has suggested that the KD may be neuroprotective, and parents and patients also perceive it as different and more "natural" than medications, the use of dietary therapy for some neurologic disorders that can be progressive has recently attracted attention (28). There is predominantly experimental literature suggesting that the KD may be an effective treatment for several neurologic conditions. Clinical trials in humans are ongoing and completed for Alzheimer's disease, autism, amyotrophic lateral sclerosis, brain tumors, and migraine, with mixed results (29–33). The diet has also been reported as helpful in two metabolic conditions not associated with epilepsy, phosphofructokinase

deficiency and glycogenosis type V (McArdle disease) (34, 35).

It is unknown and probably unlikely that the mechanisms of action that have been theorized for the effects of the KD versus epilepsy are identical to what may be helpful for these disorders. With expanding use of dietary treatments for these nontraditional uses comes responsibility of neurologists and dietitians to ensure that studies are scientific and do not overstate the results. Considering these treatments have been used for metabolic syndrome and diabetes, they may be increasingly used for other metabolic conditions beside the metabolic epilepsies discussed below.

METABOLIC EPILEPSIES AND THE DIET

GLUT-1 Deficiency Syndrome

GLUT-1 deficiency syndrome was first reported in 1991 by DeVivo and colleagues (2). In this epileptic encephalopathy, there is impaired transport of glucose across the blood–brain barrier, as often diagnosed with low CSF glucose levels (or with mutations in the SLC2A1 gene). According to a recent review, approximately 200 children have been reported to date in the medical literature (36). Children can present with early-onset severe epilepsy, but often the clinical spectrum is more complex including exercise-induced dystonia, global developmental delay (especially speech), chorea, absence epilepsy, and hemiplegia (36).

The KD is the traditional treatment of choice for GLUT-1 deficiency, allowing ketones to serve as the energy source to the brain rather than glucose. Improvements have been reported not only in seizure control but also motor and cognitive function. As children with GLUT-1 deficiency have symptom exacerbation during fasting periods, a fast to institute the KD should probably be avoided in these patients. The ideal ketogenic ratio and duration of treatment is unclear at this time. Although most children are treated with high ketogenic ratios such as 4:1, others have used the MAD with benefit (23) as well. For those children diagnosed at an early age, switching to the MAD may be beneficial for long-term tolerability and compliance. Some experts on GLUT-1 have suggested that perhaps after adolescence the critical period for brain development may have passed and the continued use of dietary treatment is no longer necessary (36).

Pyruvate Dehydrogenase Deficiency

Pyruvate dehydrogenase (PDH) deficiency involves a defect in the link between the pathways of glycolysis and the citric acid cycle by converting pyruvate into acetyl CoA (37) (Figure 6.1). In this mitochondrial deficiency the cause in approximately 25% is through an X-linked genetic mutation in the alpha unit of E1 in the PDH complex (Xp22.2–p22.1). The remainder of cases are autosomal recessive in inheritance. In this rare condition, there can be symptoms including developmental delay, lactic acidosis, seizures, and spasticity (37). Symptoms often start at a young age and the disease is then typically fatal, whereas older children may survive.

Treatments for this condition have been historically limited and thiamine, carnitine, and lipoic acid have been recommended. In 1976, Falk et al. reported the use of the KD for an 11-month-old boy with PDH deficiency (38). Other studies have followed, including the most typically cited study by Wexler and colleagues of seven boys with pyruvate dehydrogenase deficiency in 1997, with those who were treated earlier or with fewer carbohydrates having improved longevity and cognition (3).

At this time, however, there are many unanswered questions about the long-term benefit of the KD for PDH deficiency (37). One recent review has commented that the high fatty acids might (albeit theoretically) decrease any residual enzyme activity, worsen renal hyperfiltration common to these patients due to excessive protein, and increase risk of bone mineral demineralization (37). To date, no prospective study of the KD for PDH deficiency has yet been performed to our knowledge.

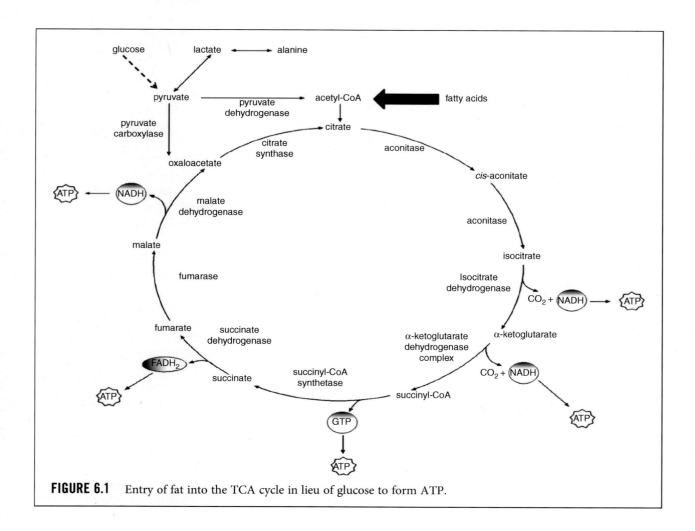

FIGURE 6.1 Entry of fat into the TCA cycle in lieu of glucose to form ATP.

Other Mitochondrial Disease

Other than PDH deficiency, the use of dietary treatments has only been recently promoted as an effective therapy for mitochondrial diseases causing epilepsy. Basic science evidence of improved mitochondrial biogenesis had suggested that this may be the case (39). It was initially believed that mitochondrial disorders would be exacerbated by the KD; however, a study by Kang and colleagues from Korea in 2007 changed this perception (40). In this study of 14 children [9 with Complex I, 1 Complex II, 3 Complex IV (including two with Leigh disease), and 1 with combined Complex I and IV defects], half became seizure-free with the diet (40). Seizure types were varied and included infantile spasms, Lennox Gastaut syndrome, and Landau–Kleffner syndrome. Interestingly, the two children with Leigh disease did not respond to the diet. Following this work, the group from Korea expanded their series 1 year later to 48 children, with improvement reported in 75% overall (41). Other research has described the beneficial effects of the KD for mitochondrial disease with features of Ohtahara syndrome (42), Landau–Kleffner syndrome (40), as well as Alpers–Huttenlocher disease (43, 44). Although not epilepsy, the KD has also been described for mice with mitochondrial myopathy with decreased numbers of cytochrome c oxidase negative muscle fibers and a return to wild-type levels (45).

Similar to PDH deficiency and GLUT-1 deficiency, questions remain about the long-term duration and safety of dietary treatment for these conditions. Due to concerns of mitochondrial stress, these children are typically not fasted to minimize oxidative stress (40). Would there be benefit from supplements such as carnitine that are often used for children with mitochondrial disorders? Would there be changes in neuroimaging and muscle biopsy results in those successfully treated over time?

Metabolic Contraindications

A child with an inability to shift metabolism from carbohydrate burning to fat would be impaired significantly by dietary treatments. As such, there are several contraindications to the use of KDs, typically metabolic conditions (12). Some of these can be associated with epilepsy as well.

A disorder of fatty acid oxidation is an absolute contraindication; these include primary carnitine deficiency, carnitine palmitoyltransferases I or II deficiency, and carnitine translocase deficiency. Additionally, short-, long-, or medium-chain acyl dehydrogenase deficiency or 3-hydroxyacyl-CoA deficiency should preclude the use of high-fat diets. In addition, pyruvate carboxylase deficiency (an enzyme within mitochondria that converts pyruvate to oxaloacetate) and porphyria are contraindications. The primary concern with pyruvate carboxylase deficiency is that of increased risk of acidosis with KDs as the buildup of acetyl-CoA in these patients (due to pyruvate being shunted towards the PDH complex) will already induce high levels of ketosis, which would be worsened by the KD (46).

DIRECTIONS FOR FUTURE RESEARCH

Currently, there are several avenues of research for neurologists and dietitians involved in dietary treatments. Despite the 2009 consensus statement, there is still some disagreement regarding the benefits of fasting at diet initiation and many centers have anecdotal experience in starting the KD as an outpatient (12). The MAD and LGIT have a fair amount of prospective, often single center, experience, yet the long-term effects of these diets and true effectiveness in comparison to the traditional KD remain unclear. As evidence grows regarding ideal epilepsy indications for dietary treatment, future research should focus on using the KD as a first-line treatment when these epilepsies are identified early and parents agree to forego (at least initially) anticonvulsants. Continued active research is currently ongoing to advance "nontraditional" uses including adults, developing countries, and nonepilepsy indications. Last, the long-term outcomes of the KD have started to be studied, but more formal, prospective examination of patients after a return to standard nutrition would address lingering concerns about long-term adverse effects.

For metabolic epilepsies, future research related to the KD is also warranted. Can the anecdotal improvement in cognition seen with dietary treatments and GLUT-1 deficiency be demonstrated objectively? Does it require long-term dietary treatment as theorized or can the alternative diets with lower ketosis be substituted over time? Can the trajectory of epilepsy and development be altered by using dietary treatments, perhaps forever and even after diets are discontinued at a later age? What is the full spectrum of mitochondrial diseases that are amenable to dietary treatment? Similarly, would early administration of this treatment be advantageous?

KEY POINTS

Dietary therapies are a useful treatment option for both children and adults with intractable epilepsy. While diets can improve seizure control in many patients with epilepsy, certain particular epilepsy syndromes may respond better to the diets than others. While often seen as a more "natural" treatment, side effects from the diets do occur and the complexity of the diets makes them difficult for some families. The recent emergence of "alternative" KDs such as the Modified Atkins and low-glycemic index diets have also led to additional options for patients, especially adolescents and adults. Dietary therapies are also valuable for certain metabolic epilepsies, specifically GLUT-1 deficiency, pyruvate dehydrogenase deficiency, and mitochondrial disorders. For these conditions, the KD may address biochemical defects, improve not only seizures but cognitive outcomes, and provide the long-term "fuel" necessary.

CLINICAL PEARLS

- Today there are four KDs available: the traditional KD, modified Atkins diet, low glycemic index treatment, and MCT diet.
- Fasting, admissions, and calorie and fluid restriction are no longer mandatory at the onset of dietary treatment.
- Several clear epilepsy indications exist including infantile spasms, Doose syndrome, tuberous sclerosis complex, and Dravet syndrome.
- Children with GLUT-1 deficiency should be treated with dietary treatment at a young age, although the ideal duration of treatment is unknown.
- Mitochondrial diseases (eg, pyruvate dehydrogenase deficiency, complex I and II deficiency) may do very well with the diet, although a fasting period is not advised.
- Those with Leigh disease (Complex IV) in limited publications do not respond as well.
- Several metabolic contraindications for dietary treatment exist, including pyruvate carboxylase deficiency and primary carnitine deficiency, and should be carefully screened for.

REFERENCES

1. Kossoff EH, Zupec-Kania BA, Rho JM. Ketogenic diets: An update for child neurologists. *J Child Neurol.* 2009;24(8): 979–988.
2. De Vivo DC, Trifiletti RR, Jacobson RI, et al. Defective glucose transport across the blood-brain barrier as a cause of persistent hypoglycorrhachia, seizures, and developmental delay. *N Engl J Med.* 1991;325(10):703–709.
3. Wexler ID, Hemalatha SG, McConnell J, et al. Outcome of pyruvate dehydrogenase deficiency treated with ketogenic diets. Studies in patients with identical mutations. *Neurology.* 1997;49(6):1655–1661.
4. Wilder RM. The effect of ketonemia on the course of epilepsy. *Mayo Clin Bull.* 1921;2:307–308.
5. Peterman MG. The ketogenic diet in the treatment of epilepsy: a preliminary report. *Am J Dis Child.* 1924;28:28–33.
6. Barborka CJ. Epilepsy in adults: results of treatment by ketogenic diet in one hundred cases. *Arch Neurol.* 1930;6:904–914.
7. Kossoff EH, McGrogan JR. Worldwide use of the ketogenic diet. *Epilepsia.* 2005;46(2):280–289.
8. Lefevre F, Aronson N. Ketogenic diet for the treatment of refractory epilepsy in children: a systematic review of efficacy. *Pediatrics.* 2000;105(4):e46.
9. Levy R, Cooper P. Ketogenic diet for epilepsy. *Cochrane Database Syst Rev.* 2003;3:CD001903.
10. Neal EG, Chaffe HM, Schwartz RH, et al. The ketogenic diet in the treatment of epilepsy in children: a randomised, controlled trial. *Lancet Neurol.* 2008;7(6):500–506.
11. Freeman JM, Vining EPG, Kossoff EH, et al. A blinded, crossover study of the ketogenic diet. *Epilepsia.* 2009;50(2): 322–325.
12. Kossoff EH, Zupec-Kania BA, Amark PE, et al. Optimal clinical management of children receiving the ketogenic diet: recommendations of the international ketogenic diet study group. *Epilepsia.* 2009;50(2):304–317.
13. Hong AM, Hamdy RF, Turner Z, et al. Infantile spasms treated with the ketogenic diet: prospective single-center experience in 104 consecutive infants. *Epilepsia.* 2010;51(8):1403–1407.
14. Kossoff EH, Hedderick EF, Turner Z, et al. A case–control evaluation of the ketogenic diet versus ACTH for new-onset infantile spasms. *Epilepsia.* 2008;49(9):1504–1509.
15. Kossoff EH, McGrogan JR, Freeman JM. Benefits of an all-liquid ketogenic diet. *Epilepsia,* 2004;45(9):1163.
16. Bergqvist AG, Schall JI, Gallagher PR, et al. Fasting versus gradual initiation of the ketogenic diet: a prospective, randomized clinical trial of efficacy. *Epilepsia.* 2005;46(11):1810–1819.
17. Kossoff EH, Laux LC, Blackford R, et al. When do seizures improve with the ketogenic diet? *Epilepsia.* 2008;49(2):329–333.
18. Huttenlocher PR. Ketonemia and seizures: metabolic and anticonvulsant effects of two ketogenic diets in childhood epilepsy. *Pediatr Res.* 1976;10(5):536–540.
19. Kossoff EH, Dorward JL. The modified Atkins diet. *Epilepsia.* 2008;49(Suppl 8):37–41.
20. Kossoff EH, Rowley H, Sinha SR, et al. A prospective study of the modified Atkins diet for intractable epilepsy in adults. *Epilepsia.* 2008;49(2):316–319.

21. Kossoff EH, Dorward JL, Molinero MR, et al. The modified Atkins diet: a potential treatment for developing countries. *Epilepsia.* 2008;49(9):1646–1647.

22. Pfeifer HH, Thiele EA. Low-glycemic-index treatment: a liberalized ketogenic diet for treatment of intractable epilepsy. *Neurology.* 2005;65(11):1810–1812.

23. Ito S, Oguni H, Ito Y, et al. Modified Atkins diet therapy for a case with glucose transporter type 1 deficiency syndrome. *Brain Dev.* 2008;30(3):226–228.

24. Nizamuddin J, Turner Z, Rubenstein JE, et al. Management and risk factors for dyslipidemia with the ketogenic diet. *J Child Neurol.* 2008;23(7):758–761.

25. McNally MA, Pyzik PL, Rubenstein JE, et al. Empiric use of oral potassium citrate reduces symptomatic kidney stone incidence with the ketogenic det. *Pediatrics.* 2009;124(2):e300–e304.

26. Vining EP, Pyzik P, McGrogan J, et al. Growth of children on the ketogenic diet. *Dev Med Child Neurol.* 2002;44(12):796–802.

27. Groesbeck DK, Bluml RM, Kossoff EH. Long-term use of the ketogenic diet. *Dev Med Child Neurol.* 2006;48(12):978–981.

28. Baranano KW, Hartman AL. The ketogenic diet: uses in epilepsy and other neurologic illnesses. *Curr Treat Options Neurol.* 2008;10(6):410–419.

29. Henderson ST. Ketone bodies as a therapeutic for Alzheimer's disease. *Neurotherapeutics.* 2008;5(3):470–480.

30. Evangeliou A, Vlachonikolis I, Mihaildou H, et al. Application of a ketogenic diet in children with autistic behavior: pilot study. *J Child Neurol.* 2003;18(2):113–118.

31. Zhao Z, Lange DJ, Voustianiouk A, et al. A ketogenic diet as a potential novel therapeutic intervention in amyotrophic lateral sclerosis. *BMC Neurosci.* 2006;7(4):29.

32. Zhou W, Mukherjee P, Kiebish MA, et al. The calorically restricted ketogenic diet, an effective alternative therapy for malignant brain cancer. *Nutr Metab (London).* 2007;4(2):5.

33. Kossoff EH, Huffman J, Turner Z, et al. Use of the modified Atkins diet for adolescents with chronic daily headache. *Cephalalgia.* 2010;30(8):1014–1016.

34. Swoboda KJ, Specht L, Jones HR, et al. Infantile phosphofructokinase deficiency with arthrogryposis: clinical benefit of a ketogenic diet. *J Pediatr.* 1997;131(6):932–934.

35. Busch V, Gempel K, Hack A, et al. Treatment of glycogenosis type V with ketogenic diet. *Ann Neurol.* 2005;58(2):341.

36. Klepper J. GLUT-1 deficiency syndrome in clinical practice. *Epilepsy Res.* 2011;100(3):272–277.

37. Weber TA, Antognetti MR, Stacpoole PW. Caveats when considering ketogenic diets for the treatment of pyruvate dehydrogenase complex deficiency. *J Pediatr.* 2001;138(3):390–395.

38. Falk RE, Cederbaum SD, Blass JP, et al. Ketogenic diet in the management of pyruvate dehydrogenase deficiency. *Pediatrics.* 1976;58(5):713–721.

39. Bough KJ, Wetherington J, Hassel B, et al. Mitochondrial biogenesis in the anticonvulsant mechanism of the ketogenic diet. *Ann Neurol.* 2006;60(2):223–235.

40. Kang HC, Lee YM, Kim HD, et al. Safe and effective use of the ketogenic diet in children with epilepsy and mitochondrial respiratory chain complex defects. *Epilepsia.* 2007;48(1):82–88.

41. Lee YM, Kang HC, Lee JS, et al. Mitochondrial respiratory chain defects: underlying etiology in various epileptic conditions. *Epilepsia.* 2008;49(4):685–690.

42. Seo JH, Lee YM, Lee JS, et al. A case of Ohtahara syndrome with mitochondrial respiratory chain complex I deficiency. *Brain Dev.* 2010;32(3):253–257.

43. Joshi CN, Greenberg CR, Mhanni AA, et al. Ketogenic diet in Alpers–Huttenlocher syndrome. *Pediatr Neurol.* 2009;40(4):314–316.

44. Cardenas JF, Amato RS. Compound heterozygous polymerase gamma gene mutation in a patient with Alpers disease. *Semin Pediatr Neurol.* 2010;17(1):62–64.

45. Ahola-Erkkilä S, Carroll CJ, Peltola-Mjösund K, et al. Ketogenic diet slows down mitochondrial myopathy progression in mice. *Hum Mol Genet.* 2010;19(10):1974–1984.

46. DeVivo DC, Haymond MW, Leckie MP, et al. The clinical and biochemical implications of pyruvate carboxylase deficiency. *J Clin Endocrinol Metab.* 1977;45(6):1281–1296.

PART II. SMALL MOLECULE DISEASES

7

Amino and Organic Acid Disorders and Epilepsy

Kimberly A. Chapman

INTRODUCTION

Disorders of small molecule metabolism can present with or be complicated by seizures, motor disturbances, and brain damage. Such disorders include the systemic organic acidemias, cerebral organic acidemias, and classical amino acidopathies. These disorders of small molecule metabolism are due to dysfunction of enzymes required for catabolism of various amino acids and fatty acids to produce energy. Dysfunction of these enzymes also results in accumulation of intermediates that may, in of themselves, be toxic to brain cells.

Organic acidemias, both systemic and cerebral, are disorders in which dysfunction of metabolic enzymes result in the accumulation of nonamino acid organic acids within a patient's urine (Table 7.1). Systemic organic acidemias have symptoms affecting more than just the brain, whereas cerebral organic acidemias have predominately findings of brain dysfunction and injury. Different disorders often have diagnostic, identifiable metabolites in urine (and plasma) such that recognition of the possibility and appropriate testing is important to diagnosis (1). Neurological symptoms include acute (cerebral edema, metabolic "strokes," encephalopathic crises) and chronic symptoms of deterioration due to accumulation of long-term brain injuries. Brain imaging, particularly MRI and now MR spectroscopy, can show resultant brain damage especially involving white matter. The basal ganglia

are especially sensitive to accumulation of organic acids or decreased energy production seen in organic acids.

Seizure activity in organic acidemias can be a result of the accumulation of toxic intermediates leading to brain edema, brain metabolic activation of neurotransmitter receptors, or due to resultant brain damage. EEGs in patients with organic acidemias can be normal, or may show slowing with focal or generalized paroxysmal activity and can be a marker of a worse prognosis (2).

Seizures seen in biochemical disorders of small molecule metabolism can be caused by direct intoxication of neurotransmitter receptors (preventing their recycling, with continuous activation, and thus increasing their post-excitatory activity), resultant energy pathway deficiency, and prevention of formation of GABA by blocking production of precursors. Moreover, secondary biochemical effects such as hyperammonemia, hypoglycemia, and metabolic acidosis from these disorders can also lead to seizures (especially due to brain damage or cerebral edema).

Moreover, most patients who have an organic acidemia who also have a seizure disorder often have worsening seizure activity with metabolic decompensation. Similarly, seizures in phenylketonuria (PKU) and maple syrup urine disease are caused by accumulation of a toxic amino acid (phenylalanine and leucine, respectively).

TABLE 7.1　Summary of Systemic Organic Acidemias, Cerebral Organic Acidemias, and Amino Acidopathies, Their Affected Enzyme, Encoding Genes, and Diagnostic Biochemical Metabolite

Metabolic Disorder	Dysfunctional Enzyme	Genes	Diagnostic Metabolites
Propionic acidemia (PA)	Propionyl CoA carboxylase (PCC)	PCCA PCCB	Propionylcarnitine (C3; P) Methylcitrate (U) 3-Hydroxypropionic acid (U)
Methylmalonic acidemia (MMA)	Methylmalonic mutase Cobalamin A Cobalamin B	MUT MMAA MMAB	Methylmalonic acid (P, U) Propionylcarnitine (C3; P) Methylcitrate (U) 3-Hydroxypropionic acid
Methylmalonic acidemia with homocysteinuria/ cobalamin C/D	Cobalamin C Cobalamin D	MMACHC MMACHD	Methylmalonic acid (P, U) Propionylcarnitine (C3; P) Methylcitrate (U) Total homocysteine (P) 3-Hydroxypropionic acid (U)
Isovaleric acidemia (IVA)	Isovaleryl dehydrogenase	IVD	Isovaleric acid (U) Isovalerylcarnitine (C5; P)
3-Methylcrotonylglycinuria (3MCC)	3-Methylcrontonyl CoA carboxylase	MCC1 MCC2	3-Hydroxyisovaleric acid (U) 3-Methylcrotonylglycine (U) Hydroxyisovalerylcarnitine (C5OH; P)
HMG-CoA lyase deficiency	3-Hydroxy-3-methylglutaryl CoA lyase	HMGCL	Hydroxyisovalerylcarnitine (C5OH; P) 3-HMG (U) 3-Methylglutaconic acid (U)
Malonic aciduria	Malonyl CoA decarboxylase	MLYCD	Malonate (U)
2-Methyl-3-hydroxybutyrl CoA dehydrogenase deficiency	2-Methyl-3-hydroxybutyryl CoA dehydrogenase	HSD17B10	2-Methyl-3-hydroxybutyrate (U) Tiglylglycine (U)
Ethylmalonic encephalopathy		ETHE1	C4 C5 Ethylmalonic acid (U) Methylsuccinic acid C4–C6 acylglycines (P)
Beta-ketothiolase deficiency	3-Methyl acetoacetate thiolase	ACAT1	C5:1 (P) 2-Methyl-3- hydroxybutyrate (U) Tiglylglycine (U) 2-Methyacetoacetate (U)
Biotinidase deficiency and holocarboxylase synthetase deficiency	Biotinidase Holocarboxylase synthetase	BTD HLCS	Propionylcarnitine (C3; P) Hydroxy-isovalerylcarnitine (C5OH, P) Biotinidase enzyme deficiency (P)

(continued)

TABLE 7.1 Summary of Systemic Organic Acidemias, Cerebral Organic Acidemias, and Amino Acidopathies, Their Affected Enzyme, Encoding Genes, and Diagnostic Biochemical Metabolite (*continued*)

Metabolic Disorder	Dysfunctional Enzyme	Genes	Diagnostic Metabolites
			Lactate (P, U)
			3-Methylcrotonylglycine (U)
			Methylcitrate (U)
			3-Hydroxypropionic acid (U)
2-Methyl butyryl CoA dehydrogenase or short/ branched-chain acyl CoA dehydrogenase deficiency	2-Methyl butyryl CoA dehydrogenase	ACADSB	2-Methylglycine (U)
			Isovalerylcarnitine (C5; P)
Glutaric acidemia I	Glutaryl CoA dehydrogenase	GCDH	Glutaric acid (U)
			3-Hydroxyglutaric acid (U)
			Glutarylcarnitine (C5-DC; P)
3-Methylglutaconic acidurias	3-Methylglutaconyl CoA hydratase (Type I)	AUH	3-Methylglutaconic acid (U)
	Barth (Type II)	TAZ	C5OH (P)
	Costeff (Type III)	OPA3	
	Type IV	TMEM70 or ATP12	
	Type V	DNAJC19	
Canavan disease	Aspartoacylase	ASPA	N-Acetylaspartic acid (U)
L-2-Hydroxyglutaric aciduria	L-2-Hydroxyglutarate dehydrogenase	L2HGDH	L-2-Hydroxyglutaric acid (U)
			Lysine (CSF)
D-2-Hydroxyglutaric aciduria	D-2-Hydroxyglutarate dehydrogenase	D2HGDH HOT	D-2-Hydroxyglutaric acid (U)
4-Hydroxybutyric aciduria	Succinate semialdehyde dehydrogenase	ALDH5A1	Gamma-hydroxybutyric acid (GABA) (U)
			Gamma-hydroxybutyric acid (GHB) (U)
Fumaric aciduria	Fumarate hydratase	FH	Fumarate (U)
		BCKDHA	Leucine (P)
Maple syrup urine disease (MSUD)	Branched-chain keto-dehydrogenase	BCKDHB	Alloisoleucine (P)
		DBT	Dicarboxylic acids (U)
Dihydrolipamide dehydrogenase	MSUD III	DLD	Leucine (P)
			Alloisoleucine (P)
			Dicarboxylic acids (U)
			Lactic acid (P, U)
Phenylketonuria (PKU)	Phenylalanine hydratase (PAH)	PAH	Phenylalanine (P)
			Low tyrosine (P)

CSF: cerebral spinal fluid; P: plasma; U: urine.

DISORDERS

CLASSICAL SYSTEMIC ORGANIC ACIDEMIAS

Classical systemic organic acidemias are characterized by nonamino acid organic acids in the urine, but also have system-wide metabolic acidosis and often other organ dysfunction. Typically, seizures in this group of disorders are related to brain damage from episodes of metabolic instability or accumulation of toxic intermediates leading to decreased cellular energy, secondary mitochondrial dysfunction, or cerebral edema during metabolic decompensation.

In organic acidopathies, the energy state of the brain is very precarious. In typical individuals, the brain uses about 20% of the oxygen and glucose available and only accounts for 2% of total body weight (3); major consumers in brain of energy include excitatory glutamatergic neurons and Na^+ dependent glutamate transporters (4). Secondary mitochondrial dysfunction due to toxin production in organic acidopathies interrupting normal brain energy availability is thought to cause the neurologic phenotype and could explain tissue-specific findings like metabolic strokes (1, 5–11). Some intermediates that accumulate in organic acidopathies may also be excitatory to neuron receptors and cause additional damage (12, 13).

There are a number of systemic organic acidopathies; this discussion of specific disorders is not all-inclusive. Those disorders chosen to be discussed are the "more" common, members of this category. Many of these are rare in the general population, but early diagnoses have significantly improved outcomes in patients.

Propionic Acidemia

Propionic acidemia (PA, MIM #606054) is an organic acidemia caused by mutations of both copies of either of the two genes that code for the enzyme propionyl CoA carboxylase (PCC; E.C. 6.4.1.3). PCC metabolizes the conversion of propionyl CoA to methylmalonyl CoA, a precursor of the tricarboxylic acid intermediate succinyl CoA. Urine organic acids are diagnostic with elevations of methylcitrate, propionylglycine, and 3-hydroxypropionic acid in the absence of elevated methylmalonic acid (Table 7.1). Moreover, propionylcarnitine (C3) can be identified to be elevated in the plasma.

Patients with PA often present with metabolic acidemia, lethargy, and vomiting (14). A subset of patients will present with neurological findings including seizures, metabolic stroke-like findings (especially basal ganglia) which can result in a movement disorder (Figure 7.1) (15). In addition, individuals with PA can have hyperammonemia which can also result in seizure activity if cerebral edema results. In the acute metabolically decompensated state, MRI may show white matter edema as well as basal ganglia changes, especially involving the lentiform nuclei and caudate (16, 17).

Individuals with PA do not often have abnormal EEGs at baseline in the absence of brain damage, hypoglycemia, or hyperammonemia during metabolic decompensation events (precipitated by fever, vomiting, or other metabolic stress) (15). However, about half of individuals with PA will develop seizures (2, 15, 18). In infancy and early childhood, generalized and myoclonic seizure are more common. As individuals age, these evolve to mild generalized or absence forms. In one series, 9/15 children had pathologic EEG epileptiform discharges. The epileptiform electrical activity sometimes preceded clinical seizures; however, all nine eventually developed seizures (18). During severe acute metabolic decompensations, EEG can show severe diffuse slowing (19). In a different study, about half of the patients with abnormal EEGs showed diffuse slowing with disorganized background or focal slow wave activity (2). There is a single report of presentation of PA with infantile spasms and hypsarrhythmia in a 6-month-old boy (20). Antiepileptic therapy is guided by seizure type as it would be for patients having similar seizures of other etiologies. In the presence of infantile spasms and hypsarrhythmia on EEG, vigabatrin lead to normalization (20).

Methylmalonic Acidemia

Any of a number of disorders can result in elevated methylmalonic acid in urine and systemic Methylmalonic acidemia (MMA) so the differential diagnosis of these disorders is based on the presence or absence of homocysteine, whether vitamin B_{12} (cobalamin) is deficient, and whether a patient responds to cobalamin. Genetic testing and enzyme activity levels can also be used to differentiate the multiple forms of MMA.

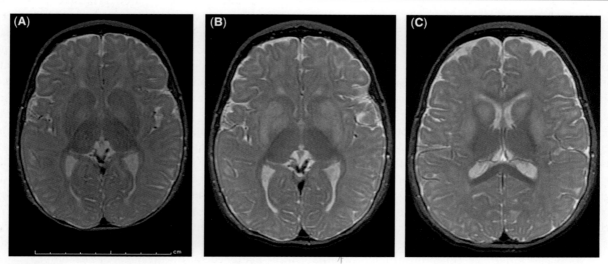

FIGURE 7.1 T2 axial images of a patient with propionic acidemia following a severe metabolic decompensation event. (A) MRI findings consistent with bilateral globus pallidus involvement. (B and C) MRI images of extension of the initial globus pallidus injury to include putamen and caudate nuclei. The child has had a subsequent movement disorder as a result of these insults.

These disorders include classical methylmalonic acidemia from dysfunction of methylmalonyl CoA mutase (MUT), but also the rarer forms from deficiency of the enzyme methylmalonyl CoA epimerase (MCEE), deficiency of the cobalamin A, cobalamin B, cobalamin C, or cobalamin D enzymes, or severe vitamin B_{12} deficiency (Table 7.1).

Classic MMA is caused by mutations in both copies of the *MUT* genes which code for the methylmalonyl CoA mutase enzyme (MUT, E.C. 5.4.99.2) and presents with lethargy, metabolic acidosis, and coma. Although much rarer than MUT deficiency, a similar presentation is seen with loss of MCEE activity. Patients will present with elevations of methylmalonic acid, 3-hydroxypropionic acid, and methylcitrate in their urine and propionylcarnitine (C3) in their plasma (Table 7.1).

Approximately 50% of patients have seizures at some point in their life (21). The type of seizures is variable and some are related to brain damage from metabolic decompensation. Patients can also have acidosis-related seizures and so prompt diagnosis and treatment of acidosis is important. EEGs can be normal, but if they show abnormalities this is thought to be a consequence of chronic brain dysfunction (2).

In one study, a third of abnormal EEGs showed multifocal spike discharges and decreased background organization, with other findings being background slowing and occasional loss of sleep spindles (2).

Since vitamin B_{12} is essential for MUT activity, mutations affecting the metabolism of vitamin B_{12} including those seen in cobalamin A deficiency (*MMAA*) and cobalamin B deficiency (*MMAB*) can result in elevated methylmalonic acid in urine and plasma. These disorders are often responsive to high doses of hydroxycobalamin.

Severe vitamin B_{12} deficiency can result in a transient elevation in methylmalonic acid in the urine which corrects with treatment. Often times, exclusively breast fed neonates whose mothers are vitamin B_{12} deficient will be identified on newborn screen (22). Their MMA levels disappear with supplementation.

Cobalamin C deficiency (*MMACHC*, MIM #277400) causes elevations of urine methylmalonic acid, often plasma elevations of total homocysteine, and results in the inability to produce methylcobalamin and *S*-adenosylcobalamin which are cofactors for MUT and the enzyme, methionine synthase (23) (Table 7.1). Infantile and early childhood disease produces feeding difficulties, neurological dysfunction (seizures, hypotonia, and developmental delay), occasional acidosis, and progressive central nervous system injury with cortical atrophy.

Cobalamin D deficiency (*MMADHC*) can present similarly to cobalamin C deficiency with increased total homocysteine in plasma and increased methylmalonic acid in urine or blood, or with only elevations in total homocysteine (Table 7.1). Some clinicians find patients with cobalamin C/D deficiency have more neurological findings than those with MUT deficiency (24). Approximately 50% patients with cobalamin C deficiency have seizures (23). If older, previously unrecognized patients with cobalamin C/D deficiency will present with extrapyramidal symptoms, dementia, delirium, and psychiatric disease (23).

In early onset cobalamin C/D deficiency, EEG can show focal and multifocal epileptiform abnormalities (24). The EEG shown in Figure 7.2, illustrates left temporal spike and wave seen in a patient with seizures. Seizure types include focal clonic, complex partial, and tonic clonic seizures. Individuals also present with status epilepticus (24). Theoretically seizures are attributed to continued elevation of homocysteine and its metabolites, which lead to a decreased epileptogenic threshold. Thus, accumulation of excitatory amino acids (glutamate and sulfur-containing amino acids such as homocysteine) propagate seizure activity in these patients (12, 13). Radiological abnormalities including white matter changes are attributed to decreased S-adenosylmethionine, an essential methyl donor in the brain (24–27).

In patients with all forms of MMA, MRI for any of the methylmalonate producing disorders can show white matter edema during metabolic decompensations

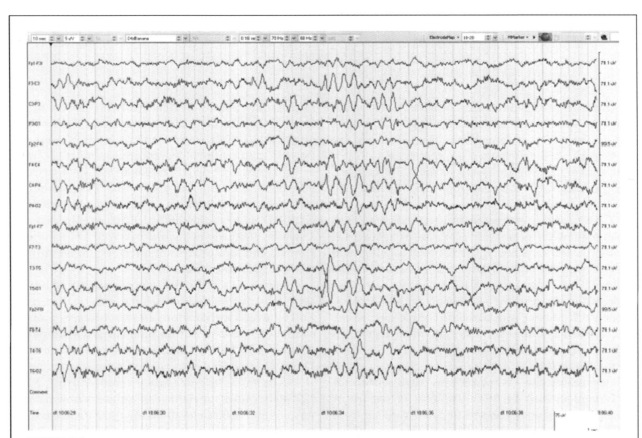

FIGURE 7.2   An EEG from a 5-year-old with cobalamin C deficiency who has left temporal spike and wave, decreased amplitude, and a background consistent with drowsiness. This patient is being treated with benzodiazapines which explains the beta wave activity.

and well as basal ganglia changes especially in the globus pallidi (16, 17). Even after biochemical recovery, permanent damage in the basal ganglia and demyelination can be seen (17).

Methylmalonyl CoA and methylmalonic acid are considered to have brain toxicity which could increase seizure potential. Methylmalonyl CoA inhibits pyruvate carboxylase which inhibits gluconeogenesis and results in hypoglycemia which in itself could lead to seizures in a systemic metabolic decompensation (28, 29). Moreover, MMA blocks transport of malate into the inner mitochondrial membrane which is a component of the tricarboxylic acid cycle (TCA) and needed to maintain TCA integrity (30). TCA is further compromised by methylmalonic acid due to its inhibition of the TCA enzyme succinyl CoA dehydrogenase as seen in rats (31). The neurological complications seen in MMA is hypothesized to be due to the compromised TCA resulting in inhibition of energy production and subsequently leading to brain damage and increased seizure risk.

Isovaleric Acidemia

Isovaleric acidemia (IVA, MIM #243500) is an organic acidopathy which is caused by dysfunction of isovaleryl CoA dehydrogenase, *IVD*) in the leucine metabolism pathway. Symptomatic patients can present with lethargy coma, odor of "sweaty feet," metabolic acidosis, and ketosis. They will have urinary elevations of isovalerylglycine and 3-hydroxyisovalerylic acid. Plasma elevations include isovalerylcarnitine (C5) which can bring a patient to care prior to symptoms due to a positive newborn screen (Table 7.1).

Some individuals identified by newborn screening may never develop metabolic acidemia; however, some individuals can have clinical disease. Newborn screening has identified a series of patients with increased plasma and urine markers of IVA who have an *IVD* genotype 932 C > T (A282V) as one or both of their mutations and have not had metabolic decompensations with metabolic acidosis (32, 33). Prior to newborn screening patients could present as infants with metabolic acidosis, vomiting, and lethargy or as older individuals with failure to thrive and developmental delay. Both these presentations had the "sweaty feet" odor without treatment (32). Treatment consists of supplemental glycine and carnitine. Some

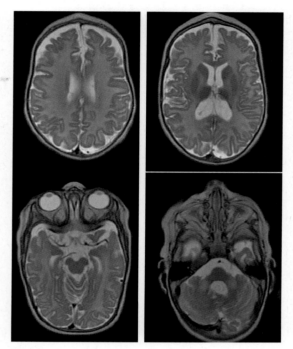

FIGURE 7.3 MRI (T2) images of a 13-month-old male with isovaleric acidemia who had been poorly controlled. Note the affected basal ganglia and white matter attenuation in the frontal regions. (Courtesy of Dr. Adeline Vanderver, Children's National Medical Center, Washington, D.C.)

will require modest dietary protein restriction to maintain biochemical stability.

In individuals with severe disease, a metabolic crisis can initiate seizure activity from resulting brain damage. MRI findings following a metabolic crisis can show white matter attenuation especially in the frontal region (see Figure 7.3). Although seizures can be seen especially in metabolic crises, for the most part, individuals with IVA have normal EEGs in the healthy state unless brain damage is present. Figure 7.4 illustrates a patient who had significant brain damage from his presenting metabolic acidosis event and has multifocal spike wave discharges as a result.

3-Methylcrotonylglycinuria

The disorder 3-methycrotonylglycinuria (3MCC, MIM #210200) can be a benign variant, but can also

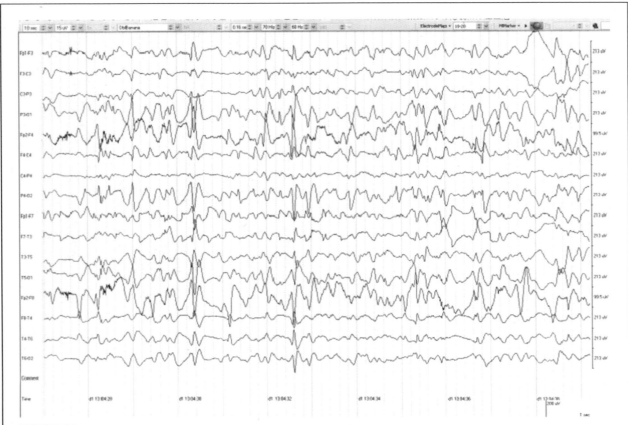

FIGURE 7.4 A 7-year-old with isovaleric acidemia who has high-amplitude multifocal spike and wave discharges in the right frontal (F4), left frontal (F7), and right frontotemporal (F8, T4) regions following brain damage from a metabolic decompensation.

lead to acidosis and seizures in selected patients. A deficiency of 3MCC (E.C. 6.4.1.4) which is an enzyme in the leucine catabolic pathway leads to increased urinary excretion of 3-hydroxyisovaleric acid, and 3-methylcrotonylglycine as well as elevated hydroxy-isovalerylcarnitine (C5OH) in the plasma (Table 7.1) (34).

With the advent of mass spectrometry-based newborn screening methods, there are a number of positive newborn screens for 3MCC in which patients have not demonstrated symptoms or the mother has had the disorder without symptoms. As a result, it is unclear who is at risk for neurological disease.

Patients can have seizures and occasionally metabolic strokes, with generalized spike and polyspike paroxysms as well as burst suppression on EEG (35). If symptomatic, patients can have generalized seizures, with EEG abnormalities especially in the neonatal period; other symptoms include decreased tone, feeding difficulty, and vomiting. In late infantile stage patients can present with a Reye-like syndrome, hepatomegaly, seizures, hyperammonemia, and hypoglycemia (36).

3-Hydroxy-3-Methylglutaric Acidemia

3-Hydroxy-3-methylglutaric acidemia (HMG CoA, MIM +246450) is due to dysfunction of 3-hydroxy-3-methylglutaryl CoA lyase (E.C. 4.1.3.4). HMG CoA results in accumulation of hydroxy-isovalerylcarnitine (C5OH) in plasma. In urine 3-hydroxy-3-methylglutaric acid, 3-methylglutaconic acid, 3-methylglutaric acid, and 3-hydroxyisovaleric acid are all elevated (Table 7.1) (37, 38).

The 3-hydroxy-3-methylglutaryl CoA lyase is the crossroads between leucine metabolism and ketogenesis. It cleaves 3-hydroxy-3-methylglutaryl CoA to acetyl CoA and acetoacetate and, if dysfunctional, clinically results in metabolic acidosis and hypoketotic hypoglycemia (39). Untreated disease results in hepatomegaly, lactic acidemia, possibly hyperammonemia, absent ketone production during metabolic acidosis, lethargy, vomiting, and coma and can progress to death. Patients often avoid high-protein foods due to feeling poorly with their consumption and this can be a hint to diagnosis.

In many cases, seizure activity in HMG CoA is related to hypoglycemia (or severe lactic acidemia) (40, 41). Some patients will develop a multifocal spike wave pattern on EEG (2).

HMG CoA is relatively more common in Saudi Arabia and is one of the most common inborn errors of metabolism seen in the Portuguese (including those in Brazil and even Japan) (41–43). The Saudi presentation especially correlates with MRI findings that show white matter lesions, dysmyelination, and mild atrophy, as well as seizures related to metabolic acidosis and hypoglycemia (41, 17).

Beta-Ketothiolase Deficiency (3-Oxothiolase Deficiency)

Beta-ketothiolase deficiency (3-oxothiolase deficiency) (MIM # 203750) is an organic acidemia which presents with metabolic acidosis, vomiting, neutropenia, thrombocytopenia, and lethargy, especially worsened by illness. Severity of symptoms can be variable (44, 45). In patients with prolonged acidosis, beta-ketothiolase deficiency can lead to developmental delay and seizures (46).

Beta-ketothiolase or 3-oxothiolase (E.C. 2.3.1.9) is required for isoleucine metabolism and its deficiency results in elevations in 2-methyl-3-hydroxybutyrate, tiglylglycine, and 2-methylacetoacetate in urine (Table 7.1) (44).

Diffuse slowing has been described on EEG in a single patient, but there are few other EEG reports available (2, 44). Patients can also develop elevated ammonias during illness and consequently have seizures related to brain edema. MRI may show increased T2 signal in the posterior lateral putamen bilaterally (17). Avoidance of fasting and mild protein restriction has allowed for improved morbidity and good developmental outcomes in patients diagnosed and treated prior to brain injury from metabolic decompensations (47).

Biotinidase or Multiple Carboxylase Deficiency

Biotinidase deficiency (MIM #253260) is caused by the inability to recycle biotin by the enzyme biotinidase (E.C. 3.5.1.12). Multiple carboxylase deficiency or holocarboxylase synthetase deficiency (MIM #253270, E.C. 6.3.4.10) is caused by the inability to load biotin onto the carboxylases. Either enzyme deficiency results in a series of nonfunctional biotin-dependent carboxylases. Untreated, these disorders present with hypotonia, ataxia, seizures, and metabolic acidosis. Elevations in urine 3-methylcrotonylglycine, 3-hydroxypropionic acid, and methylcitrate as well as elevated lactate reflect the deficient carboxylases (propionyl CoA carboxylase, 3-methylcrotonyl CoA carboxylase, and pyruvate carboxylase) (Table 7.1) (48).

Biotinidase deficiency presents between 3 and 6 months of age (when prenatal biotin stores are empty and recycling is necessary), whereas multiple carboxylase deficiency usually presents at birth due to absent functional carboxylases. Biotinidase deficiency can easily be treated with supplemental biotin and adequately treated patients do not have any symptoms and do not have any elevations in biochemical markers in their urine or plasma. Accurate and early diagnosis before symptoms with prompt treatment can prevent all neurologic symptoms in biotinidase deficiency. On the other hand, multiple carboxylase deficiency is infinitely more difficult to treat and patients have significantly increased morbidity and early death as a consequence of absence of functional carboxylases.

Seizures are predominately caused by toxic intermediates including hypoglycemia, metabolic acidosis, and hyperammonemia, leading to brain damage and cerebral edema in untreated biotinidase deficiency and in multiple carboxylase deficiency. Like many of the other systemic organic acidemias, EEGs show diffuse slowing due to these toxic intermediates (2). In untreated biotinidase deficiency and multiple carboxylase deficiency, MRI findings are consistent with the other disorders of carboxylase dysfunction such that patients have increase extracerebral space with brain atrophy, white matter changes, and basal ganglia strokes (17).

2-Methyl-3-Hydroxybutyryl CoA Dehydrogenase Deficiency

2-Methyl-3-hydroxybutyryl CoA dehydrogenase deficiency, also known as 17-beta-hydroxysteroid dehydrogenase X deficiency (HSD10, MIM #300438), leads to elevations of urinary 2-methyl-3-hydroxybutyrate and tiglylglycine without elevation of 2-methylacetoacetate (Table 7.1). It is caused by dysfunction of the enzyme 2-methyl-3-hydroxybutyryl CoA dehydrogenase (MHBD; E.C. 1.1.1.178/E.C. 1.1.1.35) which catabolizes the degradation of 2-methyl branched chain fatty acids and isoleucine in the mitochondria.

MHBD deficiency is an X-linked disorder (*HADH2* gene) and usually presents initially with delayed psychomotor development. Then there is a progressive loss of mental and motor skills. This is followed by development of choreathetoid movements, absence of directed hand movements, blindness, failure to thrive and marked hypotonia (47, 49). In addition, some patients have elevated lactate in CSF, MR spectroscopy, plasma, and urine, and so there initially is a concern for a mitochondrial disorder.

Seizures have been described in an 8-year-old with initially abnormal vision and started with myoclonic seizures at $3\frac{1}{2}$ years, associated with generalized sharp waves and background slowing on EEG (50). 17-Beta hydroxysteroid dehydrogenase also has a role in maintaining function of the gamma-amino-butyric acid (GABA)ergic neurons by deactivating neuro-steroids (47). Consequently neurologic symptoms including seizures in these patients have a trigger without requiring metabolic acidosis (47).

MRI findings are abnormal in some patients with parieto-occipital periventricular white matter changes reported similar to that seen in hypoxia-ischemia (47, 51).

Malonic Aciduria

Malonic aciduria (MIM #248360) is caused by dysfunction of malonyl CoA decarboxylase (EC 4.1.1.9) and results in developmental delay, epilepsy, recurrent vomiting, and cardiomyopathy responsive to carnitine (52). Because cardiomyopathy is a possibility, this chapter includes malonic aciduria with the systemic disorders; it can also be classified as a cerebral organic acidemia.

Individuals with malonic aciduria have diagnostic elevations of malonate in the urine and may have elevations of methylmalonic acid, ethylmalonate, succinate, adipate, suberate, and glutarate in the urine (Table 7.1). Since malonyl CoA decarboxylase is the first step in fatty acid biosynthesis (53), patients are at increased risk for hypoglycemia like those with fatty acid oxidation disorders (54).

Seizure activity is not seen in malonic aciduria unless the patient is hypoglycemic (53). However, one patient in the literature has been described with myoclonic seizures and spike/polyspike-and-wave activity on EEG and it is unclear whether he had underlying brain disease (2). On MRI, patients can have widened sulci and enlarged ventricles, as well as white matter cavitation in the posterior half of the putamen through the corona radiate and most of the centrum semiovale (17).

Ethylmalonic Acidemia

Ethylmalonic encephalopathy (MIM #602473) results in neurodevelopmental regression, pyramidal and extrapyramidal tract signs, seizures, petechiae, orthostatic acrocyanosis, chronic diarrhea, CNS malformations, and multiple lesions on MRI (55, 56). It is usually lethal in infancy or early childhood. However, there are reports of clinical heterogeneity (57). Ethylmalonic acidemia is attributed to ETHE1 gene and thought to be a mitochondrial sulfur dioxygenase (58–60). Patients have elevated ethylmalonic acid and methylsuccinic acid in their urine. They have elevated butyrylcarnitine (C4), isovalerylcarnitine (C5), and C4–C6 acylglycines in their plasma (Table 7.1).

Brain abnormalities with the most severe damage are in the deep sulci on autopsy (61). Seizures are thought to be due to these brain structural abnormalities. EEGs are often abnormal and can have multifocal slow waves and spikes, background disorganization, and may deteriorate over time (2).

2-Methylbutyryl CoA Dehydrogenase Deficiency

2-Methylbutyryl CoA dehydrogenase deficiency (MIM #610006), also known as short/branched-chain acyl CoA dehydrogenase deficiency, is an organic acidemia which can present with low glucose, intellectual disability, muscular atrophy, lethargy, apnea, and tachycardia. However, within Hmong individuals, infants have been identified by newborn screening who are asymptomatic, despite having biochemical findings and genetics consistent with 2-methylbutyryl CoA dehydrogenase deficiency (62). These children are being followed as they grow older.

2-Methylbutyryl CoA dehydrogenase (MBD) is encoded by *ACADSB* and metabolizes 2-methylbutyryl CoA to tiglyl CoA in the isoleucine pathway (63, 64). Patients have elevation in 2-methylbutyrylglycine in urine and elevations in isovalerylcarnitine (C5) in plasma, but this can be intermittent so often genetic confirmation is necessary (Table 7.1).

MRI and EEG are abnormal in symptomatic patients (47). EEG reports describe mild attenuation of background and intermittent sharp waves in central and temporal regions with illness in a patient (64).

CEREBRAL ORGANIC ACIDOPATHIES

Cerebral organic acidopathies are a category of enzyme deficiencies that produce nonamino organic acids which accumulate in a patient's urine, but have few systemic symptoms, and predominantly neurological symptoms. Obviously, categorizing several of these disorders as either systemic or cerebral organic acidopathies is complicated. In general, the pathophysiology of cerebral organic acidopathies is less due to hypoglycemia, cerebral edema, and energy deficiency pathways, but more in accord with specific toxicities functioning through neurotransmitters or activation of neuro-signaling receptors.

For cerebral organic acidopathies, astrocytes are extremely important to maintenance of brain biochemistry by several mechanisms: (1) establishment of glutamate/glutamine ratio using glutamate uptake, and synthesis of glutamate (65); (2) lactate transport to neurons; and (3) dicarboxylic acid shuttle from astrocytes to neurons to compensate for the drain of dicarboxylic acids from the tricarboxylic acid cycle (TCA) needed for glutamate synthesis (1). As a result, part of the pathology is in disruption of normal astrocyte function.

In addition, the blood–brain barrier complicates treatment and has impact on pathophysiology, especially of the cerebral organic acidopathies. It allows for sequestration of intermediates through transport mechanisms within brain tissue and prevents uptake of therapeutics. The blood–brain barrier not only brings material into the brain but also can trap intermediates such as glutaric acid or 3-hydroxyglutaric acid following

de novo synthesis which are known to damage brain cells and inappropriately activate receptors leading to their down regulation (66, 67).

Glutaric Acidemia I

Glutaric acidemia I (GA I, MIM #231670) is caused by the inability of glutaryl CoA dehydrogenase (*GCDH*; E.C. 1.3.99.7) to metabolize tryptophan, hydroxylysine, or lysine resulting in measurable glutaric acid metabolites in the urine (Table 7.1). It presents as severe progressive "post-infectious" dystonia and athetosis with striatal injury (68–70). For this reason, the indication for initial evaluation in patients with GA I can be for a newly developed movement disorder, if not identified by newborn screening. To make diagnosis of GA I more complicated, individuals may not always have abnormal biochemical findings in the healthy state, but on the other hand, they can also have elevation of glutaric acid in their urine when well fed and healthy (71, 72). Further complicating the diagnosis is that 3-hydroxyglutarate is excreted during elevated ketosis and can be misinterpreted as GA I (73).

Seizures are particularly dangerous in patients with GA I (whether idiopathic or from brain damage) in that they increase brain metabolism and increase risk for the characteristic brain damage and resulting movement disorder. Luckily they are rare outside the acute encephalopathic event (66, 69, 70). On the other hand, they can be the presenting finding with slowing of the EEG background and mixed multifocal and generalized spike and wave discharges (2, 74) (Figure 7.5). Some of the movement abnormalities do not correlate with the EEG and are not seizures but unusual dystonias (75). MRIs show increased CSF in the Sylvian fissures and in front of the temporal lobes with dilated open operculae in untreated patients (17). Many patients with treated GA I continue to have large heads with increased extracerebral CSF. In addition, the movement disorder corresponds to T2 white matter changes especially in the basal ganglia.

Glutaric acid, itself, can directly activate NMDA receptors (7, 71) resulting in inhibition of glutamate uptake from the synaptic cleft (76). In addition, patients with GA I have a depletion of the intracellular phosphate pool (10), inhibition of alpha-ketoglutarate of the tricarboxylic acid cycle and disturbance of the dicarboxylate shuttle between astrocytes and neurons resulting in

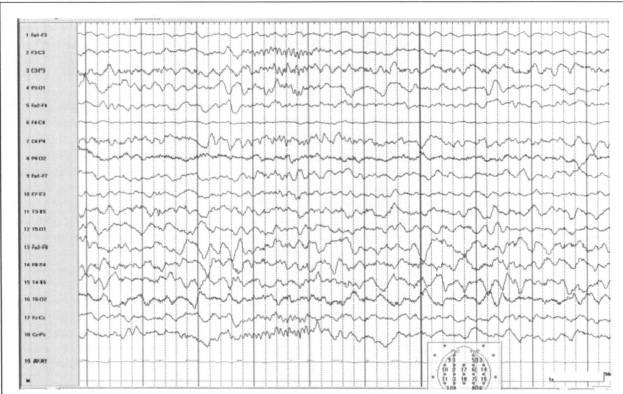

FIGURE 7.5   A 7-month-old with glutaric aciduria 1 who has right temporal focal slowing which is evident in leads 9–12 as compared to leads 5–8.

dysfunction and cell death (77). All of these mechanisms probably contribute to the neurologic phenotype.

Therapy for GA I has been shown to prevent neurological complications and centers on early identification (prior to symptoms), a low-protein diet with especially low lysine and tryptophan, carnitine supplementation and aggressive emergency management when a GA I patient is febrile or ill (70, 78, 79). If seizures occur, appropriate anticonvulsant therapy for the type of seizure is essential, but valproate should be avoided since it is thought to change acetyl CoA/CoA ratios in the mitochondria, a theoretical risk in GA I which may further impair brain cell function (70).

3-Methylglutaconic Acidurias

3-Methylglutaconic acidurias (MGA) have been divided into five types, I–V, and all have elevated 3-methylglutaconic acid in urine (Table 7.1). As a consequence,

clinical course, genetic/enzyme testing and potentially a leucine dietary challenge are used for diagnosis (80).

Type I (MIM 250950) is caused by the inability of 3-methylglutaconyl CoA hydratase, (3-MGH, E.C. 4.2.1.18), to catabolize 3-methylglutaconyl CoA to 3-hydroxy-3-methylglutaryl CoA as part of the leucine catabolic pathway. Patients with type I MGA (encoded by the *AUH* gene) can present with leukoencephalopathy, optic atrophy, ataxia, sensorineural hearing loss, and encephalopathy (epilepsy, psychosis, and depression), as well as cardiomyopathy, liver dysfunction, bone marrow failure, and exocrine pancreatic problems (80). Children may initially present with seizures or intellectual disability, but may also present with slow progression of encephalopathy (80). Adults present with ataxia and dysarthria (80, 81).

White matter lesions on MRI are usually in a supratentorial location with U structure sparing (81, 82). In a group of Saudi patients whose symptoms are consistent with type I MGA, EEGs showed mild to moderate diffuse slowing (2). There are few other reports of the exact EEG changes seen in patients with MGA, despite seizures being a known complication of type I disease.

It is unclear whether neurotoxicity is due to accumulation of cellular toxic 3-hydroxyisovaleric acid seen in CSF or whether it is due to a slow onset excitotoxicity leading to the cellular dysfunction (81). Patients have elevated 3-hydroxyisovaleric acids, 3-methylglutaconic acid, and 3-methylglutaric acid in their urine which is further elevated with high leucine diet; this is useful to differentiate type I from the other types (Table 7.1).

Type II MGA, also known as Barth syndrome (MIM 302060), shows elevated 3-methylglutaconic and 3-methylglutaric acid in the urine and decreased serum cholesterol levels (especially LDLs) (83). It is an X-linked mitochondrial disorder in which patients usually do not have seizures, but can have skeletal myopathy, cyclic neutropenia, cardiomyopathy, and mitochondrial respiratory chain dysfunction and is caused by mutations in the *TAZ* gene (84).

Type III or Costeff syndrome (MIM 258501) is an MGA which is caused by mutations in the nuclear encoded mitochondrial gene *OPA3* and presents with infantile bilateral optic atrophy, extrapyramidal symptoms, spasticity, ataxia, dysarthria, and cognitive deficiency. It is seen most commonly among those of Iraqi Jewish descent (85). Again, individuals will have elevated urine 3-methylglutaconic and 3-methylglutaric acids in their urine, but not typically seizures.

Type IV MGA (MIM 250951) is a disorder which presents predominately with psychomotor retardation, supravalvular aortic stenosis, cardiomyopathy, and poor growth. Later, Type IV MGA can progress to seizures and sensorineural hearing loss (80).

MGA, type IV is an example of genetic heterotopic variation in that several genes have been implicated. These include *TMEM70* in the Gypsy population which has the above findings, but also has hypotonia, hepatomegaly, facial dysmorphism, and microcephaly. As well, MGA, type IV has been described in individuals with ATP synthase (COX V) dysfunction due to *ATP12* mutations (one of the ATP synthase organizing proteins) (86). Finally, MEGDEL is a Leigh-like presentation with COX 1 dysfunction which has as similar findings (80). All these disorders have elevated 3-methylglutaconic and 3-methylglutaric acids in the urine. They may also have elevation in tricarboxylic acid cycle intermediates in the urine.

MGA, type V (MIM 610198) leads to cardiomyopathy, nonprogressive ataxia, and is in Canadian Dariusleut Hutterites predominately due to mutations in *DNAJC19* which codes for a mitochondrial inner membrane protein (87).

Canavan Disease

Canavan disease (MIM #271900) is caused by dysfunction of aspartoacylase (E.C.3.5.1.15) which is the enzyme that cleaves *N*-acetylaspartic acid (NAA) to acetate and L-aspartate. In patients with Canavan, NAA is elevated in urine (Table 7.1) (88). Individuals with Canavan have progressive psychomotor retardation, progressive epileptic encephalopathy, macrocephaly, leukodystrophy (particularly subcortical U-fibers), and optic atrophy (89, 90). It is predominately a demyelinating disease and suspected to be due to brain acetate deficiency (91) resulting in decreased acetyl CoA and leading to a myelination disorder. In addition, NAA is thought to play a role in maintaining cerebral water balance and its accumulation can lead to cerebral edema further causing damage (1).

Seizures start about the 2nd year of life and are treated with appropriate antiepileptic medications. Much of patient care focuses on supportive aspects since no intervention has been shown to slow progression of disease, although trials with glycerol triacetate have been attempted (92).

L-2-Hydroxyglutaric Aciduria

L-2-Hydroxyglutaric aciduria (MIM #236792) presents with progressive ataxia, mental retardation, and epilepsy. It has a classical MRI presentation with peripheral subcortical white matter loss (leukodystrophy of U-fibers), cerebellar atrophy, and symmetric T2 signal changes in dentate nuclei, globus pallidi, and thalami.

L-2-Hydroxyglutaric aciduria is caused by dysfunction of L-2 hydroxyglutarate dehydrogenase (*L2DHGH*, E.C. 1.1.99.2), an enzyme which is proposed to metabolize the conversion of L-2 hydroxyglutaric acid to alpha ketoglutarate (the TCA intermediate). It is diagnosed by elevated L-2-hydroxyglutaric acid in urine (Table 7.1).

Generalized seizures can be seen and patients have multifocal spikes (93) and burst suppression with marked epileptiform activity on EEG (94, 95).

D-2-Hydroxyglutaric Aciduria

D-2-Hydroxyglutaric aciduria (MIM 600721) is an epileptic encephalopathy in which patients can also have cyclic vomiting and cardiomyopathy. D-2-Hydroxyglutarate is the more rare of the two enantiomers (other is the L, see above), and more variable in clinical findings with severe to mild presentations (96, 97).

D-2-Hydroxyglutaric aciduria can be caused by loss of one of two enzymes: hydroxyacid-oxoacid transhydrogenase (*HOT*), which metabolizes gamma hydroxybutyrate, and D-2-hydroglutaric dehydrogenase (*D2HGD*) (98). Elevations of D-2-hydroxyglutaric acid in the urine are useful in diagnosis (Table 7.1).

Severe onset disease presents in the neonatal period with encephalopathy, cardiomyopathy, and intractable epilepsy with MRI findings of delayed or disturbed cerebral maturation. The epilepsy in mild patients can be medically controlled, whereas seizures in severe patients are intractable despite therapy with medication. Moreover, epilepsy is noted in almost all patients no matter their severity (99). Because of its rarity, EEG reports of patients are not common in the literature, but findings in one family were consistent with multiple focal synchronous discharges (97).

4-Hydroxybutyric Aciduria (Succinic Semialdehyde Dehydrogenase Deficiency)

4-Hydroxybutyric aciduria (MIM #271980) is caused by deficiency of succinate semialdehyde dehydrogenase (SSADH, E.C. 1.2.1.16) due to mutations in *ALDH5A1*. SSADH leads to developmental delay, new onset hypotonia and ataxia, decreased reflexes, and atonia. Approximately 50% of patients with SSADH will develop seizures including absence, myoclonic and generalized tonic-clonic types. EEG typically shows background slowing and spike discharges (100) and can be progressively abnormal (2). This disorder is covered in more detail in the chapter on disorders of GABA metabolism.

SSADH is considered to cause a GABA abnormality such that individuals with the disease have elevated gamma-hydroxybutyric acid (GHB) and GABA in their urine (Table 7.1) (101). If elevated, GHB activates $GABA_B$ receptors (102) and acutely activates pre- and postsynaptic release of dopamine, GABA, and glutamate (103). Chronically elevated GABA results in down regulation of $GABA_A$ receptors. In the mouse model of SSADH, down regulation of $GABA_A$ receptors lead to their hyperexcitability and subsequently to seizures (104). As a result of the GABA hyperexcitability, the success of using vigabatrin in seizures in patients with SSADH deficiency has a biological basis (105).

MR imaging shows a dentatopallidoluysian pattern with increased T2 signal in the globus pallidi, cerebellar dentate nuclei, and subthalamic nuclei with increased GABA peaks on MR spectrometry (106).

Fumaric Aciduria

Fumaric aciduria (MIM #606812) is an organic acidemia caused by loss of fumarase or fumaric hydratase (*FH*, E.C.), a component of the TCA cycle which converts fumarate to malate. Fumaric aciduria can present prenatally with polyhydramnios and cerebral ventriculomegaly. Moreover, patients have lack of or very slow development, hepatomegaly, opisthotonus, vision failure, seizures, severe intellectual disability, and relative macrocephaly (107–109). Patients have extremely elevated fumarate in urine, and can also have elevations in succinate, citrate, malate, and 2-ketoglutarate in their urine (Table 7.1) (109).

Seizures are a common complication and status epilepticus has been seen (109). Seizures are considered to be a consequence of the abnormal brain structures which have included diffuse polymicrogyria, decreased cerebral white matter, large ventricles, and open opercula as seen by MRI (109). Large head size is usually a complication of ventriculomegaly and patients with ventriculoperitoneal (VP) shunts can develop microcephaly (109).

AMINO ACIDOPATHIES

Amino acidopathies are disorders of amino acid metabolism, including maple syrup urine disease (MSUD) and phenylketonuria (PKU). Patients with these disorders may or may not have elevated organic acids in their urine and, if present, the organic acids are often related to ketones. The neurotoxicity is related to accumulation of amino acids which cannot be broken down due to the causative dysfunctional enzyme.

Maple Syrup Urine Disease

Maple syrup urine disease (MSUD, MIM 248600) is caused by mutations in both copies of the genes that code for the enzyme, branched-chain 2-keto dehydrogenase (BCKD). Infants with MSUD often present with lethargy, vomiting, bicycling movements, and potential progression to coma and death if not treated promptly (110). Neurological pathology is thought to be due to hyperleucinemia resulting in cerebral edema as well as 2-oxoisocaproic acid (which can be seen elevated in the urine) acting as a neurotoxin (111).

BCKD is created from four subunits *BCKDHA*, *BCKDHB*, *DBT*, and *DLD* (E3). Mutations in the first three have been described to cause MSUD; mutations in E3 lead to another disorder, lipoamide dehydrogenase deficiency (discussed in the next section of this chapter). BCKD is required for the initial step in degradation of the branched-chain amino acids, leucine, valine, and isoleucine. The disorder is characterized by elevated branched chains and the presence of alloisoleucine in plasma. Patients can have elevated ketoacids in their urine (so occasionally MSUD is categorized as an organic acidemia) (Table 7.1).

Seizures in MSUD are often related to hyperleucinemia and resultant brain swelling. Treatment consists of clearing systemic leucine from blood (which in theory is thought to reduce brain levels) by reversing catabolism using calories or potentially by using dialysis with hemofiltration methods. In either approach, maintaining sodium levels is essential to prevent worsening brain damage from uncontrolled tonicity changes via osmosis (112).

Any time a child has cerebral edema from hyperleucinemia, they are at increased risk for seizure activity (110). Moreover, brain damage from these episodes can further increase risk. Consequently seizures without elevated systemic branched chain amino acids have been observed in older patients (113, 114).

Dihydrolipoaminde Dehydrogenase Deficiency (E3)

Dihydrolipoaminde dehydrogenase (DLD, E.C. 1.8.1.4) is an essential subunit of the BCKD, pyruvate dehydrogenase, and alpha-ketoglutarate dehydrogenase enzymes. Mutations in this subunit (DLD) result in a disorder which has metabolic acidosis, neuroimpairment, and often fatality at an early age and is also called MSUD type III (MIM #2486000). Individuals can present with elevated liver transaminases, hypoglycemia, no ketones, hypoglycemia, and seizures (including tonic clonic type) (115). These findings reflect the

dysfunction of all three enzymes known to have DLD as a subunit in a single patient.

Phenylketonuria

Phenylketonuria (PKU, #261600) is an amino acidopathy in which individuals cannot convert phenylalanine to tyrosine due to dysfunction of phenylalanine hydroxylase (E.C. 1.14.16.1). PKU is distinguished historically as the first of the neurometabolic disorders to be described (116) and as the first treatable biochemical disorder (117). The dietary approach of restricting problematic amino acid(s) (phenylalanine) and replacement of resultant deficient amino acid(s) (tyrosine) is the model for all treatable biochemical disorders. PKU is the most commonly screened disorder by newborn screening around the world, but if not identified, it can present with microcephaly, "mousy odor," intellectual disabilities, seizures, and lethargy and so is often classified as a cerebral disorder, despite system wide dysfunction. Patients will have elevated plasma phenylalanine and low plasma tyrosine without treatment (Table 7.1).

Excessive phenylalanine and lack of tyrosine leads to decreased dopamine, norepinephrine, and serotonin levels (118, 119). Additional brain pathophysiology is thought to be due to impaired transport of large amino acids since there is an overabundance of cerebral phenylalanine to transport. Preventing large amino acid transport can lead to depletion of serotonin, catechols, histamine, carnosine, and *S*-adenosylmethionine which are required components of brain function and structure (120–122). Moreover, phenylalanine itself also competes with glycine on the NMDA receptor and glutamate at the glutamate binding site on the AMPA receptor. Any of these possibilities may explain the epilepsy seen in this patient population, alone, but probably a combination of these factors are causative (1).

Seizures seen in PKU often correlate with periods of elevated phenylalanine. EEG findings reported are generalized slowing of background activity and independent bihemispheric spike and sharp wave discharges (123).

CONCLUSION

Systemic organic acidemias, cerebral organic acidemias, and amino acidopathies can all cause seizures in affected patients. Multiple seizure types and EEG findings have been seen in these disorders. No particular EEG or seizure type is diagnostic for any one of these disorders. There should be a high level of suspicion for an organic acidemia or amino acidopathy in any patient with EEG findings of diffuse background slowing. For these patients, a urine organic acid may be diagnostic. Many of these disorders also have abnormal findings on brain MRI (both in the acute and chronic setting) and on MR spectroscopy.

CLINICAL PEARLS

1. Systemic organic acidemias, cerebral organic acidemias, and classical amino acidopathies are disorders of small molecule metabolism which are due to dysfunction of enzymes required for catabolism of various amino acids and fatty acids to produce energy.
2. Seizures are usually complications from toxic intermediates or structural damage in systemic organic acidemias and amino acidopathies.
3. Cerebral organic acidemias present with seizures or other neurologic symptoms.
4. Multiple seizure types and EEG findings have been seen in cerebral and systemic organic acidopathies as well as amino acidopathies.
5. Urine organic acids to detect nonamino acid organic acids can be diagnostically useful in patients suspected to have cerebral or systemic organic acidemias.

Special thanks to Drs Adeline Vanderver and Tammy Tsuchida at Children's National Medical Center in Washington, DC for their assistance in preparation of this chapter.

REFERENCES

1. Kolker S, Sauer SW, Hoffmann GF, et al. Pathogenesis of CNS involvement in disorders of amino and organic acid metabolism. *J Inherit Metab Dis.* 2008;31:194–204.
2. Stigsby B, Yarworth SM, Rahbeeni Z, et al. Neurophysiologic correlates of organic acidemias: A survey of 107 patients. *Brain Dev.* 1994;16(Suppl):125–144.
3. Sokoloff L. The metabolism of the central nervous system in vivo. In: J Field, HW Magoun, VE Hall eds. *Handbook of Physiology.* New York: Raven Press, 1960:161–168.
4. Erecinska M, Dagani F. Relationships between the neuronal sodium/potassium pump and energy metabolism. Effects of K+, Na+, and adenosine triphosphate in isolated brain synaptosomes. *J Gen Physiol.* 1990;95(4):591–616.
5. Okun JG, Horster F, Farkas LM, et al. Neurodegeneration in methylmalonic aciduria involves inhibition of complex II and the tricarboxylic acid cycle, and synergistically acting excitotoxicity. *J Biol Chem.,* 2002;277(17):14674–14680.
6. Heidenreich R, Natowicz M, Hainline BE, et al. Acute extrapyramidal syndrome in methylmalonic acidemia: "metabolic stroke" involving the globus pallidus. *J Pediatr.* 1988;113(6):1022–1027.
7. Kolker S, Koeller DM, Okun JG, et al. Pathomechanisms of neurodegeneration in glutaryl-CoA dehydrogenase deficiency. *Ann Neurol.* 2004;55(1):7–12.
8. Sauer SW, Okun JG, Schwab MA, et al. Bioenergetics in glutaryl-coenzyme A dehydrogenase deficiency: A role for glutaryl-coenzyme A. *J Biol Chem.* 2005;280(23):21830–21836.
9. Schwab MA, Sauer SW, Okun JG, et al. Secondary mitochondrial dysfunction in propionic aciduria: A pathogenic role for endogenous mitochondrial toxins. *Biochem J.* 2006;398(1):107–112.
10. Ullrich K, Flott-Rahmel B, Schluff P, et al. Glutaric aciduria type I: Pathomechanisms of neurodegeneration. *J Inherit Metab Dis.* 1999;22(4):392–403.
11. Zinnanti WJ, Lazovic J, Wolpert EB, et al. New insights for glutaric aciduria type I. *Brain.* 2006;129(Pt 8):e55.
12. Meldrum BS. The role of glutamate in epilepsy and other CNS disorders. *Neurology.* 1994;44(11 Suppl 8):S14–S23.
13. Telfeian AE, Connors BW. Epileptiform propagation patterns mediated by NMDA and non-NMDA receptors in rat neocortex. *Epilepsia.* 1999;40(11): 1499–1506.
14. Fenton WA, Gravel RA, Rosenblatt DS. Disorders of Propionate and Methylmalonate Metabolism. In: CR Scriver, AL Beaudert, WS Sly, et al. eds. *The Metabolic & Molecular Basis of Inherited Disease.* New York:McGraw-Hill; 2001:2165–2193.
15. Sass JO, Hofmann M, Skladal D, et al. Propionic acidemia revisited: A workshop report. *Clin Pediatr (Phila).* 2004;43(9):837–843.
16. Brismar J, Ozand PT. CT and MR of the brain in disorders of the propionate and methylmalonate metabolism. *AJNR Am J Neuroradiol.* 1994;15(8):1459–1473.
17. Brismar J, Ozand PT. CT and MR of the brain in the diagnosis of organic acidemias. Experiences from 107 patients. *Brain Dev.* 1994;16(Suppl):104–124.
18. Haberlandt E, Canestrini C, Brunner-Krainz M, et al. Epilepsy in patients with propionic acidemia. *Neuropediatrics.* 2009;40(3):120–125.
19. Johnson JA, Le KL, Palacios E. Propionic acidemia: Case report and review of neurologic sequelae. *Pediatr Neurol.* 2009;40(4):317–320.
20. Aldamiz-Echevarria Azuar L, Prats Vinas JM, Sanjurjo Crespo P, et al. [Infantile spasms as the first manifestation of propionic acidemia]. *An Pediatr (Barc).* 2005;63(6):548–550.
21. Horster F, Garbade SF, Zwickler T, et al. Prediction of outcome in isolated methylmalonic acidurias: Combined use of clinical and biochemical parameters. *J Inherit Metab Dis.* 2009;32(5):630–639.
22. Chapman KA, Bennett MJ, Sondheimer N. Increased C3-carnitine in a healthy premature infant. *Clin Chem.* 2008;54(11):1914–1917.

23. Rosenblatt DS, Aspler AL, Shevell MI, et al. Clinical heterogeneity and prognosis in combined methylmalonic aciduria and homocystinuria (cblC). *J Inherit Metab Dis.* 1997;20(4):528–538.

24. Biancheri R, Cerone R, Rossi A, et al. Early-onset cobalamin C/D deficiency: Epilepsy and electroencephalographic features. *Epilepsia.* 2002;43(6):616–622.

25. Biancheri R, Cerone R, Schiaffino MC, et al. Cobalamin (Cbl) C/D deficiency: Clinical, neurophysiological and neuroradiologic findings in 14 cases. *Neuropediatrics.* 2001;32(1):14–22.

26. Surtees R, Leonard J, Austin S. Association of demyelination with deficiency of cerebrospinal-fluid S-adenosylmethionine in inborn errors of methyl-transfer pathway. *Lancet.* 1991;338(8782–8783):1550–1554.

27. Surtees R. Demyelination and inborn errors of the single carbon transfer pathway. *Eur J Pediatr.* 1998;157(Suppl 2):S118–S121.

28. Wajner M, Coelho JC. Neurological dysfunction in methylmalonic acidaemia is probably related to the inhibitory effect of methylmalonate on brain energy production. *J Inherit Metab Dis.* 1997;20(6):761–768.

29. Oberholzer VG, Levin B, Burgess EA, et al. Methylmalonic aciduria. An inborn error of metabolism leading to chronic metabolic acidosis. *Arch Dis Child.* 1967;42(225):492–504.

30. Halperin ML, Schiller CM, Fritz IB. The inhibition by methylmalonic acid of malate transport by the dicarboxylate carrier in rat liver mitochondria. A possible explantation for hypoglycemia in methylmalonic aciduria. *J Clin Invest.* 1971;50(11):2276–2282.

31. Dutra JC, Dutra-Filho CS, Cardozo SE, et al. Inhibition of succinate dehydrogenase and beta-hydroxybutyrate dehydrogenase activities by methylmalonate in brain and liver of developing rats. *J Inherit Metab Dis.* 1993;16(1): 147–153.

32. Vockley J, Ensenauer R. Isovaleric acidemia: New aspects of genetic and phenotypic heterogeneity. *Am J Med Genet C Semin Med Genet.* 2006;142C(2):95–103.

33. Ensenauer R, Vockley J, Willard JM, et al. A common mutation is associated with a mild, potentially asymptomatic phenotype in patients with isovaleric acidemia diagnosed by newborn screening. *Am J Hum Genet.* 2004;75(6):1136–1142.

34. Baumgartner MR, Almashanu S, Suormala T, et al. The molecular basis of human 3-methylcrotonyl-CoA carboxylase deficiency. *J Clin Invest.* 2001;107(4):495–504.

35. Pinto L, Zen P, Rosa R, et al. Isolated 3-methylcrotonyl-coenzyme A carboxylase deficiency in a child with metabolic stroke. *J Inherit Metab Dis.* 2006;29(1):205–206.

36. Bannwart C, Wermuth B, Baumgartner R, et al. Isolated biotin-resistant deficiency of 3-methylcrotonyl-CoA carboxylase presenting as a clinically severe form in a newborn with fatal outcome. *J Inherit Metab Dis.* 1992;15(6):863–868.

37. Gibson KM. Assay of 3-hydroxy-3-methylglutaryl-CoA lyase. *Methods Enzymol.* 1988;166:219–225.

38. Faull KF, Bolton PD, Halpern B, et al. The urinary organic acid profile associated with 3-hydroxy-3-methylglutaric aciduria. *Clin Chim Acta.* 1976;73(3): 553–559.

39. Gibson KM, Breuer J, Nyhan WL. 3-Hydroxy-3-methylglutaryl-coenzyme A lyase deficiency: Review of 18 reported patients. *Eur J Pediatr.* 1988;148(3): 180–186.

40. Mir C, Lopez-Vinas E, Aledo R, et al. A single-residue mutation, G203E, causes 3-hydroxy-3-methylglutaric aciduria by occluding the substrate channel in the 3D structural model of HMG-CoA lyase. *J Inherit Metab Dis.* 2006;29(1):64–70.

41. Ozand PT, al Aqeel A, Gascon G, et al. 3-Hydroxy-3-methylglutaryl-coenzyme A (HMG-CoA) lyase deficiency in Saudi Arabia. *J Inherit Metab Dis.* 1991;14(2):174–188.

42. Cardoso ML, Rodrigues MR, Leao E, et al. The E37X is a common HMGCL mutation in Portuguese patients with 3-hydroxy-3-methylglutaric CoA lyase deficiency. *Mol Genet Metab.* 2004;82(4):334–338.

43. Muroi J, Yorifuji T, Uematsu A, et al. Molecular and clinical analysis of Japanese patients with 3-hydroxy-3-methylglutaryl CoA lyase (HL) deficiency. *Hum Genet.* 2000;107(4):320–326.

44. Ozand PT, Rashed M, Gascon GG, et al. 3-Ketothiolase deficiency: A review and four new patients with neurologic symptoms. *Brain Dev.* 1994;16(Suppl): 38–45.

45. Daum RS, Scriver CR, Mamer OA, et al. An inherited disorder of isoleucine catabolism causing accumulation of alpha-methylacetoacetate and alpha-methyl-beta -hydroxybutyrate, and intermittent metabolic acidosis. *Pediatr Res.* 1973;7(3): 149–160.

46. Aramaki S, Lehotay D, Sweetman L, et al. Urinary excretion of 2-methylacetoacetate, 2-methyl-3-hydroxybutyrate and tiglylglycine after isoleucine loading in the diagnosis of 2-methylacetoacetyl-CoA thiolase deficiency. *J Inherit Metab Dis.* 1991;14(1):63–74.

47. Korman SH. Inborn errors of isoleucine degradation: A review. *Mol Genet Metab.* 2006;89(4):289–299.

48. Schubiger G, Caflisch U, Baumgartner R, et al. Biotinidase deficiency: Clinical course and biochemical findings. *J Inherit Metab Dis.* 1984;7(3):129–130.

49. Zschocke J, Ruiter JP, Brand J, et al. Progressive infantile neurodegeneration caused by 2-methyl-3-hydroxybutyryl-CoA dehydrogenase deficiency: A novel inborn error of branched-chain fatty acid and isoleucine metabolism. *Pediatr Res.* 2000;48(6):852–855.

50. Sutton VR, O'Brien WE, Clark GD, et al. 3-Hydroxy-2-methylbutyryl-CoA dehydrogenase deficiency. *J Inherit Metab Dis.* 2003;26(1):69–71.

51. Poll-The BT, Wanders RJ, Ruiter JP, et al. Spastic diplegia and periventricular white matter abnormalities in 2-methyl-3-hydroxybutyryl-CoA dehydrogenase deficiency, a defect of isoleucine metabolism: Differential diagnosis with hypoxic-ischemic brain diseases. *Mol Genet Metab.* 2004;81(4):295–299.

52. Wightman PJ, Santer R, Ribes A, et al. MLYCD mutation analysis: Evidence for protein mistargeting as a cause of MLYCD deficiency. *Hum Mutat.* 2003;22(4):288–300.

53. Salomons GS, Jakobs C, Pope LL, et al. Clinical, enzymatic and molecular characterization of nine new patients with malonyl-coenzyme A decarboxylase deficiency. *J Inherit Metab Dis.* 2007;30(1):23–28.

54. Bennett MJ, Harthcock PA, Boriack RL, et al. Impaired mitochondrial fatty acid oxidative flux in fibroblasts from a patient with malonyl-CoA decarboxylase deficiency. *Mol Genet Metab.* 2001;73(3):276–279.

55. Mineri R, Rimoldi M, Burlina AB, et al. Identification of new mutations in the ETHE1 gene in a cohort of 14 patients presenting with ethylmalonic encephalopathy. *J Med Genet.* 2008;45(7):473–478.

56. Zafeiriou DI, Augoustides-Savvopoulou P, Haas D, et al. Ethylmalonic encephalopathy: Clinical and biochemical observations. *Neuropediatrics.* 2007;38(2):78–82.

57. Pigeon N, Campeau PM, Cyr D, et al. Clinical heterogeneity in ethylmalonic encephalopathy. *J Child Neurol.* 2009;24(8): 991–996.

58. Tiranti V, Briem E, Lamantea E, et al. ETHE1 mutations are specific to ethylmalonic encephalopathy. *J Med Genet.* 2006;43(4):340–346.

59. Tiranti V, Viscomi C, Hildebrandt T, et al. Loss of ETHE1, a mitochondrial dioxygenase, causes fatal sulfide toxicity in ethylmalonic encephalopathy. *Nat Med.* 2009;15(2): 200–205.

60. Tiranti V, D'Adamo P, Briem E, et al. Ethylmalonic encephalopathy is caused by mutations in ETHE1, a gene encoding a mitochondrial matrix protein. *Am J Hum Genet.* 2004;74(2): 239–252.

61. Jamroz E, Paprocka J, Adamek D, et al. Clinical and neuropathological picture of ethylmalonic aciduria—diagnostic dilemma. *Folia Neuropathol.* 2011;49(1):71–77.

62. Van Calcar SC, Gleason LA, Lindh H, et al. 2-methylbutyryl-CoA dehydrogenase deficiency in Hmong infants identified by expanded newborn screen. *WMJ.* 2007;106(1):12–15.

63. Rozen R, Vockley J, Zhou L, et al. Isolation and expression of a cDNA encoding the precursor for a novel member (ACADSB) of the acyl-CoA dehydrogenase gene family. *Genomics.* 1994;24(2):280–287.

64. Gibson KM, Burlingame TG, Hogema B, et al. 2-Methylbutyryl-coenzyme A dehydrogenase deficiency: A new inborn error of L-isoleucine metabolism. *Pediatr Res.* 2000;47(6):830–833.

65. Schousboe A, Westergaard N, Sonnewald U, et al. Glutamate and glutamine metabolism and compartmentation in astrocytes. *Dev Neurosci.* 1993;15(3–5): 359–366.

66. Kolker S, Garbade SF, Greenberg CR, et al. Natural history, outcome, and treatment efficacy in children and adults with glutaryl-CoA dehydrogenase deficiency. *Pediatr Res.* 2006;59(6):840–847.

67. Kolker S, Sauer SW, Surtees RA, et al. The aetiology of neurological complications of organic acidaemias—a role for the blood-brain barrier. *J Inherit Metab Dis.* 2006;29(6): 701–704.

68. Strauss KA, Morton DH. Type I glutaric aciduria, part 2: A model of acute striatal necrosis. *Am J Med Genet C Semin Med Genet.* 2003;121C(1):53–70.

69. Strauss KA, Puffenberger EG, Robinson DL, et al. Type I glutaric aciduria, part 1: Natural history of 77 patients. *Am J Med Genet C Semin Med Genet.* 2003;121C(1): 38–52.

70. Kolker S, Christensen E, Leonard JV, et al. Diagnosis and management of glutaric aciduria type I—revised recommendations. *J Inherit Metab Dis.* 2011;34(3): 677–694.

71. Hoffmann GF, Zschocke J. Glutaric aciduria type I: From clinical, biochemical and molecular diversity to successful therapy. *J Inherit Metab Dis.*1999;22(4):381–391.

72. Baric I, Zschocke J, Christensen E, et al. Diagnosis and management of glutaric aciduria type I. *J Inherit Metab Dis.* 1998;21(4):326–340.

73. Pitt JJ, Eggington M, Kahler SG. Comprehensive screening of urine samples for inborn errors of metabolism by electrospray tandem mass spectrometry. *Clin Chem.* 2002;48(11):1970–1980.

74. McClelland VM, Bakalinova DB, Hendriksz C, et al. Glutaric aciduria type 1 presenting with epilepsy. *Dev Med Child Neurol.* 2009;51(3):235–239.

75. Cerisola A, Campistol J, Perez-Duenas B, et al. Seizures versus dystonia in encephalopathic crisis of glutaric aciduria type I. *Pediatr Neurol.* 2009;40(6):426–431.

76. Porciuncula LO, Dal-Pizzol A, Coitinho AS, et al. Inhibition of synaptosomal [3H]glutamate uptake and [3H]glutamate binding to plasma membranes from brain of young rats by glutaric acid in vitro. *J Neurol Sci.* 2000;173(2):93–96.

77. Sauer SW, Okun JG, Fricker G, et al. Intracerebral accumulation of glutaric and 3-hydroxyglutaric acids secondary to limited flux across the blood-brain barrier constitute a biochemical risk factor for neurodegeneration in glutaryl-CoA dehydrogenase deficiency. *J Neurochem.* 2006;97(3): 899–910.

78. Kolker S, Garbade SF, Boy N, et al. Decline of acute encephalopathic crises in children with glutaryl-CoA dehydrogenase deficiency identified by newborn screening in Germany. *Pediatr Res.* 2007;62(3):357–363.

79. Bijarnia S, Wiley V, Carpenter K, et al. Glutaric aciduria type I: Outcome following detection by newborn screening. *J Inherit Metab Dis.* 2008;31(4):503–507.

80. Wortmann SB, Kluijtmans LA, Engelke UF, et al. The 3-methylglutaconic acidurias: What's new? *J Inherit Metab Dis.* 2010; 35(1):13–22.

81. Engelke UF, Kremer B, Kluijtmans LA, et al. NMR spectroscopic studies on the late onset form of 3-methylglutaconic aciduria type I and other defects in leucine metabolism. *NMR Biomed.* 2006;19(2):271–278.

82. Illsinger S, Lucke T, Zschocke J, et al. 3-methylglutaconic aciduria type I in a boy with fever-associated seizures. *Pediatr Neurol.* 2004;30(3):213–215.

83. Gibson KM, Sherwood WG, Hoffman GF, et al. Phenotypic heterogeneity in the syndromes of 3-methylglutaconic aciduria. *J Pediatr.* 1991;118(6):885–890.

84. Barth PG, Scholte HR, Berden JA, et al. An X-linked mitochondrial disease affecting cardiac muscle, skeletal muscle and neutrophil leucocytes. *J Neurol Sci.* 1983;62(1–3):327–355.

85. Costeff H, Gadoth N, Apter N, et al. A familial syndrome of infantile optic atrophy, movement disorder, and spastic paraplegia. *Neurology.* 1989;39(4):595–597.

86. De Meirleir L, Seneca S, Lissens W, et al. Respiratory chain complex V deficiency due to a mutation in the assembly gene ATP *J Med Genet.* 2004;41(2):120–124.

87. Davey KM, Parboosingh JS, McLeod DR, et al. Mutation of DNAJC19, a human homologue of yeast inner mitochondrial membrane co-chaperones, causes DCMA syndrome, a novel autosomal recessive Barth syndrome-like condition. *J Med Genet.* 2006;43(5): 385–393.

88. Al-Dirbashi OY, Rashed MS, Al-Qahtani K, et al. Quantification of N-acetylaspartic acid in urine by LC-MS/MS for

the diagnosis of Canavan disease. *J Inherit Metab Dis.* 2007; 30(4):612.

89. Canavan MM. Schilder's encephalitis periaxialis diffusa. *Arch Neurol Psychiat.* 1931;25(2):299–308.

90. van Bogaert L, Bertrand I. Sur une idiotie familiale acec degenerescence spongieuse de nevraxe. *Acta Neurol Belg.* 1949;49:572–587.

91. Arun P, Madhavarao CN, Moffett JR, et al. Metabolic acetate therapy improves phenotype in the tremor rat model of Canavan disease. *J Inherit Metab Dis.* 2010;33(3):195–210.

92. Segel R, Anikster Y, Zevin S, et al. A safety trial of high dose glyceryl triacetate for Canavan disease. *Mol Genet Metab.* 2011;103(3):203–206.

93. Barth PG, Wanders RJ, Scholte HR, et al. L-2-hydroxyglutaric aciduria and lactic acidosis. *J Inherit Metab Dis.* 1998;21(3): 251–254.

94. Chen E, Nyhan WL, Jakobs C, et al. L-2-Hydroxyglutaric aciduria: Neuropathological correlations and first report of severe neurodegenerative disease and neonatal death. *J Inherit Metab Dis.* 1996;19(3):335–343.

95. Wanders RJ, Vilarinho L, Hartung HP, et al. L-2-Hydroxyglutaric aciduria: Normal L-2-hydroxyglutarate dehydrogenase activity in liver from two new patients. *J Inherit Metab Dis.* 1997;20(5): 725–726.

96. van der Knaap MS, Jakobs C, Hoffmann GF, et al. D-2-hydroxyglutaric aciduria: Further clinical delineation. *J Inherit Metab Dis.* 1999; 22(4):404–413.

97. Wagner L, Hoffmann GF, Jakobs C. D-2-hydroxyglutaric aciduria: Evidence of clinical and biochemical heterogeneity. *J Inherit Metab Dis.* 1998;21(3):247–250.

98. Struys EA. D-2-Hydroxyglutaric aciduria: Unravelling the biochemical pathway and the genetic defect. *J Inherit Metab Dis.* 2006;29(1):21–29.

99. Van der Knaap MS, Jakobs C, Hoffmann GF, et al. D-2-hydroxyglutaric aciduria: Further clinical delineation. *J Inherit Metab Dis.* 1999;22(4):404–413.

100. Pearl PL, Capp PK, Novotny EJ, et al. Inherited disorders of neurotransmitters in children and adults. *Clin Biochem.* 2005;38(12):1051–1058.

101. Gibson KM, Gupta M, Pearl PL, et al. Significant behavioral disturbances in succinic semialdehyde dehydrogenase (SSADH) deficiency (gamma-hydroxybutyric aciduria). *Biol Psychiatry.* 2003;54(7):763–768.

102. Lingenhoehl K, Brom R, Heid J, et al. Gamma-hydroxybutyrate is a weak agonist at recombinant GABA(B) receptors. *Neuropharmacology.* 1999;38(11): 1667–1673.

103. Berton F, Brancucci A, Beghe F, et al. Gamma-Hydroxybutyrate inhibits excitatory postsynaptic potentials in rat hippocampal slices. *Eur J Pharmacol.* 1999;380(2–3):109–116.

104. Wu Y, Buzzi A, Frantseva M, et al. Status epilepticus in mice deficient for succinate semialdehyde dehydrogenase: GABAA receptor-mediated mechanisms. *Ann Neurol.* 2006;59(1): 42–52.

105. Matern D, Lehnert W, Gibson KM, et al. Seizures in a boy with succinic semialdehyde dehydrogenase deficiency treated with vigabatrin (gamma-vinyl-GABA). *J Inherit Metab Dis.* 1996;19(3):313–318.

106. Pearl PL, Gibson KM, Quezado Z, et al. Decreased GABA-A binding on FMZ-PET in succinic semialdehyde dehydrogenase deficiency. *Neurology.* 2009;73(6):423–429.

107. Zinn AB, Kerr DS, Hoppel CL. Fumarase deficiency: A new cause of mitochondrial encephalomyopathy. *N Engl J Med.* 1986;315(8):469–475.

108. Gellera C, Uziel G, Rimoldi M, et al. Fumarase deficiency is an autosomal recessive encephalopathy affecting both the mitochondrial and the cytosolic enzymes. *Neurology* 1990;40(3 Pt 1):495–499.

109. Kerrigan JF, Aleck KA, Tarby TJ, et al. Fumaric aciduria: Clinical and imaging features. *Ann Neurol.* 2000;47(5):583–588.

110. Chuang DT, Shih VE. Maple syrup urine diseae (branched-chain ketoaciduria). In: CR Scriver, AL Beaudet, WS Sly, et al. eds. *The Metabolic and Molecular Bases of Inherited Disease.* New York: McGraw-Hill, 2001:1971–2005.

111. Saudubray JM, Ogier H, Charpentier C, et al. Hudson memorial lecture. Neonatal management of organic acidurias. Clinical update. *J Inherit Metab Dis.* 1984;7(Suppl 1):2–9.

112. Strauss KA, Wardley B, Robinson D, et al. Classical maple syrup urine disease and brain development: Principles of management and formula design. *Mol Genet Metab.* 2010;99(4): 333–345.

113. Delis D, Michelakakis H, Katsarou E, et al. Thiamin-responsive maple syrup urine disease: Seizures after 7 years of satisfactory metabolic control. *J Inherit Metab Dis.* 2001;24(6):683–684.

114. Korein J, Sansaricq C, Kalmijn M, et al. Maple syrup urine disease: Clinical, EEG, and plasma amino acid correlations with a theoretical mechanism of acute neurotoxicity. *Int J Neurosci.* 1994;79(1–2): 21–45.

115. Sansaricq C, Pardo S, Balwani M, et al. Biochemical and molecular diagnosis of lipoamide dehydrogenase deficiency in a North American Ashkenazi Jewish family. *J Inherit Metab Dis.* 2006;29(1):203–204.

116. Scriver CR. The PAH gene, phenylketonuria, and a paradigm shift. *Hum Mutat.* 2007;28(9):831–845.

117. Bickel H, Gerrard J, Hickmans EM. Influence of phenylalanine intake on phenylketonuria. *Lancet.* 1953;265(6790): 812–813.

118. Huttenlocher PR. The neuropathology of phenylketonuria: Human and animal studies. *Eur J Pediatr.* 2000;159(uppl 2):S102–S106.

119. Paine RS. The variability in manifestations of untreated patients with phenylketonuria (phenylpyruvic aciduria). *Pediatrics.* 1957;20(2):290–302.

120. Pietz J, Kreis R, Rupp A, et al. Large neutral amino acids block phenylalanine transport into brain tissue in patients with phenylketonuria. *J Clin Invest.* 1999;103(8):1169–1178.

121. Matalon R, Surendran S, Matalon KM, et al. Future role of large neutral amino acids in transport of phenylalanine into the brain. *Pediatrics.* 2003;112(6 Pt 2):1570–1574.

122. McKean CM. The effects of high phenylalanine concentrations on serotonin and catecholamine metabolism in the human brain. *Brain Res.* 1972;47(2): 469–476.

123. Villasana D, Butler IJ, Williams JC, et al. Neurological deterioration in adult phenylketonuria. *J Inherit Metab Dis.* 1989;12(4):451–457.

Fatty Acid Oxidation Disorders and Epilepsy

Dietrich Matern and Dimitar K. Gavrilov

INTRODUCTION

Carbohydrates and fatty acids (FA) are the most important fuel sources providing most of the needed energy for the organism. The selection of fuel depends on the supply of substrates and the energy demands. In the fed state, excess carbohydrates, fat, and protein are stored as energy source during fasting or times of higher energy demands. The contribution of FA to the overall energy metabolism varies considerably and is organ specific. Some cells such as erythrocytes rely solely on glucose. In others, such as the brain, the preferential substrate is glucose, but ketone bodies can also be utilized. Although heart and skeletal muscle possess the machinery for oxidation of either glucose or FA, they require both even with ample glucose available (eg, postabsorptive state). The liver is the primary organ of energy homeostasis. It is the one organ capable of glycogen and ketone body synthesis and can utilize all available substrates for its own energy needs with the exception of ketone bodies. Multiple enzymes, transporters, and cofactors are involved in energy homeostasis. A central metabolic pathway is mitochondrial fatty acid beta-oxidation which is an integral part of the organism's appropriate response to energy depletion due to prolonged fasting and high energy requirements. Consequently, any disruption of this pathway is associated with potentially devastating symptoms which often include myopathies and sometimes seizures.

NORMAL MITOCHONDRIAL FATTY ACID BETA-OXIDATION

During well-fed conditions with a regular diet the preferred energy source is carbohydrates. The rising glucose concentration stimulates insulin release leading to an increase of the insulin/glucagon ratio and promotion of carbohydrate and lipid storage. During periods of decreased supply (eg, fasting) or increased demand (eg, febrile illness, reduced intake due to gastrointestinal disease or increased muscular activity), the oxidation of FA plays an important role in energy supply by providing alternative sources of acetyl-CoA and ketone bodies. This action has a glucose sparing effect and ensures normal functioning of tissues, in particular of the brain which cannot directly utilize FA. When glucose levels fall below 65 to 70 mg/dL, several counter-regulatory hormones are secreted, foremost glucagon but also norepinephrine, epinephrine, growth hormone, and cortisol (1). The resulting decrease of the insulin/glucagon ratio activates gluconeogenesis and glycogenolysis but also lipid mobilization through hormone sensitive lipase (2). The free FA are released into circulation and bound to albumin delivered to target cells.

The majority of FA stored in adipose tissue are long-chain fatty acids (LCFA) with 16 to 18 carbons (C_{16} to C_{18}). Because of their lipophilic properties it was initially thought that LCFA cross the lipid layer of the cell plasma membrane via nonprotein mediated diffusion or passive flip-flop (3). However, studies of different cell types suggest that LCFA uptake occurs in a tightly regulated, saturable, and substrate-specific manner and that up to 90% of fatty acid transport is carrier mediated (4). Inside the cytoplasm FA are bound to cytoplasmic fatty acid binding proteins (FABPc) (5). Unesterified LCFA are activated to their acyl-CoA esters by the action of a group of acyl-CoA synthetases (ACS) (6) (Figure 8.1).

Because FAO occurs within the mitochondria and the inner mitochondrial membrane is impermeable for long chain acyl-CoA esters (longer than 12–14 carbons), further transport mechanisms exist, namely the carnitine cycle. Carnitine (beta-hydroxy gamma-trimethyl-aminobutyric acid) derives primarily from dietary sources (eg, meat) with biosynthesis from methionine and lysine playing a minor role; no carnitine biosynthesis defect has been described to date. The

plasma concentration of carnitine is maintained mainly through an active process in the proximal renal tubule where more than 90% of filtered carnitine is reabsorbed. Carnitine enters the target cells against a concentration gradient with intracellular carnitine exceeding the plasma concentration up to 50-fold. At least two plasma membrane carnitine transporters have been described—a low-affinity, high-K_m transporter found in liver and a high-affinity low-K_m organic cation transporter 2 (OCTN2) expressed in muscle, kidney, and heart but also in cultured fibroblasts. The latter is deficient in primary carnitine deficiency (7). The carnitine cycle is a complex process comprised of several steps. The first and rate limiting reaction catalyzed by carnitine-palmitoyltransferase I (CPT I) is the conversion of fatty acyl-CoA esters into acylcarnitine species. CPT I is localized in the outer

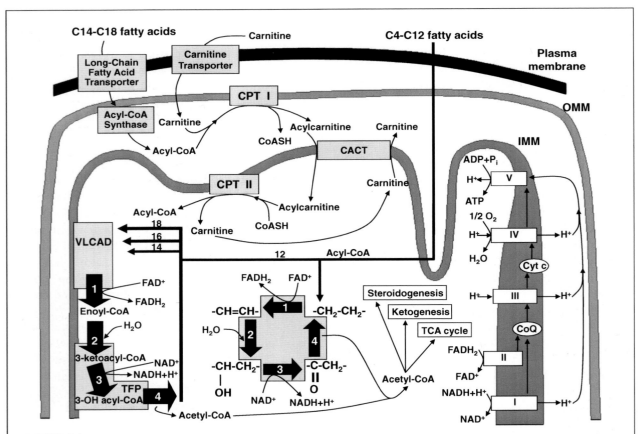

FIGURE 8.1   Schematic pathway of fatty acid transport and mitochondrial fatty acid beta-oxidation. (Adapted from Rinaldo P, Matern D, Bennett MJ. Fatty acid oxidation disorders. *Annu Rev Physiol.* 2002;64:477–502 (14)).

mitochondrial membrane and its activity is regulated by malonyl-CoA. Contrary to other enzymes of the FAO pathway CPT I exists in tissue specific isoforms. CPT that is expressed primarily in liver but also in kidney, brain, intestine and other tissues, including fibroblasts, is encoded by *CPT1A* located on chromosome 11q13.1-5 (8). The skeletal and heart muscle specific form is encoded by *CPT1B* located on chromosome 22q13.3 (8). *CPT1C* is expressed in neurons and was mapped to chromosome 19q13.33 (9). All three isoforms bind and are inhibited by malonyl-CoA but enzymatic activity has been shown only for liver and muscle CPT I, while CPT1C may play a role in dietary behavior and energy expenditure (10). CPT1C knockout mice are small and have low body weights when fed a normal chow diet (11, 12). However, when fed with a high fat diet, these mice become obese despite less food intake which confirms that CPT1C plays a significant role in nutrition, although the exact mechanisms are not yet understood (12).

The acylcarnitine species formed through the action of CPT I are exchanged for free carnitine by the action of carnitine-acylcarnitine translocase (CACT), an integral inner mitochondrial membrane protein encoded by the *CACT* gene on chromosome 3p21.31. Of note, acylcarnitine species can cross the mitochondrial membrane in the opposite direction by the action of the same transporter, providing a mechanism for removal of potentially toxic intermediary FAO metabolites from the mitochondria (13). Once inside the mitochondrial matrix CPT II replaces the carnitine moiety of the long-chain acylcarnitines with CoA. CPT II is located on the matrix side of the inner mitochondrial membrane and is encoded by *CPT2* on chromosome 1p32. Medium- and short-chain FA (less than 12 carbons), which make up only a small portion of a regular diet, appear to enter the inner mitochondrial space as free acids where they are activated to their corresponding acyl-CoA esters by different acyl-CoA synthetases (14). The activated acyl-CoA esters then undergo beta-oxidation which is a highly coordinated repetitive cycle of four chain-length specific enzymatic steps known as the beta-oxidation spiral. With completion of each cycle the acyl-CoA species are shortened by two carbon atoms as acetyl-CoA, and flavin adenine dinucleotide ($FADH_2$) and nicotinamide dinucleotide (NADH) are generated as reducing equivalents that donate electrons to the electron transport chain for production of ATP. Acetyl-CoA can be further

oxidized in the citric acid cycle, used for ketone body synthesis in the liver (and kidneys), or steroidogenesis.

The first step of mitochondrial FAO reduces the 2 to 3 bond of acyl-CoA with production of trans-2,3-enoyl-CoA species. A family of chain-length specific acyl-CoA dehydrogenases (ACAD) catalyzes this reaction. Deficiencies of very-long-chain acyl-CoA dehydrogenase (VLCAD), medium-chain acyl-CoA dehydrogenase (MCAD), short-chain acyl-CoA dehydrogenase (SCAD), and isobutyryl-CoA dehydrogenase (ACAD8) have been reported in a large number of individuals. FAD is a tightly bound prosthetic group of ACADs and the produced $FADH_2$ transfers electrons via electron-transfer flavoproteins (ETF) to ETF:ubiquinone oxidoreductase (also known as ETF dehydrogenase or ETFDH), resulting in reduction of coenzyme Q. ETF is an intramitochondrial heterodimer comprised of two subunits encoded by different genes (*ETFA* on chromosome 15q23-25 and *ETFB* on 19q13.3). ETFDH is monomer integrated in the inner mitochondrial membrane and encoded by *ETFDH* located on 4q32-qter. Both enzymes are required for electron transfer from at least nine mitochondrial flavin-containing dehydrogenases to the main respiratory chain. Multiple acyl-CoA dehydrogenase deficiency (MADD), also known as glutaric acidemia II or glutaric aciduria II, can be caused by mutation in any of the three ETF genes (15). The second step of the FAO cycle involves hydration of the double bond of the trans-2,3-enoyl-CoA producing L-3-hydroxy acyl-CoA species. This reaction involves enoyl-CoA hydratase. In the third step, L-3-hydroxyacyl-CoA is dehydrogenated at the 3-hydroxy position by L-3-hydroxyacyl-CoA dehydrogenase, producing 3-ketoacyl-CoA and NADH. The latter transfers its electrons to complex 1 of the respiratory chain. 3-Ketoacyl-CoA enters the final step of the beta-oxidation cycle where thiolitic cleavage catalyzed by 3-ketoacyl-CoA thiolase produces acetyl-CoA and a two carbon atoms shorter acyl-CoA which reenters the spiral until the final thiolitic cleavage, which results in two molecules of acetyl-CoA. The oxidation of mono- and polyunsaturated FA, normal constituents of a regular diet, requires two additional steps. Monounsaturated FA require dodecenoyl-CoA delta isomerase (DCI; also known as 3,2-*trans*-enoyl-CoA isomerase) which is encoded by *ECI1* on chromosome 16p13.3 (16). Polyunsaturated FA undergo additional reduction catalyzed by 2,4-dienoyl-CoA reductase (*DECR1* located on 8q21.3)

(17). Odd-chain FAs are oxidized until the final thiolytic cleavage produces acetyl- and propionyl-CoA, which is further metabolized by propionyl-CoA carboxylase, a biotin-dependent enzyme.

Long-chain FA (C_{16}–C_{18}), the predominant substrates for mitochondrial FAO, are metabolized by enzymes, which are bound to the inner mitochondrial membrane. The first step requires VLCAD, which is encoded by *ACADVL* located on chromosome 17p11.13-11.2. VLCAD differs from the other ACAD family members because it is membrane associated and the only homodimer (the others being tetrameric proteins situated in the mitochondrial matrix). The mitochondrial trifunctional protein (TFP) is a multienzyme complex and responsible for the subsequent three steps of the oxidation of long-chain fatty acyl-CoA. TFP is a membrane-bound heterooctamer with four alpha- and four beta-subunits. The alpha-subunit harbors the 3-hydroxyacyl-CoA dehydrogenase and enoyl-CoA hydratase activities and the beta-subunit the 3-ketoacyl-CoA thiolase activity. The subunits are encoded by different genes, *HADHA* and *HADHB*, respectively; both genes are located on 2p23 (18).

Acyl-CoA species shorter than 12 carbons are substrates for medium- and short-chain mitochondrial matrix enzymes. The first step is performed by MCAD encoded by *ACADM* on chromosome 1p31. SCAD, encoded by *ACADS* on chromosome 12q24.31, participates in the final FAO cycles. Both enzymes are homotetramers with significant similarity. The enzymes responsible for the second, third, and fourth steps of the beta-oxidation of medium- and short-chain acyl-CoA esters are also located within the mitochondrial matrix and include enoyl-CoA hydratase (also known as crotonase); medium/short-chain 3-hydroxy acyl-CoA dehydrogenase (M/SCHAD); and mitochondrial acetyl-CoA acyltransferase also known as medium-chain 3-ketoacyl-CoA thiolase (MCKAT). Mitochondrial acetoacetyl-CoA thiolase, also known as mitochondrial beta-ketothiolase (*ACAT1*), is also involved in the catabolism of the amino acid isoleucine and in ketone body metabolism.

PATHOPHYSIOLOGY OF FAO DISORDERS

During periods of decreased supply (eg, fasting) or increased demand (eg, febrile illness, reduced intake due gastrointestinal disease, cold exposure or increased muscular activity), mitochondrial FAO plays an important role in energy metabolism by providing acetyl-CoA, ketone bodies, and reducing equivalents. Although FAO disorders lead to ubiquitous energy shortage, their effects differ between organs based on available back-up mechanisms. The liver is central to energy metabolism and the main source of glucose for other tissues because enzymes required for glycogenolysis and gluconeogenesis are exclusively expressed in liver. In addition, the liver is able to synthesize ketone bodies although is not able to utilize them due to a lack of succinyl-CoA:3-oxoacid CoA transferase (SCOT). Fatty acid uptake and synthesis also occur predominantly in liver cells. Consequently, FAO defects generally impair production of acetyl-CoA and ketone bodies which then leads to a relative increase in glucose utilization jeopardizing tissues such as the brain which cannot make adequate use of FA. Because acetyl-CoA is a cofactor of pyruvate carboxylase, the rate limiting enzyme of gluconeogenesis, low levels of acetyl-CoA can limit glucose production from noncarbohydrate sources. This increase of glucose utilization along with limited glucose production and dwindling glucose reserves explains one of the hallmark features of FAO disorders: hypoglycemia with inadequate ketone production. Hypoglycemia can present as seizure-like episodes but the gravest consequence of an episode of non- or hypo-ketotic hypoglycemia is sudden unexpected death (SUD) (19–21). In addition, FA accumulating inside the mitochondria during fasting are shuttled into the cytosol causing microvesicular steatosis of the liver. Their concentration also increases in blood, an often overlooked but diagnostically helpful finding in patients with FAO defects. Furthermore, acetyl-CoA along with glutamate is a substrate for *N*-acetylglutamate synthase (NAGS) which forms *N*-acetylglutamate, a cofactor of the rate-limiting enzyme of the urea cycle, carbamoylphosphate synthetase I (CPS I). Reduced availability of acetyl-CoA, therefore, can lead to hyperammonemia due to the secondary dysfunction of CPS I. The combined presentation of hypoglycemia and hepatic encephalopathy with hyperammonemia and microvesicular steatosis constitute a Reye-like syndrome, a frequent presentation of several untreated FAO disorders (22).

Muscle can utilize various sources for energy production, the choice being determined by the duration and intensity of the physical activity. FA are the predominant substrate and glucose utilization increases with exercise intensity. The pathogenesis of muscle disease associated with FAO disorders is likely due to depletion of energy stores but also the accumulation of toxic intermediates, in particular of long-chain FA and their derivatives in long-chain FAO disorders that are often associated with rhabdomyolysis and myoglobinuria with possible renal failure as a consequence (22). The rhabdomyolysis of FAO disorders can at least in part be explained by a decreased production of ATP with subsequent impairment of Na–K–ATPase which in combination with the increased intracellular calcium initiates intracellular proteases causing cell damage (23). Furthermore, several LCFA have been shown to have detergent-like properties and progressive lipid storage myopathy could be caused by increased lipid deposition in myocytes (24).

Cardiac involvement including cardiomyopathy and conduction abnormalities has been observed in most FAO disorders (22). The high energy demand of heart muscle is normally obtained by more than 70% from FA, but when necessary can rapidly be switched to alternative sources such as carbohydrates, lactate, and ketone bodies (25). Although this metabolic flexibility and adaptive capacity of the heart muscle are well established, the role of substrate shortages as the cause of cardiomyopathy is not yet understood (13, 26). Intracellular lipid deposition or accumulation of toxic intermediates are also possible contributors to the development of cardiomyopathy or arrhythmias in FAO disorders (27).

INHERITANCE AND INCIDENCE

Inherited deficiencies have been described for almost all known enzymes involved in FAO. All of these conditions follow an autosomal recessive inheritance pattern. In many countries—at least in the developed world—most FAO disorders are identified during the first week of life through newborn screening (NBS) by acylcarnitine analysis using tandem mass spectrometry (MS/MS). Based on NBS data, the overall incidence of FAO disorders is approximately 1:9,300 live births, with a range of 1:15,000 for MCAD deficiency to 1:2 million for CPT I, CPT II, CACT, and glutaric acidemia type II (28).

CLINICAL PRESENTATION

As a rule, FAO disorders result in failure to produce sufficient energy during fasting or higher energy demands. Although residual activity and chain-length specificity of the affected enzyme play an important role in the determination of the phenotype, environmental factors such as diet, exposure to cold, exercise, or intercurrent illness (leading to decreased food intake and thus reduced glycogen stores) are the primary triggers of clinical symptoms. Accordingly, the presentation of patients is not limited to a particular age group, although it is generally accepted that an early presentation indicates a more profound enzyme deficiency. However, due to limited glycogen stores in liver and muscle, higher energy requirements, and restricted access to food, morbidity, and mortality are higher in younger patients independent of genotype. Early diagnosis and treatment are therefore crucial but patients are often overlooked because laboratory investigations can yield normal results when the patient is asymptomatic while a large number of patients have died acutely during their first episode of catabolism. Often such unfortunate patients were categorized as Sudden Infant Death Syndrome (SIDS) (21). This situation along with technological advances eventually led to the inclusion of FAO disorders, foremost MCAD deficiency, in NBS panels. This significantly altered the natural course of these conditions through presymptomatic diagnosis and preventive treatment. Not surprisingly, NBS also uncovered the presence of apparently milder variants of FAO disorders that previously remained undiagnosed.

The phenotype of late-onset variants of FAO disorders involves primarily the skeletal muscle. Patients may present with muscle weakness or pain that is typically associated with physical exercise or other causes of higher energy demands such as illness, cold exposure, dehydration or prolonged fasting. Characteristically, symptoms become evident after prolonged activity, are not relieved by resting, and can progress to rhabdomyolysis and renal failure.

DEFECTS OF THE CARNITINE CYCLE

Carnitine Uptake Defect (Primary Carnitine Deficiency; Systemic Carnitine Deficiency)

Mutations in *SLC22A5* which encodes the carnitine transporter OCTN2 cause carnitine uptake defect (CUD) (7). OCTN2 is expressed in heart and skeletal muscle and renal tubules and its deficiency is characterized by nearly undetectable plasma carnitine levels reflecting low intracellular carnitine content in muscle cells leading to impaired FAO. Prior to its inclusion in NBS programs, the clinical presentation in infants was that of a typical FAO disorder with hypoketotic hypoglycemia and a Reye-like syndrome triggered by an intermittent common illness, such as upper respiratory tract infections or gastroenteritis. In older patients involvement of heart and skeletal muscle are more prominent but combinations of these presentations also occur. Early diagnosis and carnitine supplementation are life-saving and prevent the occurrence of symptoms. A seemingly mild variant of CUD is now frequently identified in adult women through NBS of their heterozygous offspring (29, 30). Most of these women were asymptomatic or had nonspecific complaints such as decreased stamina or fasting intolerance, but one suffered syncope at 20 years of age, was diagnosed with prolonged QT interval causing ventricular tachycardia, and remained asymptomatic on carnitine supplementation (31). NBS in Minnesota revealed an incidence of CUD in newborns of 1 in 282,000 live births but a nearly 10-fold higher incidence of maternal CUD (1 in 22,500 live births).

Carnitine-Palmitoyltransferase I Deficiency

Only patients with the liver variant of carnitine-palmitoyltransferase I (CPT I) have been described. As with the other FAO disorders, the most severe form presents in early infancy with hypoketotic hypoglycemia or hepatic encephalopathy usually induced by febrile illness or prolonged fasting and poor feeding. Elevated concentrations of ammonia and liver enzymes (ALT, AST) are frequently found and coagulopathy is not uncommon. Heart and skeletal muscle are generally not affected, but renal tubular acidosis, possibly reflecting the expression of CPT1A in renal tubules, has been described (32, 33). Most of the patients not detected by NBS present in the first year of life. NBS has led to the identification of a high incidence among the Alaskan Inuit and the Canadian First Nations due to a founder effect (c.1436C > T, p.P479L) (34, 35). The clinical significance of this variant is uncertain. Most patients appear to remain asymptomatic, but recent studies have shown reduced fasting tolerance and suggested higher infant mortality

among homozygous carriers of the c.1436C > T mutation (34, 36). Another mutation, c.2129G > A (p.G710E) is common among North American Hutterites (37, 38) and is associated with the more severe phenotype unless recognized and treated early with frequent feedings of a high carbohydrate, low fat diet including medium-chain triglycerides (MCT). The prevalence of CPT IA among the general population is much lower (ca. 1:2 million live births) (28).

Carnitine-Acylcarnitine Translocase Deficiency

Carnitine-acylcarnitine translocase (CACT) is expressed in all tissues that use FAO as a source of energy and its deficiency presents early in life with cardiomyopathy and arrhythmia, liver failure, and skeletal myopathy reflected in similar laboratory findings as CPT I deficiency with additional elevation of creatine kinase, elevated long-chain acylcarnitines and low free carnitine. Patients presenting in the first days of life typically suffer higher mortality than those with later onset (39). Early, preferably presymptomatic initiation of a high carbohydrate, low-fat diet with predominantly MCTs and possibly L-carnitine supplementation facilitate effective treatment. While NBS can detect CACT deficiency with high sensitivity, the most severely affected patients may not be detected early enough to prevent metabolic decompensation or even death (7).

Carnitine-Palmitoyltransferase II Deficiency

Contrary to other FAO defects, carnitine-palmitoyltransferase II (CPT II) deficiency was first described in adolescent and adult patients who presented with muscle cramps, rhabdomyolysis and myoglobinuria following relatively intense exercise. Factors such as dehydration, excessive heat or cold exposure, and prolonged fasting can also provoke symptoms while patients remain asymptomatic when avoiding such stressors. In this adult-onset variant of CPT II deficiency, heart and liver are usually not affected. The neonatal form of CPT II deficiency presents in the first few days of life with liver failure, Reye-like encephalopathy, hypertrophic cardiomyopathy and often dysmorphism, renal cysts, and brain malformations; survival is rare (22). An intermediate variant of CPT II deficiency usually manifests before age 3 years with hypoketotic hypoglycemia during prolonged fasting or febrile illness. If not recognized and treated, a Reye-like syndrome, cardiomyopathy, and arrhythmia may ensue and prove fatal. A genotype–phenotype correlation has been observed with mutations leading to negligible enzyme activity being associated with the severe neonatal presentation (40). Adult-onset, myopathic CPT II deficiency is almost invariably caused by mutation c.338C > T (p.S113L) with high residual enzyme activity (40). Most of the patients with intermediate forms of the disease are compound heterozygotes for null and milder mutations. Treatment of the neonatal and infantile variants follows the same concept of the aforementioned FAO disorders (avoidance of fasting; high-carbohydrate, low-fat diet with predominant MCT). Medical treatment of myopathic CPT II deficiency with bezafibrate was proposed nearly a decade ago by Bastin and colleagues (41). They suggested that bezafibrate may boost residual CPT II activity through activation of the peroxisome proliferator-activated receptor alpha which participates in regulation of FAO enzyme expression. A clinical trial appears to support this hypothesis (42). Another approach to treatment was shown to be beneficial by Roe and colleagues. Treating seven patients for up to 5 years, they found that a triheptanoin-rich diet markedly improved exercise tolerance (43). The effect of triheptanoin is thought to lie in its role as a precursor of acetyl-CoA and propionyl-CoA, which when adequately available enhance Krebs cycle function and energy production. A clinical trial of this approach is currently ongoing in the United States (www.clinicaltrials.gov).

DEFECTS OF THE FAO SPIRAL

Very-Long-Chain Acyl-CoA Dehydrogenase Deficiency

Several patients with biochemical evidence of defective long-chain FAO were deemed affected with long-chain acyl-CoA dehydrogenase (LCAD) deficiency (44, 45). However, once LCAD and VLCAD genes were identified, these patients were reclassified as VLCAD deficient by molecular genetic analysis. VLCAD deficiency also has a variable phenotype, which is at least partly explained by genotype (46). Patients with the most severe variant usually present in the neonatal period and suffer high mortality due to severe nonketotic hypoglycemia, Reye-like illness, and cardiomyopathy. The intermediate phenotype presents in infancy or early childhood and is usually triggered by intercurrent febrile illness or prolonged fasting. Hypoketotic hypoglycemia, hepatomegaly, and myopathy are typical but cardiac involvement is variable. Chronic myopathy may be the only manifestation in adults with intermediate VLCAD deficiency. The late-onset variant appears to be limited to skeletal muscle involvement expressed as muscle pain, exercise intolerance, and rhabdomyolysis (46). VLCAD deficiency is included in all NBS programs in the USA and many other countries. Its early detection can significantly improve the prognosis through implementation of treatment corresponding to other long-chain FAO disorders. Treatment with a triheptanoin-rich diet was suggested by Roe and tested in three patients with early-onset VLCAD deficiency (47). A clinical trial of this approach is underway (www.clinicaltrials.gov).

Mitochondrial Trifunctional Protein Deficiency

Mitochondrial trifunctional protein (TFP) combines the last three steps of long-chain FAO and is an octamer of four alpha- and four beta-subunits, which are encoded by different genes. Most patients appear to be affected with isolated LCHAD deficiency as opposed to complete TFP deficiency. Isolated LCHAD deficiency was first described in 1989 (48) and was considered one of the more frequent FAO defects. More than 50% of patients are homozygous for a common mutation (c.1528G > C, p.E474Q) in the alpha-subunit gene (*HADHA*) (49, 50). Isolated LCHAD deficiency and the severe variant of complete TFP deficiency usually present in the first six months of life and, similar to other long-chain FAO disorders with hypoketotic hypoglycemia and a Reye-like syndrome, are precipitated by increased energy requirements due to prolonged fasting or intercurrent illness. More unique to LCHAD deficiency are occasional associations with jaundice due to cholestasis and hypocalcemia (51). Cardiomyopathy and arrhythmias are common and associated with high mortality. In fact, cardiopulmonary arrest or sudden unexpected death is frequently the first presentation, in particular where LCHAD and TFP deficiency are not included in NBS programs (51, 52). However, even where NBS affords early diagnosis and treatment, a significant number of patients will still develop symptoms, although fatal outcomes are rare (53).

A milder presentation of TFP deficiency has been described with gradual onset of clinical symptoms, including muscle hypotonia, cardiomyopathy, and failure to thrive (52). The third, and probably most common, phenotype is the late-onset myopathic form which presents similarly to adult-onset VLCAD and CPT II deficiencies (54, 55).

Unique to other FAO defects are the development of pigmentary retinitis and peripheral neuropathy in patients with isolated LCHAD and complete TFP deficiencies. Patients may develop progressive chorioretinopathy as early as 4 months of age, leading to retinal atrophy, and loss of vision (52, 56, 57). Peripheral sensorimotor polyneuropathy often occurs in association with limb-girdle myopathy and recurrent myoglobinuria (58–61). Muscle biopsies reveal muscle fiber atrophy consistent with a denervating process (54). This complication is more often observed in patients with the milder neuromyopathic phenotype of TFP deficiency than with isolated LCHAD deficiency (51).

Medium-Chain Acyl-CoA Dehydrogenase Deficiency

As implied by its name, medium-chain acyl-CoA dehydrogenase (MCAD) deficiency affects the oxidation of medium-chain fatty acyl-CoA (C_{12}–C_6) (62). Accordingly, the first few turns of the FAO spiral are intact, thereby allowing for production of some acetyl-CoA. Thus, some ketone production is expected with a few patients presenting with seemingly normal ketogenic response to fasting (63). During periods of increased energy demand, however, the lack of sufficient production of acetyl-CoA leads to insufficient production of ketone bodies and secondary inhibition of gluconeogenesis resulting in hypoketosis and increased utilization of glucose and hypoglycemia.

Before MCAD deficiency's inclusion in NBS programs the first metabolic crisis usually occurred before two years old (64); however, the first presentation can occur throughout life, whenever a patient is exposed to a significant stressor, such as common intercurrent illnesses associated with prolonged fasting and higher energy requirements leading to vomiting, lethargy, and sometimes seizures. If not already diagnosed, at least 18% of affected individuals die during their first metabolic crisis which may be in adulthood (19, 64–66). A Reye-like syndrome is often

part of the clinical presentation but hypoglycemia is not always documented. When surviving a life-threatening presentation and presumably due to resulting brain injury, long-term neurological impairment, including aphasia and attention deficit disorder, are frequent (67). Chronic muscle weakness is observed in nearly 20% of patients with a history of a severe episode (64).

NBS has significantly improved the outcome of MCAD deficiency; however, vigilance remains required because some patients present before NBS results are reported. In a cohort of 41 newborns with MCAD deficiency identified by NBS none experienced hypoglycemia, although some required treatment or hospitalization during intercurrent illness (68). NBS has also uncovered more than the expected cases of MCAD deficiency, many of which have a less pronounced biochemical phenotype.

Nearly 100 ACADM mutations are known while one mutation, c.985A > G (p.K329E), has been reported to account for 70% of alleles in individuals with MCAD deficiency based on newborn screening and clinical testing results in diverse populations (69). The milder biochemical phenotype is associated with compound heterozygosity for K329E (30%–40%) and or genotypes that do not involve the common mutation (10%–30%) (70–73). The clinical risk associated with these alterations remains uncertain, but to dismiss such cases as risk free is unwarranted (74). More importantly, it is essential to remember that environmental or circumstantial stressors are likely the most important morbidity determining factors in all MCAD cases independent of genotype or age.

Medium-Chain 3-Ketoacyl-CoA Thiolase Deficiency

Only a single case of medium-chain 3-ketoacyl-CoA thiolase (MCKAT) deficiency has been described. The Japanese male neonate died shortly after presenting at 2 days of age with vomiting, dehydration, metabolic acidosis, liver dysfunction, and rhabdomyolysis (75). Urine organic acid analysis revealed ketotic lactic aciduria and significant C_6–C_{12} dicarboxylic aciduria, with C_{10} and C_{12} species being most prominent. Although additional cases have not been reported in the literature, the lack of specific biochemical and molecular testing makes it likely that this disorder is underdiagnosed.

Short-Chain Acyl-CoA Dehydrogenase Deficiency

In short-chain acyl-CoA dehydrogenase (SCAD) deficiency ketogenesis and energy production are not significantly impaired given that primarily the dehydrogenation of butyryl(C_4)-CoA is affected (62). Of the first two patients reported both excreted significant ethylmalonic acid (EMA) and one died during the neonatal period, whereas the other suffered only one metabolic decompensation in the newborn period and remained asymptomatic thereafter (76). EMA is derived from the accumulating butyryl-CoA that is carboxylated by propionyl-CoA carboxylase to EMA. A variety of symptoms have been described in SCAD deficient patients, the most common being developmental delay and muscle hypotonia (77). Interestingly, most patients identified through NBS remain asymptomatic. Clinically ascertained patients with SCAD deficiency tend to present in childhood but van Maldegem and colleagues found during follow-up of 31 patients for one to 18 years progressive deterioration in two, no change in 12, improvement in eight, and complete recovery in nine patients (78). Furthermore, asymptomatic individuals, including adults, meeting the same biochemical and molecular criteria for SCAD deficiency as their relatives have been reported (79). The inclusion of SCAD deficiency in NBS programs therefore raised questions about the clinical significance of this condition, leading some programs to not screen for it (80). Furthermore, several clinically identified patients had normal NBS results suggesting that SCAD deficiency is the only FAO defect included in NBS that is associated with poor screening sensitivity (81). More then 40 different mutations have been described in ACADS, most being missense substitutions or in frame deletions (77). Two alterations, c.625G > A (p.G209S) and c.511C > T (p.R171W), are present in high frequency in the general population with prevalence of homozygosity of 5.5% and 0.3% respectively, and an overall frequency of these variants in either homozygous or compound heterozygous form in 7% of the population (79, 82). These alterations affect the proper folding or the (thermo)stability of the mature SCAD protein but do not cause significant deficiency of SCAD activity. Nevertheless, they have been found in homozygous or combined heterozygous genotypes of 56% of clinically ascertained patients regardless of the severity of the clinical phenotype (77) but less frequently in NBS because they are associated with butyrylcarnitine concentrations that remain below most NBS laboratory's cut off values (82). Given the uncertainty of SCAD deficiency being a disease entity in itself, it is increasingly recommended to pursue different or additional diagnoses to explain the clinical phenotype of patients with biochemical and molecular evidence of SCAD deficiency (79, 81).

Short-Chain 3-Hydroxyacyl-CoA Dehydrogenase Deficiency

Short-chain 3-hydroxyacyl-CoA dehydrogenase (SCHAD) catalyzes the third step in the FAO cycle of short- and medium-chain fatty acids (C_4–C_{14}) and therefore is sometimes referred to as medium-/short-chain 3-hydroxy acyl-CoA dehydrogenase (M/SCHAD). Curiously, it has two very different presentations. One is more consistent with that of other FAO defects with prominent liver disease, including a Reye-like syndrome (83); the other is characterized by hyperinsulinemic hypoglycemia (84). The latter phenotype is explained by the absent inhibitory action of SCHAD on glutamate dehydrogenase (GDH) in pancreatic islet cells where SCHAD is highly expressed. Activation of GDH by ADP and leucine increases insulin secretion which in the absence of SCHAD's inhibition of GDH causes hyperinsulinism and hypoglycemia (85). This phenotype appears to be associated with complete absence of the SCHAD protein whereas protein with residual enzyme activity is present in patients with the hepatic phenotype (83). Less than 20 cases with SCHAD deficiency have been described; most present during the first year of life and NBS should identify this condition based on elevated concentrations of 3-hydroxy butyrylcarnitine (C_4-OH) (86). Other typical laboratory findings include hyperinsulinemic hypoglycemia and overexcretion of urinary 3-hydroxy butyric acid (in the absence of acetoacetic acid) and 3-hydroxy glutaric acid. Patients typically respond to treatment with diazoxide; however, to avoid long-term neurological deficits treatment must be initiated early.

Glutaric Acidemia Type II

ETF and ETF-DH are involved in FAO only indirectly because they accept electrons from the FAD dependent acyl-CoA dehydrogenases (Figure 8.1). Therefore, glutaric acidemia type II (GA II), caused by either deficiency, is also known as multiple acyl-CoA dehydrogenase deficiency (MADD). The most severely affected patients present in the neonatal period with congenital anomalies, dysmorphic features reminiscent of peroxisomal disorders, hypotonia, hypoglycemia, metabolic acidosis, and often a sweaty-feet-like odor. The latter is explained by the secondary dysfunction of isovaleryl-CoA dehydrogenase (the enzyme deficient in isovaleric acidemia) which also requires ETF as electron acceptor. Due to the often severe congenital anomalies, affected patients usually do not survive the neonatal period. A second variant of GA II also presents in the newborn period, but is not associated with congenital anomalies. Affected patients may live beyond infancy but typically die during an acute metabolic decompensation and/or due to the development of a cardiomyopathy independent of treatment which includes avoidance of fasting, a diet low in fat and isoleucine, and supplementation with riboflavin and L-carnitine. Treatment with methylene blue as an alternative electron acceptor has also been proposed (15). A third phenotype presents after the neonatal period with potentially fatal episodes of vomiting, hypoglycemia, hepatomegaly, and myopathy. Treatment is identical to that of patients with severe GA II and without congenital anomalies, but significant morbidity and mortality cannot always be prevented. Other patients present as late as early adulthood, primarily with a myopathy affecting proximal muscles of the extremities and the neck. Some of these patients have a history of myalgia and cyclic vomiting typically associated with episodes of higher energy demands such as intercurrent illness. This mildest variant of GA II responds to supplements with riboflavin, a cofactor for ETF and ETF-DH (87). More recently a transient presentation of GA II was reported in the neonate of a mother who was found to be riboflavin deficient due to mutations in a riboflavin transporter (88). Finally, a clinical and biochemical phenocopy of GA II is Jamaican vomiting sickness which is caused by ingestion of an unripe Jamaican fruit (ackee) (89).

2,3-Dienoyl-CoA Reductase Deficiency

A single patient with biochemical and enzymatic evidence of 2,3-dienoyl-CoA reductase (DER) was described by Roe et al (90). The patient presented with sepsis in the first days of life, remained hypotonic with poor feeding requiring gastrostomy, and died at 4 months of age after developing respiratory acidosis which did not respond to treatment. The diagnosis was suggested by the identification of 2-*trans*,4-*cis*-decadienoylcarnitine (C10:2-carnitine) in plasma and urine by acylcarnitine analysis. No additional patient has been identified, although acylcarnitine analysis is typically included in the laboratory work up of patients presenting as the index case.

"NEW" FAO DISORDERS

ACAD9 Deficiency

ACAD9, an acyl-CoA dehydrogenase with substrate specificity toward unsaturated very long-chain acyl-CoA species is expressed in multiple tissues, including the brain (62, 91). Three patients presenting with either a Reye-like syndrome and cerebellar stroke, recurrent episodes of acute and fulminant liver disease, or cardiomyopathy were described in 2007 (92). More recently, two different groups linked ACAD9 to complex I of the respiratory chain complex and reported four more patients who presented with cardiomyopathy, encephalopathy, and persistent lactic acidosis (93, 94). Treatment with multivitamins appeared to be beneficial in these patients (94).

Long-Chain Acyl-CoA Dehydrogenase Deficiency

Although a number of patients have been described as LCAD deficient in the early 1990s, their diagnoses were revised to VLCAD deficiency when immunoblot and molecular genetic analyses revealed the true etiology (45). Nearly two decades later and given the fact that LCAD is highly expressed in type II pneumocytes, Vockley and colleagues investigated a newborn with respiratory distress syndrome of unknown cause and found lacking LCAD antigen in lung tissue and a homozygous mutation in exon 6 of ACADL that causes a splicing error (95).

Pregnancy Complications and FAO Disorders

Defects in FAO have been associated with maternal and fetal complications. In particular acute fatty liver of pregnancy (AFLP), the HELLP syndrome (hemolysis, elevated liver enzymes, and low platelets) and pree-clampsia have been observed in heterozygous mothers whose offspring were later diagnosed primarily with isolated LCHAD deficiency. Such maternal pregnancy complications were more rarely reported in other fetal FAO defects including CPT I, TFP, MCAD, and SCAD deficiencies (96). A case–control study by Browning and colleagues found 16% of pregnancies carrying a fetus with an FAO disorder were associated with maternal liver disease, with long-chain FAO defects having a 50-fold higher risk of gestational complications and other FAO disorders a 12-fold higher risk compared to pregnancies of healthy fetuses (97). HELLP syndrome and especially AFLP are serious complications of the third trimester and usually preceded by hypertension and proteinuria resembling preeclampsia. The most effective treatment is delivery of the fetus to avoid liver and renal failure, coagulopathy, and even encephalopathy and death. These complications appear to affect mostly primigravidae and have prevalences of ca. 1:15,000 (AFLP) to 1:500 (HELLP) deliveries (98).

LABORATORY DIAGNOSIS OF FAO DISORDERS

FOLLOW UP OF ABNORMAL NEWBORN SCREENING RESULTS

Five FAO disorders (CUD, VLCAD, LCHAD, TFP, and MCAD deficiencies) are included in all NBS programs in the United States. Most states also screen for an additional seven conditions (SCAD, M/SCHAD, MCKAT, CACT, CPT II, CPT Ia, and DER deficiencies). Diagnostic algorithms have been prepared by the American College of Medical Genetics to provide guidance to the rapid laboratory evaluation of newborns with presumptive positive screening results (99). The importance of prompt follow up on suggestive screening results cannot be overemphasized given the potential of acute metabolic decompensation and sudden unexpected death in these conditions. Furthermore, care needs to be taken not to consider uninformative or "normal" follow up biochemical testing results as sufficient evidence to rule out a diagnosis of several FAO disorders, in particular VLCAD deficiency (100). Normal laboratory results are not unusual in affected patients who are in stable metabolic, particularly anabolic, condition which is expected in well-fed newborns.

SYMPTOMATIC PATIENTS WITH FAO DISORDERS

Figure 8.2 provides a basic diagnostic algorithm. Of foremost importance is the consideration of an underlying FAO disorder in patients of all ages and with a variety of symptoms ranging from nonspecific muscle fatigue to life-threatening metabolic crises. Particularly during a metabolic decompensation sample collection should occur immediately along with treatment initiation, and even in newborns care providers should not rely on or wait for NBS results. The finding of hypoglycemia with a disproportionately low ketone response (low blood glucose and negative to small urine ketones on urine test strip) is highly suspicious and can be determined in most clinic environments. Of note, the absence of this finding does not rule out a possible FAO disorder, in particular those affecting the metabolism of medium and short chain fatty acids. Liver enzymes, lactate, ammonia, and creatine kinase may be markedly abnormal. Once an FAO disorder is suspected urine and blood should be sent for more specialized biochemical investigations, particularly plasma carnitine, acylcarnitine and fatty acid profiles as well as urine organic acid and acylglycine analyses (Table 8.1). The likelihood of informative results is highest when samples are collected prior to treatment initiation. As indicated above, uninformative test results cannot necessarily be considered sufficient to rule out the possibility of an underlying FAO disorder. Fasting challenges in undiagnosed patients, when well, with a history of previous suspicious metabolic decompensation but uninformative biochemical results, may be useful but should only occur under close observation and following placement of an IV line to administer dextrose in case of an acute drop in glucose. Blood should be collected for the above-mentioned investigations when blood glucose drops below 45 mg/dL or any hypoglycemic symptoms develop and before glucose or food are given. However, given the risk and effort necessary for fasting challenges, in particular when the patient is very young, in vitro methods using fibroblast cultures derived from a small skin biopsy may be more appropriate. Once obtained, fibroblast cultures can be grown for a variety of functional screening tests, enzyme, transport, and immunoassays, and as a source of DNA for molecular genetic analyses. Obvious limitations of fibroblast cultures are the possibility that the affected enzyme is not expressed in this tissue, extended turnaround time

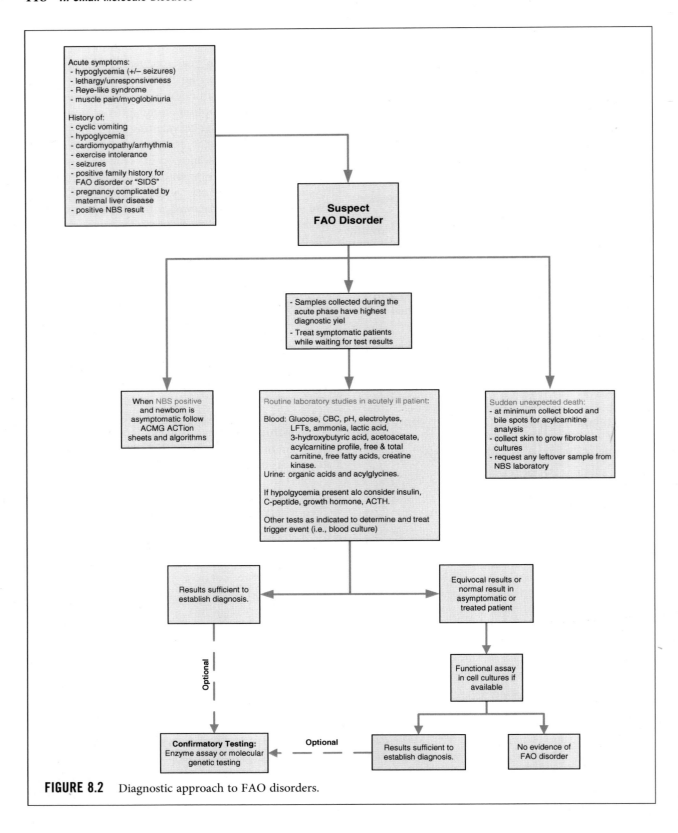

FIGURE 8.2 Diagnostic approach to FAO disorders.

TABLE 8.1   Diagnostic Laboratory Investigations With Likely Informative Results In FAO Disorders

FAO Disorders	OMIM	Plasma		Urine		WBC or Fibroblast Cultures			Newborn Screening	Prenatal Diagnosis§	Postmortem Screening (Blood, bile)
		Free Carnitine	Acylcarnitine Profile	Organic Acids	Acylglycines	Screening Assay	Enzyme Assay	Molecular Analysis			
CUD	212140	Low	N	N	N	−	+	+	+	+	+
CPT IA	255120	N/High	LCAC low	N	N	±	+	+	+	+	+
CPT II (lethal neonatal)	608836	N/Low	C16–C18	N	N	+	+	+	+	+	+
CPT II (infantile)	600649										
CPT II (myopathic)	255110								±		
CACT	212138	N/Low	C16–C18	N	N	+		+	+	+	+
Isolated LCHAD	609016	N/Low	LCOHAC ±LCAC	+	N	+	+	+	+	+	+
TFP	609015						−	+	+	+	+
VLCAD	201475	N/Low	C14:1	(+)	N	+	+	+	+	+	+
MCAD	201450	N/Low	C6 < C8 > C10	(+)	HG ±SG, OG, (PPG)	+	+	+	+	+	+
MCKAT	602199	N/Low	? (C8–C12)	(+)	N	−	−	−	±	−	−
SCAD	201470	N/Low	C4	+	EMA ± MSA	+	−	+	+	+	±
M/SCHAD (HADH)	231530	N/Low	C4-OH	(+)	N	−	−	+	±	+	±
GA II	231680	N/Low	variable#	(+)	EMA, MSA, IVG, GA, HG, OG, SG	±	+	+	+	+	+
2,4-Dienoyl-CoA reductase deficiency	222745	N/Low	C10:2	N	N	−	−	+	±	+	±
ACAD9	611126	N/Low	N	(+)	N	−	−	+	+		−

*For availability see www.genetests.org; §, prenatal diagnosis may be available but indication is questionable for treatable conditions (eg, MCAD) or conditions of uncertain significance (eg, SCAD); #, elevations of multiple acylcarnitines with chain length >C4 are typical but not observed in all cases; (+), may be normal when patient is well; EMA, ethylmalonic acid; GA, glutaric acid; HG, hexanoylglycine; IVG, isovalerylglycine; LCAC, long-chain acylcarnitines; LCOHAC, long-chain hydroxy-acylcarnitines; MSA, methylsuccinic acid; N, normal; OG, octanoylglycine; PPG, phenylpropionylglycine; SG, suberylglycine; WBC, white blood cells.

due to the time required for culturing a sufficient amount of cells for testing, and the availability of tests in only a few specialized laboratories. Liver and muscle biopsies can also be necessary to establish or confirm a diagnosis by specific enzyme assays. An intriguing alternative to these biochemical assays is the increasing availability of molecular genetic testing for most FAO disorders in blood samples. However, this approach is not yet a reasonable, cost-effective option when evaluating a patient without at least somewhat suggestive biochemical blood and urine studies. Accordingly, molecular genetic analysis in FAO disorders is primarily of value for the confirmation of a particular diagnosis that is only suggested but not proven through biochemical testing, to determine risk in an asymptomatic sibling of an affected and genotyped patient, and for prenatal diagnosis (101). Furthermore, the still frequent identification of new, previously not reported mutations commonly referred to as "variants of uncertain significance" can lead to diagnostic uncertainties, in particular in asymptomatic patients identified through NBS (73). Information about which laboratories offer biochemical and molecular genetic testing for FAO disorders can currently be found at www.genetests.org and in the near future at a new Genetic Testing Registry (www.ncbi.nlm.nih. gov/gtr). Communication between clinicians and laboratorians should be encouraged as it can be essential to ensure appropriate testing (correct test using correct specimen), a rapid diagnosis, and clarification of (equivocal) test results.

POSTMORTEM TESTING

Given that FAO disorders can manifest with sudden unexpected death, postmortem investigations to exclude these conditions in such cases are important to consider to provide closure and counseling to the surviving family members (102, 103). Tissues, including skin to grow fibroblast cultures can be collected and used for functional or specific assays (103). However, before such samples are submitted for testing, blood and bile spotted and dried on filter paper for acylcarnitine analysis represent a more economical means for postmortem diagnosis (104). In case postmortem samples were not taken or permission not given by a deceased patient's family, retrieval of the unused and potentially still available portion of the NBS sample from the relevant screening laboratory

could be arranged with the family's consent for retrospective acylcarnitine analysis (105). If neither postmortem nor leftover NBS samples are available for testing of the deceased patient, a biochemical work-up of first-degree relatives should be considered. Although this approach must take into consideration the potentially concealed biochemical phenotype, it has been effective for several FAO disorders (103).

TREATMENT

When it comes to treatment of FAO disorders, the approach can be divided based on the clinical presentation: the acutely ill patient, the asymptomatic/metabolically stable patient, and the patient with cardio/myopathic symptoms. Furthermore, every patient should be equipped with a written treatment plan for sick days and carry an emergency bracelet.

TREATMENT OF THE ACUTELY ILL PATIENT

The foremost goal of treatment of the acutely ill patient is the reversal of catabolism in a hospital setting. If the ill patient is able to tolerate oral feeds, glucose polymers by mouth and observation may be sufficient. Otherwise, intravenous glucose administration with appropriate electrolytes is required to correct hypoglycemia and stimulate insulin secretion which will suppress lipolysis. This will reduce the need for FAO thereby decreasing the accumulation of toxic fatty acid metabolites. Glucose is usually given as 10% dextrose at a rate of 10 to 12 mg/kg/min to achieve blood glucose concentrations of at least 5 mmol/L (22). A central line may be required for high concentration glucose infusions. If oral intake cannot resume within 24 hours, additional provision of amino acids is required to support anabolism. Intralipids should be avoided and for long-chain FAO disorders be given as MCT. Appropriate treatment of the condition that caused the metabolic decompensation is of course also essential.

TREATMENT OF THE ASYMPTOMATIC PATIENT

Treatment of the asymptomatic patient, nowadays typically identified through NBS, consists primarily in the avoidance of fasting and dietary modification in patients with long-chain FAO disorders. Patients with the latter should obtain fat primarily in the form of MCT with supplementation of essential long-chain fatty acids. The time interval between meals is age dependent: infants less than 6 months old should not go without feeding for more than 3 to 4 hours, between 6 and 12 months old not to exceed 4 to 8 hours, in the second year of life up to 10 hours and thereafter up to 12 hours (106, 107). During the day, however, and based on activity level and overall metabolic status, additional snacks may be required. A bedtime snack of uncooked cornstarch may be necessary to prevent hypoglycemia overnight and to avoid waking the patient for intermittent feedings. Prevention or at least delay of the development of retinopathy in patients with LCHAD and TFP deficiencies may be possible with strict adherence to a low-fat diet supplemented with MCT oil. Supplementation with docosahexanoic acid (DHA) may provide additional support in the avoidance of a retinopathy (57, 108).

Carnitine supplementation had initially been a staple in the treatment of FAO disorders. However, no significant benefit or preventive effect has been shown incontrovertibly to be facilitated by its indiscriminate use with the important exception of carnitine transporter deficiency for which L-carnitine supplementation is essential (100 mg/kg/d divided in three doses). Two exercise studies in MCAD deficient patients before and after L-carnitine supplementation suggested improved exercise tolerance with supplementation of 100 mg/kg/day (109) and statistically insignificant benefit with supplementation of 50 mg/kg/day (110). In a controlled fasting challenge of MCAD deficient patients L-carnitine supplementation had no beneficial effect (111). Treatment of a patient with CACT deficiency with a fat-restricted diet, MCT oil and L-carnitine supplementation led to reversal of symptoms which included cardiomyopathy, arrhythmia and nonketotic hypoglycemia (112). In light of these uncertainties, a pragmatic approach may be to supplement at least temporarily those patients with L-carnitine who have low plasma levels of free carnitine (100).

TREATMENT OF THE MYOPATHIC PATIENT

The simplest treatment of myopathic patients with exercise intolerance associated with muscle pain and rhabdomyolysis is avoidance of exercise. However,

because of the general health benefits of physical activity this is not recommended (107). Patients with myopathic FAO disorders should avoid extreme cold and heat, and when exercising for longer periods should take time to rest and to rehydrate. In addition, Gillingham and colleagues have shown that LCHAD and TFP patients who took MCT supplements prior to exercise had lower long-chain hydroxyacylcarnitines, higher ketones and an improved steady-state heart rate than without supplementation (113).

"NEW" TREATMENTS

Additional treatment options are currently in clinical trials (for information see: www.clinicaltrials.gov). These include supplementation with triheptanoic acid and bezafibrate as mentioned above (see CPT II deficiency, VLCAD deficiency). Gene therapy has been suggested and shown promise in studies in fibroblast cultures of a patient with MCAD deficiency and in in vivo experiments in VLCAD, LCAD, and SCAD deficient mouse models, respectively (114–117).

FOLLOW UP AND MONITORING

Once diagnosed and treated, follow up should occur based on the particular condition and the patient's age. Young patients are typically seen every few months to ensure: prevention or improvement of symptoms, such as cardiomyopathy and retinopathy; appropriate growth and development; dietary evaluation (preferably by an experienced dietitian); and continued education and support of the patient's family. The patient's history and clinical evaluation have the highest impact and including the review of educational assessments (day-care, pre-school, kindergarten, school) can provide important insight into the patient's development (118). A few laboratory parameters are considered helpful in determining the patient's metabolic status. Normal or near normal 3-hydroxyacylcarnitines in LCHAD and TFP deficient patients have been associated with improved retinal function and slower progression of the peripheral neuropathy. Creatine kinase should be checked in patients with myopathic symptoms. Monitoring and dietary supplementation of essential FA, in particular docosahexanoic acid (DHA), may help in preventing or slowing the development of the retinopathy observed in LCHAD and TFP deficiencies, but should also be included in the follow up of any patient with fat-restriction and supplementation of MCT (57). Carnitine monitoring is essential in CUD and of limited value in the other conditions. Consultation with other specialists including cardiologists, neurologists, ophthalmologists, physical, occupational and speech therapists, social workers, and others should be considered at each visit. A cardiology exam should probably occur at least once a year in patients with conditions associated with cardiac involvement (118).

CLINICAL PEARLS

1. Mitochondrial fatty acid beta-oxidation (FAO) plays an important role in energy homeostasis during times of increased demand (fever, exercise, etc.) or decreased supply (prolonged fasting) by providing acetyl-CoA and reducing equivalents.
2. FAO disorders primarily affect organs and tissues with high energy requirements and limited back-up mechanisms during periods of metabolic stress (liver, heart, brain, kidneys).
3. FAO disorders can present at any age.
4. Acute metabolic decompensation is characterized by hypoketotic hypoglycemia, a Reye-like syndrome with or without cardiomyopathy and arrhythmia, and rhabdomyolysis. Seizures may be a presenting sign.
5. Treatment aims to avoid fasting by frequent feedings of a low-fat, carbohydrate-rich diet.
6. Physical activity should not be discouraged but patients with myopathy may need to take MCT-rich snacks prior to exercising.
7. Treatment trials are currently underway for some FAO disorders (see: www.clinicaltrials.gov).
8. Informative laboratory studies are best achieved in blood and urine samples collected when the patient is symptomatic.
9. Relevant laboratory investigations include plasma glucose, free fatty acids, creatine kinase, liver function tests, ketone bodies, insulin, free and total carnitine, and acylcarnitines, as well as urine organic acid and acylglycine analyses.
10. Confirmation of a diagnosis can be achieved by enzymatic and molecular genetic studies.

REFERENCES

1. Taylor S. Insulin action, insulin resistance, and Type 2 diabetes mellitus. In: DBA Valle, B Vogelstein, KW Kinzler, et al. eds. *Scriver's Online Metabolic and Molecular Bases of Inherited Disease*; 2006.
2. Holm C, Kirchgessner TG, Svenson KL, et al. Hormone-sensitive lipase: Sequence, expression, and chromosomal localization to 19 cent-q13.3. *Science.* 1988;241:1503–1506.
3. Hamilton JA, Guo W, Kamp F. Mechanism of cellular uptake of long-chain fatty acids: Do we need cellular proteins? *Mol Cell Biochem.* 2002;239:17–23.
4. Richieri GV, Kleinfeld AM. Unbound free fatty acid levels in human serum. *J Lipid Res.* 1995;36:229–240.
5. Schaap FG, Binas B, Danneberg H, et al. Impaired long-chain fatty acid utilization by cardiac myocytes isolated from mice lacking the heart-type fatty acid binding protein gene. *Circ Res.* 1999;85:329–337.
6. Soupene E, Kuypers FA. Mammalian long-chain acyl-CoA synthetases. *Exp Biol Med (Maywood).* 2008;233:507–521.
7. Longo N, Amat di San Filippo C, Pasquali M. Disorders of carnitine transport and the carnitine cycle. *Am J Med Genet C Seminars Med Genetics.* 2006;142C:77–85.
8. Britton CH, Mackey DW, Esser V, et al. Fine chromosome mapping of the genes for human liver and muscle carnitine palmitoyltransferase I (CPT1A and CPT1B). *Genomics.* 1997;40:209–211.
9. Price N, van der Leij F, Jackson V, et al. A novel brain-expressed protein related to carnitine palmitoyltransferase I. *Genomics.* 2002;80:433–442.
10. Wolfgang MJ, Lane MD. Hypothalamic malonyl-CoA and CPT1c in the treatment of obesity. *FEBS J.* 2011;278:552–558.
11. Gao XF, Chen W, Kong XP, et al. Enhanced susceptibility of Cpt1c knockout mice to glucose intolerance induced by a high-fat diet involves elevated hepatic gluconeogenesis and decreased skeletal muscle glucose uptake. *Diabetologia.* 2009;52:912–920.
12. Wolfgang MJ, Kurama T, Dai Y, et al. The brain-specific carnitine palmitoyltransferase-1c regulates energy homeostasis. *Proc Natl Acad Sci USA.* 2006;103:7282–7287.
13. Houten SM, Wanders RJ. A general introduction to the biochemistry of mitochondrial fatty acid beta-oxidation. *J Inherit Metab Dis.* 2010;33:469–477.
14. Rinaldo P, Matern D, Bennett MJ. Fatty acid oxidation disorders. *Annu Rev Physiol.* 2002;64:477–502.
15. Frerman FE, Goodman SI. Defects of the electron transfer flavoprotein and electron transfer flavoprotein-ubiquinone oxidoreductase: Glutaric acidemia type II. In: CR Scriver, AL Beaudet, WS Sly, et al. eds. *The Metabolic and Molecular Bases of Inherited Diseases.* 8th ed. New York: McGraw-Hill; 2001:2357–2365.
16. Janssen U, Fink T, Lichter P, et al. Human mitochondrial 3,2-trans-enoyl-CoA isomerase (DCI): Gene structure and localization to chromosome 16p13.3. *Genomics.* 1994;23:223–228.
17. Helander HM, Koivuranta KT, Horelli-Kuitunen N, et al. Molecular cloning and characterization of the human

mitochondrial 2,4-dienoyl-CoA reductase gene (DECR). *Genomics.* 1997;46:112–119.

18. Yang BZ, Heng HH, Ding JH, et al. The genes for the alpha and beta subunits of the mitochondrial trifunctional protein are both located in the same region of human chromosome 2p23. *Genomics.* 1996;37:141–143.

19. Raymond K, Bale AE, Barnes CA, et al. Medium-chain acyl-CoA dehydrogenase deficiency: Sudden and unexpected death of a 45 year old woman. *Genet Med.* 1999;1:293–294.

20. Rinaldo P, Stanley CA, Hsu BY, et al. Sudden neonatal death in carnitine transporter deficiency. *J Pediatr.* 1997;131: 304–305.

21. Boles RG, Buck EA, Blitzer MG, et al. Retrospective biochemical screening of fatty acid oxidation disorders in postmortem livers of 418 cases of sudden death in the first year of life. *J Pediatr.* 1998;132:924–933.

22. Saudubray JM, Martin D, de Lonlay P, et al. Recognition and management of fatty acid oxidation defects: A series of 107 patients. *J Inherit Metab Dis.* 1999;22:488–502.

23. Fink R, Luttgau HC. An evaluation of the membrane constants and the potassium conductance in metabolically exhausted muscle fibres. *J Physiol.* 1976;263:215–238.

24. Tein I. Role of carnitine and fatty acid oxidation and its defects in infantile epilepsy. *J Child Neurol.* 2002;17(Suppl 3):3S57–3S82; discussion 3S-3.

25. Lopaschuk GD, Ussher JR, Folmes CD, et al. Myocardial fatty acid metabolism in health and disease. *Physiol Rev.* 2010;90: 207–258.

26. Huss JM, Kelly DP. Mitochondrial energy metabolism in heart failure: A question of balance. *J Clin Invest.* 2005;115:547–555.

27. Huang JM, Xian H, Bacaner M. Long-chain fatty acids activate calcium channels in ventricular myocytes. *Proc Natl Acad Sci USA.* 1992;89:6452–6456.

28. Lindner M, Hoffmann GF, Matern D. Newborn screening for disorders of fatty-acid oxidation: Experience and recommendations from an expert meeting. *J Inherit Metab Dis.* 2010;33:521–526.

29. Schimmenti LA, Crombez EA, Schwahn BC, et al. Expanded newborn screening identifies maternal primary carnitine deficiency. *Mol Genet Metab.* 2007;90:441–445.

30. El-Hattab AW, Li FY, Shen J, et al. Maternal systemic primary carnitine deficiency uncovered by newborn screening: Clinical, biochemical, and molecular aspects. *Genet Med.* 2010;12: 19–24.

31. Sarafoglou K, Tridgell AH, Bentler K, et al. Cardiac conduction improvement in two heterozygotes for primary carnitine deficiency on L-carnitine supplementation. *Clinical Genetics.* 2010;78:191–194.

32. Falik-Borenstein ZC, Jordan SC, Saudubray JM, et al. Brief report: Renal tubular acidosis in carnitine palmitoyltransferase type 1 deficiency. *N Engl J Med.* 1992;327:24–27.

33. Bergman AJ, Donckerwolcke RA, Duran M, et al. Rate-dependent distal renal tubular acidosis and carnitine palmitoyltransferase I deficiency. *Pediatr Res.* 1994;36:582–588.

34. Gessner BD, Gillingham MB, Johnson MA, et al. Prevalence and distribution of the c.1436C- > T sequence variant of carnitine palmitoyltransferase 1A among Alaska Native infants. *J Pediatr.* 2011;158:124–129.

35. Collins SA, Sinclair G, McIntosh S, et al. Carnitine palmitoyltransferase 1A (CPT1A) P479L prevalence in live newborns in Yukon, Northwest Territories, and Nunavut. *Mol Genet Metab.* 2010;101:200–204.

36. Gillingham MB, Hirschfeld M, Lowe S, et al. Impaired fasting tolerance among Alaska native children with a common carnitine palmitoyltransferase 1A sequence variant. *Mol GenetMetab.* 2011;104:261–264.

37. Prip-Buus C, Thuillier L, Abadi N, et al. Molecular and enzymatic characterization of a unique carnitine palmitoyltransferase 1A mutation in the Hutterite community. *Mol Genet Metab.* 2001;73:46–54.

38. Prasad C, Johnson JP, Bonnefont JP, et al. Hepatic carnitine palmitoyl transferase 1 (CPT1 A) deficiency in North American Hutterites (Canadian and American): Evidence for a founder effect and results of a pilot study on a DNA-based newborn screening program. *Mol Genet Metab.* 2001;73: 55–63.

39. Rubio-Gozalbo ME, Bakker JA, Waterham HR, et al. Carnitine-acylcarnitine translocase deficiency, clinical, biochemical and genetic aspects. *Mol Aspects Med.* 2004;25: 521–532.

40. Bonnefont JP, Djouadi F, Prip-Buus C, et al. Carnitine palmitoyltransferases 1 and 2: Biochemical, molecular and medical aspects. *Mol Aspects Med.* 2004;25:495–520.

41. Djouadi F, Bonnefont JP, Thuillier L, et al. Correction of fatty acid oxidation in carnitine palmitoyl transferase 2-deficient cultured skin fibroblasts by bezafibrate. *Pediatr Res.* 2003;54:446–451.

42. Bonnefont JP, Bastin J, Laforet P, et al. Long-term follow-up of bezafibrate treatment in patients with the myopathic form of carnitine palmitoyltransferase 2 deficiency. *Clin Pharmacol Ther.* 2010;88:101–108.

43. Roe CR, Yang BZ, Brunengraber H, et al. Carnitine palmitoyltransferase II deficiency: Successful anaplerotic diet therapy. *Neurology.* 2008;71:260–264.

44. Hale DE, Batshaw ML, Coates PM, et al. Long-chain acyl coenzyme A dehydrogenase deficiency: An inherited cause of nonketotic hypoglycemia. *Pediatr Res.* 1985;19:666–671.

45. Yamaguchi S, Indo Y, Coates PM, et al. Identification of very-long-chain acyl-CoA dehydrogenase deficiency in three patients previously diagnosed with long-chain acyl-CoA dehydrogenase deficiency. *Pediatr Res.* 1993;34:111–113.

46. Andresen BS, Olpin S, Poorthuis BJ, et al. Clear correlation of genotype with disease phenotype in very-long-chain acyl-CoA dehydrogenase deficiency. *Am J Hum Genet.* 1999;64:479–494.

47. Roe CR, Sweetman L, Roe DS, et al. Treatment of cardiomyopathy and rhabdomyolysis in long-chain fat oxidation disorders using an anaplerotic odd-chain triglyceride. *J Clin Invest.* 2002;110:259–69.

48. Wanders RJ, Duran M, Ijlst L, et al. Sudden infant death and long-chain 3-hydroxyacyl-CoA dehydrogenase. *Lancet.* 1989;2:52–53.

49. Ijlst L, Ruiter JP, Hoovers JM, et al. Common missense mutation G1528C in long-chain 3-hydroxyacyl-CoA dehydrogenase deficiency. Characterization and expression of the mutant protein, mutation analysis on genomic DNA and

chromosomal localization of the mitochondrial trifunctional protein alpha subunit gene. *J Clin Invest.* 1996;98:1028–1033.

50. Sims HF, Brackett JC, Powell CK, et al. The molecular basis of pediatric long chain 3-hydroxyacyl-CoA dehydrogenase deficiency associated with maternal acute fatty liver of pregnancy. *Proc Natl Acad Sci USA.* 1995;92:841–845.

51. den Boer ME, Wanders RJ, Morris AA, et al. Long-chain 3-hydroxyacyl-CoA dehydrogenase deficiency: Clinical presentation and follow-up of 50 patients. *Pediatrics.* 2002;109:99–104.

52. den Boer ME, Dionisi-Vici C, Chakrapani A, et al. Mitochondrial trifunctional protein deficiency: A severe fatty acid oxidation disorder with cardiac and neurologic involvement. *J Pediatr.* 2003;142:684–689.

53. Spiekerkoetter U, Lindner M, Santer R, et al. Management and outcome in 75 individuals with long-chain fatty acid oxidation defects: Results from a workshop. *J Inherit Metab Dis.* 2009;32:488–497.

54. Spiekerkoetter U, Bennett MJ, Ben-Zeev B, et al. Peripheral neuropathy, episodic myoglobinuria, and respiratory failure in deficiency of the mitochondrial trifunctional protein. *Muscle Nerve.* 2004;29:66–72.

55. Spiekerkoetter U, Sun B, Khuchua Z, et al. Molecular and phenotypic heterogeneity in mitochondrial trifunctional protein deficiency due to beta-subunit mutations. *Hum Mutat.* 2003;21:598–607.

56. Tyni T, Paetau A, Strauss AW, et al. Mitochondrial fatty acid beta-oxidation in the human eye and brain: Implications for the retinopathy of long-chain 3-hydroxyacyl-CoA dehydrogenase deficiency. *Pediatr Res.* 2004;56:744–750.

57. Gillingham MB, Weleber RG, Neuringer M, et al. Effect of optimal dietary therapy upon visual function in children with long-chain 3-hydroxyacyl CoA dehydrogenase and trifunctional protein deficiency. *Mol Genet Metab.* 2005;86:124–133.

58. Tein I, Donner EJ, Hale DE, et al. Clinical and neurophysiologic response of myopathy and neuropathy in long-chain L-3-hydroxyacyl-CoA dehydrogenase deficiency to oral prednisone. *Pediatr Neurol.* 1995;12:68–76.

59. Vici CD, Burlina AB, Bertini E, et al. Progressive neuropathy and recurrent myoglobinuria in a child with long-chain 3-hydroxyacyl-coenzyme A dehydrogenase deficiency. *J Pediatr.* 1991;118:744–746.

60. Bertini E, Dionisi-Vici C, Garavaglia B, et al. Peripheral sensory-motor polyneuropathy, pigmentary retinopathy, and fatal cardiomyopathy in long-chain 3-hydroxy-acyl-CoA dehydrogenase deficiency. *Eur J Pediatr.* 1992;151:121–126.

61. Poll-The BT, Bonnefont JP, Ogier H, et al. Familial hypoketotic hypoglycaemia associated with peripheral neuropathy, pigmentary retinopathy and C6-C14 hydroxydicarboxylic aciduria. A new defect in fatty acid oxidation? *J Inherit Metab Dis.* 1988;11(Suppl 2):183–185.

62. He M, Pei Z, Mohsen AW, et al. Identification and characterization of new long chain acyl-CoA dehydrogenases. *Mol Genet Metab.* 2011;102:418–429.

63. Patel JS, Leonard JV. Ketonuria and medium-chain acyl-CoA dehydrogenase deficiency. *J Inherit Metab Dis.* 1995;18:98–99.

64. Iafolla AK, Thompson RJ, Jr., Roe CR. Medium-chain acyl-coenzyme A dehydrogenase deficiency: Clinical course in 120 affected children. *J Pediatr.* 1994;124:409–415.

65. Feillet F, Steinmann G, Vianey-Saban C, et al. Adult presentation of MCAD deficiency revealed by coma and severe arrythmias. *Intensive Care Med.* 2003;29:1594–1597.

66. Wilhelm GW. Sudden death in a young woman from medium chain acyl-coenzyme A dehydrogenase (MCAD) deficiency. *J Emerg Med.* 2006;30:291–294.

67. Wilson CJ, Champion MP, Collins JE, et al. Outcome of medium chain acyl-CoA dehydrogenase deficiency after diagnosis. *Arch Dis Child.* 1999;80:459–462.

68. Wilcken B, Haas M, Joy P, et al. Outcome of neonatal screening for medium-chain acyl-CoA dehydrogenase deficiency in Australia: A cohort study. *Lancet.* 2007;369:37–42.

69. Matern D, Rinaldo P. Medium-chain acyl-coenzyme a dehydrogenase deficiency. In: RA Pagon, TD Bird, CR Dolan, et al. eds. *GeneReviews.* Seattle (WA); 2012.

70. Andresen BS, Dobrowolski SF, O'Reilly L, et al. Medium-chain acyl-CoA dehydrogenase (MCAD) mutations identified by MS/MS-based prospective screening of newborns differ from those observed in patients with clinical symptoms: Identification and characterization of a new, prevalent mutation that results in mild MCAD deficiency. *Am J Hum Genet.* 2001;68:1408–1418.

71. Hsu HW, Zytkovicz TH, Comeau AM, et al. Spectrum of medium-chain acyl-CoA dehydrogenase deficiency detected by newborn screening. *Pediatrics.* 2008;121:e1108–e1114.

72. Maier EM, Liebl B, Roschinger W, et al. Population spectrum of ACADM genotypes correlated to biochemical phenotypes in newborn screening for medium-chain acyl-CoA dehydrogenase deficiency. *Hum Mutat.* 2005;25:443–452.

73. Smith EH, Thomas C, McHugh D, et al. Allelic diversity in MCAD deficiency: The biochemical classification of 54 variants identified during 5 years of ACADM sequencing. *Mol Genet Metab.* 2010;100:241–250.

74. Dessein AF, Fontaine M, Andresen BS, et al. A novel mutation of the ACADM gene (c.145C > G) associated with the common c.985A>G mutation on the other ACADM allele causes mild MCAD deficiency: A case report. *Orphanet J Rare Dis.* 2010;5:26.

75. Kamijo T, Indo Y, Souri M, et al. Medium chain 3-ketoacyl-coenzyme A thiolase deficiency: A new disorder of mitochondrial fatty acid beta-oxidation. *Pediatr Res.* 1997;42:569–576.

76. Amendt BA, Greene C, Sweetman L, et al. Short-chain acyl-coenzyme A dehydrogenase deficiency. Clinical and biochemical studies in two patients. *J Clin Invest.* 1987;79:1303–1309.

77. Pedersen CB, Kolvraa S, Kolvraa A, et al. The ACADS gene variation spectrum in 114 patients with short-chain acyl-CoA dehydrogenase (SCAD) deficiency is dominated by missense variations leading to protein misfolding at the cellular level. *Hum Genet.* 2008;124:43–56.

78. van Maldegem BT, Duran M, Wanders RJ, et al. Clinical, biochemical, and genetic heterogeneity in short-chain acyl-coenzyme A dehydrogenase deficiency. *JAMA.* 2006;296:943–952.

79. van Maldegem BT, Wanders RJ, Wijburg FA. Clinical aspects of short-chain acyl-CoA dehydrogenase deficiency. *J Inherit Metab Dis.* 2010;33:507–11.

80. Wilcken B, Haas M, Joy P, et al. Expanded newborn screening: Outcome in screened and unscreened patients at age 6 years. *Pediatrics.* 2009;124:e241–248.

81. Waisbren SE, Levy HL, Noble M, et al. Short-chain acyl-CoA dehydrogenase (SCAD) deficiency: An examination of the medical and neurodevelopmental characteristics of 14 cases identified through newborn screening or clinical symptoms. *Mol Genet Metab.* 2008;95:39–45.

82. Nagan N, Kruckeberg KE, Tauscher AL, et al. The frequency of short-chain acyl-CoA dehydrogenase gene variants in the US population and correlation with the C(4)-acylcarnitine concentration in newborn blood spots. *Mol Genet Metab.* 2003;78:239–246.

83. Bennett MJ, Russell LK, Tokunaga C, et al. Reye-like syndrome resulting from novel missense mutations in mitochondrial medium- and short-chain l-3-hydroxy-acyl-CoA dehydrogenase. *Mol Genet Metab.* 2006;89:74–79.

84. Stanley CA. Two genetic forms of hyperinsulinemic hypoglycemia caused by dysregulation of glutamate dehydrogenase. *Neurochem Int.* 2011;59:465–472.

85. Li C, Chen P, Palladino A, et al. Mechanism of hyperinsulinism in short-chain 3-hydroxyacyl-CoA dehydrogenase deficiency involves activation of glutamate dehydrogenase. *J Biol Chem.* 2010;285:31806–31818.

86. Martins E, Cardoso ML, Rodrigues E, et al. Short-chain 3-hydroxyacyl-CoA dehydrogenase deficiency: The clinical relevance of an early diagnosis and report of four new cases. *J Inherit Metab Dis.* 2011;34:835–842.

87. Wang ZQ, Chen XJ, Murong SX, et al. Molecular analysis of 51 unrelated pedigrees with late-onset multiple acyl-CoA dehydrogenation deficiency (MADD) in southern China confirmed the most common ETFDH mutation and high carrier frequency of c.250G > A. *J Mol Med (Berl).* 2011;89: 569–576.

88. Ho G, Yonezawa A, Masuda S, et al. Maternal riboflavin deficiency, resulting in transient neonatal-onset glutaric aciduria Type 2, is caused by a microdeletion in the riboflavin transporter gene GPR172B. *Hum Mutat.* 2011;32: E1976–E1984.

89. Tanaka K, Ikeda Y. Hypoglycin and Jamaican vomiting sickness. *Progr Clin Biol Res.* 1990;321:167–184.

90. Roe CR, Millington DS, Norwood DL, et al. 2,4-Dienoylcoenzyme A reductase deficiency: A possible new disorder of fatty acid oxidation. *J Clin Invest.* 1990;85:1703–1707.

91. Zhang J, Zhang W, Zou D, et al. Cloning and functional characterization of ACAD-9, a novel member of human acyl-CoA dehydrogenase family. *Biochem Biophys Res Commun.* 2002;297:1033–1042.

92. He M, Rutledge SL, Kelly DR, et al. A new genetic disorder in mitochondrial fatty acid beta-oxidation: ACAD9 deficiency. *Am J Hum Genet.* 2007;81:87–103.

93. Nouws J, Nijtmans L, Houten SM, et al. Acyl-CoA dehydrogenase 9 is required for the biogenesis of oxidative phosphorylation complex I. *Cell Metab.* 2010;12:283–294.

94. Haack TB, Danhauser K, Haberberger B, et al. Exome sequencing identifies ACAD9 mutations as a cause of complex I deficiency. *Nat Genet.* 2010;42:1131–1134.

95. Suhrie KRS, Karunanidhi AK, Mohsen AW, et al. Long chain acyl-CoA dehydrogenase deficiency: A new inborn error of metabolism manifesting as congenital surfactant deficiency. *J Inherit Metab Dis.* 2011;34:S149.

96. Shekhawat PS, Matern D, Strauss AW. Fetal fatty acid oxidation disorders, their effect on maternal health and neonatal outcome: Impact of expanded newborn screening on their diagnosis and management. *Pediatr Res.* 2005;57: 78R–86R.

97. Browning MF, Levy HL, Wilkins-Haug LE, et al. Fetal fatty acid oxidation defects and maternal liver disease in pregnancy. *Obstetrics Gynecol.* 2006;107:115–120.

98. Riely CA. Liver disease in the pregnant patient. American College of Gastroenterology. *Am J Gastroenterol.* 1999;94: 1728–1732.

99. In: *ACMG ACT Sheets and Confirmatory Algorithms.* Bethesda (MD); 2001.

100. Arnold GL, Van Hove J, Freedenberg D, et al. A Delphi clinical practice protocol for the management of very long chain acyl-CoA dehydrogenase deficiency. *Mol Genet Metab.* 2009;96:85–90.

101. Rinaldo P, Studinski AL, Matern D. Prenatal diagnosis of disorders of fatty acid transport and mitochondrial oxidation. *Prenat Diagn.* 2001;21:52–54.

102. Olpin SE. The metabolic investigation of sudden infant death. *Ann Clin Biochem.* 2004;41:282–293.

103. Rinaldo P, Yoon HR, Yu C, Raymond K, et al. Sudden and unexpected neonatal death: A protocol for the postmortem diagnosis of fatty acid oxidation disorders. *Semin Perinatol.* 1999;23:204–10.

104. Rashed MS, Bucknall MP, Little D, et al. Screening blood spots for inborn errors of metabolism by electrospray tandem mass spectrometry with a microplate batch process and a computer algorithm for automated flagging of abnormal profiles. *Clin Chem.* 1997;43:1129–1141.

105. Matern D, Strauss AW, Hillman SL, et al. Diagnosis of mitochondrial trifunctional protein deficiency in a blood spot from the newborn screening card by tandem mass spectrometry and DNA analysis. *Pediatr Res.* 1999;46:45–49.

106. Derks TG, van Spronsen FJ, Rake JP, et al. Safe and unsafe duration of fasting for children with MCAD deficiency. *Eur J Pediatr.* 2007;166:5–11.

107. Spiekerkoetter U, Bastin J, Gillingham M, et al. Current issues regarding treatment of mitochondrial fatty acid oxidation disorders. *J Inherit Metab Dis.* 2010;33:555–561.

108. Fahnehjelm KT, Holmstrom G, Ying L, et al. Ocular characteristics in 10 children with long-chain 3-hydroxyacyl-CoA dehydrogenase deficiency: A cross-sectional study with long-term follow-up. *Acta Ophthalmol.* 2008;86:329–337.

109. Lee PJ, Harrison EL, Jones MG, et al. L-carnitine and exercise tolerance in medium-chain acyl-coenzyme A dehydrogenase (MCAD) deficiency: A pilot study. *J Inherited Metab Dis.* 2005;28:141–152.

110. Huidekoper HH, Schneider J, Westphal T, et al. Prolonged moderate-intensity exercise without and with L-carnitine supplementation in patients with MCAD deficiency. *J Inherited Metab Dis.* 2006;29: 631–636.

111. Treem WR, Stanley CA, Goodman SI. Medium-chain acyl-CoA dehydrogenase deficiency: Metabolic effects and

therapeutic efficacy of long-term L-carnitine supplementation. *J Inherited Metab Dis.* 1989;12:112–119.

112. Iacobazzi V, Pasquali M, Singh R, et al. Response to therapy in carnitine/acylcarnitine translocase (CACT) deficiency due to a novel missense mutation. *Am J Med Genet A.* 2004;126A: 150–155.

113. Gillingham MB, Scott B, Elliott D, et al. Metabolic control during exercise with and without medium-chain triglycerides (MCT) in children with long-chain 3-hydroxy acyl-CoA dehydrogenase (LCHAD) or trifunctional protein (TFP) deficiency. *Mol Genet Metab.* 2006;89:58–63.

114. Merritt JL, 2ND, Nguyen T, Daniels J, et al. Biochemical correction of very long-chain acyl-CoA dehydrogenase deficiency following adeno-associated virus gene therapy. *Mol Ther.* 2009; 17:425–429.

115. Beattie SG, Goetzman E, Conlon T, et al. Biochemical Correction of Short-Chain Acyl-Coenzyme A Dehydrogenase Deficiency After Portal Vein Injection of rAAV8-SCAD. *Hum Gene Ther.* 2008;19:579–588.

116. Beattie SG, Goetzman E, Tang Q, et al. Recombinant adeno-associated virus-mediated gene delivery of long chain acyl coenzyme A dehydrogenase (LCAD) into LCAD-deficient mice. *J Gene Med.* 2008;10: 1113–1123.

117. Schowalter DB, Matern D, Vockley J. In vitro correction of medium chain acyl CoA dehydrogenase deficiency with a recombinant adenoviral vector. *Mol Genet Metab.* 2005;85:88–95.

118. Lund AM, Skovby F, Vestergaard H, et al. Clinical and biochemical monitoring of patients with fatty acid oxidation disorders. *J Inherited Metab Dis.* 2010;33:495–500.

9

Urea Cycle Disorders and Epilepsy

Debra S. Regier, Brendan Lanpher, and Marshall L. Summar

INTRODUCTION

The urea cycle is a series of steps required to produce urea from nitrogen produced during protein catabolism. Krebs and Henseleit first described this pathway in 1932 (1). To date, six enzymes and two transporters have been identified as necessary for urea cycle activity, based on deficiencies of each leading to disease. The urea cycle converts nitrogen from ammonia and aspartate into urea, which is freely excreted by the kidney (2) (Figure 9.1). Embedded within the urea cycle is the nitric oxide cycle. Nitric oxide is generated from arginine by nitric oxide synthase (NOS), producing citrulline (3). The complete urea cycle is present only in the

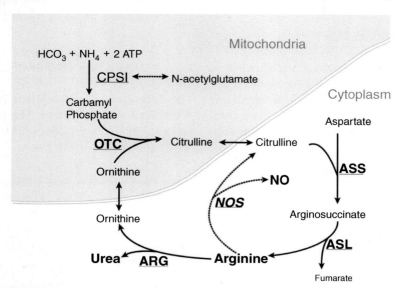

FIGURE 9.1 The urea cycle. The urea cycle is a pathway of cytosolic and mitochondrial proteins involved in the conversion of ammonia (NH_4) to urea for excretion via the kidneys. The enzymes in the pathway are as follows: carbomylphosphate synthetase (CPS1); ornithine transcarbamylase (OTC); argininosuccinic acid synthase (ASS); arginosuccinic acid lyase (ASL); arginase I (ARG); nitric oxide synthase (NOS).

liver. The proximal cycle (NAGS, CPS, OTC) is also present in the intestinal tract while the distal cycle (ASS, ASL, ARG) is active in the kidney.

Infants with severe urea cycle disorders often present at 1 to 4 days of life with encephalopathic features, such as decreased intake, lethargy, or seizures. The overall incidence of all urea cycle disorders is estimated at between 1/10,000 to 1/25,000, though patients with incomplete deficiency are likely significantly more common (4). In the absence of a functional urea cycle, nitrogen accumulates in the form of toxic ammonium. In null activity patients, this typically presents in the first days of life with hyperammonemia, resulting in CNS dysfunction with overwhelming encephalopathy and coma, brain edema, seizures, and potentially death with severe long-term neurodevelopmental sequelae if not rapidly reversed. The differential diagnosis of severe hyperammonemia includes organic acidemias, herpes-related hepatitis, and other disorders of liver function. Respiratory alkalosis and hyperventilation is classically seen in UCDs, though if encephalopathy progresses, apneas and acidosis may be seen (5). If not recognized and reversed immediately, this may progress to fatal cerebral edema and herniation. There are multiple postulated mechanisms for ammonia-related neurotoxicity.

CLINICAL CASE

A 24-hour-male infant was brought to the attention of the pediatrician on call to the well baby nursery at a large delivery hospital due to the infant appearing sleepy, with decreased breast feeding and activity compared to day of life one. The pediatrician contacted the neonatal intensive care unit, where the child was started on antibiotics after a sepsis work-up was initiated. Over the next 12 hours, the neonate demonstrated increasing lethargy with normal white blood count and C-reactive protein levels. An ammonia level was obtained and found to be greater than 1,500 (normal less than 50). The neonate was immediately transferred to a tertiary neonatal intensive care unit for emergent dialysis and intervention. The finding of elevated orotic acid in the urine supported a urea cycle defect. While arranging for emergent placement of dialysis catheters, the neurology service began continuous video EEG monitoring with initial findings of seizure activity. Due to imminent dialysis, a midazolam drip was initiated and titrated for subclinical seizures. The first doses of intravenous sodium phenylacetate and sodium benzoate were given prior to dialysis to facilitate the removal of glutamine and glycine, repositories for nitrogen, which can reduce the total body ammonia load. After hemodialysis, the neonate continued hemofiltration until the electrolytes and ammonia level stabilized. In this infant's case, total dialysis lasted five days. During dialysis, enteral feeding with low-protein formula was initiated with oral sodium phenylbutyrate started for long-term treatment. Due to inability to tolerate full oral feeds, prior to discharge home a gastrostomy tube was placed to ensure that the low protein diet and medications would be feasible for the infant.

UREA CYCLE COMPONENTS (TABLE 9.1)

The urea cycle is the sole mechanism for nitrogen detoxification and disposal. The primary enzymes are reviewed in Figure 9.1. Since the urea cycle is localized

TABLE 9.1   Urea Cycle Components

Gene Name	Gene Symbol	Location	Protein Name
Carbamylphosphate synthetase I	CPS1	2q35	Carbamoyl-phosphate synthase ammonia
Ornithine transcarbamylase	OTC	Xp21.1	Ornithine carbamoyltransferase
Argininosuccinate synthase	ASS	9q34	Argininosuccinate synthase
Argininosuccinate lyase	ASL	7cen-q11.2	Argininosuccinate lyase
Arginase	ARG1	6q23	Arginase 1
N-acetyl glutamate synthase	NAGS	17q21.3	N-acetyl glutamate synthetase
Ornithine Transporter Mitochondrial 1	ORNT1	13q14	Ornithine Transporter Mitochondrial 1

TABLE 9.2 Clinical Pearls For Urea Cycle Disorders

Symptom	Common Timing of Symptom	Laboratory/Clinical Testing	Intervention
Newborn with poor feeding	1 to 4 days of life (often before newborn screening results obtained)	• Ammonia level • Plasma Amino Acids • Urine organic acids	• Dialysis • EEG monitoring • Scavenger treatment, as appropriate • Co-factor treatment, as appropriate
Seizure activity with hyperammonemia	Usually within hours of hyperammonemia	• Continuous video EEG monitoring	• Antiepileptic medical management • Continuous drip if dialysis candidate.
Known urea cycle disorder patient with change in mental status	Any age: During acute changes in metabolic demand: illness, dehydration	• Ammonia Level • Continuous video EEG monitoring during acute phase	• Treat underlying event • Hydration • Dialysis for hyperammonemia not otherwise controlled
Child or adult with encephalopathy of unknown etiology	Any age: usually with recent history of increased metabolic demand	• Ammonia Level • Continuous video EEG monitoring during acute phase	• Treat hyperammonemia • Genetic testing for partial urea cycle activity or carrier status • Aggressive treatment of seizure activity
Child or adult with new onset seizure activity of unknown etiology	Any age: usually with recent history of increased metabolic demand	• Ammonia level • Plasma Amino Acids • Urine organic acids	• Treat Hyperammonemia • Genetic testing for partial urea cycle activity or carrier status • Aggressive treatment with antiepileptic medications

in both the mitochondria and the cytoplasm, there are two transport molecules responsible for shuttling intermediates across the mitochondrial membrane that are also critical for proper urea cycle function. There are well-described inborn errors associated with each of these enzymatic steps and transporters (6). A portion of the distal urea cycle (argininosuccinic acid synthase and arginosuccinic acid lyase) is also embedded within another metabolic cycle responsible for producing nitric oxide.

A brief review of the enzymes, transporters, and cofactor producers of the urea cycle follows:

CARBAMYL PHOSPHATE SYNTHETASE I (CPSI) DEFICIENCY

CPSI is the rate-limiting step of the urea cycle. The protein product is found in the mitochondria, though it is encoded in the nuclear genome. The mature protein is a 160 kDA monomer that converts ammonia and bicarbonate into carbamyl phosphate (7–9). The clinical presentation of CPSI deficiency is dependent on the severity of the deficiency, but is characterized by elevated ammonia and glutamine and decreased citrulline and arginine. Orotic acid is typically not elevated. CPSII is not involved in the urea cycle, but instead in the pyrimidine synthetic pathway.

N-ACETYLGLUTAMATE SYNTHASE (NAGS) DEFICIENCY

N-acetylglutamate is an essential co-factor for CPSI activity; thus, deficiency in NAGS causes decreased CPSI activity. NAGS deficiency is extremely rare, but is treatable with carbamylglutamate (10, 11). This medication has recently been used for the hyperammonemia observed in acute organic acidemias (12).

ORNITHINE TRANSCARBAMYLASE (OTC) DEFICIENCY

The most common disorder of the urea cycle is OTC deficiency. OTC catalyzes the formation of citrulline from carbamyl phosphate and ornithine. It is encoded on the X-chromosome. Hemizygous male individuals typically have severe disease. Heterozygous female individuals have a wide range of phenotypes, ranging from severe neonatal hyperammonemia to asymptomatic. Subtle neuropsychological effects are often seen in carrier female individuals. The clinical presentation includes accumulation of ammonia and glutamine, and decreased citrulline and arginine. In contrast to CPSI deficiency, in OTC deficiency excess mitochondrial carbamyl phosphate is shunted to cytoplasmic pyrimidine synthesis and leads to accumulation of orotic acid (13–20).

ARGININOSUCCINIC ACID SYNTHASE (ASS) DEFICIENCY

ASS is responsible for the condensation of citrulline and aspartate into arginosuccinate. In a second pathway, it also plays a role in cycling arginine and citrulline to produce nitric oxide (21). ASS is a cytoplasmic protein, and it requires the transport of citrulline out of the mitochondria. The aspartate required by ASS is produced in the TCA cycle or as a product of protein breakdown. Defects in ASS present with hyperammonemia, decreased arginine, and massive (10–100 times above normal) levels of citrulline (22–26).

ARGININOSUCCINIC ACID LYASE DEFICIENCY

Argininosuccinic acid is cleaved by ASL to form arginine and fumarate. It is ubiquitously expressed. The presentation of the defect is characterized by hyperammonemia, decreased arginine, citrulline accumulation (less than in ASS deficiency), and argininosuccinic acid accumulation (unique to this disorder). Patients with ASL deficiency appear to be uniquely susceptible to long-term hepatic fibrosis that may lead to cirrhosis (27–30) Patients with ASL deficiency also appear to have neuropsychological compromise out of proportion to their history of hyperammonemia, suggestive of involvement in other neurological pathways (personal observation).

ARGINASE I (ARG) DEFICIENCY

Unlike deficiencies of the other primary enzymes of the urea cycle, arginase deficiency does not typically present with severe hyperammonemia. Instead, patients with this deficiency are characterized by a gradual-onset spastic paraplegia, more in the lower than upper extremities. Patients may have short stature if untreated. There is an increased risk for seizures, and development is often slow. Hyperammonemic crises may occur with severe catabolic stress (31, 32).

ORNITHINE TRANSLOCASE DEFICIENCY (HHH SYNDROME)

The HHH syndrome (hyperornithinemia, hyperammonemia, homocitrullinemia) is caused by deficient transport of ornithine into the mitochondria. With intramitochondial ornithine depletion, ureagenesis is impaired. The accumulation of homocitrulline is caused by transcobalamination of lysine, and is diagnostic for the condition, but is not always easily identified in mildly affected patients. Patients present with episodic hyperammonemia, seizures, and developmental delay (33–35).

CITRIN DEFICIENCY (CITRULLINEMIA TYPE II)

Transportation of aspartate and glutamate across the mitochondrial membrane is thought to be facilitated by citrin, or Solute Carrier Family 25. When deficient, there is inadequate aspartate available for ASS activity; thus, ureagenesis is impaired. Levels of citrulline are elevated. This disorder is nearly exclusively reported in patients of Asian descent. There are two primary clinical phenotypes associated with citrin deficiency. Patients may present in the newborn period with cholestatic liver disease, or in adulthood with insidious neurologic disease (36–38).

NEUROPATHOLOGY AND NEUROIMAGING

Neuropathological changes found in neonates who died with urea cycle disorders include cerebral edema, intracranial hemorrhages, and generalized neuronal cell loss. In children who survived neonatal hyperammonemia and died later, neuropathology included cortical atrophy, related ventriculomegaly and cortical neuronal loss (39). Alterations in the astrocyte morphology have been demonstrated. The basal ganglia may also be affected in urea cycle disorder, in particular the lentiform nuclei. This correlates with cognitive difficulty in tasks that require attention and fine motor skills (40).

Only small series of patients with urea cycle disorders have been studied using CT or MRI (41, 42). Chronic changes observed in survivors of prolonged hyperammonemic coma include ventriculomegaly, cerebral atrophy, and symmetrical low-density white matter lesions which may be partially reversible with treatment. Proton magnetic resonance spectroscopy of the brain in patients with late-onset OTC deficiency has shown decreased myoinositol, increased glutamine, and decreased choline concentrations (43, 44). Neurological severity trended with increased levels of restricted diffusion in pre-insular and frontal regions. The most severe patients in one study showed basal ganglia and thalami restricted diffusion and two of the three most severe patients in this study had brainstem involvement prior to death. Thus, this suggests that restricted diffusion of the thalami, basal ganglia, and brainstem may serve as markers of clinical severity (41). Individuals with a mild OTC mutation or carrier status show strengths in language, rote memory, and language arts (considered gray matter correlates), and deficits in visual–spatial, tactile, and motor functions that are often accompanied by attention/executive weaknesses. This is consistent with the finding of alterations in cerebral white matter in neuropathological and neuroimaging studies in urea cycle disorders (45, 46).

NEUROCOGNITIVE OUTCOMES IN UCDs

The degree of neuropathological damage is related to the duration of hyperammonemia and whether it is acute or chronic in origin. When considering the outcomes of urea cycle disorders, it is important to separate patients into the relevant categories of neonatal onset, partial defect, and asymptomatic heterozygotes. For patients with severe neonatal urea cycle defects, the prognosis remains quite guarded. The overall mortality for UCD patients presenting in the newborn period is approximately 50%; and a significant number have cerebral palsy, epilepsy, or multiple neurodevelopmental disabilities. The outcome is correlated to the duration of hyperammonemia. The peak ammonia level is less predictive of outcome. These data come from a study published only a few years after the development of alternative pathway drugs (42, 47). There is considerable hope that with improved therapy outcomes may be improved (46, 48). Delayed recognition of hyperammonemia remains a significant barrier to rapid resolution of a crisis. In a study of 92 patients, increased cognitive impairment was observed in the neonatal-onset population, which was about one-third of the study population. Furthermore, ~30% of the neonatal onset patients had severe cognitive impairment. When siblings of neonatal onset cases of either OTC deficiency or carbamyl phosphate synthetase deficiency (but not with citrullinemia or argininosuccinic aciduria) were treated from birth, thereby averting neonatal hyperammonemic coma, IQ was within the low-normal range (49).

The patients with late-onset urea cycle disorders (partial enzyme deficiencies) can present at any age with hyperammonemic crisis; however, they have only a 4% chance of severe cognitive impairment. They do have difficulties in areas of attention and executive functioning out of proportion to other areas of cognitive development (49). Minimally symptomatic OTC-deficient heterozygous women were shown to have cognitive deficits, learning disabilities and ADHD (40, 45).

SEIZURE ACTIVITY IN UCDs

Seizures have long been associated with UCDs, thought to be caused by high levels of ammonia. Furthermore, the brain damage obtained during metabolic crisis has been thought to damage critical structures leading to epilepsy after the conclusion of the crisis. In general, the treatment of clinical and subclinical seizures should include both acute medications (versed or other drip-type medication while on dialysis and phenobarbital once stabilized) and long term medical management, often with levetiracetam or carbamazepine (personal experience, 50). In all cases, valproic acid should be avoided as a treatment based on multiple publications showing that this medication directly alters the urea cycle leading to metabolic crises (48, 51, 52, 53). It is thought that valproic acid directly alters the urea cycle in one of its steps or one of its metabolite precursors. Valproic acid is also known to reduce the levels of carnitine, leading to decreased metabolism of fatty acids through a poorly defined mechanism resulting in fatty liver disease. Presumably this leads to increased protein metabolism and increased stress on the urea cycle causing increased levels of ammonia that need to be metabolized (54).

EFFECTS OF HYPERAMMONEMIA ON THE CNS

There are multiple interrelated effects of hyperammonemia on the CNS. Ammonia and related metabolites have osmotic effects, alter neurotransmitter metabolism, alter electrophysiological activity of neurons, and effect energy metabolism.

As ammonia accumulates in the circulating plasma, it diffuses freely across the blood–brain barrier and is rapidly combined with glutamate in the astrocyte to form glutamine via glutamine synthetase. Glutamine accumulation leads to astrocyte swelling via osmosis (55, 56). This may lead to cytotoxic edema and decreased blood flow across cerebral capillaries, which, in turn, may lead to a localized decrease in blood flow and oxygen transfer to brain tissue This then stimulates the respiratory drive, leading to the respiratory alkalosis typical of hyperammonemia. In severe cases, the ammonia and glutamine accumulation may lead to severe generalized brain edema and herniation. This is a leading cause of mortality and morbidity in patients with UCDs. Inhibition of glutamine synthase has been proposed as a potential therapy for hyperammonemic encephalopathy (57).

Elevated CNS ammonia affects brain function by inhibiting chloride release from neurons, decreasing inhibitory synaptic transmission. Ammonia also diminishes the effects of calcium and voltage-dependent chloride currents. The net effect increases neuronal excitability (58, 59). This would predict propensity to seizures. Ammonia also affects the energy metabolism of the brain. Ammonia at concentrations typically seen in UCDs inhibits alpha-ketoglutarate dehydrogenase, impairing Krebs cycle function. There is also stimulation of glycolysis via phosphofructokinase. These effects explain the elevated CSF and brain lactate concentrations that have been observed in UCDs (60, 61),

As ammonia levels increase in the CSF, glutamine synthetase acts to decrease them through increased production of glutamine. In animal models of hyperammonemia, glutamine has been associated with astrocyte swelling and cerebral hypercirculation. Furthermore, this increases blood–brain barrier transport of the aromatic amino acids that act as precursors of serotonin and other key neurotransmitters. The increased serotonin may contribute to the anorexia and sleep abnormalities that are often problematic in UCD patients (62).

There are regional differences in neuronal sensitivity to hyperammonemia. It has been demonstrated that in acute hyperammonemia, the lentiform nuclei and surrounding basal ganglia are particularly at risk (63). In severe cases of neonatal hyperammonemia, postmortem studies reveal evidence of additional gray-matter injury with cortical atrophy, gliosis with Alzheimer type II astrocytes, and spongiform changes particularly affecting the grey-white junction and deep-grey nuclei (64).

In the CNS, there is evidence of compartmentalization of ammonia metabolism and shuttling of ammonia and other nitrogenous intermediates between the astrocyte and neuron. Ammonia is consumed in the CNS by the action of glutamine synthetase, which is almost exclusively expressed in astrocytes. Ammonia also freely diffuses across the blood–brain barrier in the free base form (NH_3). The equilibrium between blood and brain concentrations of ammonia is a complex interplay between ammonia uptake, local ammonia production, and metabolic trapping (65, 66). Due to these factors, it is clear that blood ammonia concentrations are a poor indicator of brain concentration, particularly in acute hyperammonemia. This likely underlies the observation that the blood ammonia level is limited as a predictor of severity of hyperammonemic episodes. Thus, EEG monitoring may more closely monitor the ammonia levels in the brain than do serum ammonia levels.

TYPES OF SEIZURE ACTIVITY OBSERVED IN UCDs

The studies performed to evaluate clinical or subclinical seizure activity in patients with UCDs has been limited based on numbers per study and the brevity of descriptions used in some of the studies, such as normal and abnormal findings. Overall, studies have shown consistent abnormal EEG findings during acute metabolic crisis with hyperammonemia. The studies are varied with regard to EEG findings during recorded interval times. In one large study from Japan evaluating 41 patients with urea cycle enzymopathies, abnormal EEG during normal levels of ammonia were statistically related to abnormalities on CT scan. Thus, this study suggested that much of the late seizure activity observed is secondary to damage obtained during acute metabolic crises (67).

OTC Deficiency

In a case study of two infants with OTC deficiency confirmed with liver biopsy, both demonstrated multifocal independent spike and sharp wave discharges at diagnosis during elevated ammonia levels (68). One patient did not have clinical seizures at birth; however, he was found in interval EEGs during preschool evaluations to have attenuation and slowing of background rhythms without epileptiform discharges. In contrast, the second infant described had clinical seizures with excessive EEG background discontinuity, absence of state changes, and multifocal independent and generalized spike-and-sharp wave discharges. Prior to death at 7 days of age, his EEG showed abnormalities in the background with superimposed ictal and interictal patterns, coincident with diffuse cerebral edema on CT scan.

Verma et al evaluated a group of patients with either OTC or SAS-L deficiency and monitored EEGs both during acute crises and during intercrisis intervals. In their group, all infants had clinical seizures prior to EEG recordings. The EEGs demonstrated epileptiform activity with multifocal spike, spike-wave, or sharp-and-slow-wave activity. Two of the 11 patients had sustained monorhythmic theta activity. In one infant, EEG normalized after beginning a protein restricted diet. Another term infant showed 10 times the normal frequency of spindle-delta brushes typically associated with prematures, consistent with the trend that secondary CNS or systemic disease in a neonate can cause regression and dyschronism leading to EEG activity more similar to an earlier gestational age (69).

ASS Deficiency (Citrullemia)

In a single study of three children with citrullenemia, EEGs showed multifocal spikes and repetitive paroxysmal activity at the time of crisis. The EEGs normalized, but this lagged behind the resolution of hyperammonemia. Follow-up several years after diagnosis showed isolated spikes which improved with dietary alterations. In one follow-up at 12 years of age, the EEG showed slowing and disorganization of the posterior basic rhythm, diffuse theta–delta frequency slowing, and occasional generalized paroxysms of sharp activity (70).

Arginosuccinic Acid Lyase (ASL) Deficiency

Two large studies have recently been published evaluating the long-term outcomes of patients with arginosuccinate lyase deficiency. In one study of 13 patients, six had EEG abnormalities and three had documented epilepsy. The abnormalities noted on EEG included

abnormal sharp irregular background activity, frequent bilateral epileptiform paroxysms, and increased slow-wave activity. The EEG was improved with increased diet compliance in two patients and normalized with compliance in one patient. The three cases of patients with seizures were late-onset patients, and seizure semiology included staring, night disturbances with vomiting and opisthotonus, and generalized tonic–clonic convulsions. One patient in the study had febrile seizures with EEG after the acute period being normal (71). In a second study performed in Austria, nine patients with ASL agreed to long-term monitoring. Four of the nine patients had abnormal EEGs without evidence of clinical seizures without abnormalities in liver function tests or ammonia levels. Diffuse slowing of background activity was observed in four and multifocal spike activity in two of the nine participants (72).

Citrin Deficiency (Citrullinemia Type II)

In a case report of a single patient with adult-onset Type II citrullinemia a Japanese group reported the findings of nonconvulsive status epilepticus after a woman presented with repeated episodes of unconsciousness and abnormal behaviors, not always associated with ammonia elevations (73). Thus, this study supports the use of EEG for monitoring metabolic patients routinely during acute clinical changes.

TREATMENT OF UCDs

The first and most critical step of successful treatment of urea cycle disorders is recognition. Neurologic monitoring is an essential part of the emergency management of UCDs. Electroencephalography should be used, as seizures can be triggered by hyperammonemia and may be under recognized. Clinical, EEG, and radiographic assessment of neurologic function is critical in determining the potential for recovery and the appropriateness of continued aggressive treatment (64). Furthermore, aggressive antiepileptic treatment may be needed. Of note, short-acting intravenous drip-type infusions should be used during the acute phase of treatment to ensure seizure activity is controlled even during dialysis treatments.

Once a patient is in a hyperammonemic crisis, there are three interdependent and concurrent goals of therapy—physical removal of ammonia, pharmacologic scavenging of excess nitrogen through stimulation of alternative routes of disposal, and reversal of the catabolic state that precipitated the crisis. Once hyperammonemic coma is recognized, central venous access is required and hemodialysis should be started immediately (74). Scavenging of excess ammonia is facilitated by the combination of sodium benzoate and sodium phenylacetate (Ammonul, Ucyclyd Pharma). These compounds trap nitrogen in safely excretable forms. Arginine supplementation also decreases ammonia load by allowing the functional parts of the cycle to incorporate some nitrogen (75, 76). Finally, reversal of catabolic state is an essential and often underappreciated component of emergency management of UCDs. Catabolism, precipitated by infections, surgeries, fasting, or other physiologic stressors, mobilizes endogenous protein stores. Intravenous fluids with a high concentration of dextrose and a lipid source should be used to provide calories. Withholding protein is emergently necessary, but must be temporary to prevent muscle breakdown and subsequent worsening of a hyperammonenic crisis. Essential amino acids will stimulate protein synthesis, an effective sink for excess nitrogen (77).

Chronic management of UCDs is predicated on avoiding triggers of catabolic crises. For this reason, systemic steroids are contraindicated, as is valproic acid. Long-term diet management is based on overall protein restriction, with provision of adequate essential amino acids to allow for normal growth. Excessive restriction of protein is at least as dangerous as an overly liberal diet, as it may lower the patient's threshold for a catabolic crisis. Specialized formulas for UCDs are enhanced in essential amino acids and have a lower overall nitrogen load per unit of protein. There are enteral forms of the scavenger medications that may be used chronically (78). Recently two studies showed that vaccines are not associated with increased metabolic events; thus, they should be administered per the routine vaccine schedule to protect these children from illness and increased risk of metabolic crises (79, 80).

For patients with severe, neonatal-onset urea cycle disorders, the definitive treatment is orthotopic liver transplant. Maximal pharmacologic management is generally inadequate to avoid decomposition in patients with severe CPSI or OTC deficiency. After transplantation, the risk for metabolic decomposition is far lower, but not eliminated. Because transplantation does not correct enzymatic deficits in other organs, patients generally continue to require supplemental citrulline or arginine (81, 82).

A frequently updated resource for physicians describing current suggestions for treatment of patients with urea cycle defects may be found at the NIH-sponsored Urea Cycle Disorders Consortium at http://www.rarediseasesnetwork.org/ucdc.

SUMMARY

The neurological abnormalities observed in patients with urea cycle defects are vast. Controlling ammonia levels by dialysis and complementary medication are needed. EEG monitoring should be initiated early, as this likely follows brain ammonia levels and may be very useful for clinical management and indicate untreated metabolic crises. Furthermore, aggressive treatment of clinical and subclinical seizure activity may be helpful in optimizing outcomes for these patients.

REFERENCES

1. Krebs HA, Henseleit K. Untersuchungen uber die harnstoffbildung im tierkorper. *Hoppe-Seyler's Z Physiol Chem.* 1932;210:325–332.
2. Brusilow SW. Urea cycle disorders: clinical paradigm of hyperammonemic encephalopathy. *Prog Liver Dis.* 1995;13:293–309.
3. Scaglia F, Brunetti-Pierri N, Kleppe S, et al. Clinical consequences of urea cycle enzyme deficiencies and potential links to arginine and nitric oxide metabolism. *J Nutr.* 2004;134(10 Suppl):2775S–2782S.
4. Nagata N, Matsuda I, Oyanagi K. Estimated frequency of urea cycle enzymopathies in Japan. *Am J Med Genet.* 1991;39(2):228–229.
5. Burton BK. Inborn errors of metabolism in infancy: a guide to diagnosis. *Pediatrics* 1998;102(6):E69.
6. Jackson MJ, Beaudet AL, O'Brien WE. Mammalian urea cycle enzymes. [Review]. *Ann Rev Genet* 1986;20:431–464.
7. Britton HG, Garcia-Espana A, Goya P, et al. A structure-reactivity study of the binding of acetylglutamate to carbamoyl phosphate synthetase I. *Eur J Biochem.* 1990;188:47–53.
8. Rubio V, Cervera J. The carbamoyl-phosphate synthase family and carbamate kinase: structure–function studies. [Review]. *Biochem Soc Trans.* 1995;23:879–883.
9. Summar ML, Hall LD, Eeds AM, et al. Characterization of genomic structure and polymorphisms in the human carbamyl phosphate synthetase I gene. *Gene* 2003;311:51–57.

10. Tuchman M, Caldovic L, Daikhin Y, et al. *N*-carbamylglutamate markedly enhances ureagenesis in *N*-acetylglutamate deficiency and propionic acidemia as measured by isotopic incorporation and blood biomarkers. *Pediatr Res.* 2008;64(2):213–217.

11. Caldovic L, Morizono H, Panglao MG, et al. Null mutations in the *N*-acetylglutamate synthase gene associated with acute neonatal disease and hyperammonemia. *Hum Genet* 2003;112(4): 364–368.

12. Daniotti M, la MG, Fiorini P, et al. New developments in the treatment of hyperammonemia: emerging use of carglumic acid. *Int J Gen Med.* 2011;4:21–28.

13. Oexle K. Biochemical data in ornithine transcarbamylase deficiency (OTCD) carrier risk estimation: logistic discrimination and combination with genetic information. *J Hum Genet.* 2006;51(3):204–208.

14. Tuchman M, Jaleel N, Morizono H, et al. Mutations and polymorphisms in the human ornithine transcarbamylase gene. *Hum Mutat* 2002;19(2):93–107.

15. Schwab S, Schwarz S, Mayatepek E, et al. Recurrent brain edema in ornithine-transcarbamylase deficiency. *J Neurol.* 1999;246(7): 609–611.

16. Yeh SJ, Hou WL, Tsai WS, et al. Ornithine transcarbamylase deficiency. *J Formosan Med Assoc.* 1997;96(1):43–45.

17. Maestri NE, Clissold D, Brusilow SW. Neonatal onset ornithine transcarbamylase deficiency: a retrospective analysis [see comments]. *J Pediatr.* 1999;134(3):268–272.

18. Tuchman M, McCullough BA, Yudkoff M. The molecular basis of ornithine transcarbamylase deficiency. *Eur J Pediatr.* 2000;159(Suppl 3):S196–S198.

19. Tuchman M, Morizono H, Rajagopal BS. The biochemical and molecular spectrum of ornithine transcarbamylase deficiency. *J Inherit Metab Dis.* 1998;21(Suppl 1):40–58.

20. Gordon N Ornithine transcarbamylase deficiency: a urea cycle defect. *Eur J Paediatr Neurol.* 2003;7(3):115–121.

21. Solomonson LP, Flam BR, Pendleton LC, et al. The caveolar nitric oxide synthase/arginine regeneration system for NO production in endothelial cells. *J Exp Biol.* 2003;206(Pt 12):2083–2087.

22. Berning C, Bieger I, Pauli S, et al. Investigation of citrullinemia type I variants by in vitro expression studies. *Hum Mutat.* 2008;29(10):1222–1227.

23. Sanjurjo P, Rodriguez-Soriano J. Management of neonatal citrullinemia. *J Pediatr.* 1993;123(5):838–839.

24. Balsekar MV, Ambani LM, Bhatia RS, et al. Citrullinemia: early diagnosis & successful management of an otherwise lethal disorder. *Indian Pediatr.* 1989;26(6):589–592.

25. Oyanagi K, Itakura Y, Tsuchiyama A, et al. Citrullinemia: quantitative deficiency of argininosuccinate synthetase in the liver. *Tohoku J Exp Med.* 1986;148(4):385–391.

26. Tokatli A, Coskun T, Ozalp I Citrullinemia. Clinical experience with 23 cases. *Turk J Pediatr.* 1998;40(2):185–193.

27. Gerrits GP, Gabreels FJ, Monnens LA, et al. Argininosuccinic aciduria: clinical and biochemical findings in three children with the late onset form, with special emphasis on cerebrospinal fluid findings of amino acids and pyrimidines. *Neuropediatrics* 1993;24(1):15–18.

28. Zimmermann A, Bachmann C, Baumgartner R. Severe liver fibrosis in argininosuccinic aciduria. *Arch Pathol Lab Med* 1986;110(2):136–140.

29. Parsons HG, Scott RB, Pinto A, et al. Argininosuccinic aciduria: long-term treatment with arginine. *J Inherit Metab Dis.* 1987;10(2):152–161.

30. Reid SV, Pan Y, Davis EC, et al. A mouse model of argininosuccinic aciduria: biochemical characterization. *Mol Genet Metab.* 2003;78(1):11–16.

31. Crombez EA, Cederbaum SD. Hyperargininemia due to liver arginase deficiency. *Mol Genet Metab.* 2005;84(3):243–251.

32. Iyer R, Jenkinson CP, Vockley JG, et al. The human arginases and arginase deficiency. *J Inherit Metab Dis* 1998;21(Suppl 1):86–100.

33. Camacho JA, Mardach R, Rioseco-Camacho N, et al. Clinical and functional characterization of a human ORNT1 mutation (T32R) in the hyperornithinemia–hyperammonemia–homocitrullinuria (HHH) syndrome. *Pediatr Res.* 2006;60(4): 423–429.

34. Smith L, Lambert MA, Brochu P, et al. Hyperornithinemia, hyperammonemia, homocitrullinuria (HHH) syndrome: presentation as acute liver disease with coagulopathy. *J Pediatr Gastroenterol Nutr.* 1992;15(4):431–436.

35. Fecarotta S, Parenti G, Vajro P, et al. HHH syndrome (hyperornithinaemia, hyperammonaemia, homocitrullinuria), with fulminant hepatitis-like presentation. *J Inherit Metab Dis.* 2006;29(1):186–189.

36. Saheki T, Kobayashi K, Iijima M, et al. Pathogenesis and pathophysiology of citrin (a mitochondrial aspartate glutamate carrier) deficiency. *Metab Brain Dis.* 2002;17(4):335–346.

37. Saheki T, Kobayashi K, Iijima M, et al. Adult-onset type II citrullinemia and idiopathic neonatal hepatitis caused by citrin deficiency: involvement of the aspartate glutamate carrier for urea synthesis and maintenance of the urea cycle. *Mol Genet Metab.* 2004;81(Suppl 1):S20–S26.

38. Saheki T, Kobayashi K, Iijima M, et al. Metabolic derangements in deficiency of citrin, a liver-type mitochondrial aspartate-glutamate carrier. *Hepatol Res.* 2005;33(2):181–184.

39. Butterworth RF Effects of hyperammonaemia on brain function. [Review] [75 refs]. *J Inherit Metab Dis.* 1998;21(Suppl 1):6–20.

40. Gyato K, Wray J, Huang ZJ, et al. Metabolic and neuropsychological phenotype in women heterozygous for ornithine transcarbamylase deficiency. *Ann Neurol* 2004;55(1):80–86.

41. Bireley WR, Van Hove JL, Gallagher RC, et al. Urea cycle disorders: brain MRI and neurological outcome. *Pediatr Radiol.* 2011;42(4):455–462.

42. Msall M, Batshaw ML, Suss R, et al. Neurologic outcome in children with inborn errors of urea synthesis. Outcome of urea-cycle enzymopathies. *N Engl J Med.* 1984;310(23): 1500–1505.

43. Choi CG, Yoo HW. Localized proton MR spectroscopy in infants with urea cycle defect. *AJNR Am J Neuroradiol* 2001;22(5):834–837.

44. Takanashi J, Kurihara A, Tomita M, et al. Distinctly abnormal brain metabolism in late-onset ornithine transcarbamylase deficiency. *Neurology* 2002;59(2):210–214.

45. Gropman AL, Fricke ST, Seltzer RR, et al. 1H MRS identifies symptomatic and asymptomatic subjects with partial ornithine transcarbamylase deficiency. *Mol Genet Metab.* 2008;95(1–2): 21–30.

46. Gropman AL, Batshaw ML Cognitive outcome in urea cycle disorders. *Mol Genet Metab* 2004;81(Suppl 1):S58–S62.

47. Msall M, Monahan PS, Chapanis N, et al. Cognitive development in children with inborn errors of urea synthesis. [Review] [16 refs]. *Acta Paediatr Jap.* 1988;30(4):435–441.

48. Summar ML, Dobbelaere D, Brusilow S, et al. Diagnosis, symptoms, frequency and mortality of 260 patients with urea cycle disorders from a 21-y, multicentre study of acute hyperammonaemic episodes. *Acta Paediatr.* 2008;97(10):1420–1425.

49. Krivitzky L, Babikian T, Lee HS, et al. Intellectual, adaptive, and behavioral functioning in children with urea cycle disorders. *Pediatr Res.* 2009;66(1):96–101.

50. Ficicioglu C, Mandell R, et al. Argininosuccinate lyase deficiency: longterm outcome of 13 patients detected by newborn screening. *Mol Genet Metab.* 2009;98(3):273–277.

51. Summar ML, Barr F, et al. Unmasked adult-onset urea cycle disorders in the critical care setting. *Crit Care Clin.* 2005; 21(4 Suppl):S1–S8.

52. Dealberto MJ, Sarazin FF. Valproate-induced hyperammonemic encephalopathy without cognitive sequelae: a case report in the psychiatric setting. *J Neuropsychiatry Clin Neurosci.* 2008;20(3):369–371.

53. Thakur V, Rupar CA, Ramsay DA, et al. Fatal cerebral edema from late-onset ornithine transcarbamylase deficiency in a juvenile male patient receiving valproic acid. *Pediatr Crit Care Med.* 2006;7(3):273–276.

54. Perrott J, Murphy NG, et al. L-carnitine for acute valproic acid overdose: a systematic review of published cases. *Ann Pharmacother.* 2010;44(7–8):1287–1293.

55. Norenberg MD, Jayakumar AR, Rama Rao KV, et al. New concepts in the mechanism of ammonia-induced astrocyte swelling. *Metab Brain Dis.* 2007;22(3–4):219–234.

56. Norenberg MD. A light electron microscopic study of experimental portal-systemic (ammonia) encephalopathy. Progression and reversal of the disorder. *Lab Invest.* 1977;36(6):618–627.

57. Tanigami H, Rebel A, Martin LJ, et al. Effect of glutamine synthetase inhibition on astrocyte swelling and altered astroglial protein expression during hyperammonemia in rats. *Neuroscience.* 2005;131(2):437–449.

58. Rose C. Effect of ammonia on astrocytic glutamate uptake/ release mechanisms. *J Neurochem.* 2006;97(Suppl 1):11–15.

59. Bachmann C Mechanisms of hyperammonemia. *Clin Chem Lab Med.* 2002;40(7):653–662.

60. Felipo V, Butterworth RF Mitochondrial dysfunction in acute hyperammonemia. *Neurochem Int.* 2002;40(6):487–491.

61. Tsacopoulos M Metabolic signaling between neurons and glial cells: a short review. *J Physiol Paris.* 2002;96(3–4):283–288.

62. Colombo JP. Urea cycle disorders, hyperammonemia and neurotransmitter changes. *Enzyme.* 1987;38(1–4):214–219.

63. Eather G, Coman D, Lander C, et al. Carbamyl phosphate synthase deficiency: diagnosed during pregnancy in a 41-year-old. *J Clin Neurosci.* 2006;13(6):702–706.

64. Gropman AL, Summar M, Leonard JV. Neurological implications of urea cycle disorders. *J Inherit Metab Dis.* 2007;30(6):865–879.

65. Marcaggi P, Coles JA. Ammonium in nervous tissue: transport across cell membranes, fluxes from neurons to glial cells, and role in signalling. *Prog Neurobiol.* 2001;64(2): 157–183.

66. Giaume C, Tabernero A, Medina JM Metabolic trafficking through astrocytic gap junctions. *Glia.* 1997;21(1):114–123.

67. Nagata N, Matsuda I, Matsuura T, et al. Retrospective survey of urea cycle disorders: Part 2. Neurological outcome in forty-nine Japanese patients with urea cycle enzymopathies. *Am J Med Genet.* 1991;40(4):477–481.

68. Brunquell P, Tezcan K, DiMario FJ, Jr. Electroencephalographic findings in ornithine transcarbamylase deficiency. *J Child Neurol.* 1999;14(8):533–536.

69. Verma NP, Chheda RL, Nigro MA, et al. Electroencephalographic findings in Rett syndrome. *Electroencephalogr Clin Neurophysiol.* 1986;64(5):394–401.

70. Engel RC, Buist NR. The EEGs of infants with citrullinemia. *Dev Med Child Neurol.* 1985;27(2):199–206.

71. Ficicioglu C, Mandell R, Shih VE. Argininosuccinate lyase deficiency: longterm outcome of 13 patients detected by newborn screening. *Mol Genet Metab.* 2009;98(3):273–277.

72. Mercimek-Mahmutoglu S, Moeslinger D, Haberle J, et al. Long-term outcome of patients with argininosuccinate lyase deficiency diagnosed by newborn screening in Austria. *Mol Genet Metab.* 2010;100(1):24–28.

73. Funabe S, Tanaka R, Urabe T, et al. [A case of adult-onset type II citrullinemia with repeated nonconvulsive status epilepticus]. *Rinsho Shinkeigaku.* 2009;49(9):571–575.

74. Summar M, Pietsch J, Deshpande J, et al. Effective hemodialysis and hemofiltration driven by an extracorporeal membrane oxygenation pump in infants with hyperammonemia. *J Pediatr.* 1996;128(3):379–382.

75. Summar M. Current strategies for the management of neonatal urea cycle disorders. *J Pediatr.* 2001;138(1 Suppl): S30–S39.

76. Brusilow SW, Danney M, Waber LJ, et al. Treatment of episodic hyperammonemia in children with inborn errors of urea synthesis. *New Engl J Med.* 1984;310:1630–1634.

77. Singh RH, Rhead WJ, Smith W, et al. Nutritional management of urea cycle disorders. *Crit Care Clin.* 2005;21(4 Suppl): S27–S35.

78. Singh RH. Nutritional management of patients with urea cycle disorders. *J Inherit Metab Dis* 2007;30(6):880–887.

79. Morgan TM, Schlegel C, Edwards KM, et al. Vaccines are not associated with metabolic events in children with urea cycle disorders. *Pediatrics* 2011;127(5):e1147–e1153.

80. Klein NP, Aukes L, Lee J, et al. Evaluation of immunization rates and safety among children with inborn errors of metabolism. *Pediatrics.* 2011;127(5):e1139–e1146.

81. Morioka D, Kasahara M, Takada Y, et al. Current role of liver transplantation for the treatment of urea cycle disorders: a review of the worldwide English literature and 13 cases at Kyoto University. *Liver Transpl.* 2005;11(11):1332–1342.

82. McBride KL, Miller G, Carter S. Developmental outcomes with early orthotopic liver transplantation for infants with neonatal-onset urea cycle defects and a female patient with late-onset ornithine transcarbamylase deficiency. *Pediatrics.* 2004;114(4):e523–e526.

10

Mitochondrial Diseases and Epilepsy

Sumit Parikh, Lynne A. Wolfe, and Andrea L. Gropman

INTRODUCTION

Epilepsy is one of the most common neurological disorders worldwide, with a prevalence of 0.5% to 1% in the general population (1). Epilepsy is characterized by recurrent, unprovoked epileptic seizures that result from excessive, synchronous, abnormal firing patterns of neurons typically located predominantly in the cerebral cortex. The burst firing neurons associated with epileptic discharges could lead to a large number of changes with events of cascades at the cellular level, such as activation of glutamate receptors, changes in composition and distribution of glutamate and gamma-aminobutyric acid receptors, cytokine activation, and oxidative stress as well as changes in plasticity and activation of late cell death pathways (2, 3) and ultimately mitochondrial dysfunction.

PATHOGENESIS OF SEIZURES IN MITOCHONDRIAL DYSFUNCTION

Bioenergetic failure in neuronal mitochondria disrupts the clearance of excitatory neurotransmitters, principally glutamate, increasing neuronal excitability and, ultimately, risk for epileptiform discharges. This seizure activity, in turn, exerts oxidative stress on neuronal mitochondria, perpetuating bioenergetic failure and hypometabolism, and ultimately compromising the active transport-mediated maintenance of ionic gradients. Loss of effective neuronal repolarization in epileptogenic zones disrupts the coordinated activity of neuronal assemblies, increasing the risk for further seizure activity.

Since mitochondria are the primary site of reactive oxygen species (ROS), this makes them uniquely vulnerable to oxidative damage that may affect neuronal excitability as well as seizure susceptibility.

Mitochondrial dysfunction may lead to acquired epilepsy. Additionally, a number of mitochondrial syndromes feature epilepsy as a core component on presentation, or with progression of disease. Compelling evidence for mitochondrial dysfunction in acquired epilepsy comes from the observation that metabolic and bioenergetic changes occur following acute seizures and during chronic epilepsy. After an acute prolonged seizure such as in status epilepticus, there is an increase in cellular glucose uptake and metabolism. As a result, increased cerebral blood flow occurs as a compensatory action. Lactate builds up due to the increased rate of glycolysis which exceeds pyruvate utilization. Mitochondria may also alter neurotransmitter metabolism based on the loss of mitochondrial *N*-acetyl aspartate in human epileptic tissue (4, 5).

Oxidative stress is one of the possible mechanisms in the pathogenesis of epilepsy, both acquired and from genetic mitochondrial dysfunction. Oxidative stress is caused by the peroxidation of cellular proteins, membrane lipids, and nuclear DNA (6). Impaired mitochondrial oxidative phosphorylation results in excessive free radical generation and a deficient antioxidant system (7).

Mitochondrial dysfunction disrupts intracellular calcium homeostasis leading to membrane depolarization and subsequent neuronal loss (8). Both the excessive generation of free radicals as well as a deficient antioxidant system is associated with an increased risk of seizure recurrence (9, 10). Human and animal studies support the concept of antioxidant supplementation for the prevention of progressive deterioration in some epilepsies (11). Hence, antioxidant therapy may be beneficial for epilepsy patients according to the brain oxidative status. This chapter will focus on epilepsy as a core feature of several genetic mitochondrial syndromes. We introduce the idea of mitochondrial dysfunction in epilepsy, and the ability to use magnetic resonance spectroscopy (MRS) to detect this is discussed in Chapter 3 of this book.

OVERVIEW OF MITOCHONDRIAL DISORDERS

Mitochondria are intracellular organelles responsible for generating energy in the form of ATP. Mitochondria are composed of about 3,000 proteins with about 300 necessary for oxidative phosphorylation. Since only 13 proteins are encoded by mitochondrial DNA (mtDNA), most mitochondrial proteins are actually encoded by the nuclear DNA (nDNA). They must then be transcribed, translated, targeted to mitochondria, imported, then folded, and assembled into final active conformation (12, 13).

There are a total of five enzyme complexes in the inner mitochondrial membrane that carry on oxidative phosphorylation: (1) Complex I (NADH: ubiquinone oxidoreductase), Complex II (succinate: ubiquinone oxidoreductase, also known as succinate dehydrogenase), (2) Complex III (ubiquinol: cytochrome C reductase), (3) Complex IV (cytochrome C oxidase also known as COX), and (4) Complex V (ATP synthase) (12).

Complex I has approximately 45 polypeptides, seven encoded from mtDNA and the others encoded by nuclear DNA. It is the largest of all the complexes. Complex I mtDNA mutations affect mostly tRNA's that cause LHON (Leber hereditary optic neuropathy) and MELAS (mitochondrial encephalomyopathy lactic acidosis and stroke-like episodes) in adults. In children with isolated Complex I deficiency, the assembly factors NDUFV1 and NDUFS4 are most commonly found with a Leigh syndrome phenotype. Patients with Complex I deficiency may be expected to have

increased reactive oxidation species that antioxidants such as ubiquinol, vitamin E and/or vitamin C may help remove. To date there is no evidence-based clinical research to suggest these diminish symptoms or prevent progression of disease (6, 13, 17).

Complex II is the smallest complex, consisting of five polypeptides, all encoded by nuclear DNA. It is unique because it is the only complex that interacts with both the TCA cycle and the electron transport chain. In addition, it is the only complex completely encoded by nuclear DNA. Complex II catalyzes oxidation of succinate to fumarate in the TCA cycle. In the electron transport chain, Complex II reduces ubiquinone to ubiquinol by taking electrons from fumarate through three iron–sulfur clusters and cytochrome b. Complex II does not generate proton flux as Complex I, III, and IV do therefore it does not directly contribute to ATP generation. Multiple phenotypes including myoclonic seizures, movement disorders and paragangliomas have been reported in patients with Complex II deficiency (13).

Complex III is made up of 11 subunits, with only the cytochrome b subunit encoded by mtDNA. Three subunits including; cytochrome b, cytochrome c1 and its iron–sulfur, pump protons into the mitochondrial matrix. Complex III is associated with multiple clinical presentations that affect multiple systems and result in early death in most patients. Mutations in the *BCS1L* gene can cause Leigh syndrome or GRACILE syndrome (growth retardation, aminoaciduria, cholestasis, iron overload, lactic acidosis and early death) (13.)

Complex IV has 13 polypeptides, the three subunits made up by copper redox centers, cytochromes and heme are encoded by mtDNA. Ten smaller subunits are nuclear encoded. Complex IV transfers electrons to oxygen that is reduced to water as protons are pumped across the inner mitochondrial membrane. Complex IV deficiency can cause Leigh syndrome, fatal infantile cardiomyopathy or a renal tubulopathy. Current research in the sco2 knock-out mouse suggests that AICAR, a AMP-dependent kinase agonist, may be a viable treatment for some patients with Complex IV deficiency (13).

Complex V contains 17 subunits of which two are encoded by mtDNA. The majority of patients with Complex V deficiency have mutations in the mtDNA *ATPase6* gene. Phenotypes most commonly associated with Complex V deficiency include LHON and neuropathy ataxia retinitis pigmentosa (NARP). TMEM70 nuclear mutations cause an early fatal syndrome that includes dysmorphic features, encephalopathy, and cardiomyopathy (13).

ATP production begins with the oxidation of glucose into pyruvate via glycolysis. Pyruvate is transported into the mitochondrial matrix where the pyruvate dehydrogenase complex converts it into acetyl-CoA for the generation of energy-rich molecules such as NADH, FADH, GTP, and ATP. Within the tricarboxylic acid (TCA) cycle, electrons generated are transferred to Complex I of the electron transport chain through NADH and to Complex II through FADH to ubiquinone (CoQ). CoQ transports electrons to Complex III and then to Complex IV via cytochrome c causing oxidation of molecular oxygen to water. Pumping protons from Complexes I, III, and IV, across the inner mitochondrial membrane, generates an electrochemical proton gradient that allows protons to flow back from the inter-membrane space into the mitochondrial matrix through Complex V generating ATP from ADP and inorganic phosphate in Complex V (12, 13, 17).

Approximately 4 million children are born each year in the United States and up to 4,000 can be expected to develop a mitochondrial disease. Many are affected by multiple electron transport chains complex deficiencies (13, 17). Additionally, in the United States, more than 50 million adults suffer from diseases in which mitochondrial dysfunction is involved. Mitochondrial dysfunction is found in diseases as diverse as cancer, infertility, diabetes, heart disease, blindness, deafness, kidney disease, liver disease, stroke, migraine, dwarfism, and also medication toxicity. Mitochondrial dysfunction is also involved in normal aging and age-related neurodegenerative diseases such as Parkinson and Alzheimer diseases (12, 13).

Mitochondrial disorders should be considered any time a progressive multisystem disorder is suspected and sometimes for isolated symptoms such as optic atrophy, sensorineural deafness, cardiomyopathy, pseudo-intestinal obstruction, neuropathy, myopathy, liver disease, early strokes, and seizures (13, 14). Besides the generation of energy, mitochondria also function in fatty acid and amino acid oxidation, heme and pyrimidine synthesis, calcium homeostasis, and apoptosis (12, 13).

The worldwide incidence of mitochondrial diseases was estimated at 11.5/100,000 (1:8,500) in 2000. In 2006, the incidence of oxidative phosphorylation (electron chain transport defects) was predicted to be approximately 1:5,000 (15). In 2008, the incidence of "at-risk" carriers of mitochondrial DNA mutations in the United Kingdom was estimated at 1:10,000 adults, the equivalent of 1:200 persons (15, 16).

MITOCHONDRIAL INHERITANCE

About 20% of mitochondrial diseases are inherited maternally as little or no mtDNA is transferred from sperm to the fertilized egg. Mitochondrial diseases can also occur sporadically or be inherited in an autosomal dominant or recessive manner. More than 200 mtDNA point mutations or deletions have been associated with mitochondrial disease (17). Approximately 100 nDNA mutations affecting mitochondrial metabolism have also been described mostly since 2006 (12, 17). It is now known that mitochondrial disease can occur across the lifespan since the regulation of many mitochondrial proteins is developmental and may also be impacted by environmental toxins. Carrier proteins normally acting as chaperones and mitochondrial fusion/fission abnormalities have also been described as the causes for mitochondrial diseases (15). Additionally, there can be tissue specific mtDNA changes that are difficult to detect with only noninvasive blood or urine studies. Finally, the clinical presentation of some mitochondrial disorders such as LHON (Leber's Hereditary Optic Neuropathy) and sensorineural deafness may be impacted by gene–gene interactions (15).

MITOCHONDRIAL DISORDERS AND EPILEPSY

Neurons represent some of the body's most metabolically demanding cells and are highly dependent on ATP produced via mitochondrial oxidative phosphorylation. Thus it is not surprising that seizures and epilepsy are a common occurrence in patients with mitochondrial disease. Some studies have shown that upwards of 60% of patients with biochemically confirmed mitochondrial disease have epilepsy, many of whom have seizures that are refractory to treatment (18). While myoclonic epilepsy has most commonly been linked to mitochondrial disease, almost any seizure type is seen and most patients typically have more than one seizure type (17). Unexplained myoclonic epilepsy or epilepsia partialis continua with other associated neurologic abnormalities are common enough findings in mitochondrial disease that their presence should lead one to begin a mitochondrial evaluation.

TYPES OF EPILEPSY IN MITOCHONDRIAL DISORDERS

Outside of myoclonic epilepsy, patients with mitochondrial disease frequently have partial or secondarily generalized clinical events with behavioral arrest and a tonic or clonic motor component to their ictal activity.

The EEG typically shows focal- or multiregional discharges, reported in over 60% of mitochondrial patients in one series (19). Atypical absence, primary generalized and atonic events can also occur, although isolated generalized epilepsy is rare in mitochondrial disease. Infantile spasms may occur, particularly in Leigh syndrome (20). It is possible that mitochondrial diseases remain under diagnosed in children with West syndrome (21). Central dopamine and folate deficiency may occur in mitochondrial patients and may provoke epilepsy in some individuals (22, 23).

EPILEPSY ALONE IS RARE AS A SYMPTOM OF MITOCHONDRIAL DISORDERS

Rarely do patients with mitochondrial disease present with isolated epilepsy. Recently, mutations in the mtDNA tRNA have been shown to present as an isolated epilepsy phenotype with complex partial seizures, focal status, and myoclonias. These patients eventually, however, develop cognitive impairment and other neurologic symptoms (24).

Here we will review the various mitochondrial syndromes and the types of epilepsy associated with them.

MITOCHONDRIAL DNA (mtDNA) DISORDERS

Mitochondria are the only structures of our bodies that carry their own separate DNA—the mitochondrial DNA (mtDNA)—a compact 37 gene volume that is maternally inherited and responsible for creating part of the machinery needed to create functional mitochondria. Some of the earliest recognized forms of mitochondrial disease were due to defects in the mtDNA, with well-defined phenotypes and clustering of the patient's symptoms into various categories or syndromes. While we now understand that most patients with mitochondrial disease do not present syndromically or with maternally inherited disease, these initially described conditions, often designated by acronyms, remain an important cause of mitochondrial disease and epilepsy. A selected subset of over 10 known mtDNA syndromes is described below.

MYOCLONIC EPILEPSY, LACTIC ACIDOSIS, AND STROKE (MELAS)

MELAS is a mitochondrial disorder due to one of several mtDNA point mutations with the 3243 mutation seen most commonly, affecting the formation of mitochondrial tRNA-leucine (15).

Classically, MELAS presents in childhood with the sudden onset of stroke-like episodes. Children may be asymptomatic prior to this event or have varying degrees of underlying developmental disabilities. The strokes typically occur in a nonvascular distribution and manifest as seizures. These seizures are often focal at onset, with secondary generalization. Focal status or EPC may occur. Strokes often occur in the occipital lobes and seizures may present as visual auras or hallucinations with occipital headaches. Patients may present with occipital status epilepticus (25). Worsening of headaches in these patients may imply break-through epileptic events. Myoclonic seizures frequently develop over time. Nonepileptic photic, action or postural myoclonus may also occur. The disease progresses with associated cognitive decline, hearing loss and myopathy. Lactic acidosis is a common finding, especially during times of acute deterioration. Other features of mitochondrial disease such as short stature, retinal degeneration, and optic atrophy can occur. These findings are not specific to MELAS and may be seen in any mitochondrial disease.

MYOCLONIC EPILEPSY WITH RAGGED-RED FIBERS (MERRF)

MERRF is a mitochondrial disorder due to one of several mutations in the mtDNA, with the A > G8344 mutation seen most commonly. Symptoms typically begin in the adolescent or young adult years with myoclonic epilepsy. Ataxia eventually develops. Affected individuals may have short stature, and develop hearing loss, optic atrophy, myopathy, and cognitive decline (15). Due to the prominence of myoclonus and eventual neurologic decline, MERRF is classified as one of the progressive myoclonus epilepsy

(PME) syndromes. Lactic acidosis and ragged red fibers on muscle biopsy histology are characteristic findings though they are not always present early in the disease course.

Electroencephalogram findings may include background slowing, focal epileptiform discharges, and atypical spike or sharp and slow-wave discharges that have a variable association with the myoclonic jerks. Suppression of these discharges during sleep is characteristic. As with many of the PMEs, giant somatosensory evoked potentials are observed (19).

mtDNA DELETION SYNDROMES

Large-scale deletions of the mtDNA lead to three syndromes with overlapping symptoms, including Kearns–Sayre syndrome (KSS), chronic progressive external ophthalmoplegia (CPEO), and Pearson's syndrome (15). Patients with KSS have a combination of short stature, retinopathy, cardiac conduction defects, ataxia and ophthalmoplegia with ptosis. Symptoms begin in childhood and progress over time (17). Most patients with Pearson's syndrome present in childhood with sideroblastic anemia and pancreatic insufficiency and most CPEO patients predominantly have ptosis and ophthalmoplegia. However, a subset of these patients often develops some of the symptoms seen in KSS. Epilepsy is extremely rare in these conditions. CPEO can be seen in mitochondrial disorders due to other mutations, however, in which case epilepsy may be a more common occurrence.

MITOCHONDRIAL DISORDERS DUE TO MUTATIONS IN nDNA

Nuclear (nDNA) genes are involved in guiding mitochondrial assembly, subunit formation, fusion/fission and mtDNA replication. Defects in these genes may lead to syndromic or nonsyndromic mitochondrial disease.

DISORDERS OF mtDNA DEPLETION

mtDNA replicaton is an essential and complex process involving the coordinated efforts of a variety of nDNA genes. Mutations in any one of these genes (*DGUOK, MPV17, POLG, RRM2B, SUCLA2, SUCLG1, TK2,* and *PEO1*) leads to defective mtDNA replication or disruption in maintaining mitochondrial nucleotide pools, culminating in mtDNA depletion in various cells and eventual mitochondrial disease (15). Mutations in the

POLG1 was one of the first identified mtDNA replication genes and mutations here have become a critical and frequent finding in many patients with mitochondrial disease.

POLG1 DISEASE, INCLUDING CHILDHOOD ONSET EPILEPSIA PARTIALIS CONTINUA AND ALPERS DISEASE

Mutations in POLG1 are now linked to a wide array of growing mitochondrial disease phenotypes. While many of these phenotypes do not have seizures as their primary or only feature, a phenotype with EPC as the initial and often only manifestation is known as a form with progressive myoclonus epilepsy (26).

POLG1 mutations have also been identified as the principal cause of Alpers disease (27). Alpers or Alpers–Huttenlocher disease is characterized by a rapidly progressive encephalopathy with intractable seizures and diffuse neuronal degeneration. Seizures are often partial complex or myoclonic though they can evolve to include multiple types (28). Varying amounts of liver disease are also present. Symptoms may begin at any age and liver disease may not be present for years. Encephalopathy and liver disease can stabilize with partial resolution of symptoms. Disease onset or worsening after exposure to valproate are characteristic of this condition (29).

POLG1 disease, as with MELAS, may mimic an occipital-lobe epilepsy syndrome or cause status epilepticus (28).

In a child with previously normal development, an explosive onset of focal epilepsy, EPC, status epilepticus, or prominent occipital epileptiform discharges, *POLG1*-related mitochondrial disease should be considered and valproate should be avoided until this diagnosis is excluded. There is discussion as to whether select patients should receive *POLG1* testing prior to initiating valproate therapy (30). Status epilepticus in POLG1-related disease is often difficult to treat.

POLG1-related mitochondrial disease may also lead to a phenotype of myoclonic epilepsy myopathy sensory ataxia (MEMSA). Symptoms typically begin in late adolescence to young adulthood with cerebellar ataxia due to a sensory polyneuropathy. Epilepsy, often focal, begins in the subsequent years. Seizures are often refractory to treatment. Recurrent bouts of status epilepticus may occur. Patients often develop cognitive decline and a myopathy over time (31).

OTHER mtDNA DEPLETION SYNDROMES

POLG2 and *TWINKLE* related mitochondrial diseases may also present with recurrent status epilepticus (28, 32). Mutations in *SUCLA2* and *SUCLG1* lead to infant onset hypotonia, muscle atrophy, a hyperkinetic movement disorder, and epilepsy including infantile spasms or generalized convulsions. Seizures typically start prior to age 3 years. A unique finding in these patients is an elevation in methylmalonic acid in plasma and urine (33, 35). Mutations in *DGUOK, MPV17, TK2* are not typically associated with epilepsy (31, 34, 35).

LEIGH SYNDROME

Leigh syndrome (subacute necrotizing encephalomyopathy) is a clinical and radiologic subtype of mitochondrial disease. Patients typically present with acute to subacute neurologic regression and neuroimaging findings of varying amounts of bilateral, symmetric basal ganglia, thalamic, mid-brain, and brainstem lesions that fluctuate in severity. The disease progresses with fluctuating but worsening hypotonia, spasticity, eye movement abnormalities, and brain-stem failure. The MRI eventually also shows varying degrees of white matter disease along with cortical and cerebellar atrophy in addition to the brainstem, midbrain, and subcortical findings (36).

Leigh syndrome can occur in mitochondrial disorders due to nDNA or mtDNA mutations (36). This phenotype can occur due to certain nonmitochondrial metabolic disorders as well.

Both focal and generalized epilepsy have been described in Leigh syndrome (36). Patients with infantile spasms and EEG hypsarrhythmia have been described as well (37, 38). In addition, there have been cases of epilepsia partialis continua. EEG features do not appear to be distinctive enough to contribute to the clinical diagnosis of Leigh syndrome (38).

Biochemical Defects in Mitochondrial Function

Owing to limitations in genetic technology and knowledge, many patients with mitochondrial disease often receive a biochemical diagnosis due to abnormalities found in enzyme analysis of mitochondrial function in muscle tissue. In these circumstances, the patient often does not have a readily identifiable syndromic mitochondrial disease. These individuals often have their mitochondrial disease designated as Complex I–V disease, labeled by the mitochondrial electron-transport-chain (ETC) component(s) most impaired on biochemical analysis of muscle tissue. A mitochondrial disease diagnosis is often made utilizing a combination of clinical, laboratory, and biochemical findings with the aid of various clinical diagnostic criteria (12, 13, 17, 39). In some instances, a genetic diagnosis of the nDNA or mtDNA is eventually established with mutations in various genes involved in encoding ETC structural or assembly protein components.

In patients with biochemically confirmed mitochondrial disease, a variety of epilepsy subtypes have been noted. These include neonatal status epilepticus, infantile spasms, refractory status, focal status, myoclonic events, and complex partial seizures. Ohtahara syndrome has been described (17, 38). Most of these patients rarely have epilepsy as their only symptom and present with other symptoms or neuroimaging or laboratory abnormalities indicative of mitochondrial disease (17, 31, 38).

TREATMENT

Although efficacy varies, epilepsy in mitochondrial disease is typically difficult to treat. All anticonvulsants and nonmedical treatments have been attempted including the ketogenic diet and vagus nerve stimulator. The ketogenic diet and vagus nerve stimulator have had modest and mixed success though are safe in many mitochondrial patients (40, 41).

The ketogenic diet, based on the intake of high-fat dietary content with low carbohydrate and protein, leads to a switch from glucose metabolism to the generation and metabolism of ketone bodies. Preliminary data suggest that the mechanism of action of the ketogenic diet may involve decreasing mitochondrial dysfunction in epileptogenic cells (40).

Recent evidence suggests that chronic administration of a ketogenic diet may alter mitochondrial function by chronically decreasing production of reactive oxygen species. This, in turn, increases the expression of uncoupling proteins, promoting mitochondrial biogenesis, as well as stimulating glutathione synthase biosynthesis, and activating the NF E2-related factor 2 pathway by redox signaling. The end result is cellular adaptation, induction of protective proteins, and overall improvement of the mitochondrial redox state (39, 40). These findings raise the possibility that targeting mitochondrial dysfunction may provide a future therapeutic approach for treatment of seizures.

IV infusions of arginine may benefit some patients with MELAS and other mitochondrial cytopathies in the setting of status epilepticus, although this therapy has been better studied for the indication of acute metabolic strokes (42, 43). Levetiracetam may be beneficial for myoclonic seizures, especially in MERRF syndrome.

Whether or not utilization of valproic acid is safe in mitochondrial patients remains unsettled, although it is contraindicated in most patients with *POLG1* mutations and may aggravate symptoms in other mitochondrial cytopathies including *TWINKLE* gene mediated disease and MELAS (29, 30). Magnesium infusions may help treat refractory status epilepticus in patients with POLG1 mutations (44).

Surgical management of mitochondrial epilepsy is typically contraindicated since these patients often have multiple regions of epileptiform discharges along with the potential for other regions of the brain to become epileptogenic. The exception to this rule may be in patients with coexisting focal malformations of cortical development.

Although multiple combinations of B vitamins, antioxidants, creatine, carnitine, and other supplements have been used alone or in combinations known as a Mitochondrial Cocktail, to date there is limited evidence to support these strategies and clinical trials are needed. Specific to mitochondrial-related seizure management, we have learned to look for POLG1 mutations before using valproic acid formulations to avoid having patients develop Alper syndrome. Likewise, seizures in POLG disease may respond to magnesium even if resistant to most antiepileptic medications. MERRF-related myoclonic epilepsy may respond best to levetiracetam. Current recommendations for patients with mitochondrial disease in general include eating a well-balanced diet with supplemental gastrostomy tube feedings as necessary, avoidance of obesity, endurance-based exercise, and early recognition and treatment of infections, seizures, cardiac rhythm disturbances, or cardiomyopathy.

FUTURE DIRECTIONS

Methods that allow for the detection of brain oxidative status may be important for predicting the prognosis of epilepsy in patients with mitochondrial disorders.

KEY POINTS

- A mitochondrial disease diagnosis is often made utilizing a combination of clinical, laboratory, and biochemical findings with the aid of various clinical diagnostic criteria. Patients with mitochondrial disorders often present with epilepsy.
- Bioenergetic failure in neuronal mitochondria disrupts the clearance of excitatory neurotransmitters, principally glutamate, increasing neuronal excitability and, ultimately, the risk for epileptiform discharges.
- Surgical management of epilepsy is rarely successful in patients with mitochondrial disorder since they tend to have multifocal epileptiform discharges.
- In a child with previously normal development, an explosive onset of focal epilepsy, EPC or status epilepticus, and at times a predominance of occipital epileptiform discharges, *POLG1*-related mitochondrial disease should be considered.
- Valproic acid is contraindicated in patients with POLG1 mutations.

CLINICAL PEARLS

- All of the five complexes of the electron chain are comprised of nuclear encoded and mtDNA encoded subunits except complex II which is solely derived from nDNA encoded proteins. This is important from a diagnostic viewpoint.
- Outside of myoclonic epilepsy, most patients with mitochondrial disease have partial or secondarily generalized clinical events with behavioral arrest, and a tonic or clonic motor component to their clinical seizure activity.
- Avoid valproic acid in a patient suspected of a POLG1 mutation.

REFERENCES

1. Hauser WA, Annegers JF, Kurland LT. Prevalence of epilepsy in Rochester, Minnesota: 1940–1980. *Epilepsia.* 1991;32(4):429–445.
2. Haut SR, Velísková J, Moshé SL. Susceptibility of immature and adult brains to seizure effects. *Lancet Neurol.* 2004;3(10): 608–617.
3. Henshall DC, Simon RP. Epilepsy and apoptosis pathways. *J Cereb Blood Flow Metab.* 2005;25(12):1557–1572.
4. Savic I, Thomas AM, Ke Y, et al. *In vivo* measurements of glutamine + glutamate (Glx) and *N*-acetyl aspartate (NAA) levels in human partial epilepsy. *Acta Neurol Scand.* 2000;102(3):179–188.

5. Vielhaber S, Niessen HG, Debska-Vielhaber G, et al. Subfield-specific loss of hippocampal *N*-acetyl aspartate in temporal lobe epilepsy. *Epilepsia*. 2008;49(1):40–50.

6. Floyd RA, Carney JM. Free radical damage to protein and DNA: mechanisms involved and relevant observations on brain undergoing oxidative stress. *Ann Neurol*. 1992;32(Suppl): S22–S27.

7. Peternel S, Pilipović K, Zupan G. Seizure susceptibility and the brain regional sensitivity to oxidative stress in male and female rats in the lithium-pilocarpine model of temporal lobe epilepsy. *Prog Neuropsychopharmacol Biol Psychiatry*. 2009; 33(3): 456–462.

8. Waldbaum S, Patel M. Mitochondrial dysfunction and oxidative stress: a contributing link to acquired epilepsy? *J Bioenerg Biomembr*. 2010;42(6):449–455.

9. Jesberger JA, Richardson JS. Oxygen free radicals and brain dysfunction. *Int J Neurosci*. 1991;57(1–2):1–17.

10. Kürekçi AE, Alpay F, Tanindi S, et al. Plasma trace element, plasma glutathione peroxidase, and superoxide dismutase levels in epileptic children receiving antiepileptic drug therapy. *Epilepsia*. 1995;36(6):600–604.

11. Wu Y, Liu Y, Han Y, et al. Pyridoxine increases nitric oxide biosynthesis in human platelets. *Int J Vitam Nutr Res*. 2009;79(2):95–103.

12. Calvo SE, Mootha VK. The mitochondrial proteome and human disease. *Annu. Rev. Genom Hum Genet*. 2010;11:25–44.

13. Koene S, Smeitink JAM. *Mitochondrial Medicine: A Clinical Guideline*. Nijemgen, The Netherlands: Khondrion; 2011.

14. Johns DR. Mitochondrial DNA and disease. *N Engl J Med*. 1995;333:638–644.

15. DiMauro S. A history of mitochondrial diseases. *J Inherit Metab Dis*. 2010;34(2):261–276.

16. Elliot H, Samules DC, Eden JA, et al. Pathogenic mitochondrial DNA mutations are common in the general population. *Am J Hum Genet*. 2008;83:254–260.

17. DiMauro S, Schon EA. Mitochondrial disorders in the nervous system. *Annu Rev Neurosci*. 2008;31:91–123.

18. Khurana DS, Salganicoff L, Melvin JJ, et al. Epilepsy and respiratory chain defects in children with mitochondrial encephalopathies. *Mol Genet Metab*. 2008;39:8–13.

19. Canafoglia L, Franceschetti S, Antozzi C, et al. Epileptic pheotypes associated with mitochondrial disorders. *Neurology*. 2001;56(10):1340–1346.

20. Sadier LG, Connolly MB, Applegarth D, et al. Spasms in children with definite and probable mitochondrial disease. *Eur J Neurol*. 2004;11(2):103–110.

21. Blanco-Barca O, Pintos-Martinez E, Alonso-Martin A, et al. Mitochondrial encephalopathies and West's syndrome: a frequently under-diagnosed association. *Rev Neurol*. 2004;39(7): 618–623.

22. Garcia-Cazorla A, Quadros EV, Nascimento A, et al. Mitochondrial diseases associated with cerebral folate deficiency. *Neurology*. 2008;70(16):1360–1362.

23. Raemaekers VT, Weis J, Sequeira JM, et al. Mitochondrial complex I encephalopathy and cerebral 5-methyltetrahydrofolate deficiency. *Neuropediatrics*. 2007; 38(4):184–187.

24. Zsurka G, Hampel KG, Nelson I, et al. Severe epilepsy as the major symptom of new mutations in the mitochondrial tRNA (Phe) gene. *Neurology*. 2010;74(6):507–512.

25. Karkare S, Merchant S, Solomon G, et al. MELAS A3243G mutation presenting with occipital status epilepticus. *J Child Neurol*. 2009;24(12):1564–1567.

26. Engelsen BA, Tzoulis C, Karlson B, et al. POLG1 mutations cause a syndromic epilepsy with occipital lobe predilection. *Brain*. 2008;131(Part 3):818–828.

27. Chan SS, Copeland WC. DNA polymerase gamma is the only known DNA polymerase in human mitochondria and is essential for mitochondrial DNA replication and repair. *Biochim Biophys Acta*. 2009; 1787(5):312–319.

28. Wolf NI, Rahman S, Schmitt B, et al. Status epilepticus in children with Alpers disease caused by POLG1 mutations: EEG and MRI features. *Epilepsia*. 2009;50(6):1596–1607.

29. McFarland R, Hudson G, Taylor RW, et al. Reversible valproate heptotoxicity due to mutations in mitochondrial DNA polymerase gamma (POLG1). *Arch Dis Child*. 2008;93(2):151–153.

30. Saneto RP, Lee IC, Loenig MK, et al. POLG DNA testing as an emerging standard of care before instituting valproic acid therapy for pediatric seizure disorders. *Seizure*. 2010;19(3):140–146.

31. Finsterer J. Inherited mitochondrial neuropathies. *J Neurol Sci*. 2011;15:304(1–2):9–16.

32. Lonnqvist T, Paetua A, Valanne L, et al. Recessive twinkle mutations cause severe epileptic encephalopathy. *Brain*. 2009;132(Pt 6):1553–1562.

33. Cohen BH, Chinnery PF, Copeland WC. POLG-related disorders. 1993. In: RA Pagon, TD Bird, CR Dolan, K Stephens eds. *GeneReviews [Internet]*. University of Washington: Seattle, WA; 1993–2010.

34. Dimmock DP, Zhang Q, Dionisi-Vici C, et al. Clinical and molecular features of mitochondrial DNA depletion due to mutations in deoxyguanosine kinase. *Hum Mutat*. 2008;29(2):330–331.

35. Spinazzola A, Invernizzi F, Carrara F, et al. Clinical and molecular features of mitochondrial DNA depletion syndromes. *J Inherit Metab Dis*. 2009;32(2):143–158.

36. DiMauro S, DiVivo DC. Genetic heterogeneity of Leigh syndrome. *Ann Neurol*. 1996;40(1):5–7.

37. DiMauro S, Ricci E, Hirano M, et al. Epilepsy in mitochondrial encephalopathies. *Epilepsy Res Suppl*. 1991;4:173–180.

38. El Sabbagh S, Lebre AS, Bahi-Buisson N, et al. Epileptic phenotypes in children with respiratory chain disorders. *Epilepsia*. 2010;51(7):1225–1235.

39. Wolf NI, Smeitink JA. Mitochondrial disorders: a proposal for consensus diagnostic criteria in infants and children. *Neurology*. 2002;59(9):1402–1405.

40. Bough K. Energy metabolism as part of the anticonvulsant mechanism of the ketogenic diet. *Epilepsia*. 2008;49(Suppl 8):91–93.

41. Schiff M, Benit P, Coulibaly A, et al. Mitochondrial response to controlled nutrition in health and disease. *Nutr Rev*. 2011;69(2):65–75.

42. Koga Y, Akita N, Junko N, et al. Endothelial dysfunction in MELAS improved by L-arginine supplementation. *Neurology*. 2006;66:1766–1769.

43. Koga Y, Povalko N, Nishioka J, et al. MELAS and L-arginine therapy: pathophysiology of stroke-like episodes. *Ann NY Acad. Sci*. 2010;104–110.

44. Visser NA, Braun KP, Leiten FS, et al. Magnesium treatment for patients with refractory status epilepticus due to POLG1-mutations. *J Neurol*. 2011;258(2):218–222.

Pyridoxine-Dependent Epilepsy and Related Conditions

Sidney M. Gospe, Jr.

INTRODUCTION

Pyridoxine-dependent epilepsy (PDE) may be considered as the prototypical form of a metabolic neonatal epilepsy which is unresponsive to anticonvulsants but which is specifically treated with a vitamin or cofactor. First described in 1954, our understanding of this inherited epileptic encephalopathy has improved greatly since the reporting of various clinical phenotypes during the 1980s and 1990s, and the subsequent discovery of mutations in the *ALDH7A1* gene which encodes the protein antiquitin (ATQ) in 2006. This chapter reviews our current understanding of PDE together with two related disorders: folinic acid-responsive seizures, which is allelic to PDE, and pyridoxal phosphate-responsive neonatal epileptic encephalopathy, a metabolic epilepsy in which pyridoxine treatment is ineffective while administration of the active cofactor pyridoxal-5′-phosphate (PLP) is curative.

PYRIDOXINE-DEPENDENT EPILEPSY (ATQ DEFICIENCY)

HISTORICAL ASPECTS

In the original description of PDE, and in what is frequently thought of as the typical form of the disorder, patients present with neonatal seizures which are intractable to treatment with conventional anticonvulsants and which only come under control once pharmacologic doses of pyridoxine are administered

and then continued on a regular basis. PDE was first described in 1954 by Hunt and colleagues in their report of a newborn with pharmacoresistant seizures that finally came under control after the institution of scheduled treatment with a parenteral multivitamin preparation (1). With the methodical elimination of various components of this product, it was eventually discovered that pyridoxine (vitamin B_6) was the factor responsible for controlling the baby's seizures. In this same report, the heritability of PDE was suggested, as one of the mother's previous pregnancies resulted in a newborn who succumbed from intractable seizures. An autosomal recessive pattern of inheritance was subsequently demonstrated. In the more than 5 decades since the first description of PDE, more than 200 cases have been reported (2–7), with the majority of these publications appearing over the past 25 years focusing on atypical clinical presentations (8–11), neurodevelopmental features (12–16), electroencephalographic (EEG) characteristics (17–22), and imaging findings (13, 21, 23). The most recent reports have focused on the biochemical abnormality underlying PDE and the associated mutations in the *ALDH7A1* gene (15, 24–32).

EPIDEMIOLOGY

PDE is considered to be a rare disease, and only a few epidemiologic studies have been published (12, 13, 33–35). For example, a study from the United

Kingdom and the Republic of Ireland reported a point prevalence of 1:687,000 for definite and probable cases of PDE (33), while a survey conducted in the Netherlands reported an estimated birth incidence of 1:396,000 (34). PDE is quite likely under-diagnosed and a higher birth incidence is suspected. This notion is supported by a study from a German center where pyridoxine administration is part of a standard treatment protocol for neonatal seizures and a birth incidence of probable cases of 1:20,000 was reported (35). In addition, in a hospital-based study from India, six of 81 children with intractable seizures responded to the vitamin (36).

CLINICAL DESCRIPTION

Patients with PDE must receive regular pharmacologic doses of pyridoxine. If not treated in this manner, the disorder frequently results in death from status epilepticus. This particular clinical scenario has been reported retrospectively in children who expired prior to the birth and subsequent diagnosis of PDE in a younger sibling (2, 7). A variety of clinical presentations of PDE have been reported. Universally, all patients with PDE have clinical seizures which either recur serially or evolve into status epilepticus despite treatment with large doses of one or more conventional anticonvulsants. In most instances, the institution of either parenteral or oral pyridoxine rapidly results in seizure control and improvement in the encephalopathy. PDE may present within hours of birth as an epileptic encephalopathy that may mimic hypoxic-ischemic encephalopathy (2, 7, 13, 33). In a few instances neonatal lactic acidosis, hypoglycemia, electrolyte disturbances, hypothyroidism and diabetes insipidus have been reported (27, 37). In addition, mothers may report having experienced unusual fetal movements that likely represent intrauterine fetal seizures. While PDE may also present with seizures at various times during the first 2 months of life, the presentation of the epileptic encephalopathy after this age is considered to be late-onset and therefore atypical (7, 10, 38). Together with the late-onset cases, other atypical forms of PDE have been described, including patients whose seizures first respond to anticonvulsants but who then develop a recurrence weeks to months later in which seizures become intractable, and infants whose seizures are not controlled by initial large doses of pyridoxine but which then do respond at a subsequent time to a second trial (2, 8–10, 38). Pyridoxine treatment must continue, or clinical seizures will reappear, generally within days. Patients with PDE are not pyridoxine-deficient, and it is important to educate parents, therapists, teachers and others providing services to these patients about this important clinical point.

SEIZURE SEMIOLOGY

A variety of clinical features and semiology of seizures have been reported in patients with PDE. The condition may present with a neonatal encephalopathy which includes gastrointestinal symptoms such as emesis and abdominal distention, neurologic irritability, hyperalertness, sleeplessness, facial grimacing and abnormal eye movements associated with recurrent partial motor seizures, generalized tonic seizures or myoclonus. Subsequently, complex partial seizures, infantile spasms and other myoclonic seizures as well as a mixed seizure pattern may develop. In untreated cases, it is not uncommon for status epilepticus to develop at some point. Similar seizure types may occur in patients with late-onset PDE, along with infantile spasms as an initial clinical presentation, generalized clonic seizures, atonic seizures, visual seizures (described as intermittent loss of vision, flashing lights, and visual hallucinations sometimes followed by a generalized convulsion) and recurrent status epilepticus (7, 12, 13, 15, 16, 20, 33). Importantly, in all cases there is a high risk of status epilepticus developing after the discontinuation of pyridoxine supplementation. With adherence to a regimen of daily lifelong pharmacological doses of pyridoxine, the prognosis for seizure control in most individuals with PDE is generally excellent, with only an occasional breakthrough seizure which may occur during an acute illness such as when the patient is febrile or experiences gastroenteritis leading to a temporary reduction in pyridoxine bioavailability. However, some patients managed compliantly with appropriate doses of pyridoxine may still experience recurrent seizures and will therefore require treatment with one or more anticonvulsant medications. It has been hypothesized that in these cases a secondary cause of epilepsy, such as mesial temporal sclerosis, hydrocephalus or other brain dysgenesis, may be responsible (2, 12, 39).

ASSOCIATED NEURODEVELOPMENTAL DISABILITIES

A spectrum of neurodevelopmental disabilities have been reported in patients with PDE. Deficits in expressive language are common, and affected patients have also been described with nonverbal cognitive deficits, as well as motor developmental delay associated with mild hypotonia (2, 7, 12). Severely affected patients have been described with cerebral palsy and a significant intellectual handicap. Behavioral features typical for either obsessive–compulsive disorder or autistic spectrum disorder have been reported in some adolescent and adult cases (12). It has been suggested that the early diagnosis and effective treatment of PDE results in a more favorable neurodevelopmental outcome, and that individuals with late-onset PDE more frequently have a better prognosis (including a few cases with reportedly normal development). However, the neurodevelopmental profile of PDE is likely multifactorial, and would include the time of clinical onset (fetal, neonatal, or late-onset), the length of time to diagnosis and effective treatment, compliance with pyridoxine therapy, associated brain dysgenesis, and the presently undiscovered correlation between *ALDH7A1* genotype and neurodevelopmental phenotype (2, 7, 12, 15, 16, 27, 32, 40, 41). Few neuropsychologic evaluations of PDE patients have been reported in the literature. From these formal psychometric assessments, a characteristic behavioral profile has been suggested which includes a reduction in the cognitive/verbal IQ, particularly in measures of expressive language, together with a low normal motor/performance IQ (2, 12–14).

CLINICAL DIAGNOSTIC STUDIES

Reports of the ictal and interictal EEG characteristics of patients with PDE have been inconsistent and it therefore remains difficult to define a specific pattern of EEG abnormalities (17–22, 42). In patients with PDE, it is not uncommon for an EEG to be performed after several seizures have been observed as well as after anticonvulsant medications, typically phenobarbital, have been instituted. The EEG may be affected by one or both of these factors and therefore confound a PDE-specific pattern. Considering this important caveat, abnormal background activity along with a variety of paroxysmal features has been described. These include generalized and multifocal epileptiform activity, discontinuous patterns including burst-suppression, bursts of high-voltage slow waves, and hypsarrhythmia in patients with infantile spasms. While electrographic seizures are characteristically recorded during an accompanying clinical seizure in PDE patients, some behavioral changes considered to be clinical seizures (such as facial grimacing and abnormal eye movements) may not have an EEG correlate (20). It is important to emphasize that in some untreated patients, as well as in many pyridoxine-treated patients, is it not uncommon for the interictal EEG to be normal or to demonstrate only minimal epileptiform activity. In addition, the immediate and long-term responses of the EEG to the administration of pyridoxine are varied. While classically parenteral pyridoxine administration results in a dramatic termination of electrographic seizures which correlates with a striking clinical improvement, recent studies indicate that this response may be incomplete or delayed, or a transient worsening of the EEG may actually develop (18, 20). Therefore, clinicians must realize that a clinical diagnosis of PDE should not be made solely by examining the minute-to-minute effects of pyridoxine administration on either the ictal or interictal EEG. A definitive diagnosis of PDE must be based on clinical effectiveness of pyridoxine therapy together with biochemical and/or genetic confirmation.

Various neuroimaging findings have been described in PDE cases, but it is not uncommon for affected patients to have normal imaging studies. Therefore, none of these imaging features may be concluded to be pathognomonic of the disease. Thinning of the isthmus of the corpus callosum, mega cisterna magna, and neuronal migration abnormalities have been reported in several patients, while varying degrees of cerebral atrophy have been described in late-diagnosed or inadequately treated patients. Progressive hydrocephalus necessitating shunting has also been reported (2, 13, 21, 23, 27).

NEUROCHEMISTRY AND NEUROGENETICS

The term pyridoxine encompasses the six vitamers of vitamin B_6: the alcohol pyridoxine (referred to as pyridoxol in older literature), the aldehyde pyridoxal, the amine pyridoxamine, and their respective 5'-phosphorylated esters (Figure 11.1). Though vitamin B_6 is an essential nutrient, these compounds are present in both animal- and plant-derived foods, and therefore clinical pyridoxine-deficiency states are uncommon (43, 44). After ingestion, the phosphorylated esters,

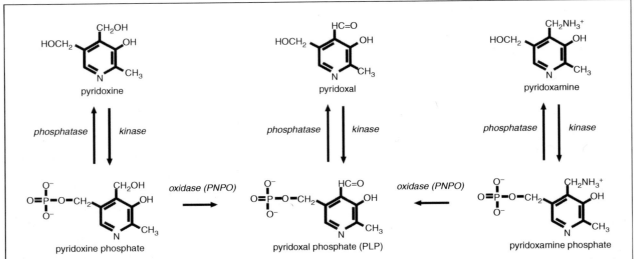

FIGURE 11.1   The six vitamin B_6 vitamers and the enzymatic reactions leading to their interconversion. Reproduced with permission from the *Chang Gung Medical Journal* (Gospe SM. Neonatal vitamin-responsive epileptic encephalopathies. *Chang Gung Med J.* 2010;33:1–12) (5).

either from foods or commercially prepared supplements, are dephosphorylated by a phosphatase, and then absorbed. After absorption, pyridoxine, pyridoxamine and pyridoxal may by phosphorylated by a kinase and the six vitamers are systemically distributed. Importantly, both pyridoxine phosphate and pyridoxamine phosphate are converted to the active cofactor pyridoxal phosphate (PLP) by pyridox(am)ine 5'-phosphate oxidase, and PLP is also formed by the direct phosphorylation of pyridoxal. PLP plays numerous metabolic roles in over 140 reactions making up at least 4% of all classified enzyme activities including transamination of amino acids, decarboxylation reactions, modulation of the activity of steroid hormones and regulation of gene expression (45, 46). Of neurologic significance, abnormalities of pyridoxine homeostasis may result in alterations in dopaminergic, serotonergic, glutaminergic, and GABAergic neurotransmission.

In 2006, mutations in the *ALDH7A1* gene which encodes ATQ, an aldehyde dehydrogenase that functions within the cerebral lysine catabolism pathway (Figure 11.2), were demonstrated to underlie PDE (28). Over 60 *ALDH7A1* mutations have now been reported in patients with both homozygous and compound heterozygous *ALDH7A1* genotypes. These reports have included primarily patients with neonatal-onset PDE together with a few individuals with late-onset PDE

(15, 24, 26–28, 30–32, 41). Importantly, affected patients have elevations in alpha-aminoadipic semialdehyde (AASA) in plasma, urine and cerebrospinal fluid (CSF), and detection of elevated levels of this organic acid is a sensitive marker for PDE (27, 47, 48). While AASA was first thought to be a specific biomarker for PDE, recent research has demonstrated that AASA is also elevated in patients with molybdenum cofactor deficiency and isolated sulfite oxidase deficiency (50). In patients with elevated levels of AASA, these latter two conditions may be differentiated from PDE by measuring urinary sulfite/sulfocysteine levels. While the biochemical finding of elevated plasma, urine and CSF levels of AASA in PDE patients persists even after years of effective treatment, elevations of the indirect biomarker pipecolic acid (PA) may also be detected in plasma and CSF, but in some patients normalize after effective long-term therapy (25, 28, 29, 49).

AASA is in equilibrium with Δ^1-piperidine-6-carboxylate (P6C) which through a Knoevenagel condensation reaction with PLP inactivates the cofactor (28). Therefore, accumulation of AASA results in an intracellular reduction in PLP; importantly, while patients with PDE are not systemically pyridoxine-deficient, from a cellular physiology perspective they are PLP-deficient. Reduced levels of PLP in the cerebrospinal fluid (CSF) have been documented in a few patients

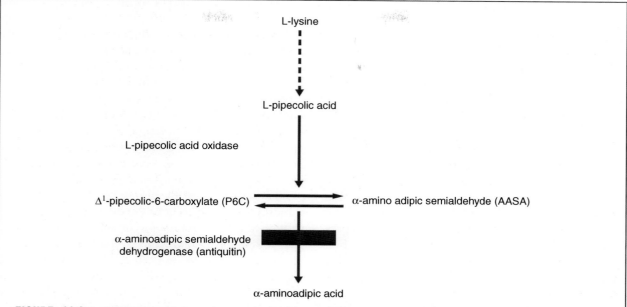

FIGURE 11.2 Cerebral lysine metabolic pathway. Bar indicates the site of the block of alpha-aminoadipic semialdehyde dehydrogenase (ATQ) in pyridoxine-dependent seizures. Reproduced with permission from the *Chang Gung Medical Journal* (Gospe SM. Neonatal vitamin-responsive epileptic encephalopathies. *Chang Gung Med J.* 2010;33:112) (5).

with PDE (51). This PLP deficiency likely affects the function of glutamic acid decarboxylase, the enzyme that converts the excitatory neurotransmitter glutamic acid into the inhibitory neurotransmitter GABA. An imbalance between these excitatory and inhibitory neurotransmitters may be responsible for the development of encephalopathy and intractable epileptic seizures. It is also possible that altered GABA signaling may be implicated in the abnormal neurogenesis, proliferation and migration noted in some cases (52). It is likely that dysfunction of other PLP-dependent enzymes also plays a role in the pathophysiology of PDE. For example, some of the white matter and other developmental abnormalities noted on neuroimaging could be secondary to dysfunction of serine palmitoyl transferase which catalyses the rate limiting step in the synthesis of sphingolipids (53), sphingosine-1-phosphate (S1P) lyase which degrades S1P, a molecule that regulates proliferation, differentiation, migration and apoptosis (54), or serine racemase which plays a role in neuronal migration (27, 55). Also, elevations of threonine, glycine, and 3-methoxytyrosine in CSF, indicative of dysfunction of

threonine hydratase, glycine cleavage enzyme and aromatic L-amino acid decarboxylase, respectively, have been noted in some PDE patients (27). Lastly, the role of PA in the pathophysiology of PDE needs to be considered. PA can act as a modulator of GABA (11, 56), and build-up of PA in brain could contribute to an increased risk of seizures and developmental abnormalities. No definite genotype–phenotype correlation has yet to be described. Genotypes that result in some degree of residual activity of ATQ may have an overall better outcome, while those patients with the highest urinary levels of AASA may have a worse overall prognosis (27, 32).

CLINICAL AND LABORATORY DIAGNOSTIC STEPS

The clinical diagnosis of PDE is made by careful observation, where an infant with anticonvulsant-resistant seizures is administered a trial of pyridoxine that results in a cessation of these events. The most convincing clinical demonstration of the effectiveness of pyridoxine is to administer parenteral pyridoxine while the patient is actively experiencing seizures and is undergoing continuous EEG monitoring (2–6). In some patients with PDE, both clinical and electrographic evidence of pyridoxine's effectiveness may be demonstrated, generally within minutes of a single dose of 20 to 100 mg. However, in some instances higher doses are required, and electrographic changes may not be noted in all patients who subsequently are shown to have genetically confirmed PDE (22). Therefore, if a patient does not respond to an initial 100 mg dose, up to 500 mg of intravenous pyridoxine should be administered in sequential 100 mg doses every 5 to 10 min before concluding that the infant's clinical and electrographic seizures are not immediately responsive to the vitamin. Ideally this trial should take place within an intensive care unit setting, as profound CNS depression with associated changes in the EEG have been noted in some PDE patients after the initial treatment with pyridoxine (2, 3, 9). An alternate clinical diagnostic approach should be used for patients who are experiencing frequent short anticonvulsant-resistant seizures. In this circumstance, oral pyridoxine (up to 30 mg/kg/d) is administered, and patients with PDE should have a resolution of clinical seizures within 3 to 7 days (2, 4–6).

As patients with PDE have a lifelong dependence on pyridoxine supplementation, the definitive clinical confirmation of the diagnosis requires additional steps. Specifically, the various anticonvulsants which the patient is receiving should be sequentially withdrawn, and the patient must then demonstrate persistent control of seizures on pyridoxine monotherapy. At some point pyridoxine must then be withdrawn, which should result in a recurrence of seizures; once pyridoxine is reintroduced then control of seizures should return. Given the clinical scenario that frequently evolves prior to the initial pyridoxine trial, many parents and clinicians have been reluctant to take the confirmatory step of withdrawing pyridoxine. Therefore, past epidemiologic studies and case series have reported such instances as possible (rather than definite) PDE cases (2, 12, 33). However, one needs to be cautious in diagnosing all patients treated in this manner with PDE. Patients have been reported with seizures that cease in response to pyridoxine therapy, but in whom seizures do not recur once the vitamin is discontinued. The term pyridoxine-responsive seizures (PRS) has been coined to describe this particular condition (2, 33). Therefore, some patients with possible PDE may actually have PRS.

The recent discovery of the biochemical and genetic abnormalities which underlie PDE has led to a fundamental change in our approach to diagnose the disorder. In PDE patients, documentation of elevated levels of PA in plasma samples, taken either prior to treatment or within several months after therapy is instituted, can serve as indirect confirmatory evidence of PDE (29, 49). The demonstration of elevated levels of AASA in plasma, cerebrospinal fluid, or urine is a more specific biochemical confirmation of the inborn error of metabolism that underlies PDE (25, 27, 28, 48). A diagnosis of PDE may also be accomplished via testing of the *ALDH7A1* gene in patients clinically suspected to have the disorder. The demonstration of either homozygous or compound heterozygous mutations in both *ALDH7A1* alleles will confirm the diagnosis (24, 27, 28, 30–32, 41). Therefore, by taking one or both of these measures, the withdrawal of pyridoxine to clinically verify the diagnosis is no longer necessary. Both biochemical and genetic testing is recommended, as a few individuals with elevated PA and/or AASA levels have not demonstrated mutations of one or both *ALDH7A1* alleles (24, 30), and definite PDE patients treated for an extended period of time may have a normalization of PA levels (29, 30).

TREATMENT

Patients with PDE require lifelong pyridoxine treatment to prevent recurrent seizures. While the recommended daily allowance for pyridoxine is 0.5 mg for infants and 2 mg for older children and adults, patients with PDE generally require higher (ie, pharmacologic) doses. For PDE patients, the optimal dose of pyridoxine has not been firmly established; in most cases daily administration of 50 to 200 mg (given once daily or in two divided doses) is generally effective in preventing seizures (3). As individuals with PDE are at an increased risk of seizure recurrence when experiencing a febrile illness, particularly gastroenteritis, the pyridoxine dose may be doubled for several days during this period. Once diagnosed, it is not uncommon for PDE patients to remain on the same amount of pyridoxine for many years, despite continued growth that effectively reduces the mg/kg/d dose. In a study of six children with PDE, an increase in the daily pyridoxine dose resulted in an improvement in IQ scores, with the expressive language scores showing the smallest change (2, 13).

Any additional increase in IQ was generally not seen with doses higher than 15 to 18 mg/kg/d. As megavitamin therapy with pyridoxine is known to cause a dorsal root ganglionopathy (57), and a sensory neuropathy has been reported in a few PDE patients (39, 41), parents and clinicians must be cautioned about the overzealous use of pyridoxine. Therefore, it is suggested that patients with PDE should receive approximately 15–18 mg/kg/d. Some patients may still experience seizures with these doses, and in those circumstances pyridoxine may be increased to 30 mg/kg/d with a maximum daily dose of 500 mg. When patients require these high doses of pyridoxine, a secondary cause of seizures, such as cerebral dysgenesis, may be present. In this circumstance one or more anticonvulsants may be required for optimal seizure control. Fortunately, in most instances, patients with PDE do not require the concurrent use of anticonvulsants. However, some patients may be prescribed certain anticonvulsants, specifically for their psychotropic effects, as well as neuroleptics and mood stabilizers for the management of associated neurodevelopmental and behavioral symptoms (12). As deficits in expressive language are expected in PDE patients, these children should be offered early intervention services that focus on language. Older patients will benefit from special education and a variety of physical, occupational, and speech therapy services.

While the neurodevelopmental outcome of PDE patients is multifactorial, a prompt diagnosis and institution of specific treatment is important. As PDE is an autosomal recessive disorder, there is a 25% recurrence risk in subsequent pregnancies. Therefore, it has been suggested that during each future pregnancy, mothers should take a daily pyridoxine dose of 50 to 100 mg during the last half of gestation (2, 40). In some cases, affected newborns treated prenatally with pyridoxine followed by postnatal therapy had a better neurodevelopmental outcome when compared with their older affected siblings (2, 47). However, this has not been universally observed, again suggesting that genotype may play a role in the neurodevelopmental outcome of PDE (41). Previously, for at risk infants who received both *in utero* and subsequent postnatal pyridoxine therapy, parents and health care providers were faced with the decision of whether or not to withdraw pyridoxine supplementation in order to determine if the newborn will experience seizures, and thereby meeting the clinical criteria for PDE. Now that

biochemical and *ALDH7A1* gene testing have become more clinically available, these at risk newborns treated prenatally with pyridoxine may be tested for PDE biomarkers and/or genotype, so that pyridoxine therapy may be either maintained or safely discontinued. Prenatal and postnatal pyridoxine use is not necessarily without risk in babies who do not have ATQ deficiency. An encephalopathy with seizures developed in a newborn treated with prophylactic pyridoxine who had a family history of PDE. The pyridoxine was withdrawn after ATQ deficiency was ruled-out and the encephalopathy resolved (58). This case emphasizes the importance of an expeditious evaluation of at risk neonates either via biochemical testing or targeted genotyping.

FOLINIC ACID-RESPONSIVE SEIZURES

In 1995, Hyland and colleagues reported the first cases of a neonatal epileptic encephalopathy in which intractable neonatal seizures responded to treatment with folinic acid (5-formyltetrahydrofolate), a form of folic acid that can cross the blood–brain barrier (59). Over the following decade a total of seven cases folinic acid-responsive seizures were reported (60–62). Each of these infants presented with encephalopathy and anticonvulsant-resistant seizures within the first 5 days of life. In the first case, by chance it was discovered that folinic acid given at a dose of 2.5 mg twice daily led to marked improvement in seizure control (59, 62). Over time, some breakthrough seizures developed that responded to higher daily doses. A family history of a deceased older sibling with intractable neonatal seizures was documented in this infant as well as in two other cases; therefore, the familial nature of this vitamin-responsive neonatal epileptic encephalopathy was established. During the course of the diagnostic evaluation of these first described cases, cerebrospinal fluid (CSF) analysis of neurotransmitter metabolites via high performance liquid chromatography (HPLC) with electrochemical detection was conducted. Analysis of the chromatograms revealed a previously unrecognized pattern of peaks that included two unidentified substances, a pattern that was also noted in subsequently diagnosed cases (59–62). Importantly, these cases point out the utility of conducting a metabolic analysis of CSF in infants with unexplained epileptic encephalopathy.

In some of the reported cases of folinic acid-responsive seizures, the patients had actually demonstrated a variable degree of clinical response to pyridoxine. In 2009, Gallagher and colleagues described two infants with an epileptic encephalopathy whose seizures responded to a combination of pyridoxine followed by the addition of folinic acid who not only had the characteristic pattern of peaks present on CSF analysis, but who also had AASA and PA elevations in CSF as well as mutations in *ALDH7A1* (63). This discovery led to a retrospective analysis of CSF and DNA specimens from the seven previously reported cases of folinic acid-responsive seizures, and similar biochemical and genetic abnormalities were demonstrated; hence, folinic acid-responsive seizures are allelic to PDE. While the identity of the two characteristic CSF peaks remains unknown, as does the biochemical mechanism of folinic acid resulting in improved seizure control, the discovery that these two vitamin-responsive disorders are identical now changes our approach to the diagnosis and management of infants with epileptic encephalopathy. As noted in some of these recent cases, as well as in some earlier reports (2, 9), patients with PDE may show initial unresponsiveness or only partial responsiveness to the administration of pyridoxine. While this may have been due to the specific pyridoxine treatment protocol that was used in each case, it is possible that with an earlier simultaneous administration of both pyridoxine and folinic acid, a more rapid clinical diagnosis of a vitamin-responsive epileptic encephalopathy may have been made. In addition, a low lysine diet, similar to the treatment of glutaric aciduria type I (another disorder of lysine metabolism) (6, 64), together with continuous combination therapy with both pyridoxine and folinic acid may lead to a better long-term outcome (63). These are presently unanswered questions that will require the development of multicenter collaborative clinical trials.

PYRIDOXAL PHOSPHATE-RESPONSIVE NEONATAL EPILEPTIC ENCEPHALOPATHY (PNPO DEFICIENCY)

In 2002, Kuo and Wang first described a neonatal epileptic encephalopathy that clinically responded to PLP rather than to pyridoxine (65). Subsequently, additional cases along with metabolic alterations in CSF, plasma and urine that suggested dysfunction in several PLP-dependent enzymes were reported. These biochemical findings included increases in CSF L-DOPA and 3-methoxytyrosine, along with decreased CSF levels of homovanillic acid and 5-hydroxyindoleacetic acid and urinary excretion of vanillacetic acid, all indicative of aromatic L-amino acid decarboxylase dysfunction; increased plasma and CSF levels of threonine consistent with threonine dehydratase dysfunction; and increased plasma and CSF glycine levels, an indication of reduced glycine cleavage enzyme activity (66). Clayton and colleagues suggested that this disorder was secondary to a deficiency of pyridox(am)ine 5'-phosphate oxidase which converts both pyridoxine phosphate and pyridoxamine phosphate to PLP. Patients with this enzyme deficiency would only be able to generate PLP through dietary sources of pyridoxal and PLP, therefore being PLP-dependent. This hypothesis was subsequently confirmed when mutations in the *PNPO* gene, which encodes the enzyme, were demonstrated along with an autosomal recessive mode of inheritance (67).

Subsequently, some additional infants with PLP-dependent seizures were reported and a clinical and biochemical phenotype began to emerge (20, 68–71). Reports of fetal seizures are common, and affected neonates are frequently born premature and present with encephalopathy and seizures. In addition to the metabolic disturbances listed above (which are not uniformly present in all cases), PLP levels in the CSF are reduced, and lactic acidosis and hypoglycemia may also be present. Similar to cases of PDE, the semiology of clinical seizures includes myoclonus, clonic movements and ocular, facial and other automatisms. The seizures in these infants are resistant to anticonvulsants and pyridoxine, but come under clinical control with the enteral administration of PLP (a parenteral preparation is not available). A burst suppression pattern, characteristic of Ohtahara Syndrome and nonketotic hyperglycemia which may present in a similar fashion, is present on the EEG. However, as with cases of PDE, not all clinical events interpreted as seizures have an electrographic correlate. PLP treatment results in significant improvement in the EEG, but may first show a transient worsening with significant electrographic depression, another similarity with PDE. Brain imaging studies reported from these patients show cerebral atrophy and abnormal patterns of myelination. Left untreated, infants with PNPO deficiency either die or survive with severe neurodevelopmental disabilities. With early diagnosis and treatment, affected patients may have near normal development (69). Clinicians caring for a newborn with an epileptic encephalopathy, particularly one who was born prematurely, should include PNPO deficiency in their differential diagnosis.

NOT ALL EPILPETIC ENCPEPHALOPATHIES RESPONSIVE TO PYRIDOXINE VITAMERS ARE DUE TO ANTIQUITIN OR PNPO DEFICIENCY

Epileptic encephalopathies possibly not due to either ATQ or PNPO dysfunction but which are responsive to either pyridoxine or PLP have been reported. Of great interest is that clinicians in Japan and Taiwan commonly use these vitamers for the treatment for infantile spams (West Syndrome) as well as for some other epileptic conditions (44, 72, 73). For example, simultaneous treatment with both PLP and low-dose ACTH has produced a high rate of remission of infantile spasms (72). In 2005, Wang and colleagues compared the effectiveness of both pyridoxine and PLP in the treatment of patients between the ages of 8 months and 15 years with intractable idiopathic epilepsy (73). Seizures were completely controlled by PLP in 11 of 94 children. Of these 11 patients, six had a recurrence of seizures when pyridoxine was substituted for PLP but recovered seizure control when PLP therapy was resumed. The metabolic and genetic nature of these pyridoxine and PLP responders is not known. Some of the PLP responders could represent unreported phenotypes of PNPO deficiency, or a late onset PLP-responsive epileptic condition not due to PNPO dysfunction, as recently reported by Veerapandiyan and colleagues (74). In addition, some of the pyridoxine responders could represent cases of PDE. It is also possible, as suggested by Baxter (75), that both pyridoxine and PLP may have an anticonvulsant effect in these patients, and that these vitamers were not treating a specific metabolic defect. One might propose a similar hypothesis regarding the activity of pyridoxine in the successful treatment of infantile spasms in patients without *ALDH7A1* mutations (24), as well as in patients whose epileptic condition is rigorously defined as PRS (2, 33, 75).

DIAGNOSTIC AND TREATMENT PATHWAY

For these vitamin-responsive epileptic encephalopathies, prompt diagnosis and institution of disease-specific management leads to a more favorable outcome in many instances. At presentation, these patients are cared for by pediatricians, neonatologists, critical care specialists and neurologists, and these clinicians must consider ATQ deficiency and PNPO deficiency as possible etiologies of neonatal epileptic encephalopathy. When confronted with the clinical problem of a newborn with seizures which are not responding to therapeutic doses and levels of first-line anticonvulsants and in whom there is no clear infectious, traumatic, cerebrovascular or marked structural cause, immediate steps should be instituted both to conduct biochemical and genetic testing and to begin therapy with one or more of the three important cofactors discussed in this chapter (Table 11.1). DNA should be banked for possible future gene testing of either *ALDH7A1* or *PNPO*, depending on clinical course and the results of biochemical testing of urine, plasma, and possibly CSF. Biochemical tests that should be considered include assays of AASA in plasma or urine or an assay of pipecolic acid in plasma. An elevation of either compound would be supportive of a diagnosis of PDE. While analysis of CSF for amino acids, neurotransmitter metabolites and PLP may be considered, other than the HPLC peaks characteristic of ATQ deficiency (63), other abnormal findings are not specific for either PDE or PNPO deficiency (27, 51). The patient should be managed within a neonatal or pediatric intensive care unit, and if the infant is clinically in status epilepticus or having frequent recurrent seizures, continuous EEG monitoring should be considered. The clinical and electrographic effects of one or more (up to five) 100 mg test doses of pyridoxine given intravenously should be recorded. As not all patients with PDE will have an immediate response to parenteral pyridoxine, the patient should be started on enteral PLP (as this will treat both ATQ deficiency and PNPO deficiency) at 30 mg/kg/d in three or four divided doses, along with folinic acid at 3–5 mg/kg/d. Both the PLP and folinic acid should be continued for 3 to 5 days and the infant's course should be followed closely. Toxic effects of these substances should not be expected to occur with only a few days of administration. If the patient has either PDE or PNPO deficiency, this treatment regimen should result in clinical improvement. If either of these metabolic disorders is then confirmed by biochemical and/or genetic testing, then chronic therapy with pyridoxine 15 to 18 mg/kg/d and folinic acid 3 to 5 mg/kg/d (for PDE), or PLP 30 to 50 mg/kg/d divided in four to six doses (for

TABLE 11.1   **Proposed Diagnostic And Treatment Steps For Anticonvulsant-Resistant Neonatal Epileptic Encephalopathy (See Text)**

Diagnostic studies	• CSF for neurotransmitter metabolites, the presence of ATQ deficiency-specific peaks on HPLC is diagnostic • Blood for alpha-aminoadipic semialdehyde (AASA) or pipecolic acid • Urine for AASA • Bank DNA for future confirmatory testing of either *ALDH7A1* or *PNPO* genes
Therapeutic trials	• Pyridoxine 100 to 500 mg intravenously (continuous EEG monitoring recommended if infant is experiencing status epilepticus or frequent clinical seizures) • PLP 30 mg/kg/day divided in three or four doses enterally, for 3 to 5 days • Folinic acid 3 to 5 mg/kg/day enterally, for 3 to 5 days
Chronic therapy	• For confirmed PDE: pyridoxine 15 to 30 mg/kg/day (maximum daily dose of 500 mg), and folinic acid 3 to 5 mg/kg/d • For confirmed PNPO Deficiency: PLP 30 to 50 mg/kg/day divided in four to six doses

PNPO deficiency) should be instituted. Pharmaceutical grade preparations of PLP are not readily available in hospital formularies in the United States and Europe and this can lead to a delay in instituting a therapeutic trial with this cofactor (43,69). Given our increasing recognition and understanding of both PDE and PNPO deficiency, over time the ready availability of PLP should improve. Tertiary care centers that include neonatal and pediatric intensive units should consider adding PLP to their formulary.

FUTURE DIRECTIONS FOR RESEARCH

A number of unanswered questions remain regarding the pathophysiology of ATQ deficiency and PNPO deficiency and the management of the two disorders.

• What are the toxic compounds responsible for the brain dysgenesis, neonatal epileptic encephalopathy, and developmental impairment in PDE? Specifically, what roles do PA, AASA, P6C, the P6C-PLP complex, and reduced PLP levels play in the disorder?
• Are certain brain regions more susceptible to the neurotoxic effects of these substances and/or to PLP depletion due to a regional expression of *ALDH7A1*?
• Is there a biochemical signature for PDE other than the peaks noted on HPLC analysis of CSF and the elevation of AASA in urine and plasma? Is there a pattern of organic acids and amino acids that would reliably differentiate PDE from PNPO deficiency?

• Are there genotype–phenotype correlations that can help predict the neurodevelopmental outcome and/or guide treatment?
• For the treatment of PDE, what is the optimal dose of pyridoxine supplementation?
• Why do some patients require the addition of folinic acid to obtain adequate control of seizures and encephalopathy, and what is the mechanism? What is the role of folinic acid in the treatment of PDE? Should all patients diagnosed with PDE be treated with both pyridoxine and folinic acid; in particular will the two medications together improve developmental outcome?
• Will a lysine-restricted diet improve the neurodevelopmental prognosis of patients with PDE? Would this dietary therapy be required throughout life, or only during infancy and childhood?
• Could both PDE and PNPO deficiency be added to newborn screening programs thereby allowing for early detection and initiation of specific therapy?

Given the rarity of these disorders, an international collaborative approach will be necessary to answer these important questions.

KEY POINTS

• PDE (ATQ deficiency) is characterized by anticonvulsant-resistant seizures which typically present in the newborn period and which only come under control with the use of pharmacologic doses of pyridoxine (vitamin B_6). Pyridoxine supplementation is a lifelong requirement.

- The disorder may mimic neonatal hypoxic–ischemic encephalopathy.
- Neurodevelopmental disability is common, but may be improved in some circumstances by early diagnosis and treatment (including in utero fetal treatment).
- PDE is definitively diagnosed by detecting increased levels of AASA in urine or plasma followed by documenting mutations in the *ALDH7A1* gene.
- PDE is an autosomal recessive disorder with a 25% recurrence risk.
- Folinic acid-responsive seizures have also been shown to be due to ATQ deficiency.
- Some neonatal epileptic encephalopathies respond to PLP rather than to pyridoxine. One particular condition is due to mutations in the *PNPO* gene, is autosomally recessively inherited, and can be successfully treated with daily supplements of PLP.
- Pediatricians, neonatologists, neurologists, and other clinicians who care for patients with neonatal seizures must be familiar with these two conditions, and know the steps required to initiate and continue therapy, and to confirm a diagnosis.

CLINICAL PEARLS

Comparison of Clinical and Metabolic Features of PDE (ATQ Deficiency) and PLP-responsive Epileptic Encephalopathy (PNPO Deficiency)

	ATQ Deficiency	PNPO Deficiency
Prenatal signs	Occasional in utero fetal seizures	Fetal distress and in utero fetal seizures
Prematurity	Uncommon	Frequent
Postnatal signs	Seizures, gastrointestinal symptoms, encephalopathy with hyperalertness, sleeplessness	Seizures, encephalopathy
Blood chemistry	Normal, but hypoglycemia and lactic	Hypoglycemia and lactic acidosis common

(continued)

	ATQ Deficiency	PNPO Deficiency
	acidosis have been noted	
Blood and CSF amino acids	Inconsistent elevations of glycine, threonine, and taurine	Inconsistent elevations of glycine, threonine, and taurine
Urine vanillactic acid	Absent	Present
CSF neurotransmitter metabolites	3-Methoxytyrosine may be elevated	Elevated L-DOPA and 3-methoxytyrosine; decreased homovanillic acid and 5-hydroxyindoleacetic acid
Blood and CSF pipecolic acid	Elevated	Normal
Blood, CSF, and urine alpha-aminoadipic semialdehyde (AASA)	Elevated	Normal

Modified from Hoffmann, Schmitt, Windfuhr, et al. (69), and Mills, Footitt, Mills, et al. (27).

REFERENCES

1. Hunt AD, Stokes J, McCrory WW, et al. Pyridoxine dependency: report of a case of intractable convulsions in an infant controlled by pyridoxine. *Pediatrics.* 1954;13:140–145.
2. Baxter P. Pyridoxine dependent and pyridoxine responsive seizures. In: P Baxter, ed. *Vitamin Responsive Conditions in Paediatric Neurology.* London: MacKeith Press, 2001:109–165.
3. Gospe SM, Jr. Current perspectives on pyridoxine-dependent seizures. *J Pediatr.* 1998;132:919–923.
4. Gospe SM, Jr. Pyridoxine-dependent epilepsy and antiquitin deficiency: clinical and molecular characteristics and recommendations for diagnosis, treatment and follow-up. *Mol Genet Metab.* 2011;104: 48–60.
5. Gospe SM, Jr. Neonatal vitamin-responsive epileptic encephalopathies. *Chang Gung Med J.* 2010;33:1–12.
6. Stockler S, Plecko B, Gospe SM, Jr., et al. Pyridoxine dependent epilepsy and antiquitin deficiency: clinical and molecular characteristics and recommendations for diagnosis, treatment and follow-up. *Mol Genet Metab.* 2011;104: 48–60.
7. Haenggeli CA, Girardin E, Paunier L. Pyridoxine-dependent seizures clinical, therapeutic aspects. *Eur J Pediatri.* 1991;150:452–455.

8. Bankier A, Turner M, Hopkins IJ. Pyridoxine dependent seizures—a wider clinical spectrum. *Arch Dis Child.* 1983;58: 415–418.

9. Bass NE, Wyllie E, Cohen B, et al. Pyridoxine-dependent epilepsy: the need for repeated pyridoxine trials and the risk of severe electrocerebral suppression with intravenous pyridoxine infusion. *J Child Neurol.* 1996;11:422–424.

10. Coker S. Postneonatal vitamin B$_6$-dependent epilepsy. *Pediatrics.* 1992;90:221–223.

11. Gutierrez MC, Delgado-Coello BA. Influence of pipecolic acid on the release and uptake of [3H]-GABA from brain slices of mouse cerebral cortex. *Neurochem Res.* 1989;14: 405–408.

12. Basura GJ, Hagland SP, Wiltse AM, et al. Clinical features and the management of pyridoxine-dependent and pyridoxine-responsive seizures: review of 63 North American cases submitted to a patient registry. *Eur J Pediatr.* 2009;168:697–704.

13. Baxter P, Griffiths P, Kelly T, et al. Pyridoxine-dependent seizures: demographic, clinical, MRI and psychometric features, and effect of dose on intelligence quotient. *Dev Med Child Neurol.* 1996;38: 998–1006.

14. Baynes K, Tomaszewski Farias S, et al. Pyridoxine-dependent seizures and cognition in adulthood. *Dev Med Child Neurol.* 2003;45:782–785.

15. Kluger G, Blank R, Paul K, et al. Pyridoxine-dependent epilepsy: normal outcome in a patient with late diagnosis after prolonged status epilepticus causing cortical blindness. *Neuropediatrics.* 2008;39:276–279.

16. Ohtsuka Y, Hattori J, Ishida T, et al. Long-term follow-up of an individual with vitamin B$_6$-dependent seizures. *Dev Med Child Neurol.* 1999;41:203–206.

17. Mikati MA, Trevathan E, Krishnamoorthy KS. Pyridoxine-dependent epilepsy: EEG investigation and long-term follow-up. *Electroenceph Clin Neurophys.* 1991;78:215–221.

18. Naasan G, Yabroudi M, Rahi A, et al. Electroencephalographic changes in pyridoxine-dependant epilepsy: new observations. *Epileptic Disord.* 2009;11:293–300.

19. Nabbout R, Soufflet C, Plouin P, et al. Pyridoxine dependent epilepsy: a suggestive electroclinical pattern. *Arch Dis Child Fetal Neonatal Ed.* 1999;81:F125–F129.

20. Schmitt B, Baumgartner M, Mills PB, et al. Seizures and paroxysmal events: symptoms pointing to the diagnosis of pyridoxine-dependent epilepsy and pyridoxine phosphate oxidase deficiency. *Dev Med Child Neurol.* 2010;52:e133–142.

21. Shih JJ, Kornblum H, Shewmon DA. Global brain dysfunction in an infant with pyridoxine dependency: evaluation with EEG, evoked potentials, MRI, and PET. *Neurology.* 1996;47:824–826.

22. Bok LA, Maurits NM, Willemsen MA, et al. The EEG response to pyridoxine-IV neither identifies nor excludes pyridoxine-dependent epilepsy. *Epilepsia.* 2010;51:2406–2411.

23. Gospe SM, Jr., Hecht ST. Longitudinal MRI findings in pyridoxine-dependent seizures. *Neurology.* 1998;51: 74–78.

24. Bennett CL, Chen Y, Hahn S, et al. Prevalence of ALDH7A1 mutations in 18 North American pyridoxine-dependent seizure (PDS) patients. *Epilepsia.* 2009;50: 1167–1175.

25. Bok LA, Struys E, Willemsen MA, et al. Pyridoxine-dependent seizures in Dutch patients: diagnosis by elevated urinary alpha-aminoadipic semialdehyde levels. *Arch Dis Child.* 2007;92: 687–689.

26. Kanno J, Kure S, Narisawa A, et al. Allelic and non-allelic heterogeneities in pyridoxine dependent seizures revealed by ALDH7A1 mutational analysis. *Mol Genet Metab.* 2007;91:384–389.

27. Mills PB, Footitt EJ, Mills KA, et al. Genotypic and phenotypic spectrum of pyridoxine-dependent epilepsy (ALDH7A1 deficiency). *Brain.* 2010;133:2148–2159.

28. Mills PB, Struys E, Jakobs C, et al. Mutations in antiquitin in individuals with pyridoxine-dependent seizures. *Nat Med.* 2006;12:307–309.

29. Plecko B, Hikel C, Korenke G-C, et al. Pipecolic acid as a diagnostic marker of pyridoxine-dependent epilepsy. *Neuropediatrics.* 2005;36:200–205.

30. Plecko B, Paul K, Paschke E, et al. Biochemical and molecular characterization of 18 patients with pyridoxine-dependent epilepsy and mutations of the antiquitin (ALDH7A1) gene. *Hum Mutat.* 2007;28:19–26.

31. Salomons GS, Bok LA, Struys EA, An intriguing, et al. "silent" mutation and a founder effect in antiquitin (ALDH7A1). *Ann Neurol.* 2007;62:414–418.

32. Scharer G, Brocker C, Vasiliou V, et al. The genotypic and phenotypic spectrum of pyridoxine-dependent epilepsy due to mutations in ALDH7A1. *J Inherit Metab Dis.* 2010;33: 571–581.

33. Baxter P. Epidemiology of pyridoxine dependent and pyridoxine responsive seizures in the UK. *Arch Dis Child.* 1999;81:431–433.

34. Been JV, Bok JA, Andriessen P, et al. Epidemiology of pyridoxine-dependent seizures in The Netherlands. *Arch Dis Child.* 2005; 90:1293–1296.

35. Ebinger M, Schutze C, Konig S. Demographics and diagnosis of pyridoxine-dependent seizures. *J Pediatr.* 1999;134:795–796.

36. Ramachandrannair R, Parameswaran M. Prevalence of pyridoxine dependent seizures in south Indian children with early onset intractable epilepsy: a hospital based prospective study. *Eur J Paediatr Neurol.* 2005;9:409–413.

37. Mercimek-Mahmutoglu S, Horvath GA, Coulter-Mackie M, et al. Atypical presentation of antiquitin deficiency in a female with neonatal seizures, hypoglycemia, hyperlacticacidemia and intractable myoclonic epilepsy. *J Inherit Metab Dis.* 2010;33:S158.

38. Goutières F, Aicardi J. Atypical presentations of pyridoxine-dependent seizures: a treatable cause of intractable epilepsy in infants. *Ann Neurol.* 1985;17: 117–120.

39. McLachlan RS, Brown WF. Pyridoxine dependent epilepsy with iatrogenic sensory neuronopathy. *Can J Neurol Sci.* 1995;22: 50–51.

40. Baxter P, Aicardi J. Neonatal seizures after pyridoxine use [letter]. *Lancet.* 1999; 354:2082–2083.

41. Rankin PM, Harrison S, Chong WK, et al. Pyridoxine-dependent seizures: a family phenotype that leads to severe cognitive deficits, regardless of treatment regime. *Dev Med Child Neurol.* 2007; 49:300–305.

42. Baxter P. Pyridoxine-dependent seizures: a clinical and biochemical conundrum. *Biochim Biophys Acta.* 2003; 1647:36–41.

43. Gospe SM, Jr. Pyridoxine-dependent seizures: new genetic and biochemical clues to help with diagnosis and treatment. *Curr Opin Neurol.* 2006;19:148–153.

44. Wang HS, Kuo MF. Vitamin B6 related epilepsy during childhood. *Chang Gung Med J.* 2007;30:396–401.

45. Bender DA. Vitamin B$_6$. *Nutritional Biochemistry of the Vitamins*. Cambridge: Cambridge University Press; 2003:232–269.
46. Percudani R, Peracchi A. A genomic overview of pyridoxal-phosphate-dependent enzymes. *EMBO Rep.* 2003;4:850–854.
47. Bok LA, Been JV, Struys EA, et al. Antenatal treatment in two Dutch families with pyridoxine-dependent seizures. *Eur J Pediatr.* 2010;169:297–303.
48. Sadilkova K, Gospe SM, Jr., Hahn SH. Simultaneous determination of alpha-aminoadipic semialdehyde, piperideine-6-carboxylate and pipecolic acid by LC-MS/MS for pyridoxine-dependent seizures and folinic acid-responsive seizures. *J Neurosci Methods.* 2009;184:136–141.
49. Plecko B, Stöckler-Ipsiroglu S, Paschke E, et al. Pipecolic acid elevation in plasma and cerebrospinal fluid of two patients with pyridoxine-dependent epilepsy. *Ann Neurol.* 2000;48: 121–125.
50. Mills PB, Footitt EJ, Ceyhan S, et al. Urinary AASA excretion is elevated in patients with molybdenum cofactor deficiency and isolated sulphite oxidase deficiency. *J Inherit Metab Dis.* 2012 March 9 [Epub ahead of print].
51. Footitt EJ, Heales SJ, Mills PB, et al. Pyridoxal 5′-phosphate in cerebrospinal fluid; factors affecting concentration. *J Inherit Metab Dis.* 2011;34:529–538.
52. Wang DD, Kriegstein AR. Defining the role of GABA in cortical development. *J Physiol.* 2009;587:1873–1879.
53. Hanada K. Serine palmitoyltransferase, a key enzyme of sphingolipid metabolism. *Biochim Biophys Acta.* 2003;1632: 16–30.
54. Ikeda M, Kihara A, Igarashi Y. Sphingosine-1-phosphate lyase SPL is an endoplasmic reticulum-resident, integral membrane protein with the pyridoxal 5′-phosphate binding domain exposed to the cytosol. *Biochem Biophys Res Commun.* 2004;325:338–343.
55. Kim PM, Aizawa H, Kim PS, et al. Serine racemase: activation by glutamate neurotransmission via glutamate receptor interacting protein and mediation of neuronal migration. *Proc Natl Acad Sci USA.* 2005;102: 2105–2110.
56. Charles AK. Pipecolic acid receptors in rat cerebral cortex. *Neurochem Res.* 1986;11:521–525.
57. Schaumburg H, Kaplan J, Windebank A, et al. Sensory neuropathy from pyridoxine abuse. A new megavitamin syndrome. *N Engl J Med.* 1983;309:445–448.
58. Hartmann H, Fingerhut M, Jakobs C, et al. Status epilepticus in a newborn treated with pyridoxine due to familial recurence risk for antiquitin deficiency-pyridoxine toxicity? *Dev Med Child Neurol.* 2011;53(12), 1150–1153.
59. Hyland K, Buist NR, Powell BR, et al. Folinic acid responsive seizures: a new syndrome? *J Inherit Metab Dis.* 1995;18: 177–181.
60. Frye RE, Donner E, Golja A, et al. Folinic acid-responsive seizures presenting as breakthrough seizures in a 3-month-old boy. *J Child Neurol.* 2003;18:562–569.
61. Nicolai J, van Kranen-Mastenbroek VH, Wevers RA, et al. Folinic acid-responsive seizures initially responsive to pyridoxine. *Pediatr Neurol.* 2006;34:164–167.
62. Torres OA, Miller VS, Buist NM, et al. Folinic acid-responsive neonatal seizures. *J Child Neurol.* 1999;14: 529–532.
63. Gallagher RC, Van Hove JL, Scharer G, et al. Folinic acid-responsive seizures are identical to pyridoxine-dependent epilepsy. *Ann Neurol.* 2009;65:550–556.
64. Kolker S, Christensen E, Leonard JV, et al. Guideline for the diagnosis and management of glutaryl-CoA dehydrogenase deficiency (glutaric aciduria type I). *J Inherit Metab Dis.* 2007;30:5–22.
65. Kuo MF, Wang HS. Pyridoxal phosphate-responsive epilepsy with resistance to pyridoxine. *Pediatr Neurol.* 2002;26: 146–147.
66. Clayton PT, Surtees RAH, DeVile C, et al. Neonatal epileptic encephalopathy. *Lancet.* 2003;361:1614.
67. Mills PB, Surtees RAH, Champion MP, et al. Neonatal epileptic encephalopathy caused by mutations in the PNPO gene encoding pyridox(am)ine 5′-phosphate oxidase. *Human Mol Genet.* 2005;14:1077–1086.
68. Bagci S, Zschocke J, Hoffmann GF, et al. Pyridoxal phosphate-dependent neonatal epileptic encephalopathy. *Arch Dis Child Fetal Neonatal Ed.* 2008;93: F151–152.
69. Hoffmann GF, Schmitt B, Windfuhr M, et al. Pyridoxal 5′-phosphate may be curative in early-onset epileptic encephalopathy. *J Inherit Metab Dis.* 2007;30:96–99.
70. Ormazabal A, Oppenheim M, Serrano M, et al. Pyridoxal 5′-phosphate values in cerebrospinal fluid: reference values and diagnosis of PNPO deficiency in paediatric patients. *Mol Genet Metab.* 2008;94:173–177.
71. Ruiz A, Garcia-Villoria J, Ormazabal A, et al. A new fatal case of pyridox(am)ine 5′-phosphate oxidase (PNPO) deficiency. *Mol Genet Metab.* 2008;93:216–218.
72. Takuma Y. ACTH therapy for infantile spasms: a combination therapy with high-dose pyridoxal phosphate and low-dose ACTH. *Epilepsia.* 1998;39(Suppl.5), 42–45.
73. Wang H-S, Chou M-L, Hung P-C, et al. Pyridoxal phosphate is better than pyridoxine for controlling idiopathic intractable epilepsy. *Arch Dis Child.* 2005;90: 512–515.
74. Veerapandiyan A, Winchester SA, Gallentine WB, et al. Electroencephalographic and seizure manifestations of pyridoxal 5′-phosphate-dependent epilepsy. *Epilepsy Behav.* 2011;20: 494–501.
75. Baxter P. Pyridoxine or pyridoxal phosphate for intractable seizures? *Arch Dis Child.* 2005;90:441–442.

12

Tetrahydrobiopterin Deficiencies and Epilepsy

Nenad Blau and Thomas Opladen

INTRODUCTION

Tetrahydrobiopterin (BH_4) deficiencies are disorders affecting phenylalanine homeostasis, and catecholamine and serotonin biosynthesis (1). The minimum requirements for the normal reaction(s) are the apoenzymes [phenylalanine-4-hydroxylase (PAH), tyrosine-3-hydroxylase (TH), or tryptophan-5-hydroxylase (TPH)], oxygen, iron (II), the corresponding aromatic (amino acids (phenylalanine, tyrosine, or tryptophan), and BH_4 (2). The fully functioning hydroxylating system consists of the two additional BH_4-regenerating enzymes: pterin-4α-carbinolamine dehydratase (PCD) and dihydropteridine reductase (DHPR). BH_4 is synthesized from guanosine triphosphate (GTP) catalyzed by three enzymes: GTP cyclohydrolase I (GTPCH), 6-pyruvoyl-tetrahydropterin synthase (PTPS), and sepiapterin reductase (SR) (3). The first two steps are clinically relevant; the third one can be catalyzed by alternative short-chain keto-reductases (eg, aldose and carbonyl reductase) (Figure 12.1). BH_4 deficiency comprises a heterogeneous group of disorders caused by mutations in one of the genes encoding enzymes involved in the biosynthesis (GTPCH, PTPS, or SR) or regeneration (PCD or DHPR) of BH_4 (4). Phenotypically, it presents mostly with hyperphenylalaninemia (HPA) and deficiency of the neurotransmitter precursors, L-dopa and 5-hydroxytryptophan, and thus can be detected through neonatal phenylketonuria (PKU) screening programs (5). However, some variants may present without HPA (eg, SR deficiency or GTPCH deficiency) (6) and some with normal neurotransmitter homeostasis (mild peripheral forms). Brain nitric oxide synthase (NOS) may also be affected by a deficit of the essential cofactor BH_4 (7). The genes of the corresponding enzymes are located and characterized in normal and mutant genomes. *GCH1* coding for GTPCH (six exons) is on chromosome 14q22.1–q22.2 and harbors mutations, most of them associated with non-HPA Dopa-responsive dystonia (DRD, Segawa disease). *PTS* coding for PTPS (six exons) maps to human chromosome 11q22.3–q23.3 and harbors mutations associated with HPA, some having a mild phenotype. *SPR* coding for SR (three exons) maps to chromosome 2p14–p12 and harbors mutations associated with a severe neurotransmitter deficiency without HPA and with accumulation of presumably neurotoxic dihydrobiopterin and sepiapterin in CNS. *PCBD* (four exons) is on chromosome 10q22, with mutations associated with benign transient HPA. *QDPR* (seven exons) maps to chromosome 4p15.3 and harbors mutations associated with HPA and neurotransmitter deficiency (4).

Treatment of BH_4 deficiencies requires restoration of normal blood phenylalanine concentration by BH_4 supplementation (5–10 mg/kg/d) or diet and replacement therapy with the neurotransmitter precursors L-dopa (+ carbidopa) and 5-hydroxytryptophan, and supplements of folinic acid in DHPR deficiency (8). Treatment should be initiated as early as possible and continued for a lifetime.

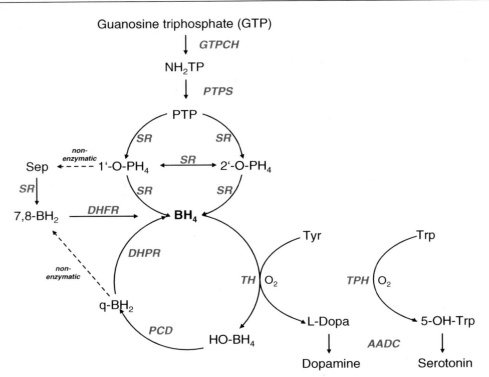

FIGURE 12.1 Tetrahydrobiopterin metabolism and its function in the biosynthesis of dopamine and serotonin. 7,8-BH$_2$, 7,8-dihydrobiopterin; DHFR, Dihydrofolate reductase; DHPR, dihydropteridine reductase; L-dopa, 3,4-dihydroxyphenylalanine; GTPCH, GTP cyclohydrolase I; HO-BH$_4$, hydroxyl-4a-tetrahydrobiopterin; NH$_2$TP, dihydroneopterin triphosphate; 5-OH-Trp, 5-hydroxytryptophan; 1′-O-PH$_4$ and 2′-O-PH$_4$, Oxo intermediates; PCD, pterin-4a-carbinolamine dehydratase; PTP, 6-pyruvoyl-tetrahydropterin; PTPS, 6-pyruvoyl-tetrahydroptrin synthase; Sep, sepiapterin; SR, sepiapterin reductase; TH, tyrosine hydroxylase; TPH, tryptophan hydroxylase; Trp, tryptophan; Tyr, tyrosine; q-BH$_2$, quinonoid dihydrobiopterin.

CLINICAL PHENOTYPES

Epileptic seizures are not a primary clinical hallmark of BH$_4$ deficiencies, particularly not in the newborn period. Only about 10% of neonates with PTPS deficiency may present with seizures, while in infants and children with PTPS and DHPR deficiency seizures are quite common (40–45% of all untreated patients) (Figure 12.2) (9).

Generally, patients with BH$_4$ deficiencies can be divided into two groups, those with a severe neonatal presentation and those with a rather mild course of the disease. This applies particularly for PTPS and DHPR deficiencies. The clinical signs and symptoms result from deficiencies of dopamine (eg, immobility, parkinsonism, somnolence, dystonia, hypertonia,

hypersalivation, oculogyric crises), noradrenaline (eg, axial hypotonia, cerebral symptoms), serotonin (depression, insomnia, temperature instability), and folates (myelin formation, basal ganglia calcifications, seizures). In untreated BH$_4$-deficient patients presenting with HPA, high brain phenylalanine levels additionally compromise biosynthesis of biogenic amines in the CNS. Phenylalanine is known to be a competitive inhibitor of both TH and TPH and potentiates the effect of BH$_4$ deficiency on catecholamines and serotonin biosynthesis. High phenylalanine concentrations during the prenatal period may also inhibit the rate of protein synthesis, which may affect early dendritic proliferation and myelination (10).

Infants affected by PTPS deficiency, the most common form of BH$_4$ deficiency, are frequently born

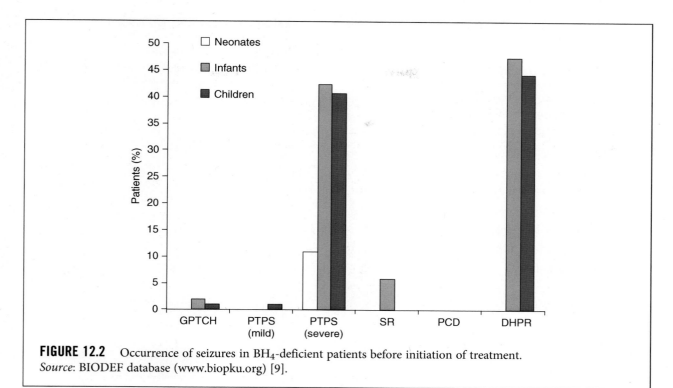

FIGURE 12.2 Occurrence of seizures in BH$_4$-deficient patients before initiation of treatment. *Source*: BIODEF database (www.biopku.org) [9].

small for gestational age (11). In the neonatal period they may show abnormal signs such as poor sucking, impaired tone and microcephaly. Later they present characteristic extrapyramidal symptoms due to lack of dopamine in the basal ganglia (12) including axial hypotonia, increased limb tone, postural instability, hypokinesia, choreic or dystonic limb movements, gait difficulties, hypersalivation due to swallowing difficulties, and oculogyric crises. Ataxia, hyperreflexia, hypothermia as well as episodes of hyperthermia (in the absence of infections), drowsiness, irritability, disturbed sleep patterns, and convulsions (grand mal or myoclonic) are often seen particularly in late-diagnosed untreated patients.

GTPCH and PTPS Deficiencies

Clinical signs and symptoms are comparable in patients with the GTPCH and PTPS deficiency (Table 12.1)

GPTCH-deficient patients develop particularly muscular hypotonia and movement disorders during the course of disease. Less frequent symptoms include muscular hypertonia and vegetative symptoms. Convulsions are seen in less than a fifth of GTPCH-deficient

patients (9). One additional prominent symptom, observed in many cases of severe GTPCH and PTPS deficiency, is mental retardation, including impaired cognitive and verbal skills. As this neurological impairment is not very amenable to therapy, it must be considered that prenatal or early development of the brain is affected. A possible reason for this finding is the involvement of NOS in long-term potentiation in the hippocampus by acting as a retrograde messenger (13).

PTPS deficiency is the most common form of all BH$_4$ deficiencies (55%) and is associated with the occurrence of preterm birth and low birth weight (9, 11). In the neonatal period PTPS deficient patients may show abnormal signs such as poor sucking, impaired tone, and microcephaly. Later they present characteristic extrapyramidal symptoms due to lack of dopamine in the basal ganglia (12) including axial hypotonia, increased limb tone, postural instability, hypokinesia, choreic or dystonic limb movements, gait difficulties, hypersalivation due to swallowing difficulties, and oculogyric crises. Ataxia, hyperreflexia, hypothermia as well as episodes of hyperthermia (in the absence of infection), drowsiness, irritability, disturbed sleep patterns, and convulsions (grand mal or

TABLE 12.1 Signs and Symptoms Associated With Classical Forms of BH_4 Deficiency (Presenting With HPA)

Signs and Symptoms	GTPCH def.	PTPS def.	PCD def.	DHPR def.
Progressive psychomotor retardation despite treatment for PKU	+	+		+
Feeding difficulties	+	+		+
Hypotonia/hypertonia	+	+	+*	+
Dystonia	+	+		
Temperature instability	+	+		+
Hypersalivation	+	+		+
Seizures—myoclonic	+	+		+
Lethargy and irritability		+		+
Choreoathetosis		+		+
Rash—eczema		+		+
Lighter pigmentation	+	+		+
Frequent infections		+		+
Sudden death		+		+
Basal ganglia calcifications				+

*Early neonatal period; + frequently present.

myoclonic) are often seen particularly in late-diagnosed untreated patients

A number of follow-up studies document the occurrence of myoclonic seizures in PTPS-deficient patients in relation to the age of patients and the age of diagnosis and treatment start (14–19).

Al Aqeel et al. (14) described neurological manifestations of 10 patients with PTPS deficiency, all of them with truncal hypotonia, limb spasticity and deep tendon reflexes at the age of diagnosis 4 months to 4 years and with myoclonic seizures more often than once a month in two patients (ages 4 months and 4 years) and more often than once a week in two patients (age 5 and 18 months). All other PTPS-deficient patients were seizure-free at the time of diagnosis.

In another study Lee et al. (17) investigated initial clinical manifestation in 10 Taiwanese patients with PTPS deficiency. The eight patients with severe form and a homogenous genotype (P87S and N52S alleles; age 11 months to 10 years and 3 months) have all seizures more than 10 times per day, while the two moderate form patients (age 7 years and 1 month and 20 years and 8 months) were seizure-free before the start of treatment. A marked decrease of frequency of seizures was observed after the onset of therapy (BH_4, 1–2 mg/kg/d; L-dopa/carbidopa, 8–15 mg/kg/d; and 5-hydroxytryptophan, 5 mg/kg/d) in the group of patients with the severe form of disease.

A single case report by Demos et al. (20) describes a PTPS-deficient patient with seizures characterized by head drops, tonic seizures, or generalized tonic–clonic seizures, which occurred weekly at the age of 8 years. At the age of 10 years a combined BH_4/L-dopa/carbidopa/5-hydroxytryptophan therapy was started resulting in cessation of seizures without antiepileptic medication.

The largest study described was by Jäggi et al. (18). They investigated 26 patients with PTPS deficiency, 17 of them diagnosed before the age of two months after birth. In 10 patients (6 early and 4 late diagnosed) development was delayed, while in 14 patients (9 early and 5 late diagnosed) no developmental delay was noted. Five patients (age 1 month to 6 years 10 months) presented with seldom occurring oculogyric crises, while another five patients (age 1 month to 3 years) presented with seizures requiring anticonvulsive therapy. In all of them anticonvulsives were replaced by the standard therapy (see above), resulting in neurological improvement.

DHPR Deficiency

In addition to the clinical signs and symptoms described in patients with GTPCH and PTPS deficiency (Table 12.1), patients with DHPR deficiency present with cerebral folate deficiency (depletion of 5-methyltetrahydrofolate in CSF) and many show calcifications of basal ganglia. EEG alterations are variable and more frequent than in other BH_4-deficient variants (incl. paroxysmal activity being epileptic discharges, sharp waves and hypsarrhythmia) (1). These patients need supplementation with folinic acid (leucovorine; 5-formyltetrahydrofolate) and, if started early, basal calcifications can be reversed under folate therapy (21). There is only a single retrospective report on a relative large number of DHPR-deficient patients. Jäggi at all (18) reported on 10 patients with DHPR deficiency, four of them diagnosed before the age of 2 months. Six patients (age 6 months to 2 years and 2 months) presented all with severe epilepsy requiring anticonvulsive medication, while four patients (age 3 weeks to 1 month) were seizure-free without medication. Introduction of the standard therapy (see above, except BH_4) plus folinic acid improved the neurological status, but some still needing antiepileptic drugs. Thus, DHPR deficiency seems to be more severe than other forms of BH_4 deficiency. One of the reasons may be the fact that in this group of patients BH_4 cannot be substituted, due to the enzyme defect in its regeneration. One would need to give one mole of BH_4 per mole of phenylalanine and this will result in accumulation of high amounts of dihydrobiopterin (BH_2). BH_2 has a negative effect on several enzymes including PAH, TH, TPH and NOS. The clinical course of illness in DHPR deficiency is similar to that seen in severe forms of PTPS deficiency. In addition, extensive neuronal loss, calcifications, and abnormal vascular proliferation were noted in cortex, basal ganglia, and thalamus (22–24).

SR DEFICIENCY

SR deficiency is a defect in the last step in the biosynthesis of BH_4 (25). In contrast to other forms of BH_4 deficiency it presents without HPA, cannot be diagnosed through newborn screening and as a consequence all thus far diagnosed patients were diagnosed late. Due to severe biogenic amine neurotransmitter deficiency, the clinical picture is severe (Table 12.2), with a progressive course leading to psychomotor handicap. Similarly to patients with DHPR deficiency (see above), accumulation of BH_2 accounts for the severity of the disease. Clinical hallmarks of SR deficiency, seen in most cases in infancy or childhood, are motor and language delay, axial hypotonia, dystonia, weakness, oculogyric crises and diurnal fluctuation of symptoms. Misdiagnoses of cerebral palsy are quite frequent and most patients benefit from L-dopa/carbidopa and 5-hydroxytryptophan substitution (6, 26). A recent retrospective study of 47 patients with SR deficiency (6) showed that the common clinical findings of SR deficiency, aside from oculogyric crises and diurnal fluctuation, are rather nonspecific and mimic cerebral palsy with hypotonia or dystonia. Features of SR deficiency, present in more than 65% of patients, include motor and speech delay, axial hypotonia, dystonia, weakness and oculogyric crises with diurnal fluctuation and sleep benefit. Frequent clinical features, present in 45% to 65% include: dysarthria, parkinsonian features (bradykinesia, rigidity, tremor, or masked facies), hyper-reflexia, psychiatric, and/or behavioral abnormalities, sleep disturbance, mental retardation, autonomic signs and limb hypertonia. Only two infants and three children presented with seizures (6).

TABLE 12.2 Signs and Symptoms Associated With SR Deficiency (Presenting Without HPA)

Signs and Symptoms	SR Deficiency
Dystonia (lower limbs, trunk, arms, neck)	+
Diurnal fluctuation of symptoms	+/−
Parkinsonism (associated with tremor, rigidity, bradykinesia)*	+/−
Spasticity	+
Oculogyric crises	+/−
Hypersalivation	+/−
Lethargy	+/−
Seizures	+/−
Psychomotor retardation	+
Response to L-Dopa	+

*In adolescence or adulthood; + frequently present;
+/− sometimes present.

PCD Deficiency

PCD deficiency is a benign form of BH_4 deficiency with transient HPA in the early neonatal period and occasionally only mild hypotonia of the trunk (27) (Table 12.1).

LABORATORY DIAGNOSIS OF BH₄ DEFICIENCY

Classical BH_4 deficiencies present with HPA and laboratory diagnosis starts with the newborn screening for PKU. A few simple tests (pterins in dried blood spots or urine, DHPR activity in blood, and BH_4 loading test) discriminate between classical PKU and cofactor defects (28) and additional investigations on neurotransmitter metabolites in CSF serve to define the disease.

Typical pterin profiles are described in Table 12.3: neopterin and biopterin are very low in GTPCH deficiency; neopterin and monapterin (isomer of neopterin) are very high in PTPS deficiency, with only traces of biopterin; neopterin is normal or slightly increased and biopterin is very high in DHPR deficiency; and neopterin is initially high, biopterin is in the subnormal range, and primapterin (7-substituted biopterin) is present in PCD deficiency. Patients with classical PKU excrete generally more neopterin and biopterin in urine than normal controls. This is due to the activation of GTPCH by phenylalanine via GTPCH feedback regulatory protein (GFRP) (1).

To distinguish between the different variants of BH_4 deficiency, that is, severe and mild forms, quantification of neopterin, biopterin, and the neurotransmitter metabolites, 5-hydroxyindoleacetic acid (5HIAA) and homovanillic acid (HVA), in CSF is essential

(29). In patients with DHPR deficiency, measurement of 5-methyltetrahydrofolic acid (5MTHF) is important due to its connection with folate metabolism. As already mentioned, SR deficiency present without HPA and thus cannot be detected through the newborn screening for PKU. The CSF metabolites HVA and 5HIAA are extremely low and high total biopterin results from accumulation of BH_2. Elevated sepiapterin levels are found in CSF. Biochemical investigations of CSF and fibroblast cultures as well as DNA testing and phenylalanine loading test (30) are of diagnostic value. Table 12.4 summarizes common biochemical findings in CSF derived from patients with different forms of BH_4 deficiency.

TREATMENT OF PATIENTS WITH BH₄ DEFICIENCY

The prognosis of BH_4 deficiency is closely related to the degree of HPA and the level of impaired biogenic amine production. Therefore, combination therapy must be promptly instituted following diagnosis. The goals of treatment include: (1) control of HPA; and (2) correction of neurotransmitter deficiencies (8). In addition, in infants with DHPR deficiency, tetrahydrofolate homeostasis must be restored.

In patients with GTPCH and PTPS deficiency, administration of BH_4 appears to be the most efficient therapy in controlling blood phenylalanine levels. A small daily dose (2−5 mg/kg/d) is sufficient in synthesis defects, whereas larger daily doses (20 mg/kg/d, given in three to four doses) are used in very few DHPR-deficient patients. Most DHPR-deficient patients are on a low-phenylalanine diet (31).

TABLE 12.3   Biochemical Findings in Urine and Dried Blood Spots (DBS) Associated With BH₄ Deficiencies

Enzyme defect	Neopterin (DBS or Urine)	Biopterin (DBS or Urine)	Primapterin (Urine)	DHPR Activity (DBS)	BH₄ Challenge* (20 mg/kg)
GTPCH	↓	↓	n	n	+
PTPS	↑	↓	n	n	+
SR	n	n	n	n	na
PCD	↑	(↓)	↑	n	+
DHPR	n-↑	n-↑	n	↓	+
PKU	(↑)	(↑)	n	n	−/+*

*Positive in patients with BH₄-responsive PAH; n = normal; + positive; na = not applicable; DBS = dried blood spot.

TABLE 12.4 Neurotransmitter Metabolites, Pterins, and Folates in CSF of Patients With Different Forms of BH$_4$ Deficiency

Enzyme Defect	5HIAA	HVA	Neopterin	Biopterin	Sepiapterin	5MTHF	Phe
With HPA							
arGTPCH	↓	↓	↓	↓	n	n	↑
PTPS	↓	↓	↑	↓	n	n	↑
PCD	n	n	(↑)	n	n	n	↑
DHPR	↓	↓	n	↑*	n	↓	↑
Without HPA							
SR	↓	↓	n	↑*	↑	n	n

*Dihydrobiopterin and fully oxidized biopterin; n = normal; 5HIAA = 5-hydroxyindoleacetic acid; HVA = homovanillic acid; 5MTHF = 5-methyltetrahydrofolic acid.

L-Dopa and 5-hydroxytryptophan administrations in combination represent a common therapeutic approach to all BH$_4$-deficiency variants. Carbidopa, an inhibitor of peripheral aromatic amino acid decarboxylase, reduces the therapeutic requirements of L-Dopa and its side effects on the periphery. The optimal dosage of each component can be determined only on a clinical basis and should be adjusted to the requirements of each patient while assessing for adverse effects. Diurnal fluctuations are also often observed and may require changes in the schedule of drug administration. Daily doses and the number of administrations have to be individually adjusted to a patient's age and requirements. Satisfying results have been obtained in recent cases with the concurrent administration of a selective MAO-B or COMT inhibitors, which facilitate reduction of the dosage of administered precursors by inhibiting their catabolism (31). Administration of folinic acid (10 − 20 mg/d) is recommended to restore normal CSF folate levels in patients with DHPR deficiency. This therapy may reverse both the demyelinating processes and the calcification of the basal ganglia in these patients. Patients with SR deficiency respond effectively to low dose L-Dopa/carbidopa, but need additional 5-hydroxytryptophan substitution (9, 31).

SUMMARY

Inherited disorders in BH$_4$ metabolism can be divided into two groups: those associated with hyperphenylalaninemia (GTPCH deficiency, PTPS deficiency, PCD deficiency, and DHPR deficiency; all inherited autosomal recessively) and those presenting without hyperphenylalaninemia (GTPCH deficiency type Segawa and SR deficiency). Patients are diagnosed by different analytical and biochemical approaches depending upon the enzyme defect and the mode of inheritance. Typical signs and symptom of late diagnosed patients are psychomotor retardation, impaired muscle tone (axial hypotonia and hypertonia of extremities), hypersalivation, swallowing difficulties, ptosis, and epileptic seizures. Treatment includes substitution with neurotransmitter precursors L-Dopa (+carbidopa), 5-hydroxytryptophan, MAO and COMT inhibitors, and BH$_4$. DHPR-deficient patients require additional supplementation with folinic acid.

CLINICAL PEARLS

- Tetrahydrobiopterin deficiencies may present *with* and *without* hyperphenylalaninemia (HPA).
- Late diagnosis and treatment are frequently associated with psychomotor retardation.
- Neuroradiologic investigations are essential in patients with DHPR deficiency.
- Sepiapterin reductase deficiency presents without hyperphenylalaninemia and cannot be diagnosed through the neonatal screening for PKU.
- CSF investigations are essential for the diagnosis of BH$_4$ deficiency presenting without HPA.
- Substitution therapy with BH$_4$ and neurotransmitter precursors should be started as early as possible.

This work was supported by the Swiss National Science Foundation grant to NB.

REFERENCES

1. Blau N, Thöny B, Cotton RGH, et al. Disorders of tetrahydrobiopterin and related biogenic amines. In: CR Scriver, AL Beaudet, WS Sly, D Valle, B Childs, B Vogelstein eds. *The Metabolic and Molecular Bases of Inherited Disease.* New York: McGraw-Hill; 2001:1725–1776.

2. Blau N, Van Spronsen FJ, Levy HL. *Phenylketonuria Lancet.* 2010;376:1417–1427.

3. Werner ER, Blau N, Thöny B. Tetrahydrobiopterin: Biochemistry and pathophysiology. *Biochem J* 2011;438: 397–414.

4. Thöny B, Blau N. Mutations in the BH$_4$-metabolizing genes GTP cyclohydrolase I, 6-pyruvoyl-tetrahydropterin synthase, sepiapterin reductase, carbinolamine-4a-dehydratase, and dihydropteridine reductase genes. *Hum Mutat.* 2006;27:870–878.

5. Blau N, Hennermann JB, Langenbeck, et al. Diagnosis, classification and genetics of phenylketonuria and tetrahydrobiopterin (BH$_4$) deficiencies. *Mol Genet Metab.* 2011;104:S2-9.

6. Friedman J, Roze E, Abdenur JE, et al. Sepiapterin reductase deficiency: a treatable mimic of cerebral palsy *Ann Neurol.* 2012; in press.

7. Zorzi G, Thöny B, Blau N. Reduced nitric oxide metabolites in CSF of patients with tetrahydrobiopterin deficiency. *J Neurochem.* 2002;80:362–364.

8. Blau N, Burgard P. Disorders of phenylalanine and tetrahydrobiopterin. In: N Blau, Hoffmann, J Leonard, J Clarke eds. *Physician's Guide to the Treatment and Follow-up of Metabolic Diseases.* Heidelberg: Springer; 2006:25–34.

9. Opladen T, Hoffmann FG, Blau N. An international survey of patients with tetrahydrobiopterin deficiencies presenting with hyperphenylalaninaemia. *J Inherit Metab Dis.* 2012. DOI: 10.1007/s10545-012-9506-x

10. Feillet F, van Spronsen FJ, MacDonald A, et al. Challenges and pitfalls in the management of phenylketonuria. *Pediatrics.* 2010;126:333–341.

11. Smith I, Dhondt JL. Birthweight in patients with defective biopterin metabolism. *Lancet.* 1985;1:818.

12. Allen RJ, Young W, Bonacci J, et al. Neonatal dystonic Parkinsonism, a "stiff baby syndrome," in biopterin deficiency with hyperprolactinemia detected by newborn screening for hyperphenylalaninemia, and responsiveness to treatment. *Ann Neurol.* 1990;28:434.

13. Dawson VL, Dawson TM. Physiological and toxicological actions of nitric oxide in the central nervous system. *Adv Pharmacol.* 1995;34:323–342.

14. al Aqeel A, Ozand PT, Gascon G, et al. Reynolds, Biopterin-dependent hyperphenylalaninemia due to deficiency of 6-pyruvoyl tetrahydropterin synthase. *Neurology.* 1991;41: 730–737.

15. Dudesek A, Röschinger W, Muntau AC, et al. Molecular analysis and long term follow-up of patients with different forms of 6-pyruvoyltetrahydropterin synthase deficiency. *Eur J Pediatr.* 2001;160:267–276.

16. Chien YH, Chiang SC, Huang A, et al. Treatment and outcome of Taiwanese patients with 6-pyruvoyl-tetrahydropterin synthase gene mutations. *J Inherit Metab Dis.* 2001;24: 815–823.

17. Lee NC, Cheng LY, Liu TT, et al. Long-term follow-up of Chinese patients who received delayed treatment for 6-pyruvoyl-tetrahydropterin synthase deficiency. *Mol Genet Metab.* 2006;87:128–134.

18. Jäggi L, Zurflüh MR, Schuler A, et al. Outcome and long-term follow-up of 36 patients with tetrahydrobiopterin deficiency. *Mol Genet Metab.* 2008;93:295–305.

19. Leuzzi V, Carducci C, Pozzessere S, et al. Blau, Phenotypic variability, neurological outcome and genetics background of 6-pyruvoyltetrahydropterin synthase deficiency. *Clin Genet.* 2010;77:249–257.

20. Demos MK, Waters PJ, Vallance HD, et al. Connolly, 6-Pyruvoyl-tetrahydropterin synthase deficiency with mild hyperphenylalaninemia. *Ann Neurol.* 2005;58: 164–167.

21. Biasucci G, Valsasina R, Giovannini M, et al. Neuroradiological improvement after one year of therapy in a case of DHPR deficiency. In: HC Curtius, S Ghisla, N Blau eds. *Chemistry and Biology of Pteridines 1989.* Berlin: Walter de Gruyter; 1990:438–444.

22. Kaufman S, Holtzman NA, Milstien S, et al. Phenylketonuria due to a deficiency of dihydropteridine reductase. *N Engl J Med.* 1975;293:785–790.

23. Ponzone A, Spada M, Ferraris S, et al. Dihydropteridine reductase deficiency in man: From biology to treatment. *Med Res Rev* 2004;24:127–150.

24. Smith I, Hyland K, Kendall B. Clinical role of pteridine therapy in tetrahydrobiopterin deficiency. *J Inherit Metab Dis.* 1985;8:39–45.

25. Bonafé L, Thöny B, Penzien JM, et al. Mutations in the sepiapterin reductase gene cause a novel tetrahydrobiopterin-dependent monoamine neurotransmitter deficiency without hyperphenylalaninemia. *Am J Hum Genet.* 2001;69:269–277.

26. Dill P, Kocygit-Wagner M, Weber P, et al. Sepiapterin reductase deficiency caused by a new mutation of the SPR gene in a 7 months old girl: case report and review of the literature. *J Inerit Metab Dis.* 2010;33: S162.

27. Blau N, Kierat L, Curtius HC, et al. Hyperphenylalaninaemia presumably due to carbinolamine dehydratase deficiency: loading tests with pterin derivatives. *J Inherit Metab Dis.* 1992;15:409–412.

28. Opladen T, Abu Seda B, Rassi A, et al. Diagnosis of tetrahydrobiopterin deficiency using filter paper blood spots: further development of the method and 5 years experience. *J Inherit Metab Dis.* 2011;34:819–826.

29. Hyland K, Surtees RAH, Heales SJR, et al. Cerebrospinal fluid concentrations of pterins and metabolites of serotonin and dopamine in a pediatric reference population. *Pediatr Res.* 1993;34:10–14.

30. Opladen T, Okun JG, Burgard P, et al. Phenylalanine loading in pediatric patients with dopa-responsive dystonia: revised test protocol and pediatric cut-off values. *J Inerit Metab Dis.* 2010;33:697–703.

31. Ponzone A, Ferraris S, Baglieri S, et al. Treatment of tetrahydrobiopterin deficiencies. In: N Blau ed. *PKU and BH$_4$: Advances in Phenylketonuria and Tetrahydrobiopterin.* Heilbronn: SPS Verlagsgesellschaft; 2006:612–637.

Disorders of GABA Metabolism and Epilepsy

Phillip L. Pearl, Cornelis Jakobs, and K. Michael Gibson

INTRODUCTION

Epilepsy is an important problem in both succinic semi-aldehyde dehydrogenase (SSADH) deficiency, a disorder of GABA catabolism, and GABA-transaminase (GABA-T) deficiency, a disorder of GABA synthesis. There is a paradox to this, as GABA is the major inhibitory neurotransmitter of the brain. Insights from these rare diseases may thus shed considerable light on the pathophysiology of epilepsy and the complex role of GABA.

SSADH is an autosomal recessive disorder that has been reported in approximately 450 people. In the absence of SSADH, the breakdown of GABA to succinic acid is altered to a resultant buildup of GABA as well as GHB (Figure 13.1). Detection of elevated GHB in physiologic fluids, typically identified on analysis of urine organic acids, is the most effective laboratory screening method for the diagnosis (1). Most patients present with developmental delay with a mean age of diagnosis of 2 years, although newly diagnosed adult cases are now well described. Clinical features include intellectual deficiency with prominent impairment in expressive language, hypotonia, hyporeflexia, and ataxia. Epilepsy is present in approximately half of affected individuals. Neuroimaging demonstrates increased T2-weighted MRI signal in the globus pallidus (Figure 13.2), cerebellar dentate nucleus and subthalamic nucleus. Cerebral and cerebellar atrophy may also be present.

A transgenic murine model of SSADH deficiency expresses a characteristic phenotype with failure-to-thrive, ataxia, and a progressive seizure disorder characterized by a transition from absence to generalized convulsive seizures and ultimately fatal status epilepticus in the first months of life (2). The transition from absence to convulsive activity could be analogized to the human epilepsy syndromes of generalized childhood absence or juvenile absence epilepsy as well as juvenile myoclonic epilepsy.

CASE VIGNETTE

A 5-year-old boy presented with severe hyperactivity and new onset generalized seizures. Neurological examination revealed a minimally verbal, nondysmorphic boy with mild hypotonia, hyporeflexia, and wide-based gait. Psychoeducational testing showed mild intellectual disability (Wechsler Intelligence Scales for Children: verbal 55, performance 65) and deficient adaptive behaviors. EEG revealed intermittent generalized spike-wave discharges with activation during sleep and mild background slowing in the awake state. Valproate was begun but was associated with lethargy. Cranial MRI showed T2-weighted hyperintensities in the globus pallidus bilaterally. Urine organic acids revealed 4-hydroxybutyric aciduria, and subsequent SSADH enzymatic activity was nondetectable. The patient was treated with lamotrigine with fair seizure control, and has had persistent problems with expressive aphasia, obsessive–compulsive disorder, and anxiety. Now age 31, the patient lives in a group home with other young

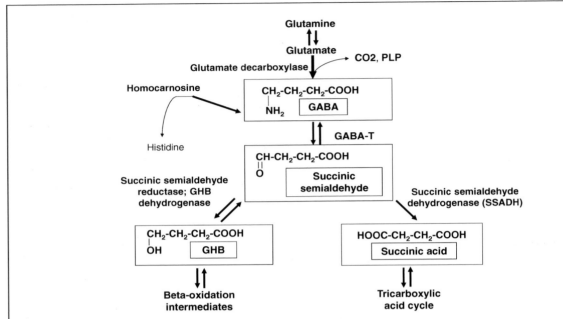

FIGURE 13.1   GABA degradation pathway. GABA is normally converted via GABA-transaminase into succinate semialdehyde, which is then broken down to succinic acid by succinate semialdehyde dehydrogenase (SSADH). In the absence of SSADH, succinate semialdehyde is converted to GHB rather than succinic acid, and this leads to a build up of both GHB and GABA in the brain.

adults, most of who have been diagnosed with cerebral palsy, intellectual disabilities, or autism.

Human SSADH deficiency is usually characterized by a relatively nonprogressive encephalopathy manifest in the first 2 years of life by hypotonia and developmental delay associated with mild ataxia and hyporeflexia. Virtually constant characteristics are intellectual disability and profound expressive language deficits. Psychiatric symptoms tend to be the most disabling and are characterized by inattention and hyperactivity,

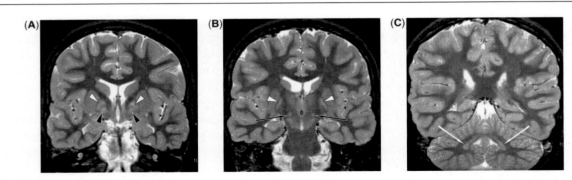

FIGURE 13.2   Dentatopallidoluysian pattern in SSADH deficiency. Coronal short tau inversion recovery sections from MRI in a patient with SSADH deficiency showing bilateral symmetric homogeneous signal abnormalities in each globuspallidus pars lateralis (white arrow, A and B), pars medialis (black arrow, A), subthalamic nucleus (black arrows, B), and dentate nucleus (white arrows, C). (Reprinted with permission from Pearl et al. *Neurology.* 2009;73:423–429.)

TABLE 13.1 Clinical Features of SSADH Deficiency (n = 84)

	Number	Percentage
Developmental delay	77	91.7
Mental retardation	76	90.5
Hypotonia	60	71.4
Behavior problems	61	72.6
Seizures	36	42.9
Ataxia	58	69.0

TABLE 13.3 Seizure Activity in Patients With SSADH Deficiency (n = 36)

	Number	Percentage
Generalized tonic–clonic	21	58.3
Absence	19	52.8
Myoclonic	9	25.0
Unspecified	6	16.7
Other (atonic, partial)	12	33.3

and sometimes aggression in early childhood, and anxiety and obsessive–compulsive behaviors in adolescence and adulthood (3, 4). Intermittent decompensation as seen in other metabolic disorders is not the usual presentation, although there is a subgroup (approximately 10% of reported patients) with a more severe phenotype including a degenerative course characterized by regression and prominent extrapyramidal manifestations (5). Genotype–phenotype correlations have not explained varying degrees of severity.

A clinical database using systematic questionnaires of 84 patients indicates that developmental delay is a universal presentation. Common clinical features include intellectual disability, behavior problems, and motor dysfunction (Tables 13.1 and 13.2). In order to address the long-term outlook, we reported on 33 patients (52% males) over 10 years of age (3). The

mean age of this patient cohort was 17.1 years ±6.4 years (range 10.1–39.6 years). The mean age when symptoms first appeared was 11 months (range 0–44 months) and the mean age at diagnosis was 6.6 years, although some individuals were not diagnosed until the mid-20s.

Nearly half of patients develop epilepsy, usually with generalized tonic–clonic and atypical absence seizures (Table 13.3) (6). The epilepsy may be difficult to control, with some patients having sporadic but recurrent episodes of generalized convulsive status epilepticus. SUDEP (Sudden Unexpected Death in Epilepsy Patients) has occurred, including one patient diagnosed with SSADH deficiency only retrospectively based on family history, neuropathology, and subsequent gene sequencing of postmortem tissue (7). Electroencephalographic findings include background slowing abnormalities (usually generalized and sometimes multifocal), and occasionally photosensitivity and electrographic status epilepticus of sleep (Table 13.4) (Figure 13.3).

TABLE 13.2 Neuropsychiatric Disturbances in Patients With SSADH Deficiency (n = 55)

	Number	Percentage
Aggression	10	18.2
Anxiety	18	32.7
Hallucinations	5	9.1
Hyperactivity	26	47.3
Inattention	36	65.5
Obsessive–compulsive disorder	20	36.4
Sleep disturbances	27	49.1
Pervasive developmental disorders/autism	5	9.1

TABLE 13.4 EEG Findings in Patients With SSADH Deficiency (n = 44)

	Number	Percentage
Normal EEG	21	47.7
Abnormal EEG	23	52.3
Background abnormal/slowing	13	29.5
Spike discharges	11	25.0
Electrographic status epilepticus during slow-wave sleep	1	2.27
Photosensitivity	3	6.82

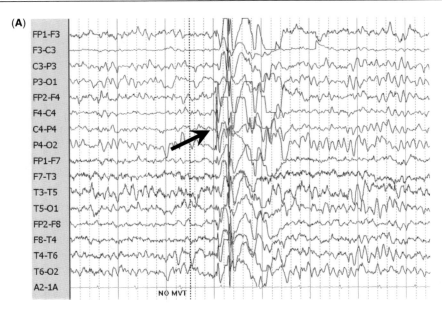

Sensitivity: 15 µV/mm

High Frequency Setting: 70 Hz

Low Frequency Setting: 1.00 Hz

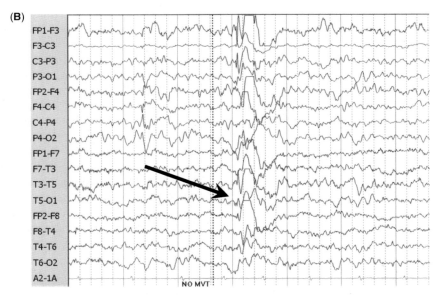

Sensitivity: 15 µV/mm

High Frequency Setting: 70 Hz

Low Frequency Setting: 1.00 Hz

FIGURE 13.3   EEG abnormalities in SSADH deficiency. (A) EEG of 3-year-old girl with SSADH deficiency. Note diffuse spike-wave paroxysm with lead-in over right hemisphere. (B) Same recording as Panel A, showing left sided spike-wave paroxysm.

Sleep disorders may include excessive daytime somnolence and disorders of initiating and maintaining sleep. Overnight polysmonography has shown prolonged latency to stage REM and reduced stage REM (8). Decreased daytime mean sleep latency is reported in half of patients studied with multiple sleep latency tests, indicating excessive daytime somnolence. Overall, there appears to be a reduction in REM sleep in the disorder. Similarly, animal models have demonstrated that hyperGABAergic states, that is, via inhibition of GABA transaminase, are associated with reduction of REM sleep and prolongation of the transition phase between sleep stages NREM and REM (9).

RADIOGRAPHIC FINDINGS

There is a characteristic pallidodentatoluysian pattern of increased T2-weighted signal intensity involving the globus pallidi, cerebellar dentate nuclei, and subthalamic nuclei bilaterally (10). Other findings include cerebral atrophy, cerebellar atrophy, delayed myelination, and T2-hyperintensities in subcortical white matter, thalamus, and brainstem (11, 12). While the pallidal hyperintensity is usually homogeneous and equally affects the internal and external portions, occasional patients have heterogeneous and asymmetric involvement. Magnetic resonance spectroscopy will show normal spectra for routine single- and multivoxel studies of *N*-acetyl aspirate, choline, and lactate, but specialized protocols that allow editing for small molecules have shown elevated levels of GABA and related glx peak compounds (including GHB and homocarnosine) in patients but not obligate heterozygotes (13). Fluorodeoxyglucose PET studies have shown decreased cerebellar glucose metabolism in patients with cerebellar atrophy demonstrated on structural MRI (1, 14).

LABORATORY AND BIOCHEMICAL FINDINGS

Laboratory screening is done with urine organic acids, which consistently show elevated GHB as well as 4,5-dihydroxyhexanoic acid and a general dicarboxylic aciduria. Routine laboratory tests including plasma amino acids and studies of bioenergetics and mitochondrial screening are typically normal. SSADH deficiency is then confirmed through either enzymatic quantification or Aldh5A1 gene sequencing. Gamma-hydroxybutyric acid is elevated in all physiologic fluids, with CSF showing a two- to fourfold increase in GABA and 30-fold increase of GHB in CSF (15, 16). There are also elevated levels of homocarnosine and a trend toward low glutamine levels, implicating dysfunction of the neuronal–glial shuttle wherein glutamine is synthesized only in astroglia with subsequent glutamate and GABA formation in neurons.

PATHOPHYSIOLOGY OF EPILEPSY IN SSADH DEFICIENCY

The epilepsy and EEG phenotypes in SSADH deficiency, specifically generalized tonic–clonic and absence seizures, and generalized spike-wave paroxysms, raise fundamental issues regarding the relationship between GABA and epilepsy. Altered $GABA_A$ and $GABA_B$ mechanisms have been long associated with absence seizures. Typical absence seizures usually present as staring episodes associated with three-per-second, generalized spike-wave discharges on EEG. Atypical absence seizures are relatively similar but are associated with a 1.5 to 2.5 Hz spike-wave and occur in the setting of a symptomatic neurodevelopmental disorder. Absence seizures are associated with altered thalamocortical circuitry involving a network of three neural cell centers: thalamic relay, thalamic reticular, and cortical pyramidal neurons (Figure 13.4). Thalamic relay neurons activate cortical pyramidal neurons in either a tonic mode, leading to the waking state or stage REM sleep, or a burst mode utilizing T-type calcium channels and producing non-REM sleep. The thalamic reticular neurons hyperpolarize thalamic relay neurons via $GABA_B$ receptors and cause burst firing during wakefulness, which may lead to absence seizures. The thalamic reticular neurons are in turn inhibited by neighboring reticular neurons through $GABA_B$ receptors. Thus, both $GABA_A$ and $GABA_B$ receptors are involved in the circuitry that produces absence seizures, with the former mediating the inhibitory postsynaptic potentials regulating thalamocortical behavior and the latter synchronizing thalamocortical circuitry (17).

$GABA_B$ mediated activity is responsible for physiologic deinactivation of T-type calcium channels that lead to the spike discharge in absence seizures. Hence, excessive $GABA_B$ activity may exacerbate absence seizures, as seen with administration of

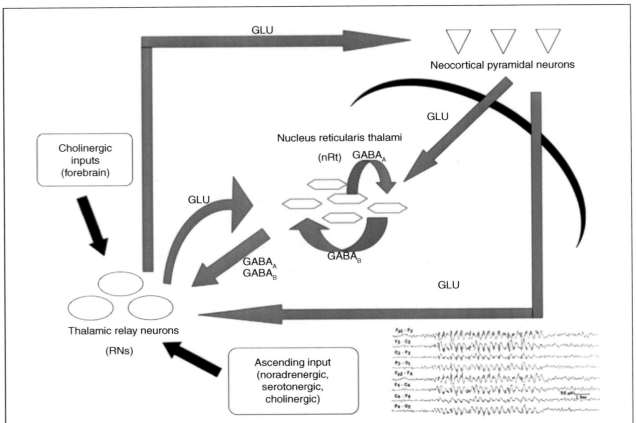

FIGURE 13.4 Thalamocortical circuitry. The thalamocortical circuit consists of thalamic relay neurons, thalamic reticular neurons and neocortical pyramidal neurons. Thalamic relay neurons activate the pyramidal neurons in either a tonic or burst mode to produce awake or REM sleep, and non-REM sleep via T-type calcium channels, respectively. Thalamic reticular neurons regulate this mode of firing by hyperpolarizing the relay neurons through GABABR. Neighboring reticular neurons in turn may inhibit reticular neurons through GABAAR activity. Additional inputs from the forebrain and neurotransmitters may also affect the mode of cortical pyramidal neuron firing by affecting the thalamic relay neurons. A disruption in the thalamocortical circuitry, and in particular, a disruption of the GABA receptor activity on the thalamic relay neurons may cause absence seizures through increased burst firing of the pyramidal neurons during the awake state.

vigabatrin, raising overall GABA levels, or more specifically baclofen, a GABA$_B$ receptor agonist. Further, decreased GABAergic activity could potentially be associated with a transition from absence to generalized convulsive seizures later in life. Brain positron emission tomography using the benzodiazepine receptor antagonist FMZ in SSADH-deficient patients show a significant reduction in FMZ binding compared to parent heterozygote and healthy controls in multiple regions: basal ganglia, amygdala, hippocampus, cerebellar vermis, and cerebral cortex (Figure 13.5). This in vivo finding is consistent with overuse-dependent downregulation of GABA$_A$R activity in patients with SSADH deficiency.

Neurophysiologic studies utilizing transcranial magnetic stimulation in SSADH deficient subjects versus controls show loss of long interval intracortical inhibition and reduction in the cortical silent period, consistent with diminished GABA$_B$R cortical activity (10). Hence, there is evidence of desensitization of both GABA$_A$ and GABA$_B$ receptor activity in patients, suggesting less GABA-mediated inhibition and potentially subsequent predisposition to convulsive seizures.

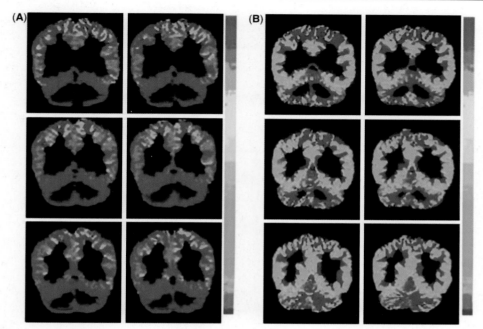

FIGURE 13.5 Decreased GABA$_A$ binding on FMZ-PET in SSADH deficiency. FMZ-PET shows marked reduction of cortical binding potential of [11C]-flumazenil in patient with SSADH deficiency (A) versus heterozygote control (B). (Reproduced with permission from Pearl et al. *Neurology.* 2009;73:423–429.)

MURINE MODEL

The murine model of SSADH deficiency has been instrumental in studying the seizure and electrocorticographic characteristics and responses to antiepileptic drugs, in addition to demonstrating multiple neurotransmitter alterations. In addition to accumulation of both GABA and GHB, there is dysregulation of multiple amino acids including glutamate, glutamine, alanine, aspartate, serine, taurine, cystathionine, methionine, homocarnosine, and arginine (18). Absence seizures may be artificially induced in the SSADH null mouse model using baclofen, a GABA$_B$R agonist, or GHB, which acts via both GHB and GABA$_B$ receptor mediated mechanisms to produce 7 Hz spike-wave discharges in thalamocortical circuitry (2, 19). Absence seizures are abolished in the mouse model with the use of the GABA$_B$R antagonist CGP35348 (2) or the antiepileptic ethosuximide, which causes voltage-dependent blockade of T-type calcium currents. It has also been demonstrated that although the increase in whole-brain GABA content in SSADH null mice does not change spontaneous inhibitory postsynaptic

currents, a measure of synaptic GABAergic connections, it does increase tonic inhibition in the neocortex through presumed extrasynaptic GABA$_A$ receptors (20). This implies that the increased extracellular GABA levels may act through extrasynaptic GABA$_A$ receptors to cause excessive cortical GABAergic neurotransmission, thus exacerbating in absence seizure production in SSADH deficiency.

A transition from absence to generalized convulsive seizures has been demonstrated in the SSADH null mouse. Compared to an uneventful electrocorticograph baseline in P16 wild-type mice, the P16 SSADH null mice display 250–300 μV, 5–7 Hz spike- and-wave discharges (SWD) lasting 3 to 6 sec duration (Figure 13.6). This activity was accompanied by a frozen stare and vibrissal twitching, consistent with absence seizures. In P20 SSADH null mice a generalized 600 μV discharge at 5 Hz followed by 1.5 to 2 Hz SWD is observed, indicative of tonic–clonic seizures. The latter were considered to be the cause of mortality due to the subsequent development of convulsive status epilepticus (2).

While the mechanism for induction of absence seizures by GHB or baclofen invokes increased GABA$_B$

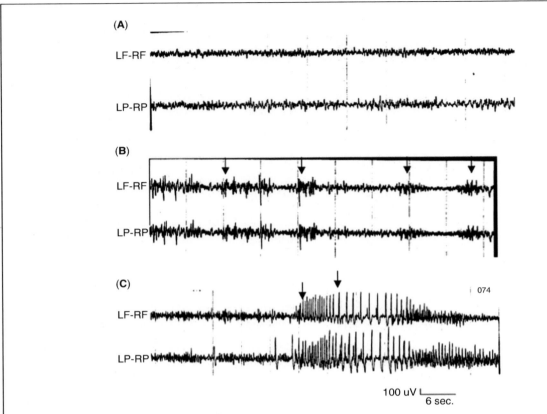

FIGURE 13.6   Transition from absence to tonic-clonic seizures in P20 SSADH (–/–) mice. (A) Baseline electrocorticogram (ECoG) recordings in P16 wild-type (+/+) mice show uneventful 35 to 50 μV and 5 to 7 Hz oscillations. (B) ECoG of P16 SSADH (–/–) mice reveals 250 to 300 μV, 5 to 7 Hz spike-and-wave discharges (SWD) lasting 3 to 6 s duration. This was associated with frozen stare and vibrissal twitching, suggesting absence seizures. (C) ECoG recording in P20 SSADH (–/–) mice show a transition from absence to a generalized 600 μV at 5 Hz followed by 1.5 to 2 Hz SWD associated with tonic-clonic seizures (arrow). LF = left frontal, RF = right frontal, LP = left parietal, RP = right parietal. (Reproduced with permission from: Cortez et al. *Pharmacol Biochem Behav.* 2004;79:547–553.)

activity, the subsequent evolution to generalized tonic–clonic seizures may be postulated to be overuse-dependent downregulation of both GABA$_A$ and GABA$_B$ receptors, resulting in a breakdown of GABA-mediated inhibition, and thus rendering an epileptogenic state.

Decreased binding of an experimental GABA$_A$R antagonist has been demonstrated in the cortex, hippocampus and thalamus of P19 SSADH null mice compared to wild-type mice before the onset of tonic-clonic seizures (21). There is specific downregulation of the GABA$_A$R subunit β2 demonstrated through immunohistochemical staining of the SSADH null mouse brain. Spontaneous rhythmic activity was recorded in two thirds of SSADH null mice, compared to no spontaneous discharges in the wild-type model. Extracellular field recordings in hippocampal CA1 pyramidal layers of P14 SSADH null mice show larger evoked postsynaptic field potentials and an increased number of population spikes. Additionally, a significant reduction in input resistance of hippocampal neurons is seen in P14 but not P9 SSADH null mice. These findings suggest a hyperexcitable state in the pyramidal cells of SSADH-deficient mice after the second week of life. GABA$_A$R-mediated IPSPs are also noted to be reduced in hippocampal neurons in both P8 and P14 SSADH null mice. It is hypothesized that this demonstrated decrease in surface $GABA_AR$ activity in SSADH deficient mice may, again, be related to overuse-dependent receptor downregulation in the presence of increased GABA levels and prolonged occupancy of $GABA_A$ receptors (21).

There is parallel evidence for $GABA_B$ downregulation in the mouse model (22). Decreased binding of an experimental $GABA_BR$ antagonist is seen throughout the brain, and particularly in the hippocampus of both P7 and P14 SSADH deficient mice when compared to wild type. Moreover, there is a significant decrease in $GABA_B$-mediated synaptic potentials in both P7 and P14 SSADH null mice compared to wild-type mice. Parallel to the data for $GABA_A$ receptors, there is animal evidence for use-dependent $GABA_B$ downregulation, which may mediate the development of generalized convulsive seizures.

TREATMENT STRATEGIES AND CLINICAL TRIALS

Treatment for SSADH deficiency remains symptomatic, including targeted antiepileptic drug therapy. Options include anxiolytic agents or selective serotonin reuptake inhibitors (SSRIs) and related medications for obsessive–compulsive disorder. Appropriate antiepileptics are chosen for generalized epilepsy other than avoidance (when possible) of valproate due to its ability to inhibit any residual SSADH enzymatic activity (23). Hence, worsening of the patient in the vignette provided (*vide supra*) was attributed in retrospect to the metabolic diagnosis. Antiepileptics used successfully for maintenance therapy have been lamotrigine, levetiracetam, and topiramate.

Vigabatrin, an irreversible inhibitor of GABA-transaminase, is a logical choice because it will inhibit the conversion of GABA to GHB, but there is the downside of exacerbating elevated GABA levels (24–26). A video-manuscript report of two adolescent brothers demonstrates exercise-induced paroxysmal dyskinesias, manifest by a prominently lurching gait, which showed some improvement following vigabatrin therapy (27). In clinical use, however, vigabatrin has not been a reliable therapeutic for these patients, and there have been many reports of lack of effect or, worse, worsening of symptoms ranging from seizure control to alertness. Further, safety concerns persist regarding retinal toxicity of vigabatrin, especially in this patient population that is unable to report visual field defects. In clinical trials, 30% of patients treated with

vigabatrin for epilepsy report visual field defects following 1 year of treatment (28–30). MRI signal changes caused by vigabatrin, particularly prominent in the GABA-rich thalamus and basal ganglia, pose additional concerns, especially given the existing signal abnormalities in the globus pallidus in this condition (31).

Current clinical trials are focused on the amino acid taurine and an experimental GABA-B receptor antagonist. Taurine, a neuromodulator which interacts with $GABA_A$ and $GABA_B$ receptors, has led to lengthened survival in the SSADH mutant mouse using either intraperitoneal or oral application (32). Taurine is associated with an observed safe level in humans at 3 g/d, and higher dosages have been tested without significant adverse effects. In a single case report available as an abstract, taurine was reported to improve gait, coordination and energy of a $2\frac{1}{2}$-year-old boy with SSADH deficiency (33). The patient was given 4 g/d ($\sim$200 mg/kg) over 1 year. Higher doses were associated with insomnia. At 9 months teachers reported improved behavior, peer interactions, increased level of activity and coordination. At 12 months, the boy's MRI was interpreted as improved. No correlation was found between improved behavior and urine GHB levels. The case was neither controlled nor blinded, and an ongoing clinical trial has thus far not confirmed efficacy based on adaptive behavior measures (34).

Animal work in the SSADH mutant model has suggested benefit from treatment with SGS 742, a $GABA_B$ receptor antagonist, and a clinical trial is anticipated depending on access to the compound. Earlier studies had shown promise with a similar compound, CGP-35348 (32, 35). SGS 742 improves electrocorticographic epileptiform activity in the mutant mouse model. Phase II human studies in adults with mild cognitive impairment have shown significantly improved attention, reaction time, visual information processing, and working memory as well as a good safety profile (36).

GABA Transaminase (GABA-T) Deficiency

GABA-transaminase is the initial key enzyme involved in GABA degradation. Deficiency of this enzyme was initially reported in two of four siblings in a single Flemish family (37). Only the female, who died at age 2 years, was confirmed enzymatically. An older brother, who had died previously at 1 year of age, had similar clinical symptomatology. Since then, one other confirmed patient of an unrelated family has been reported (38).

All patients manifested with seizures and a profound neurodevelopmental disorder. Other findings are hypotonia, hyperreflexia, lethargy, and accelerated growth. The latter is attributable to the growth hormone promoting effects of GABA.

Clinical findings in the index family were neonatal seizures and a high-pitched cry. Linear growth and head circumference were accelerated, with normal height and head circumference noted of both parents. At 2 years the female patient was 4 cm over the 97th percentile in height, and with head circumference in the 75th percentile. The male patient showed a rapid increase in head circumference, from the 50th to 97th percentiles, during the last 6 weeks of his life. The first child of these parents died at the age of 5 days from an unknown cause; the second child is healthy. EEG of the female patient was normal at 2 weeks of age, but at 7 months revealed predominantly low-voltage beta-frequency activity with intermittent epileptiform discharges, and at 2 years showed generalized epileptiform paroxysms. Visual-, auditory-, and somatosensory-evoked potentials were absent at the age of 2 years. CT in both siblings revealed severe cerebral atrophy with ventricular and sulcal enlargement (37, 39–43).

The subsequently reported patient was a 6,745 g newborn female born to nonconsanguineous Japanese parents. The patient was evaluated at 7 months for hyperreflexia, psychomotor retardation, hypotonia, and bilateral intermittent esotropia. At 8 months of age the patient experienced her first seizure, which was a febrile event followed by respiratory distress and requirement for mechanical ventilation. She then developed medically refractory myoclonic seizures. EEG at 8 months revealed diffuse spike and wave activity with one to two second periods of background suppression. By 11 months the patient demonstrated a neurodegenerative course with opisthotonus, and generalized dystonia. Free GABA was elevated in serum, CSF, and cortical tissue, and GABA-T activity was diminished. Cranial CT was normal; MRI suggested a mild delay in myelination, but no structural abnormalities. This patient was still alive at 28 months (38).

Of note, plasma amino acid concentrations in the male of the index family were normal. Hence, the diagnosis of GABA-transaminase deficiency may reside in some cases in accurate determination of CSF GABA. Proton magnetic resonance spectroscopy was used to detect significantly increased GABA concentration in the basal ganglia of the more recent published case, although this requires special editing on MR spectroscopy that is not typically available on clinical studies. Definitive diagnosis can be made by measurement of GABA-transaminase activity in liver, whole blood lymphocytes, or Epstein–Barr virus transformed cultured lymphoblasts (44).

Both confirmed patients were compound heterozygotes. In the index proband, an A-to-G transition at nucleotide 754 of the human GABA-T gene was identified in lymphoblast cDNA (c.754A > G), resulting in substitution of an invariant arginine at amino acid 220 by lysine (p.Arg220Lys) (45). This mutation results in destabilization of the binding of the co-factor pyridoxal-5′-phosphate to GABA-T. The second allele in this patient was later identified as c.1433T > C, causing the substitution p.Leu478Pro. In the second family, gene sequencing of the patient showed the transition c.275G > A that causes the substitution p.Arg92Gly, and an unspecific exon deletion around nucleotides 199 to 316 of the GABA-T coding region (38).

CONCLUSIONS

The disorders of GABA metabolism, SSADH deficiency and GABA-transaminase deficiency, are both associated with epilepsy. SSADH deficiency is characterized by developmental delay, hypotonia, cerebellar ataxia, and hyporeflexia in early childhood. Epilepsy affects approximately half of patients, and generalized epileptiform abnormalities are common. The severity of the epilepsy is variable, although some patients have experienced repeated status epilepticus and SUDEP has been reported. ESES has been documented, and a less common but more severe phenotype includes active myoclonic seizures. In the murine model, early absence seizures transition into generalized convulsive seizures, and ultimately lethal status epilepticus in the first months of life. Correlation of murine and human data suggest that absence seizures are related to excessive GHB and $GABA_B$-mediated activity, and generalized convulsive seizures may be an effect of overuse-dependent downregulation of $GABA_A$ and $GABA_B$ receptor activity. The latter would result in a hyperexcitable state and thus epileptogenesis in this hyper-GABAergic disorder. GABA-transaminase deficiency appears to be extremely rare and is associated with neonatal or infantile myoclonic seizures and a profound encephalopathy. A clinical clue would be growth acceleration related to GABA-promoting effects on growth hormone secretion.

CLINICAL PEARLS

- SSADH deficiency, a disorder of GABA degradation, manifests typically as a nonprogressive encephalopathy with developmental delay, hypotonia, intellectual deficiency, mild ataxia, hyporeflexia, psychiatric manifestations (especially ADHD and obsessive compulsive disorder), and epilepsy.
- SSADH deficiency is screened via urine organic acids for the detection of 4-hydroxybutyric acid.
- The SSADH animal model serves as a substrate to study generalized epilepsy in a hyper-GABA'ergic state.
- Human and animal investigations in SSADH deficiency indicate the presence of overuse-dependent downregulation of GABA receptor activity which may result in epileptogenesis.

This work is supported by National Institutes of Health NS 40270/HD58553 (KMG, PLP), Pediatric Neurotransmitter Disease Association (KMG, PLP), Delman Fund for Pediatric Neurology Research (PLP).

REFERENCES

1. Pearl PL, Gibson KM, Acosta MT, et al. Clinical spectrum of succinic semialdehyde dehydrogenase deficiency. *Neurology.* 2003;60:1413–1417.
2. Cortez MA, Wu Y, Gibson KM, et al. Absence seizures in succinic semialdehyde dehydrogenase deficient mice: a model of juvenile absence epilepsy. *Pharmacol Biochem Behav*, 2004;79:547–553.
3. Knerr I, Gibson KM, Jakobs C, et al. Neuropsychiatric morbidity in adolescent and adult succinic semialdehyde dehydrogenase deficiency patients. *CNS Spectr.* 2008;13:598–605.
4. Pearl PL, Gibson KM. Clinical aspects of the disorders of GABA metabolism in children. *Curr Opin Neurol.* 2004;17:107–113.
5. Pearl PL, Capp PK, Novotny EJ, et al. Inherited disorders of neurotransmitters in children and adults. *ClinBiochem.* 2005; 38:1051–1058.
6. Pearl PL, Jakobs C, Gibson KM. Disorders of beta- and gamma-amino acids in free and peptide-linked forms. In: D Valle, A Beaudet, B Vogelstein, KW Kinzler, SE Antonarakis, A Ballabio , eds. *Online Molecular and Metabolic Bases of Inherited Disease.* Online: www.ommbid.com, 2007.
7. Knerr I, Gibson KM, Murdoch G, et al. Neuropathology in succinic semialdehyde dehydrogenase deficiency. *Pediatr Neurol.* 2010;42:255–258.
8. Pearl PL, Shamin S, Theodore WH, et al. Polysomnographic abnormalities in succinic semialdehyde dehydrogenase (SSADH) deficiency. *Sleep.* 2009;36: 1645–1648.
9. Scherschlicht R. Role for GABA in the control of the sleep-wakefulness cycle. In: A Wauquier, J Gaillard, JM Monti, et al., eds. *Sleep: Neurotransmitters and Neuromodulators.* New York: Raven Press; 1985:237–249.
10. Pearl PL, Gibson KM, Cortez MA, et al. Succinic semialdehyde dehydrogenase deficiency: Lessons from mice and men. *J Inherit Metab Dis.* 2009;32:342–352.
11. Yalçinkaya C, Gibson KM, Gündüz E, et al. MRI findings in succinic semialdehyde dehydrogenase defiency. *Neuropediatrics.* 2000;31:45–46.
12. Ziyeh S, Berlis A, Korinthenberg R, et al. Selective involvement of the globus pallidus and dentate nucleus in succinic semialdehyde dehydrogenase deficiency. *Pediatr Radiol.* 2002;32:598–600.
13. Novotny EJ, Fulbright RK, Pearl PL, et al. Magnetic resonance spectroscopy of neurotransmitters in human brain. *Ann Neurol.* 2003;54(Suppl 6), S25–S31.
14. Al-Essa MA, Bakheet SM, Patay ZJ, et al. Clinical, fluorine-18 labeled 2-fluoro-2-deoxyglucose positron emission tomography (FDG PET), MRI of the brain and biochemical observations in a patient with 4-hydroxybutyric aciduria; a progressive neurometabolic disease. *Brain Dev.* 2000;22:127–131.
15. Gibson KM, Schor DS, Gupta M, et al. Focal neurometabolic alterations in mice deficient for succinate semialdehyde dehydrogenase. *J Neurochem* 2002;81:71–79.
16. Pearl PL, Novotny EJ, Acosta MT. Succinic semialdehyde dehydrogenase deficiency in children and adults. *Ann Neurol.* 2003;54:S73–S80.
17. Chang BS, Lowenstein DH. Epilepsy. *N Engl J Med.* 2003;349:1257–1266.
18. Gupta M, Polinsky M, Senephansiri H, et al. Seizure evolution and amino acid imbalances in murine succinate semialdehyde dehydrogenase (SSADH) deficiency. *Neurobiol Dis.* 2004; 16:556–562.
19. Snead OC, III. The gamma-hydroxybutyrate model of absence seizures: correlation of regional brain levels of gamma-hydroxybutyric acid and gamma-butyrolactone with spike wave discharges. *Neuropharmacology.* 1991;30: 161–167.
20. Drasbek KR, Vardya I, Delenclos M, et al. SSADH deficiency leads to elevated extracellular GABA levels and increased GABAergic neurotransmission in the mouse cerebral cortex. *J Inherit Metab Dis.* 2008; 31:662–668.
21. Wu Y, Buzzi A, Frantseva M, et al. Status epilepticus in mice deficient for succinate semialdehyde dehydrogenase GABA$_A$ receptor-mediated mechanisms. *Ann Neurol.* 2006;59:42–52.
22. Buzzi A, Wu Y, Frantseva MV, et al. Succinic semialdehyde dehydrogenase deficiency: GABA$_B$ receptor-mediated function. *Brain Res.* 2006;1090:15–22.
23. Shinka T, Ohfu M, Hirose S, et al. Effect of valproic acid on the urinary metabolic profile of a patient with succinic semialdehyde dehydrogenase deficiency. *J Chromatogr B.* 2003;792:99–106.
24. Escalera GI, Ferrer I, Marina LC, et al. Succinic semialdehyde dehydrogenase deficiency: decrease in 4-OH-butyric acid

levels with low doses of vigabatrin. *An Pediatr (Barc)*. 2010;72:128–132.

25. Pearl PL, Gropman A. Monitoring gamma-hydroxybutyric acid levels in succinate-semialdehyde dehydrogenase deficiency. *Ann Neurol*. 2004;55:599.

26. Ergezinger K, Jeschke R, Frauendienst-Egger G, et al. Monitoring of 4-hydroxybutyric acid levels in body fluids during vigabatrin treatment in succinic semialdehyde dehydrogenase deficiency. *Ann Neurol*. 2003;54: 686–689.

27. Leuzzi V, Di Sabato ML, Deodato F, et al. Vigabatrin improves paroxysmal dystonia in succinic semialdehyde dehydrogenase deficiency. *Neurology*. 2007;68:1320–1321.

28. Krauss GL, Johnson MA, Miller NR. Vigabatrin-associated retinal cone system dysfunction—Electroretinogram and ophthalmologic findings. *Neurology*. 1998;50:614–618.

29. Spence SJ, Sankar R. Visual field defects and other opthalmological disturbances associated with vigabatrin. *Drug Saf*. 2001; 24:385–404.

30. Vanhatalo S, Nousiainen I, Eriksson K, et al. Visual field constriction in 91 Finnish children treated with vigabatrin. *Epilepsia*. 2002;43:784–756.

31. Pearl PL, Vezina LG, Saneto RP, et al. Cerebral MRI abnormalities associated with vigabatrin therapy. *Epilepsia*. 2009;50(2): 184–194.

32. Gupta M, Greven R, Jansen EE, et al. Therapeutic intervention in mice deficient for succinate semialdehyde dehydrogenase (gamma-hydroxy butyric aciduria). *J Pharmacol Exp Ther*. 2002;302:180–187.

33. Saronwala A, Tournay A, Gargus JJ. Taurine treatment of succinate semialdehyde dehydrogenase (SSADH) deficiency reverses MRI-documented globus lesions and clinical syndrome. *Am Coll Med Genet*, 15th Ann Clinical Genet Meeting, March 12–16, 2008, Phoenix, AZ, USA, p. 103.[Abstract].

34. Pearl PL, Theodore WH, McCarter R, et al. Open label trial of taurine in SSADH deficiency. Abstract in press: Child Neurol Soc Proceedings 2011.

35. Hogema BM, Gupta M, Senephansiri H, et al. Pharmacologic resuce of lethal seizures in mice deficient in succinate semialdehyde dehydrogenase. *Nat Genet*. 2001;29:212–216.

36. Froestl W, Gallagher M, Jenkins H, et al. SGS742: the first GABA(B) receptor antagonist in clinical trials. *Biochem Pharmacol*. 2004;68:1479–1487.

37. Jaeken J, Casaer P, de Cock P, et al. Gamma-aminobutyric acid-transaminase deficiency: a newly recognized inborn error of neurotransmitter metabolism. *Neuropediatrics*. 1984;15: 165–169.

38. Tsuji M, Aida N, Obata T, et al. A new case of GABA transaminase deficiency facilitated by proton MR spectroscopy. *J Inherit Metab Dis*. 2010;33:85–90.

39. Gibson KM, Nyhan WL, Jaeken J. Inborn errors of GABA metabolism. *Bioessays*. 1986;4:24–27.

40. Nutzenadel W. Disorders of beta-alanine, 4-aminobutyrate (GABA), carnosine, and homocarnosine. In: J Fernandes, J-M Saudubray, K Tada, eds. *Inborn Metabolic Diseases: Diagnosis and Treatment*. New York: Springer-Verlag, 1990: 337–343.

41. Gibson KM. Gamma-aminobutyric acid (GABA) transaminase deficiency. In: ML Buyse, ed. *Birth Defects Encyclopedia*. Cambridge, MA: Blackwell Scientific, 1990:766–767.

42. Jakobs C, Jaeken J, Gibson KM. Inherited disorders of GABA metabolism. *J Inherit Metab Dis*. 1993;16:704–715.

43. Scriver CR, Gibson KM. Disorders of beta- and gamma-amino acids in free and peptide-linked forms. In: CR Scriver, AL Beaudet, WS Sly, D Valle, eds. *The Metabolic and Molecular Basis of Inherited Disease*. 7th ed. New York: McGraw-Hill, 1995.

44. Gibson KM, Sweetman L, Nyhan WL, et al. Demonstration of 4-aminobutyric acid aminotransferase deficiency in lymphocytes and lymphoblasts. *J Inherit Metab Dis*. 1985;8:204–208.

45. Medina-Kauwe LK, Tobin AJ, De Meirleir L, et al. 4-Aminobutyrate aminotransferase (GABA-transaminase) deficiency. *J Inherit Metab Dis*. 1999;22:414–427.

Glucose Transporter Type I Deficiency Syndrome and Epilepsy

Amanda Wai-Yun Pong and Darryl C. De Vivo

INTRODUCTION

Brain energy metabolism in the nonfasting state is entirely dependent on a constant glucose supply. Glucose transport across the blood–brain barrier in humans is the unique function of the glucose transporter type I (1). The Glut1 transporter resides at the endothelial cell of the brain microvasculature where it is highly expressed and participates in the facilitated diffusion of glucose across the blood-brain barrier. Additionally, the Glut1 transporter supplies glucose from the interstitium to astrocytes, oligodendrocytes, and glial cells in the brain (2).

The metabolic demand of the brain in infancy outstrips that of the older child and the adult. Hence, a disproportionately large 80% of whole-body glucose utilization is used by the neonatal brain for growth and development. This energy supply is provided specifically by glucose transport via Glut1 for aerobic metabolism, and creates the necessary fuel to balance excitatory and inhibitory neuronal populations, thus preventing epileptic activity and enabling appropriate brain maturation (2).

The discovery of the human condition of Glut1 deficiency was made in 1991 when De Vivo et al identified two children with Glut1 deficiency syndrome (OMIM 138140) (3). Both children presented with early-onset refractory seizures, movement disorder, acquired microcephaly, ataxia, and psychomotor delay. The laboratory signature of hypoglycorrhachia in the setting of normoglycemia and low-to-normal CSF lactate led De Vivo to treat the children with the ketogenic diet (KD), providing an alternate source of brain energy. Their excellent response to the KD led to the *in vitro* examination of 3-OMG uptake using erythrocytes, which also express *GLUT1* gene. The 3-OMG RBC uptake assays in the Glut1 deficiency patients demonstrated decreased values compared to their unaffected parental controls, implicating a defect in glucose transport.

EPIDEMIOLOGY

Although awareness of this syndrome has increased in the medical community, the exact incidence and prevalence of Glut1 DS are yet unknown. We suspect that the condition is significantly under-diagnosed, and posit several barriers to making a Glut1 DS diagnosis. First, is the lack of newborn screening, which exists for other treatable metabolic conditions of infancy, such as phenylketonuria. Development of a newborn screen relies on the presence of a testable compound accessible in a routine blood smear, which does not exist in the case of Glut1 DS. The utility of genetic sequencing is complicated by the myriad of over 100 potential mutations in the condition, and limited by the current cost of technology.

Second, the main diagnostic procedure, the fasting lumbar puncture is often delayed, deferred, or inaccurately interpreted, with low CSF glucose values assessed as lab-error related or clinically unimportant. The acquisition of simultaneous blood and CSF glucose and lactate values is an integral part of the evaluation. CSF lactate values are expected to be low to normal (less than 2.2 mM). In our experience, timely performance of the fasting lumbar puncture and associated blood testing are often the main impediment to early diagnosis and prevention of neurodevelopmental consequences of nontreatment.

GENETICS

The genetic defect underlying Glut1 DS (MIM 606777) is in the *SLC2A1* gene, on chromosome 1p35–31.3, consisting of 10 exons spanning 35 kilobases (MIM 138140). By the year 2010, there were over 100 reported mutations in the literature, including missense, nonsense, deletion, insertion, and splice site mutations (4). Most cases arise *de novo*; transmission in more mildly affected individuals, or those with mosaicism, shows autosomal dominant inheritance and rarely autosomal recessive inheritance (5, 6).

Recent work by our group has demonstrated that the pattern of inheritance is determined by the degree of haploinsufficiency and the pathogenicity of the mutation (7). Compound heterozygotes, for example, may inherit a mutated allele from an unaffected parent, and have a de novo mutation, resulting in a haploinsufficient state (7). The erythrocyte 3-O-methyl-D-glucose uptake assay is a surrogate measure of Glut1 haploinsufficiency that uses the Glut1 transporter on red blood cells to examine rate of glucose uptake.

Knock-out mouse models of Glut1 DS have shown similar phenotypic expressions as humans, with acquired microencephaly, seizures, and movement disorders/motor delays (8). Mutations in the glucose transporter type 1 have been shown to account for a monogenic form of dystonia and dyskinesia, paroxysmal exertion-induced dyskinesia 2 (PED, DYT18) with or without epilepsy (9). Missense mutations in *SLC2A1* with decreased glucose uptake in functional assays have also been identified in individuals with slowly progressive spastic paraparesis combined with PED (paroxysmal choreoathetosis/spasticity, DYT9) (10).

DIAGNOSTIC GENETIC TESTING

Diagnostic genetic testing for an individual presenting with epilepsy, movement disorders, and developmental delay in the setting of hypoglycorrhachia and normoglycemia is offered on a commercial basis in the United States. Glut1 DS represents one scenario in which identification of a genetic mutation in an epilepsy condition has important and direct impact on treatment choice and ultimately, the prognosis. With early diagnosis and institution of the KD, the progressive symptoms of acquired microcephaly/brain hypotrophy, refractory epilepsy, ataxia, and developmental regression may be mitigated (11).

Approximately 5% to 10% of patients with a phenotype consistent with Glut1 DS will receive negative genetic testing via current available sequencing methods. The yield of confirmatory testing will likely increase as newer molecular diagnostics are developed (12). There is, as above, no newborn screening method developed for Glut1 DS. With increased surveillance, earlier testing, and improved treatment outcomes, genetic counseling provides an important intervention for affected individuals as they mature into reproductive stages (13).

CLINICAL DIAGNOSIS

The diagnosis of Glut1 DS rests on clinical grounds, and confirmatory genetic testing is also available commercially and on a research basis. The clinical hallmarks are early onset epilepsy that is refractory to standard antiepileptic drugs (AEDs). Diagnosis is achieved through a fasting assessment of cerebrospinal fluid, showing hypoglycorrhachia (less than 40 mg/dL) and normal or low CSF lactate values (less than 2.2 mM) in the setting of normoglycemia (~70–110 mg/dL). Left untreated, patients develop subsequent acquired microcephaly, with motor and cognitive impairments. Ataxia and paroxysmal movement disorders are also prominent features.

The initial cutoff value for diagnosing hypoglycorrhachia was a glucose concentration of 40 mg/dL (or 2.2 mM) for suspected Glut1 DS cases. In the past, particular significance has been placed on the ratio of CSF glucose to serum glucose, with the cutoff value for Glut1 DS set at less than .4, while normal is greater than .6 (14). In our practice, we have given greater emphasis to the absolute CSF glucose value. However, with the increasing recognition of milder allelic variants, higher CSF glucose values of 41 to 52 mg/dL are now being described (15–19). In our experience, the CSF glucose values in 150 cases of Glut1 DS always have been less than 60 mg/dL, and the vast majority (greater than 90%) of values have been less than 40 mg/dL (unpublished observations; [20]). These observations also indicate that the normal range for CSF glucose has never been defined properly. A low CSF glucose concentration also can be found in other neurological conditions such as infectious meningitis, hypoglycemic states, subarachnoid hemorrhage, and meningeal carcinomatosis, and must be ruled out clinically by assessing cell count and imaging findings (21–25).

Although not a strict diagnostic requirement, brain imaging characteristics in Glut1 DS deserve attention due to the frequent use of neuroimaging in assessing patients with epilepsy. De Vivo et al's first Glut1 DS patient had MRI showing mild delay in myelination at 7.5 months of age, and subsequent cases have demonstrated normal or minor, nonspecific abnormalities with slight brain hypotrophy at various ages in childhood (3, 26–27). One group has reported a case in which brain hypotrophy noted at age 5 years before KD initiation was replaced by normal brain growth at 7 years on the KD, a finding that underscores the importance of appropriate early diagnosis and treatment (26). Second, findings on ^{18}F-fluorodeoxyglucose positron emission tomography (FDG-PET) show constant decrease in cortical uptake with relative increase in caudate and lentiform nuclei, as demonstrated in a study of 14 Glut1 DS patients (28, 29). In particular, there was more severe hypometabolism at the thalamus, cerebellum, and mesial temporal lobes, not associated with coexistence of epilepsy (28). These abnormalities present in infancy and persist through adulthood, and are not rectified with ketosis.

MANAGEMENT

The gold standard treatment for Glut1 DS is the KD, which provides alternative fuel for brain metabolism and development in this progressive metabolic condition. The response to KD is rapid and dramatic, and is often followed by weaning of previously instituted AEDs. In our experience, better neurodevelopmental and epilepsy results are obtained with maintenance of the betahydroxybutyrate (BHB) levels around 5 mM, rather than the standard 2 to 3 mM (30). For this reason, we recommend BHB measurements from finger stick, not urine dips (falsely reassuring). Ideally, the KD should be maintained through adolescence, to provide adequate fuel support through the brain maturation process.

In theory, particular AEDs may be associated with clinical exacerbation in Glut1 DS, based on their effects on the Glut1 transporter. Common antiepileptic agents known to inhibit the Glut1 transporter *in vitro*, that is, phenobarbital, valproate, and benzodiazepines, are relatively contraindicated in Glut1 DS (31, 32). Valproate both worsens hypocarnitinemia and inhibits fatty acid oxidation and should not be combined with the KD. Finally, as hypocarnitinemia may be seen in patients treated with the KD, oral L-carnitine supplementation at a dose of 100 mg/kg/d, up to a maximum of 2 g/d, should be considered for Glut1 DS patients on the KD (33).

Patients with Glut1 DS require frequent monitoring for neurodevelopmental progress and treatment of epilepsy and movement disorders. At our institution, we have developed a semiquantitative tool, the Columbia Neurological Score, to assess 12 domains of neurological function to define a patient's clinical trajectory. This yields a "CNS score" based on the 12 domains: (1) height, weight, and head circumference; (2) general medical exam; (3) funduscopic exam; (4) cranial nerves; (5) stance and gait; (6) involuntary movements; (7) sensation; (8) cerebellar function; (9) muscle bulk, tone, and strength; (10) tendon reflexes, (11) Babinski signs; and (12) other findings. The CNS score ranges from 0 to 76 (normal); scores of 40 to 49 indicate severe impairment, 50 to 59 moderate, 60 to 69 mild, and 70 to 76 minimal. This tool provides a high inter-rater reliability and has been demonstrated to correlate with other measures of disease severity (34).

Management of Glut1 DS patients is multifaceted and often involves a multidisciplinary team approach, with neurologists fluent in aspects of epilepsy, movement disorders, and neurodevelopment, ketogenic dieticians, geneticists and genetic counselors, and therapists. The application of video EEG to determine the nature of paroxysmal events and to follow treatment outcomes is essential to guide treatment. Close monitoring of blood parameters on the KD and AEDs is essential to avoid unintended side effects. KD support can prolong the duration of KD use, by providing resources for creative and feasible dietary options. Longitudinal follow-up with genetics is important to guide families through diagnosis and prognosis, evaluation of family members, and to assist with reproductive decisions (13). Involvement of physical, speech and occupational therapists should be ordered as needed to treat neurodevelopmental delays. Prognosis depends largely on early identification and rectification of metabolic encephalopathy with the KD and appropriate therapies.

MOVEMENT DISORDERS

Two decades since the seminal paper by De Vivo et al, the phenotypic spectrum of Glut1 deficiency has expanded, although the salient clinical features remain those initially described (3). All manner of episodic movement disorders have been described in Glut1 DS, including dysarthria, opsoclonus, choreoathetosis, myoclonus, spasticity and weakness, independent of seizure activity (35). Characteristic exacerbation of these symptoms with fatigue, dietary noncompliance with KD, and excitement has been noted (35). By 2008, a literature review of 100 published cases revealed three cases of ataxia without epilepsy (20). Alternating Hemiplegia of Childhood (AHC), which is genetically associated in a small number of cases with mutations in *ATP1A2* and *CACNA1A*, is now a recognized phenotypic presentation of GLUT1 deficiency due to *SLC2A1* mutations (35). As in many cases of AHC, these children experience hemiplegic, tonic, dystonic episodes starting before 18 months, with subsequent progressive ataxia and cognitive impairment (35). Paroxysmal exertion-induced dyskinesia 2 or DYT18 is yet another new phenotype associated with mutations in *SLC2A1* (36).

EPILEPSY

The most common symptom across all presentations of Glut1 DS remains epilepsy, affecting approximately 90% of our patient population; the seizures are often early in onset and refractory to standard antiepileptic medications. Accordingly, one aim of this chapter is to review the current understanding of the epilepsy component of this condition, highlighting the semiology, neurophysiology, and treatment response aspects of epilepsy in Glut1 DS.

The long-recognized wide variation in seizure semiology seen in Glut1 DS has led to its designation as "the great mimicker." As with many genetic entities, variable penetrance and variable expressivity represent challenges to the diagnostician.

The initial two cases described by De Vivo et al epitomize the key clinical and electrographic characteristics now well-described in the Glut1 DS literature (3, 15). Both patients manifested early onset of refractory epilepsy at age 2 months, characterized by loss of responsiveness, and focal myoclonic or horizontal roving eye movements that correlated with seizure activity on the EEG. The initial EEG tracings revealed a right frontal focus in one case and progressed from normal to generalized spike and waves in the second. Failed medication trials included the typical agents used in infancy, including phenobarbital and benzodiazepines, and later valproate and carbamazepine. Both patients experienced complete resolution on the KD, within 4 and 7 days of ketosis, followed by weaning of standard AEDs. As is often the case with newly discovered conditions, the index cases represent the severe end of the spectrum, prior to identification of a gold standard preventive treatment. Both children ultimately showed mild delays in spite of seizure freedom.

Literature review of the subsequent 2 decades provides 109 cases of Glut1 DS patients with documented epilepsy and associated clinical features. Although De Vivo et al's index cases presented in early infancy, the average age of seizure onset as described in 102 cases was 12 months, likely reflecting identification of milder cases over time (4, 11, 16, 30, 37–42). Confirmed cases of Glut1 DS now span the globe in North America, Australia, China, Japan, and Europe, and collectively re-iterate the classic presentation with early seizures described as brief, subtle myoclonic limb jerking, staring and eye rolling, pallor, loss of responsiveness, with hypotonia, and at times head bobbing (4, 15, 30, 37, 43, 44). Possible nonepileptic paroxysmal events include periodic confusion, ataxia, weakness, headache, and sleep changes, which may require characterization with EEG (15).

Later in childhood, mixed seizure types prevail. One of the largest series to focus on epilepsy in this condition was published from our group in 2003, and describes the often mixed seizure types and EEG findings. Of the 20 children with confirmed Glut1 DS, generalized tonic or clonic seizures prevailed (14/20), followed by absence (10), partial (9), myoclonic (6), and astatic (4). In another series of 15 patients, followed prospectively for 2 to 5 years, Klepper et al described absence (7/15), myoclonic (7/15), generalized tonic clonic (4/15), and tonic (2/15) seizures, in addition to seizures associated with episodic irregular eye movements (9/15) and cyanosis (3/15), at the time of Glut1 DS diagnosis. The average age of onset of seizures was prior to 9 months in 11/15 or 73%. The authors noted that the presence of episodic irregular eye movements and the aggravation of symptoms and EEG features with fasting constitute evidence for Glut1 deficiency (38).

Most recently, our group described the epilepsy features of the largest cohort of Glut1 DS patients. Of the 87 patients, 78 (90%) had epilepsy, with average age of onset at 8 months, but often delayed Glut1 DS diagnosis at 6.5 years. Seizure types included generalized tonic-clonic (53%), absence (49%), complex partial (37%), myoclonic (27%), drop (26%), tonic (12%), simple partial (3%), and spasms (3%). 68% (53/78) demonstrated variable focal and multifocal seizure types and electroencephalographic features. Effects of AEDs on seizure freedom were reviewed showing insufficient evidence to recommend specific AEDs as alternatives to the KD (39).

The potential for misclassification of symptomatic generalized seizures resulting from neuroglycopenia is hardly a new concept. In 2003, Leary et al noted that the most common EEG abnormality in their childhood aged patients was the 2.5 to 4 Hz generalized spike-wave, the hallmark of idiopathic generalized epilepsies (IGE) (11). Shortly after, Oguni et al recognized that the infantile phenomenon of myoclonic seizures could easily be misinterpreted as benign myoclonic epilepsy in infancy, prior to the development of other symptoms (44). An illustrative case was indeed reported by Roulez-Perez in 2008, when a child with occasional myoclonic seizures in infancy and short absences was given a diagnosis of idiopathic generalized epilepsy. She was treated with valproate, ethosuximide, and clobazam with only minimal improvement. The correct diagnosis was established at age 10 years after identification of periodic confusion before meals, atypical features on EEG, and learning difficulties (41). She did well on the KD, but showed mild delays.

Newer work has focused on early absence epilepsy in Glut1 DS, yet another syndrome easily misdiagnosed as idiopathic generalized epilepsy (39, 45). Suls et al. studied 34 patients with early onset absence epilepsy before 4 years, and found 4/34 cases with *SLC2A1* mutations by direct sequencing (less than 12%). These cases showed inconsistent treatment responses ranging from easily controlled to refractory, and had normal development prior to seizure onset. The authors concluded that the seizure phenotype of mutation-positive cases could not be distinguished from mutation-negative early-onset cases, or from classic CAE, except for the earlier age of onset (45).

Variability of phenotype and particularly of seizure expression within a family may also be seen in Glut1 DS, as evidenced by subsequent work by the same group (39). From the probands with early onset absence, Mullen et al identified two families with SLC2A1 mutations and identified 15 subjects with mutations (45). Of these, 12/15 were found to have epilepsy with various seizure types: 10/12 had absence seizures with onset between 3 and 34 years, and 3/12 patients had nonconvulsive status epilepticus. One sibling pair was reported to have myoclonic astatic epilepsy (MAE) with absence, GTC seizures, and atonic seizures at age 4 years and intellectual delay. Temporal-lobe epilepsy and complex partial epilepsy with multifocal epileptiform discharges on EEG were reported in two patients. Finally, isolated febrile seizures were found in one mutation carrier without further development of symptoms or delay. Of note, seven family members were identified with subtle PED, and two mutation carriers were unaffected (39).

NEUROPHYSIOLOGY

Neurophysiological features of Glut1 DS were first systematically studied by Boles et al in 1999, who performed repeated studies on two children prior to and during KD treatment (46). Not surprisingly, they found both normal recordings and generalized, 2 to 2.5 Hz paroxysmal spike-wave discharges in both patients. One patient had more frequent interictal discharges and absence seizures while not in ketosis, suggesting improvement with delivery of ketones across the blood–brain barrier. In 2002, Von Moers et al elucidated the relationship between epileptiform activity and feeding, which by increasing serum glucose concentrations may facilitate increased passage of glucose via the deficient glucose transporter. Two children with subsequently confirmed Glut1 mutations were studied on EEG prior to breakfast, and 1 and 2 hours after. The epileptiform activity at each interval was quantified as 48%, 0 and 0 (Patient 1) and 28%, 13 and 10 (Patient 2). Based on the dramatic decrease or abolishment of epileptiform activity after a normal meal, the authors suggested using pre- and postprandial EEG recordings as a simple screening test for Glut1 DS. Seizures were reported as myoclonic jerks of the shoulders and arms or nodding of the head, and corresponded with some of the generalized paroxysms of spike-waves. Subsequently, both children were placed on the KD with significant reduction in seizures and improvements in development (47).

Subsequent larger case series have recapitulated the findings of generalized spike-waves on EEG, but also demonstrated frequent focal and multifocal ictal and interictal findings (11). Leary et al, in their case series of 20 patients described above, reviewed 24 continuous 24-hour EEG recordings and found a mixed picture of background abnormalities: generalized 2.5 to 4 Hz spike-waves (41%), generalized slowing or attenuation (34%), no abnormalities (34%), focal spike-waves (13%), and focal slowing or attenuation (9%) (11, 48). The authors noted a trend toward increased focal versus generalized abnormalities in those under 2 years of age, due to immaturity of myelination, but this did not reach statistical significance ($P < .10$). Differences in EEG abnormalities prior to and after KD were also not statistically significant ($P > .10$) (11).

A recent study from our group evaluated moment-to-moment neuropsychological and neurophysiological function in response to hyperglycemia in Glut1 DS, which leads to saturation of the glucose transporter (49). Six children were recorded on video EEG 2 hours before until 6 hours after oral glucose loading. These tracings revealed continuous background slowing, generalized spike-waves, and focal frontal and central spike waves bilaterally in the pre-loading state. In the first 30 min to 3 hours after glucose loading, there were marked improvements in background activity, seizures, and certain neuropsychological tasks (coordination and attention), all of which returned to baseline after 180 min. These findings underscore the critical minute-to-minute dependence of specific neurological functions on glucose transport across the blood–brain barrier.

Seizure activation with hyperventilation and photic stimulation has been reported in two cases prior to initiation of KD. These children experience activation of upward eye deviation, behavioral arrest, and head drop correlating to less than 3 sec of generalized spike-waves on EEG (41). This phenomenon has not yet been replicated on a larger scale.

The tendency towards mixed seizure types in individuals with Glut1 DS is mirrored by the not infrequent occurrence of mixed EEG findings. EEG recordings may range from normal to abnormal, with generalized, focal or multifocal spike-waves, slowing or attenuation (11). Abnormalities may depend on neurodevelopmental state, perhaps with increased focal or multifocal findings in infants due to prematurity of myelination, and have been shown to vary in response to feeding status, ketosis, or overall metabolic state. Ultimately, Glut1 DS is a unique genetic condition whose EEG and seizure phenotype is not restricted to generalized seizure types or EEG features, and variation of expression may be seen in an individual or across affected family members (39).

FUTURE DIRECTIONS

Our knowledge about the clinical and molecular aspects of Glut1 DS has evolved rapidly over the past two decades since its discovery in humans. Nonetheless, many important areas for future research and clinical advances remain largely untapped.

The ultimate goal in Glut1 DS, as with all metabolic diseases, is to make an early, correct diagnosis and to apply this knowledge to institute the best available treatment in the hopes of preventing neurodevelopmental deficits. Development of a newborn screen for Glut1 DS would be an ideal mechanism by which to facilitate this goal, but limitations exist at a technological level, as described above. The search for other biomarkers for the condition is moving at a rapid pace, including the work by De Vivo et al to develop the erythrocyte uptake assay as a gold standard diagnostic test. The merits of this functional assay include its ability to discern a degree of haploinsufficiency at a functional level, rather than detecting, as a genetic test would, the presence or absence of a known mutation. The functionality of the assay correlates with the relative pathogenicity of the disease-causing mutation. Further work in this area will enable the medical community to better determine disease status in mutation-negative, phenotype-positive individuals.

In the treatment arena, we anticipate the development of further agents to provide fuel for brain metabolism. Triheptanoin, an anapleurotic 7-carbon fatty acid used in disorders of long-chain fatty acid metabolism, is one such agent under investigation by Roe and Mochel (50). Thioctic acid is under investigation as an antioxidant that translocates GLUT1 from intracellular pools across the plasma membrane in vitro (2, 11, 51). The therapeutic role of other agents transported across the blood–brain barrier by Glut1, such as the oxidized version of vitamin C, remain to be determined (51, 52). Supplemental agents, such as acetylcholinesterase inhibitors, are used on occasion with the aim of improving cognitive deficits in a subpopulation of Glut1 DS patients at our institution. Basic practices, such as breast feeding, may also be shown as beneficial or protective, by maintaining a high fat, ketotic, environment for neurodevelopment. Newer therapies may focus on rectifying imbalances associated with other roles of the Glut1 transporter, that is, in the movement of dehydroascorbic acid, glycopeptides, galactose, and other elements (11). Finally, greater elucidation of specific AED effects on the Glut1 transporter are needed in the future, to identify agents as inhibitors of the Glut1 transporter, which should be avoided in this condition.

KEY POINTS

Glut1 DS is a unique, treatable, metabolic encephalopathy resulting in various clinical presentations. The gold standard treatment is the KD, which provides an alternative fuel source for brain development. Most commonly, the disorder presents, after a normal pregnancy in early infancy, with refractory epilepsy. Seizure types may include focal or multifocal clonic or myoclonic seizures, with staring, loss of responsiveness, head nodding, and irregular episodic horizontal eye movements. Untreated patients experience delays in motor and cognitive realms, with acquired microcephaly and progressive spasticity and ataxia. In childhood, absence, myoclonic, tonic, or clonic seizures prevail, and patients may experience nonconvulsive status epilepticus. Variability in phenotype may be explained by Glut1 haploinsufficiency, as measured by the erythrocyte glucose uptake assay. MRI findings may be normal initially, but show hypotrophy over time. Neurophysiological studies may also be normal, but more often show generalized, focal or multifocal slowing and epileptiform discharges, which may vary over time and improve with glucose loading or treatment with KD. FDG-positron emission tomography shows lifelong decreased cortical uptake, with relative increase in the caudate and lentiform nuclei.

In the two decades since the identification of Glut1 DS in humans, forms of the condition with more prominent motor manifestations have been discovered, including many without epilepsy. KD remains the gold standard for nonepileptic forms of Glut1 DS. These individuals may manifest dysarthria, opsoclonus, choreoathetosis, myoclonus, spasticity and weakness, symptoms that may fluctuate according to metabolic status. Alternating hemiplegia of childhood and paroxysmal exertion-induced dyskinesia 2 have been associated with mutations in the SLC2A1 gene. With ever growing awareness of this treatable metabolic encephalopathy, we anticipate further discoveries of yet milder phenotypes, in step with the evolution of newer genetic testing platforms and novel therapies.

CLINICAL PEARLS

- Glut1 deficiency syndrome is a metabolic encephalopathy with wide phenotypic variability
- The condition results from deficits in the glucose transporter type1 at the blood–brain barrier, which is the exclusive purveyor of glucose to the brain tissue.
- Most patients have mutations in the *SLC2A1* gene on chromosome 1p35. Inheritance is mainly autosomal dominant and less commonly autosomal recessive; compound heterozygotes have been identified.
- Glut1 haploinsufficiency generally parallels disease severity, and may be assessed on a research basis with the erythrocyte glucose uptake assay.
- The classic phenotype comprises neuroglycopenia, with infantile onset epilepsy, acquired microcephaly, motor and cognitive delay, and spasticity, when untreated.
- Various other phenotypes, including children with milder delays and mixed seizure disorders, often with early onset absence epilepsy, have also been described.
- Movement disorders with paroxysmal ataxia, dysarthria, choreoathetosis, myoclonus, and opsoclonus have also been identified as Glut1 related.

- Ninety percent of children with the condition will have epilepsy.
- Seizure types encompass focal or generalized myoclonic, tonic, clonic, astatic, complex partial, absence, and nonconvulsive status epilepticus.
- Epilepsy may occur without accompanying motor or cognitive symptoms of Glut1 DS, and may be misclassified as idiopathic generalized epilepsy without appropriate diagnostic testing or lumbar puncture.
- Diagnosis is via clinical history and fasting lumbar puncture with concomitant fasting serum glucose.

FLOWCHART FOR DIAGNOSIS AND TREATMENT OF GLUCOSE TRANSPORTER TYPE I DEFICIENCY SYNDROME (DE VIVO DISEASE)

Clinical Features

    ±epilepsy refractory to standard AEDs

    ±paroxysmal movement disorder

    ±acquired developmental delay

    ±acquired microcephaly

    ±ataxia

Fasting Lumbar Puncture and Bloodwork

    Hypoglychorrhachia (less than 60 mg/dL) with normoglycemia

    Low or normal CSF lactate (less than 2.2 mM)

Confirmatory genetic testing

    Molecular analysis

    Erythrocyte glucose uptake assay

Test results supportive of the diagnosis

    Electroencephalography findings with variability based on prandial status

    Positron emission topography with diffusely diminished cortical uptake

    MRI normal or hypotrophy

Treatment

    KD (ratio determined by age and other factors)

    Avoid inhibitors of GLUT1 transporter: barbiturates, valproate, phenobarbital, theophyllines, methylxanthines

Follow-up

    Maintain betahydroxybuyrate levels at ~5 mM with KD

    Maintain KD through childhood

Hypoglycorrhachia with normoglycemia and low to normal CSF lactate are diagnostic.

- EEG findings include normal background features, focal or generalized slowing or attenuation, or generalized, focal or multifocal spike and waves. EEG findings may vary depending on metabolic and treatment status.
- MRI findings may be normal or nonspecific. Diffuse hypotrophy may be apparent over time, particularly without KD treatment.
- Treatment with KD is the gold standard for all forms of Glut1 DS. Treatment should be titrated according to blood betahydroxybutyrate levels around 5 mM, rather than the standard 2 to 3 mM.
- Epilepsy is often refractory to standard anticonvulsants, but responds rapidly and dramatically to the KD.
- KD provides an alternative fuel source for brain development and promotes neurocognitive development.
- Prognosis is dependent on early identification of underlying metabolic condition and initiation of treatment with KD.
- Genetic counseling for families with affected children is recommended.

REFERENCES

1. Mueckler M, et al. Sequence and structure of a human glucose transporter. *Science.* 1985;229(4717):941–945.
2. De Vivo DC, et al. Glucose transporter protein syndromes. *Int Rev Neurobiol.* 2002;51:259–288.
3. De Vivo DC, et al. Defective glucose transport across the blood–brain barrier as a cause of persistent hypoglycorrhachia, seizures, and developmental delay. *N Engl J Med.* 1991;325(10): 703–709.
4. Ito Y, et al. Clinical presentation, EEG studies, and novel mutations in two cases of GLUT1 deficiency syndrome in Japan. *Brain Dev.* 2005;27(4):311–317.
5. Wang D, Kranz-Eble P, De Vivo DC. Mutational analysis of GLUT1 (SLC2A1) in Glut1 deficiency syndrome. *Hum Mutat.* 2000;16(3):224–231.
6. Klepper J, et al. Autosomal recessive inheritance of GLUT1 deficiency syndrome. *Neuropediatrics.* 2009;40(5): 207–210.
7. Rotstein M, et al. Glut1 deficiency: inheritance pattern determined by haploinsufficiency. *Ann Neurol.* 2010;68(6):955–958.
8. Wang D, et al. A mouse model for Glut1 haploinsufficiency. *Hum Mol Genet.* 2006;15(7):1169–1179.
9. Bruggemann N, Klein C. Genetics of primary torsion dystonia. *Curr Neurol Neurosci Rep.* 2010;10(3):199–206.
10. Weber YG, et al. Paroxysmal choreoathetosis/spasticity (DYT9) is caused by a GLUT1 defect. *Neurology.* 2011;77(10): 959–964.

11. Leary LD, et al. Seizure characterization and electroencephalographic features in Glut1 deficiency syndrome. *Epilepsia.* 2003;44(5):701–707.

12. Pong AW, Pal DK, Chung WK. Developments in molecular genetic diagnostics: an update for the pediatric epilepsy specialist. *Pediatr Neurol.* 2011;44:317–327.

13. Pal DK, Pong AW, Chung WC. Genetic evaluation and genetic counseling for epilepsy. *Nat Rev Neurol.* 2010;6(8):445–453.

14. Sedel F, et al. Epilepsy and inborn errors of metabolism in adults: a diagnostic approach. *J Inherit Metab Dis.* 2007;30(6): 846–854.

15. Brockmann K. The expanding phenotype of GLUT1-deficiency syndrome. *Brain Dev.* 2009;31(7):545–552.

16. Suls A, et al. Paroxysmal exercise-induced dyskinesia and epilepsy is due to mutations in SLC2A1, encoding the glucose transporter GLUT1. *Brain.* 2008;131(Pt 7):1831–1844.

17. Weber YG, et al. GLUT1 mutations are a cause of paroxysmal exertion-induced dyskinesias and induce hemolytic anemia by a cation leak. *J Clin Invest.* 2008;118(6):2157–2168.

18. Zorzi G, et al. Paroxysmal movement disorders in GLUT1 deficiency syndrome. *Neurology.* 2008;71(2):146–148.

19. De Vivo DC, Wang D, Glut1 deficiency: CSF glucose. How low is too low? *Rev Neurol.* 2008;164(11):877–880.

20. Joshi C, et al. GLUT1 deficiency without epilepsy: yet another case. *J Child Neurol.* 2008:23(7):832–834.

21. Javadekar BB, Vyas MD, Anand IS. CSF/blood glucose ratio and other prognostic indices in pyogenic meningitis. *J Indian Med Assoc.* 1997:95(1):9–11.

22. Saez-Llorens X, McCracken GH. Bacterial meningitis in children. *Lancet.* 2003;361(9375):2139–2148.

23. Dubos F, et al. Serum procalcitonin and other biologic markers to distinguish between bacterial and aseptic meningitis. *J Pediatr.* 2006;149(1):72–76.

24. Lindquist L, et al. Value of cerebrospinal fluid analysis in the differential diagnosis of meningitis: a study in 710 patients with suspected central nervous system infection. *Eur J Clin Microbiol Infect Dis.* 1988;7(3):374–380.

25. Silver TS, Todd JK. Hypoglycorrhachia in pediatric patients. *Pediatrics.* 1976:58(1):67–71.

26. Perez-Duenas B, et al. Childhood chorea with cerebral hypotrophy: a treatable GLUT1 energy failure syndrome. *Arch Neurol.* 2009;66(11):1410–1414.

27. Wang D, et al. Glut1 deficiency syndrome: Clinical, genetic, and therapeutic aspects. *Ann Neurol.* 2005;57(1):111–118.

28. Pascual JM, et al. Imaging the metabolic footprint of Glut1 deficiency on the brain. *Ann Neurol.* 2002;52(4):458–464.

29. Pascual JM, et al. Brain glucose supply and the syndrome of infantile neuroglycopenia. *Arch Neurol.* 2007;64(4):507–513.

30. Fujii T, et al. Three Japanese patients with glucose transporter type 1 deficiency syndrome. *Brain Dev.* 2007;29(2): 92–97.

31. Klepper J, Voit T. Facilitated glucose transporter protein type 1 (GLUT1) deficiency syndrome: impaired glucose transport into brain—a review. *Eur J Pediatr.* 2002;161(6):295–304.

32. Wong HY, et al. Sodium valproate inhibits glucose transport and exacerbates Glut1-deficiency in vitro. *J Cell Biochem.* 2005;96(4):775–785.

33. De Vivo DC, et al. L-Carnitine supplementation in childhood epilepsy: current perspectives. *Epilepsia.* 1998;39(11): 1216–1225.

34. Kaufmann P, et al. Cerebral lactic acidosis correlates with neurological impairment in MELAS. *Neurology.* 2004;62(8): 1297–1302.

35. Rotstein M, et al. Glut1 deficiency and alternating hemiplegia of childhood. *Neurology.* 2009;73(23):2042–2044.

36. Schneider SA, et al. GLUT1 gene mutations cause sporadic paroxysmal exercise-induced dyskinesias. *Mov Disord.* 2009; 24(11):1684–1688.

37. Fung EL, et al. First report of GLUT1 deficiency syndrome in Chinese patients with novel and hot spot mutations in SLC2A1 gene. *Brain Dev.* 2011;33(2):170–173.

38. Klepper J, et al. Seizure control and acceptance of the ketogenic diet in GLUT1 deficiency syndrome: a 2- to 5-year follow-up of 15 children enrolled prospectively. *Neuropediatrics.* 2005;36(5): 302–308.

39. Mullen SA, et al. Absence epilepsies with widely variable onset are a key feature of familial GLUT1 deficiency. *Neurology.* 2010;75(5):432–440.

40. Leen WG, et al. Glucose transporter-1 deficiency syndrome: the expanding clinical and genetic spectrum of a treatable disorder. *Brain.* 2010;133(Pt 3):655–670.

41. Roulet-Perez E, et al. Glut1 deficiency syndrome masquerading as idiopathic generalized epilepsy. *Epilepsia.* 2008;49(11): 1955–1958.

42. Takahashi S, et al. Molecular analysis and anticonvulsant therapy in two patients with glucose transporter 1 deficiency syndrome: a successful use of zonisamide for controlling the seizures. *Epilepsy Res.* 2008;80(1):18–22.

43. Ito S, et al. Modified Atkins diet therapy for a case with glucose transporter type 1 deficiency syndrome. *Brain Dev.* 2008;30(3): 226–228.

44. Oguni H. Symptomatic epilepsies imitating idiopathic generalized epilepsies. *Epilepsia.* 2005;46(Suppl 9):84–90.

45. Suls A, et al. Early-onset absence epilepsy caused by mutations in the glucose transporter GLUT1. *Ann Neurol.* 2009;66(3): 415–419.

46. Boles RG, et al. Glucose transporter type 1 deficiency: a study of two cases with video-EEG. *Eur J Pediatr.* 1999;158(12):978–983.

47. von Moers A, et al. EEG features of glut-1 deficiency syndrome. *Epilepsia.* 2002;43(8):941–945.

48. Pong AW, Geary BR, Engelstad KM, Natarajan A, Yang H, De Vivo DC. Glucose transporter type I deficiency syndrome: Epilepsy phenotypes and outcomes. Epilepsia. 2012 Jul 19. doi: 10.1111/j.1528-1167.2012.03592.x. [Epub ahead of print].

49. Akman CI, et al. Acute hyperglycemia produces transient improvement in glucose transporter type 1 deficiency. *Ann Neurol.* 2010;67(1):31–40.

50. Roe CR, Mochel F. Anaplerotic diet therapy in inherited metabolic disease: Therapeutic potential. *J Inherit Metab Dis.* 2006;29(2–3):332–340.

51. Klepper J, et al. Defective glucose transport across brain tissue barriers: a newly recognized neurological syndrome. *Neurochem Res.* 1999;24(4):587–594.

52. Klepper J, Vera JC, De Vivo DC. Deficient transport of dehydroascorbic acid in the glucose transporter protein syndrome. *Ann Neurol.* 1998;44(2):286–287.

15

DEND Syndrome: Developmental Delay, Epilepsy, and Neonatal Diabetes, a Potassium Channelopathy

Carolina Lahmann and Frances Ashcroft

INTRODUCTION

Potassium channels are crucial regulators of excitation in most tissues, their activation hastening membrane repolarization and damping down electrical activity. Many potassium channels are also specialized for specific functions. One of these is the ATP-sensitive potassium (K_{ATP}) channel, which couples the metabolic state of the cell to plasma membrane excitability and thus to a variety of cellular functions (1–3). At low levels of metabolic activity, K_{ATP} channels are open, allowing the flux of potassium ions out of the cell. This clamps the membrane potential at a hyperpolarized level and thereby inhibits cellular activity (Figure 15.1A). Increased metabolic activity causes K_{ATP} channel closure and leads to a membrane depolarization that stimulates electrical activity and cell functions (Figure 15.1B). As a consequence, K_{ATP} channels are involved in many physiological functions including regulation of neuronal and cardiac excitability, control of smooth muscle tone, glucose uptake by skeletal muscle, and insulin secretion from pancreatic beta-cells.

In recent years, the discovery that mutations in the K_{ATP} channel are associated with various metabolic syndromes has highlighted the physiological importance of this channel. This chapter will discuss how the most severe gain-of-function mutations lead to developmental delay, epilepsy and neonatal diabetes, a condition known as DEND syndrome (4).

THE K_{ATP} CHANNEL

The K_{ATP} channel is composed of four pore-forming potassium channel (Kir6.x) subunits and four regulatory sulphonylurea receptor (SUR) subunits (Figure 15.2) (5–7). Kir6.2 is found in most tissues except for smooth muscle, where Kir6.1 serves as the pore (6). Three main SUR isoforms exist: SUR1 is expressed in neurons, atrial myocytes, and various endocrine tissues including pancreatic beta-cells (6–10), SUR2A in ventricular and skeletal muscle (10), and SUR2B in smooth muscles and a small population of neurons (9, 11). Association of Kir6.2 with different SUR subtypes endows the K_{ATP} channel with different sensitivities to modulation by metabolism and pharmacological agents.

The characteristic feature of the K_{ATP} channel is that it is regulated by cellular metabolism, with increased metabolism closing, and reduced metabolism opening, the channel. Such metabolic regulation is mediated by changes in intracellular concentrations of adenine nucleotides, which interact with the channel in complex ways. Specifically, binding of ATP, and to a lesser extent ADP, to Kir6.2 results in channel closure (12, 13). Adenine nucleotides also interact with the intracellular domains of SUR but in contrast to Kir6.2, Mg^{2+} is required for this interaction. Binding of MgADP, or the binding and hydrolysis of MgATP to MgADP, to SUR elicits channel opening

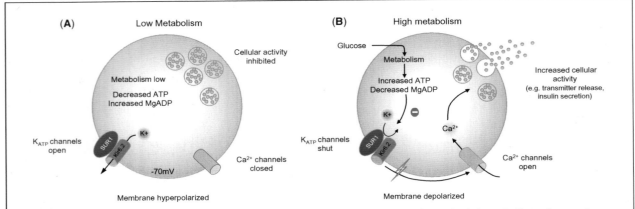

FIGURE 15.1 Schematic representation of the metabolic regulation of K$_{ATP}$ channels. (A) Under low plasma glucose conditions, K$_{ATP}$ channels are open and keep the membrane potential hyperpolarized. (B) When plasma glucose levels increase, cellular metabolism increases, causing a rise in the intracellular ATP and a decrease in MgADP. This leads to K$_{ATP}$ channel closure, membrane depolarization, electrical activity and cellular function.

(14–17). Under physiological conditions, the balance between ATP-mediated inhibition at Kir6.2 and MgATP/MgADP-mediated activation at SUR sets the level of K$_{ATP}$ channel activity in the cell.

In glucose-sensing tissues, K$_{ATP}$ channel activity is modulated by changes in the blood glucose concentration. In the pancreatic beta-cell, for example, K$_{ATP}$ channels are open at low plasma glucose, inhibiting

insulin secretion (18). By contrast, when plasma glucose levels rise, metabolism increases, closing K$_{ATP}$ channels and initiating a cascade of intracellular events that results in insulin secretion (Figure 15.1B). In other tissues, such as the heart, K$_{ATP}$ channels are thought to only open in response to severe metabolic stress (ie, hypoxia, ischemia), when intracellular ATP levels are considerably depleted. It appears that this

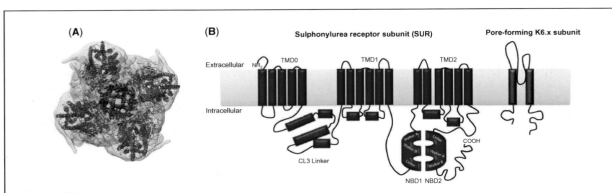

FIGURE 15.2 (A) Top view of an electron density map of the K$_{ATP}$ channel complex with models of Kir6.2 (blue), SUR1 (minus TMD0)(red) placed within the map. ATP molecules are shown in green. From Mikhailov et al. (68). (B) Membrane topology of Kir6.x and the sulphonylurea receptor. Some of the motifs within the nucleotide binding domains (NBD) that are involved in ATP-binding and hydrolysis have been labelled (Walker A, Walker B, linker "signature sequence").

different metabolic sensitivity is determined by the SUR subunit, with SUR1 rendering the channel far more sensitive to opening when metabolism decreases. The electrical activity of neurons with Kir6.2/SUR1 channels, for example, shows much greater metabolic sensitivity than that of neurons with Kir6.2/SUR2B channels (9).

The sulphonylurea receptor subunit also endows the channel with sensitivity to a range of potassium channel openers and inhibitors (19). Sulphonylurea drugs, such as glibenclamide and tolbutamide, close the channel, and have been used for over half a century to stimulate insulin secretion in patients with type 2 diabetes. As their name indicates, K-channel openers activate the K_{ATP} channel. These drugs show subunit specificity, with diazoxide opening SUR1-containing channels, and pinacidil opening SUR2-containing channels.

ACTIVATING K_{ATP} CHANNEL MUTATIONS CAUSE DIABETES AND EPILEPSY

In 2004, it was discovered that gain-of-function mutations in the *KCNJ11* gene, which encodes Kir6.2, are a common cause of neonatal diabetes (ND) (20). Subsequently, activating mutations in the *ABCC8* gene (encoding SUR1) were also described in ND patients (21, 22). Neonatal diabetes is a rare inherited disorder with an estimated incidence of 1 in 100 to 200,000 live births (4, 23, 24). It is characterized by severe hyperglycemia within the first 6 months of life, which results from an almost complete loss of insulin secretion. The diabetes can either be permanent (PNDM) or follow a remitting–relapsing pattern (TNDM).

Right from the start it was recognized that although most ND patients experience diabetes in isolation, some also have neurological features. These symptoms are associated with certain mutations and are not a secondary consequence of insulin-induced hypoglycemia. About 3% of ND patients exhibit marked developmental delay, involving failure to achieve motor and intellectual milestones appropriate to their age, muscle hypotonia, epilepsy, and dysmorphic features (4). This spectrum of symptoms is known as *DEND syndrome*, being an abbreviation of *d*evelopmental delay, *e*pilepsy, and *n*eonatal *d*iabetes. Rather more patients (~20%) present with an intermediate condition (*iDEND syndrome*), which is characterized by neonatal diabetes coupled with delayed

speech and walking, muscle hypotonia, and attention deficit. Although it was originally thought that these patients did not suffer epilepsy, there is accumulating evidence that a small number of them may experience mild and isolated seizures.

More than 40 different mutations in *KCNJ11*(Kir6.2) and a large number in *ABCC8* (SUR1) are now known to cause ND. Thirteen different mutations cause DEND syndrome and three lead to iDEND syndrome, with the Kir6.2-V59M mutation being the most common cause of the latter (23, 24) (Table 15.1). All *KCNJ11* mutations are dominantly acting heterozygous mutations that largely arose *de novo* during embryogenesis. The picture is more heterogeneous in the case of *ABCC8* mutations. Both dominant and recessively acting mutations have been described, as well as compound heterozygosity, uniparental disomy, and even compound heterozygosity for both an activating and inactivating mutation (25).

FUNCTIONAL EFFECTS ON THE CHANNEL

All gain-of-function ND mutations in Kir6.2 exert their effects by 'locking' the K_{ATP} channel in a permanently open state, even under hyperglycemic conditions (4, 24). This leads to an increased whole-cell K_{ATP} current, membrane hyperpolarization and reduced electrical activity (Figure 15.3A). In all cases, the increased K_{ATP} channel activity is caused by a reduction in the sensitivity of the channel to ATP inhibition, which can be achieved directly or indirectly. Mutations that cluster around the putative ATP-binding site of Kir6.2 are thought to impair ATP binding directly. Other mutations increase the time that the channel spends in the open state in both the absence and presence of ATP; as this molecule predominantly stabilizes the closed state of the channel, any mutation that reduces the amount of time spent in the closed state will secondarily decrease the channel sensitivity to ATP. Some Kir6.2 mutations are also thought to enhance Mg-nucleotide activation. The location of all known DEND and iDEND mutations in Kir6.2 is given in Figure 15.3B.

Few ND mutations in SUR1 have been functionally characterized, but they too appear to impair the ability of ATP to inhibit the channel (21, 22, 25). They do so either by increasing the MgATP activation or by stabilizing the open state conformation of the channel. Interestingly only two mutations in SUR1 have been

TABLE 15.1   Kir6.2 and SUR1 Gain-of-Function Mutations Associated With DEND Syndrome Cause Different Types of Epileptic Seizures

Mutation	Type of Epilepsy	Therapy (seizures)	Reference
Kir6.2-R50G	Tonic spasms	No information	(44)
Kir6.2-R50P	Hypertonic seizures; generalized epilepsy	Sodium valproate	(26)
Kir6.2-Q52R	Infantile spasms	Partially responded to vigabatrin	(20, 39, 50)
Kir6.2-G53D	Generalized epilepsy	No information	(46)
Kir6.2-G53D	Seizures during infancy	No information	(41)
Kir6.2-V59G	Myoclonic epilepsy	Responded to anti-epileptics (not clear if vigabatrin or sodium valproate)	(20)
Kir6.2-F60Y/V64L	Generalized tonic–clonic seizures	Seizures ceased with glibenclamide	(30)
Kir6.2-C166F	Infantile spasms	Refractory to antiepileptics and corticosteroids. Initially responded to tolbutamide	(40)
Kir6.2-C166Y	Infantile spasms	Sodium valproate and clobazam	(41, 42)
Kir6.2-C166Y	Tonic spasms	No information	(44)
Kir6.2-I167L	Infantile spasms; myoclonic episodes and absence states	Improved with glibenclamide	(31)
Kir6.2-I296L	Generalized complex seizures	Incompletely controlled with anti-epileptics (not clear if vigabatrin or sodium valproate)	(20, 39, 50)
Kir6.2-G334D	Myoclonic epilepsy	Sodium valproate	(28)
SUR1-I49F	Infantile spasms	Unresponsive to antiepileptic drugs. No improvement with glibenclamide	(43)
SUR1-F132L	Nonspecific generalized epileptiform activity	Phenobarbitone/phenytoin	(22)
Kir6.2-V59M (iDEND)	Absence seizures	Sodium valproate	(47)
Kir6.2-V59M (iDEND)	Myoclonic epilepsy; partial seizures	Seizures resolved spontaneously	(48)
Kir6.2-V59M (iDEND)	Epilepsy (no further information)	No information	(49)

described to cause DEND syndrome and only one has been described for iDEND syndrome (Table 15.1).

Of the 13 DEND mutations that have been described to date (Table 15.1), only those at residues R50, G53, and G334 in Kir6.2 are thought to affect ATP binding directly (26–28); the remainder (at residues Q52, V59, F60, C166, I167, and I296 in Kir6.2; and F132 in SUR1) act by stabilizing the open state of the channel (22, 29–33). The preponderance of mutations that act via changes in channel open probability reflects the much greater reduction in channel ATP sensitivity such mutations produce. Nevertheless, it is not the molecular mechanism that dictates the clinical phenotype. It is the magnitude of the decrease in the ability of MgATP to block the channel current in inside-out patches that is crucial. The greater the

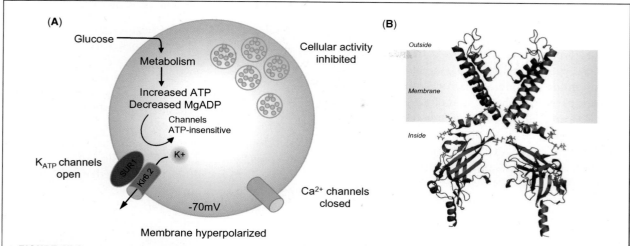

FIGURE 15.3 Gain-of-function mutations in the K_{ATP} channel can cause neonatal diabetes. (A) Activating mutations in Kir6.2 or SUR1 prevent K_{ATP} channel closure when ATP levels rise in response to metabolism. Thus, the beta-cell membrane remains hyperpolarized even when plasma glucose levels are elevated, preventing insulin secretion. (B) Structural model of Kir6.2 (69) viewed from the side. For clarity, only two transmembrane domains and two separate cytosolic domains are shown. Residues mutated in DEND syndrome are shown in magenta.

decrease in ATP sensitivity, the greater the increase in the whole-cell K_{ATP} current and more severe the clinical phenotype (34).

It is likely that the greater number of Kir6.2 mutations (compared to SUR1 mutations) associated with epilepsy is because Kir6.2 mutations generally produce a greater reduction in ATP sensitivity. However, it should not be forgotten that Kir6.2 can couple to SUR2B in some neurons, so that a wider population of neurons (9) might be affected by a Kir6.2 mutation than an SUR1 mutation. There is also a suggestion that SUR1 may couple to a nonselective cation channel (possibly TRPM4) in endothelial cells (35), which might also result in phenotypic differences between SUR1 and Kir6.2 mutations. However, this interaction has been questioned (36).

DEND SYNDROME AND EPILEPSY

A total of 11 activating *KCNJ11* mutations and two *ABCC8* mutations have been reported to cause DEND syndrome (to date). The majority of these patients suffer from generalized seizures that begin during the first 12 months of life; infantile spasms, myoclonic seizures, and tonic–clonic seizures have

been described (Table 15.1). The case histories of these patients are discussed below.

Infantile Spasms

Infantile spasms (IS) is a devastating epileptic condition that usually presents between the age of 3 and 10 months and is characterized by the abrupt onset of clustering head and arm jerks that last for seconds (37). It is usually accompanied by developmental delay or loss of already acquired developmental skills (38). In most cases, this condition is associated with a characteristic electroencephalogram (EEG) pattern known as hypsarrhythmia (37). This is an interictal pattern of very high voltage, asynchronous spike and sharp wave discharges, which usually change to lower-amplitude slow waves or to a sudden flattening (electrodecremental period) during clinical attacks.

IS is the most common type of seizure described in DEND patients, being diagnosed in four patients with activating *KCNJ11* mutations (Q52R, C166F, C166Y, I167L) and one patient with an *ABCC8* mutation (I49F) (20, 31, 39–43). Two of these patients (Kir6.2-I167L and SUR1-I49F) started developing subtle neonatal seizures at two months of age, which evolved into full infantile spasms by 3 months of age.

The other three patients (Kir6.2-Q52R, Kir6.2-C166F, Kir6.2-C166Y) developed IS abruptly, at around 3 to 4 months of age. EEG recordings of all five patients showed a typical hypsarrhythmia pattern.

Most patients with IS are treated either with corticosteroids (mainly adrenocorticotropin hormone [ACTH]) or with vigabatrin, and 60% to 80% of infants on ACTH and 50% to 60% of infants on vigabatrin become spasm-free (38). However, with one exception, all DEND patients with IS failed to respond to treatment with ACTH, vigabatrin or classical antiepileptics. The exception was the Kir6.2-C166Y patient, who responded to a combination of sodium valproate and clobazam (42). Interestingly, antiepileptic treatment attenuated the infantile spasms of the I167L patient, but daily myoclonic episodes and absence states ensued (31).

Two additional DEND patients with activating mutations in *KCNJ11* (R50G and C166Y) were reported to suffer from tonic spasms, but there is no published information about their EEG pattern, diagnosis or treatment (44).

Myoclonic Seizures

Myoclonic seizures are characterized by brief, sudden, involuntary jerks that can affect the whole body or may be confined to specific locations (45). These jerks are associated with abnormal EEG activity, which may consist of spikes, multispikes and spike-wave complexes. Myoclonic seizures have been described in two patients with activating *KCNJ11* mutations—V59G[1] and G334D (20, 28). These patients presented with generalized myoclonic seizures at 2 and 4 months of age (respectively), which was 2 to 3 months after diabetes was diagnosed. EEG recordings showed multifocal sharp waves and slow delta waves in both patients. Seizures in the Kir6.2-G334D patient were effectively managed with sodium valproate. In the case of the Kir6.2-V59G patient, seizures were stated to respond to antiepileptic drugs, though it was not clear which drug the patient received.

---

[1]Note that in the original paper (Gloyn et al, 2004) this patient was incorrectly stated to carry the Kir6.2-Q52R mutation, and vice versa (Please refer to the correction published on the 30th of September, 2004).

Generalized Tonic–Clonic or Tonic Seizures

Generalized tonic–clonic seizures are characterized by an initial phase during which patients experience continuous body stiffening ("tonic" phase) followed by a phase of rhythmic jerking of the body ("clonic" phase). To date, three patients with activating *KCNJ11* mutations (R50P, G53D, F60Y/V64L) (26, 27, 30) have been reported to suffer from generalized tonic–clonic or tonic seizures. Interestingly, all three mutations lie within the ATP-binding site.

The Kir6.2-R50P patient started developing seizures after presenting with ketoacidosis at the age of 3 months (26). He was reported to be unconscious for 6 days and to suffer from hypertonic seizures of all limbs during this time. These seizures were accompanied by an EEG pattern of diffusely abnormal electrical activity. Subsequently, the patient continued to suffer from generalized seizures, but these are reported to be well controlled with sodium valproate. In this case, it is hard to be certain whether the epilepsy was due to the ketoacidosis or to the mutation.

One patient with the Kir6.2-G53D mutation was diagnosed with diabetes at 3 months of age, and treated with insulin, but he had poor glycemic control and episodes of hypoglycemia (46). He started developing seizures at the age of 5 years, during episodes of hypoglycemia. Thus, it is not clear whether the seizures were triggered by the hypoglycemic attacks or by the mutation, particularly as the EEG did not show any abnormal electrical activity. However, another patient with the Kir6.2-G53D mutation has also been reported to suffer from seizures during infancy, which were accompanied by an abnormal EEG (41). This makes it more likely that the G53D mutation is causal for the epilepsy.

Two other patients with activating K_{ATP} mutations (I296L in *KCNJ11* and F132L in *ABCC8*) have been reported to suffer from generalized epileptic seizures (20, 22, 39). The Kir6.2-I296L patient presented with screaming attacks at 11 months of age, which were accompanied by frontal spikes on the EEG. These attacks evolved into secondary generalized complex partial seizures at a later age, which were partially controlled with anti-epileptic drugs (20, 39). The SUR1-F132L patient was diagnosed with diabetes at 13 weeks of age and was treated with insulin. He had poor glycemic control and was admitted with ketoacidosis 3 times during his first 2 years of life. During his second year, he started developing intermittent fine distal and athetoid involuntary movement disorders, which later evolved into severe muscle spasms. At this time, an EEG revealed nonspecific generalized epileptiform activity, which was controlled with a high-dose phenobarbitone and phenytoin combination (22).

iDEND SYNDROME AND EPILEPSY

Although iDEND syndrome was first described as neonatal diabetes, developmental delay and muscle weakness without epilepsy (4), it has since become apparent that some iDEND patients also suffer from seizures. However, these seizures are usually milder than those reported in DEND cases and they do not occur during the first 12 months of life. To date, epilepsy has been reported in three iDEND patients, all of whom carry the V59M mutation in *KCNJ11*, which is the most common mutation associated with this syndrome.

One patient presented at 5 weeks of age with diabetes, marked developmental delay and muscle weakness, but no epilepsy. Neurological assessment at 12 and 23 months of age indicated he had not experienced any overt epileptic seizures and had a normal EEG. However, shortly before his fourth birthday, the patient started developing absence states and diminished concentration and a 24-hr EEG revealed diffuse spike waves with frequency of 3 to 4 Hz. He was diagnosed with generalized absence epilepsy and his seizures were treated effectively with a low dose of sodium valproate (47).

In the case of the other two patients with Kir6.2-V59M mutations, one started experiencing what appeared to be partial seizures at 5 years of age. An EEG indicated she was suffering from myoclonic epilepsy. Interestingly, the seizures resolved spontaneously without any treatment (48). The third patient was reported to experience epilepsy, but without indication as to the type of epilepsy or whether any treatment was administered (49). There are also anecdotal reports of other Kir6.2-V59M patients experiencing epilepsy. One patient was diagnosed with partial complex seizures, while another patient was diagnosed with myoclonic absence seizures at the age of 6 years, after presenting with fluttering eyelids and staring spells.

Epilepsy is not uncommon in young children and neurological problems can be a secondary consequence of severe hypoglycemia. Thus one cannot rule out the possibility that in any individual patient, their epilepsy is unrelated to the ND mutation they carry. Nevertheless, the fact that there is a strong correlation between the functional effect of the mutation and the severity of the clinical phenotype, that patients with the same mutation show similar symptoms and develop epilepsy at around the same age, and that they fail to respond to classical treatment, is a strong argument that K_{ATP} channel mutations can indeed cause epilepsy. Additional evidence comes from the fact that the symptoms of some patients can be alleviated by blocking their open K_{ATP} channels.

SULPHONYLUREA THERAPY

Sulphonylurea drugs are potent and highly selective blockers of the K_{ATP} channel that act by binding to the SUR subunit and closing the K_{ATP} channel in an ATP-independent manner (19) (Figure 15.4). The discovery that many ND patients have activating K_{ATP} channel mutations immediately suggested that their open channels might be closed by sulphonylureas. This proved to be the case for many mutations. Because sulphonylureas bypass the defective metabolic regulation of the mutant K_{ATP} channels they restore insulin secretion in ND, and they do this so effectively that the diabetes of more than 90% of ND patients can be controlled with these drugs (50). Indeed, sulphonylurea therapy provides better glycemic control than insulin, reducing mean blood glucose levels, fluctuations in blood glucose levels and the frequency of hypoglycemic episodes (50, 51). Nevertheless, some mutations are less sensitive to sulphonylurea block, and patients with these mutations have been unable to switch to sulphonylurea therapy (34). These include those with the Q52R, C166Y, I296L, and G334D mutations in Kir6.2, all of which cause DEND syndrome.

It was also hoped that sulphonylureas might help control the neurological problems in DEND and iDEND patients. The extent to which sulphonylureas penetrate the blood–brain barrier and the relationship between their concentration in plasma and the cerebrospinal fluid (CSF) is unclear. Nevertheless, transition to sulphonylureas has been attempted for all DEND patients diagnosed to date because of the possibility of enhanced glycemic control. However, only five out of 13 reported patients have been successfully weaned off insulin (26, 30, 31, 43, 46). The lack of response in the other patients is likely to be because

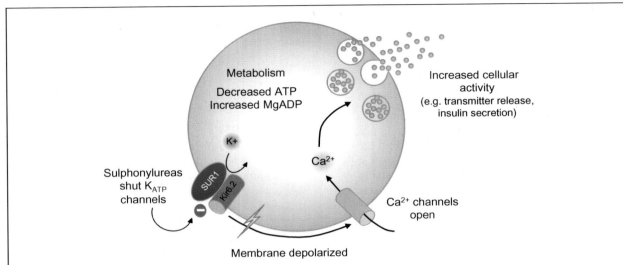

FIGURE 15.4   Sulphonylureas stimulate insulin secretion. Sulphonylureas bind directly to the K_{ATP} channel and trigger its closure in an ATP-independent manner. This triggers depolarization of the beta-cell, leading to opening of voltage-gated Ca^{2+} channels, Ca^{2+} influx, and insulin secretion.

they carried mutations that are less sensitive to sulphonylurea block.

In those DEND patients that successfully switched to sulphonylurea treatment (who carry the Kir6.2-R50P, Kir6.2-G53D, Kir6.2-F60Y/V64L, Kir6.2-I167L, and SUR1-I49L mutations), considerably better glycemic control was reported, both in terms of a reduction in blood glucose fluctuations and a decrease in HbA1C levels (26, 30, 31, 43, 46). Furthermore, a significant improvement in the epilepsy of the Kir6.2-I167L patient was reported: after 6 months on a high dose of the sulphonylurea glibenclamide, no seizures were observed during a 24-hr EEG and hypsarrhythmia was no longer present (31). A similar improvement was observed in a patient with a dual Kir6.2-F60Y/V64L mutation after transfer to sulphonylureas (30). In the case of the other three patients, no improvement in terms of neurological function or seizure control was observed.

Interestingly, the neurological function of the Kir6.2-C166F patient, who did not respond to antiepileptic drugs, improved when put on a combination of ACTH and tolbutamide (40). Even though the patient could not be weaned off insulin, approximately 25% less was required to control her diabetes. In addition, the frequency of IS was reduced and the

hypsarrhythmia in the EEG disappeared after 12 days on the combined treatment. Furthermore, the patient was successfully weaned off ACTH and the epileptic seizures were appropriately managed with tolbutamide. Unfortunately, the epilepsy started deteriorating approximately 3 months after initiation of tolbutamide therapy and the patient later died (40).

The improved control of epilepsy afforded by sulphonylurea therapy in these patients may indicate that sulphonylureas are able to cross the blood–brain barrier, at least to a limited extent, and reduce K_{ATP} channel hyperactivity in neurons. This idea is supported by the fact that improved motor function and enhanced cognition has been reported in a number of iDEND and DEND patients after initiation of sulphonylurea therapy (27, 47, 52).

All three iDEND patients with epilepsy successfully transferred to sulphonylureas. It is interesting that in all cases their seizures began *after* transfer. In one patient, absence seizures started developing two years after initiation of glibenclamide therapy (47), which also occurred with the other two (anecdotal) reports of epilepsy in iDEND patients. Why this is the case is not clear, particularly as motor and behavioral improvements were observed in all three patients.

It is important to emphasize that reports that sulphonylureas can ameliorate epilepsy should be treated with caution because of the very few number of patients involved, and the fact that some childhood epilepsies spontaneously remit. It is also not known if the sulphonylurea concentration in the CSF reaches a level high enough to close K_{ATP} channels and restore normal neurological function. Likewise, it is unclear if the reported development of absence seizures in iDEND children treated with sulphonylureas might be unrelated to drug therapy and may even have been worse in the absence of the drug, or if it is caused by drug therapy. It seems possible that it may be necessary to balance the effects of the drug on K_{ATP} channels in inhibitory and excitatory neurons, or in different brain regions.

THE NEURONAL K_{ATP} CHANNEL

K_{ATP} channels are widely expressed in the brain, including regions such as the hypothalamus, hippocampus, substantia nigra, cerebral cortex, thalamus, and cerebellum (8). In glucose responsive neurons, K_{ATP} channels have been shown to be involved in sensing central glucose levels and triggering pancreatic glucagon secretion (53). A considerable body of work has shown that K_{ATP} channels also play an important role in preventing excitotoxicity linked to metabolic stress (eg, ischemia, hypoxia, hypoglycemia). *In vitro* and *in vivo* experiments indicate that K_{ATP} channels are usually closed under normal conditions and open only in response to metabolic stress (9, 54–57). They thus appear to act as "metabolic gatekeepers," adjusting neuronal electrical activity to the available energy (58).

The discovery that mice genetically engineered to lack Kir6.2 had an increased susceptibility to generalized seizures triggered by hypoxia (54), led to the suggestion that K_{ATP} channels are involved in controlling seizure propagation. This is supported by the fact that transgenic mice selectively overexpressing SUR1 in the forebrain are significantly less susceptible to kainite-induced seizures (a common animal model of epilepsy) (59).

These studies provide evidence to support a role for K_{ATP} channel activation in *preventing* epileptic activity. The question thus remains as to why gain-of-function mutations in the genes encoding the K_{ATP} channel result in exactly the opposite phenotype.

POTENTIAL MECHANISMS

One possibility is that K_{ATP} channel activation impairs the excitability of inhibitory neurons more strongly than that of excitatory neurons, resulting in a reduction in inhibitory tone. Epilepsy is believed to result from an imbalance between excitatory and inhibitory activity in neuronal circuits, which can result either from excessive excitation or reduced inhibition. It is therefore important to know the relative density of K_{ATP} channels in excitatory and inhibitory neurons in different brain regions. However, there is only limited information on this topic.

Various *in vitro* studies have shown that in the rat hippocampus K_{ATP} channel subunits are preferentially expressed by inhibitory interneurons, that K_{ATP} currents are larger and more frequent in these cells, and that pharmacological activation of K_{ATP} channels by diazoxide markedly suppresses electrical activity of CA1 inhibitory interneurons but has no effect on excitatory CA1 pyramidal cells (60). A small reduction in electrical activity was also seen in CA3 pyramidal cells, which have a higher density of K_{ATP} channels than CA1 cells, although not as great as in interneurons. This suggests that, *in vivo*, activating K_{ATP} channel mutations would preferentially hyperpolarize hippocampal interneurons, resulting in increased excitation of the hippocampal neuronal network. If this idea is correct, it would imply that, in contrast to traditional antiepileptic drugs, which act by reducing neuronal excitability, sulphonylureas can exert an antiepileptic effect by activation of inhibitory neurons.

Evidence that ion channel mutations that impair interneuron firing can cause seizures comes from analysis of Dravet syndrome. Also known as severe myoclonic epilepsy of infancy (SMEI), this disorder is characterized by the development of generalized seizures associated with elevated body temperature during the first year of life, which later progress to prolonged spontaneous seizures and status epilepticus (61, 62). Patients are also developmentally delayed and suffer from ataxia and cognitive impairment, which contribute to their reduced life expectancy. Genetic testing of SMEI patients showed that this condition is mainly caused by heterozygous loss-of-function mutations in the $Na_v1.1$ voltage-gated sodium channel (63). Generation of mice lacking $Na_v1.1$ produced a similar phenotype: knockout animals exhibited temperature-induced seizures that later evolved to spontaneous seizures as well as ataxia, spasticity, and reduced life expectancy (64, 65). Functional studies showed this was due to a significant reduction in sodium currents in inhibitory interneurons, but not in excitatory neurons (65). The smaller sodium currents led to a reduction in the firing frequency of GABAergic interneurons, impairing inhibitory tone.

Coexpression of heterozygous $Na_v1.1$ loss-of-function with heterozygous loss-of-function for $Na_v1.6$, which is mainly expressed by excitatory neurons, in transgenic mice reversed the seizure susceptibility of $Na_v1.1$ heterozygotes (66). This supports the idea that SMEI $Na_v1.1$ mutations cause epilepsy by reducing neuronal inhibition. Furthermore, it was possible to pharmacologically reduce the seizure susceptibility of $Na_v1.1$ heterozygous mice with a combination of tiagabine and clonazepam (67). This treatment re-balanced excitation and inhibition by enhancing GABAergic neurotransmission because tiagabine increases GABA concentrations in the synaptic cleft by inhibiting its reuptake while clonazepam potentiates the response of activated postsynaptic $GABA_A$ receptors.

Considerable work is still required to understand the role of the K_{ATP} channel in epilepsy. However, if activating K_{ATP} channel mutations work in a similar way to SMEI mutations, by suppressing GABA release from inhibitory neurons, it may be possible to treat DEND patients with combination therapies that enhance GABA transmission. An example may be a combination of sulphonylureas to stimulate GABA release, and GABA uptake blockers to facilitate GABAergic transmission. This may be of value in patients with medically refractory seizures.

KEY POINTS

1. Activating mutations in the ATP-sensitive potassium channel are associated with neonatal diabetes.
2. 3% of patients with these mutations exhibit marked motor and mental developmental delay, muscle hypotonia, dysmorphic features and epilepsy (DEND syndrome), in addition to diabetes.
3. DEND patients suffer from generalized seizures that begin before 12 months of life—infantile spasms, myoclonic seizures and tonic-clonic seizures have been described.

4. Patients with a milder form of DEND, known as intermediate DEND syndrome, can also experience seizures. These are usually milder and start at a later age.
5. Sulphonylurea drugs, which block the K_{ATP} channel, have been successfully used to treat neonatal diabetes caused by most K_{ATP} mutations.
6. It is not yet clear whether sulphonylureas can improve seizures in DEND and iDEND patients.
7. The cellular mechanism by which K_{ATP} channel mutations cause epilepsy is not well understood, but it could involve impaired excitability of inhibitory neurons.

Studies in our laboratory are supported by the Wellcome Trust and the Royal Society. CL holds an OXION/Clarendon Fund PhD studentship and FMA a Royal Society Research Professorship.

REFERENCES

1. Ashcroft SJ, Ashcroft FM. Properties and functions of ATP-sensitive K-channels. *Cell. Signal.* 1990;2(3):197–214.
2. Seino S, Miki T. Physiological and pathophysiological roles of ATP-sensitive K$^+$ channels. *Prog. Biophys. Mol. Biol.* 2003; 81(2):133–176.
3. Nichols CG. K_{ATP} channels as molecular sensors of cellular metabolism. *Nature.* 2006;440(7083):470–476.
4. Hattersley AT, Ashcroft FM. Activating mutations in Kir6.2 and neonatal diabetes: new clinical syndromes, new scientific insights, and new therapy. *Diabetes.* 2005;54(9):2503–2513.
5. Clement JP, Kunjilwar K, Gonzalez G, et al. Association and stoichiometry of K_{ATP} channel subunits. *Neuron.* 1997;18(5): 827–838.
6. Sakura H, Ammälä C, Smith PA, et al. Cloning and functional expression of the cDNA encoding a novel ATP-sensitive potassium channel subunit expressed in pancreatic beta-cells, brain, heart and skeletal muscle. *FEBS Lett.* 1995;377(3):338–344.
7. Aguilar-Bryan L, Nichols CG, Wechsler SW, et al. Cloning of the beta-cell high-affinity sulphonylurea receptor: a regulator of insulin secretion. *Science.* 1995:268:423–425.
8. Karschin C, Ecke C, Ashcroft FM, et al. Overlapping distribution of K_{ATP} channel-forming Kir6.2 subunit and the sulfonylurea receptor SUR1 in rodent brain. *FEBS Lett.* 1997;401(1):59–64.
9. Liss B, Bruns R, Roeper J. Alternative sulfonylurea receptor expression defines metabolic sensitivity of K_{ATP} channels in dopaminergic midbrain neurons. *EMBO J.* 1999;18:833–846.
10. Flagg TP, Kurata HT, Masia R, et al. Differential structure of atrial and ventricular K_{ATP}: atrial K_{ATP} channels require SUR1. *Circ Res.* 2008;103(12):1458–1465.
11. Isomoto S, Kondo C, Yamada M, et al. (1996). A novel sulfonylurea receptor forms with BIR (Kir6.2) a smooth muscle type

ATP-sensitive K$^+$ channel. *J Biol Chem.* 1996;271(40): 24321–24324.

12. Tucker SJ, Gribble FM, Zhao C, et al. Truncation of Kir6.2 produces ATP-sensitive K$^+$ channels in the absence of the sulphonylurea receptor. *Nature.* 1997;387(6629):179–183.

13. Tanabe K, Tucker SJ, Matsuo M, et al. Direct photoaffinity labeling of the Kir6.2 subunit of the ATP-sensitive K$^+$ channel by 8--azido-ATP. *J. Biol. Chem.* 1999;274(7):3931–3933.

14. Matsuo M, Tanabe K, Kioka N, et al. Different binding properties and affinities for ATP and ADP among sulfonylurea receptor subtypes, SUR1, SUR2A, and SUR2B. *J. Biol. Chem.* 2000;275(37):28757–28763.

15. Nichols CG, Shyng SL, Nestorowicz A. Adenosine diphosphate as an intracellular regulator of insulin secretion. *Science.* 1996;272:1785–1787.

16. Gribble FM, Tucker SJ, Ashcroft FM. The essential role of the Walker A motifs of SUR1 in K_{ATP} channel activation by Mg-ADP and diazoxide. *EMBO J.* 1997;16:1145–1152.

17. Gribble FM, Tucker SJ, Haug T, Ashcroft FM. MgATP activates the beta cell K_{ATP} channel by interaction with its SUR1 subunit. *Proc Natl Acad Sci USA.* 1998;95:7185–7190.

18. Ashcroft FM, Harrison DE, Ashcroft SJ. Glucose induces closure of single potassium channels in isolated rat pancreatic beta-cells. *Nature.* 1984;312(5993):446–448.

19. Gribble FM, Reimann F. Sulphonylurea action revisited: the post-cloning era. *Diabetologia.* 2003;46(7):875–891.

20. Gloyn AL, Pearson ER, Antcliff JF, et al. Activating mutations in the gene encoding the ATP-sensitive potassium-channel subunit Kir6.2 and permanent neonatal diabetes. *N. Engl. J. Med.* 2004;350(18):1838–1849.

21. Babenko AP, Polak M, Cavé H, et al. Activating mutations in the ABCC8 gene in neonatal diabetes mellitus. *N. Engl. J. Med.* 2006;355(5):456–466.

22. Proks P, Arnold AL, Bruining J, et al. A heterozygous activating mutation in the sulphonylurea receptor SUR1 (ABCC8) causes neonatal diabetes. *Hum Mol Genet.* 2006; 15(11):1793–1800.

23. Flanagan SE, Clauin S, Bellanné-Chantelot C, et al. Update of mutations in the genes encoding the pancreatic beta-cell K_{ATP} channel subunits Kir6.2 (KCNJ11) and sulfonylurea receptor 1 (ABCC8) in diabetes mellitus and hyperinsulinism. *Hum Mutat.* 2009;30(2):170–180.

24. Ashcroft FM. The Walter B. Cannon Physiology in Perspective Lecture, 2007. ATP-sensitive K-channels and disease: from molecule to malady. *Am J Physiol: Endocrinol Metab.* 2007;293: E880–E889.

25. Ellard S, Flanagan SE, Girard CA, et al. Permanent neonatal diabetes caused by dominant, recessive, or compound heterozygous SUR1 mutations with opposite functional effects. *Am J Hum Genet.* 2007;81(2): 375–382.

26. Shimomura K, Girard CA, Proks P, et al. Mutations at the same residue (R50) of Kir6.2 (KCNJ11) that cause neonatal diabetes produce different functional effects. *Diabetes.* 2006;55(6):1705–1712.

27. Koster JC, Kurata HT, Enkvetchakul D, et al. DEND mutation in Kir6.2 (KCNJ11) reveals a flexible N-terminal region critical for ATP-sensing of the K_{ATP} channel. *Biophys J.* 2008; 95(10):4689–4697.

28. Masia R, Koster JC, Tumini S, et al. An ATP-binding mutation (G334D) in KCNJ11 is associated with a sulfonylurea-insensitive form of developmental delay, epilepsy, and neonatal diabetes. *Diabetes.* 2007;56(2):328–336.

29. Proks P, Antcliff JF, Lippiat J, et al. Molecular basis of Kir6.2 mutations associated with neonatal diabetes or neonatal diabetes plus neurological features. *Proc Natl Acad Sci USA.* 2004;101:17539–17544.

30. Mannikko R, Jefferies C, Flanagan SE, et al. Interaction between mutations in the slide helix of Kir6.2 associated with neonatal diabetes and neurological symptoms. *Hum Mol Genet.* 2010;19(6):963–972.

31. Shimomura K, Hörster F, de Wet H, et al. A novel mutation causing DEND syndrome: a treatable channelopathy of pancreas and brain. *Neurology.* 2007;69(13):1342–1349.

32. Proks P, Girard C, Haider S, et al. A novel gating mutation at the internal mouth of the Kir6.2 pore is associated with DEND syndrome. *EMBO Rep.* 2005;6:470–475.

33. Trapp S, Proks P, Tucker SJ, et al. Molecular analysis of K_{ATP} channel gating and implications for channel inhibition by ATP. *J Gen Physiol.* 1998;112:333–349.

34. McTaggart JS, Clark RH, Ashcroft FM. The role of the K_{ATP} channel in glucose homeostasis in health and disease: more than meets the islet. *J Physiol.* 2010;58:3201–3209.

35. Simard JM, Tsymbalyuk O, Ivanov A, et al. Endothelial sulfonylurea receptor 1-regulated NC Ca-ATP channels mediate progressive hemorrhagic necrosis following spinal cord injury. *J Clin Invest.* 2007;117(8):2105–2113.

36. Sala-Rabanal M, Wang S, Nichols CG. On potential interactions between non-selective cation channel TRPM4 and sulfonylurea receptor SUR1. *J Biol Chem.* 2012;287(12):8746–8756.

37. Lux AL, Osborne JP. A proposal for case definitions and outcome measures in studies of infantile spasms and West syndrome: consensus statement of the West Delphi group. *Epilepsia.* 2004;45(11):1416–1428.

38. Kossoff EH. Infantile spasms. *Neurologist.* 2010;16(2):69–75.

39. Sumnik Z, Kolouskova S, Wales JKH, et al. Sulphonylurea treatment does not improve psychomotor development in children with KCNJ11 mutations causing permanent neonatal diabetes mellitus accompanied by developmental delay and epilepsy (DEND syndrome). *Diabet Med.* 2007;24(10):1176–1178.

40. Bahi-Buisson N, Eisermann M, Nivot S, et al. Infantile spasms as an epileptic feature of DEND syndrome associated with an activating mutation in the potassium adenosine triphosphate (ATP) channel, Kir6.2. *J Child Neurol.* 2007;22(9):1147–1150.

41. Flanagan SE, Edghill EL, Gloyn AL, et al. Mutations in KCNJ11, which encodes Kir6.2, are a common cause of diabetes diagnosed in the first 6 months of life, with the phenotype determined by genotype. *Diabetologia.* 2006;49(6):1190–1197.

42. Manna Della T, Battistim C, Radonsky V, et al. Glibenclamide unresponsiveness in a Brazilian child with permanent neonatal diabetes mellitus and DEND syndrome due to a C166Y mutation in KCNJ11 (Kir6.2) gene. *Arq Bras Endocrinol Metabol.* 2008;52(8):1350–1355.

43. Zwaveling-Soonawala N, Hagebeuk EE, Slingerland AS, et al. Successful transfer to sulfonylurea therapy in an infant with developmental delay, epilepsy and neonatal diabetes (DEND)

syndrome and a novel ABCC8 gene mutation. *Diabetologia.* 2011;54(2):469–471.

44. Suzuki S, Makita Y, Mukai T, et al. Molecular basis of neonatal diabetes in Japanese patients. *J Clin Endocrinol Metab.* 2007; 92(10):3979–3985.

45. Leppik IE. Classification of the myoclonic epilepsies. *Epilepsia.* 2003;44:2–6.

46. Gurgel LC, Crispim F, Noffs MHS, et al. Sulfonylrea treatment in permanent neonatal diabetes due to G53D mutation in the KCNJ11 gene: improvement in glycemic control and neurological function. *Diabetes Care.* 2007;30(11):108.

47. Slingerland AS, Nuboer R, Hadders-Algra M, et al. Improved motor development and good long-term glycaemic control with sulfonylurea treatment in a patient with the syndrome of intermediate developmental delay, early-onset generalised epilepsy and neonatal diabetes associated with the V59M mutation in the KCNJ11 gene. *Diabetologia.* 2006;49(11):2559–2563.

48. Jones AG, Hattersley AT. Reevaluation of a case of type 1 diabetes mellitus diagnosed before 6 months of age. *Nat Rev Endocrinol.* 2010;6(6):347–351.

49. Tonini G, Bizzarri C, Bonfanti R, et al. Early-Onset Diabetes Study Group of the Italian Society of Paediatric Endocrinology and Diabetology. Sulfonylurea treatment outweighs insulin therapy in short-term metabolic control of patients with permanent neonatal diabetes mellitus due to activating mutations of the KCNJ11 (Kir6.2) gene. *Diabetologia.* 2006;49(9):2210–2213.

50. Pearson ER, Flechtner I, Njølstad PR, et al. Neonatal Diabetes International Collaborative Group. Switching from insulin to oral sulfonylureas in patients with diabetes due to Kir6.2 mutations. *N Engl J Med.* 2006;355(5):467–477.

51. Ashcroft FM. New uses for old drugs: neonatal diabetes and sulphonylureas. *Cell Metab.* 2010;11(3):179–181.

52. Mlynarski W, Tarasov AI, Gach A, et al. Sulfonylurea improves CNS function in a case of intermediate DEND syndrome caused by a mutation in KCNJ11. *Nat Clin Pract Neurol.* 2007; 3(11):640–645.

53. Miki T, Liss B, Minami K, et al. ATP-sensitive K$^+$ channels in the hypothalamus are essential for the maintenance of glucose homeostasis. *Nat Neurosci.* 2001;4(5):507–512.

54. Yamada K, Ji JJ, Yuan H, et al. Protective role of ATP-sensitive potassium channels in hypoxia-induced generalized seizure. *Science.* 2001;292(5521):1543–1546.

55. Bancila V, Nikonenko I, Dunant Y, et al. Zinc inhibits glutamate release via activation of pre-synaptic K channels and reduces ischaemic damage in rat hippocampus. *J Neurochem.* 2004; 90(5):1243–1250.

56. Haller M, Mironov SL, Karschin A, Richter DW. Dynamic activation of K_{ATP} channels in rhythmically active neurons. *J Physiol.* 2001;537:69–81

57. Tanner GR, Lutas A, Martinez-Francois JR, et al. Single K_{ATP} channel opening in response to action potential firing in mouse dentate granule neurons. *J Neurosci.* 2011;31(23): 8689–8696.

58. Liss B, Roeper J. A role for neuronal K_{ATP} channels in metabolic control of the seizure gate. *Trends Pharmacol. Sci.* 2001; 22(12):599–601.

59. Hernández-Sánchez C, Basile AS, Fedorova I, et al. Mice transgenically overexpressing sulfonylurea receptor 1 in forebrain resist seizure induction and excitotoxic neuron death. *Proc Natl Acad Sci USA.* 2001;98(6):3549–3554.

60. Griesemer D, Zawar C, Neumcke B. Cell-type specific depression of neuronal excitability in rat hippocampus by activation of ATP-sensitive potassium channels. *Eur Biophys J.* 2002;31(6):467–477.

61. Engel J. International League Against Epilepsy (ILAE). A proposed diagnostic scheme for people with epileptic seizures and with epilepsy: report of the ILAE Task Force on Classification and Terminology. *Epilepsia.* 2001;42(6):796–803.

62. Dravet C, Bureau M, Oguni H, et al. Severe myoclonic epilepsy in infancy: Dravet syndrome. *Adv Neurol.* 2005;95:71–102.

63. Claes L, Del-Favero J, Ceulemans B, et al. De novo mutations in the sodium-channel gene SCN1A cause severe myoclonic epilepsy of infancy. *Am J Hum Genet.* 2001;68(6):1327–1332.

64. Kalume F, Yu FH, Westenbroek RE, et al. Reduced sodium current in Purkinje neurons from Nav1.1 mutant mice: implications for ataxia in severe myoclonic epilepsy in infancy. *J Neurosci.* 2007;27(41):11065–11074.

65. Yu FH, Mantegazza M, Westenbroek RE, et al. Reduced sodium current in GABAergic interneurons in a mouse model of severe myoclonic epilepsy in infancy. *Nat Neurosci.* 2006;9(9): 1142–1149.

66. Martin MS, Tang B, Papale LA, et al. The voltage-gated sodium channel Scn8a is a genetic modifier of severe myoclonic epilepsy of infancy. *Hum Mol Genet.* 2007;16(23):2892–2899.

67. Catterall WA, Kalume F, Oakley JC. NaV1.1 channels, epilepsy. *J Physiol.* 2010;588:1849–1859.

68. Mikhailov MV, Campbell JD, de Wet H, et al. Ashcroft FM. 3-D structural and functional characterization of the purified K_{ATP} channel complex Kir6.2-SUR1. *EMBO J.* 2005;24(23): 4166–4175.

69. Stansfeld PJ, Hopkinson R, Ashcroft FM, et al. PIP(2)-binding site in Kir channels: definition by multiscale biomolecular simulations. *Biochemistry.* 2009;48(46):10926–10933.

16

Hyperammonemia/Hyperinsulinism and Epilepsy

Nicholas S. Abend and Andrea Kelly

INTRODUCTION

Inborn errors of metabolism invariably provide insights into normal physiology; the trek toward clearly defining these normal pathways, however, is not always straightforward. The hyperinsulinism/ hyperammonemia syndrome (HI/HA) is one such example. This metabolic disorder has clarified the role of amino acids and the enzyme glutamate dehydrogenase (GDH) in insulin secretion but has posed new challenges regarding the role of GDH in ammonia metabolism and toxicity, as well as the role of GDH in the brain. Given the potential contribution of hypoglycemia and hyperammonemia to disturbances in the central nervous system (CNS), a review of hyperinsulinism and the features of HI/HA is worthwhile before discussing the CNS manifestations of this disorder.

HYPERINSULINISM

Hypoglycemia arises from disturbances in either normal fasting adaptation (gluconeogenesis, glycogenolysis, fatty acid oxidation, ketogenesis) or its hormonal regulation (insulin, growth hormone, cortisol, catecholamines). Hyperinsulinism refers to the congenital and acquired disorders of hypoglycemia that arise from dysregulated insulin secretion. This excess insulin interrupts normal fasting adaptation: glucose cannot be accessed from glycogen stores, amino acids cannot

be converted into glzucose, and alternative fuels (free fatty acids and ketones) cannot be generated. Without provision of glucose or other carbohydrate, hypoglycemia ensues. In the absence of glucose or alternative fuels, namely ketones and lactate, short-term and long-term neurocognitive sequelae can occur.

CONGENITAL HYPERINSULINISM

Hyperinsulinism is the most common cause of persistent hypoglycemia in infancy. Genetic defects in the pathways of insulin secretion are responsible for the excess insulin secretion in the congenital forms of hyperinsulinism. Glucose is the major stimulant for insulin secretion (Figure 16.1). In the classically defined pathway, glucose enters the beta-cell through the GLUT-2 transporter and is phosphorylated by glucokinase (GK). Further metabolism of glucose produces ATP and leads to an increase in the beta-cell ATP to ADP ratio. The increase closes the ATP-sensitive potassium (K_{ATP}) channel, composed of the sulfonylurea receptor regulatory subunit (SUR1) and the inwardly rectifying potassium pore ($KIR_{6.2}$). Beta-cell membrane depolarization ensues triggering opening of voltage-dependent calcium channels and calcium influx. Ultimately, insulin is released (1). A K_{ATP} channel-independent pathway amplifies glucose-stimulated insulin secretion (2).

Amino acids stimulate insulin secretion through the mitochondrial enzyme GDH (Figure 16.1). This

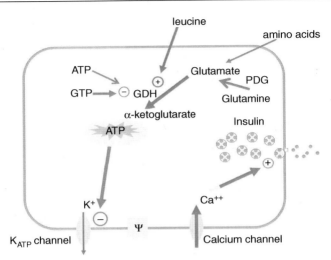

FIGURE 16.1   Pathways of insulin secretion. Glucose enters the beta-cell through the GLUT-2 glucose transporter, is phosphorylated by glucokinase (GK)—considered the beta-cell "glucosensor," and enters the TCA cycle to generate ATP. With an increase in the ATP to ADP ratio, the K_{ATP} channel closes, the beta-cell membrane depolarizes, voltage-dependent calcium channels (VDCC) open, and calcium influx occurs to effect insulin secretion. This process is referred to as the K_{ATP} channel-dependent pathway. Amino acids can stimulate insulin secretion through this K_{ATP} channel pathway via *GDH*. This process occurs through oxidation of the amino acid glutamate by GDH and ATP generation in the TCA. GDH is allosterically activated by the amino acid leucine. HI/HA causing-*GDH* mutations impair normal inhibition of GDH by GTP. This loss of inhibitory regulation permits unrestrained GDH activity and leads to leucine-sensitivity, protein-induced hypoglycemia, and fasting hypoglycemia. Diazoxide opens the K_{ATP} channel to suppress insulin secretion. Mutations in GK and K_{ATP} also cause congenital hyperinsulinism.

enzyme is responsible for oxidative deamination of glutamate to alpha -ketoglutarate (3–7). Subsequent catabolism of alpha-ketoglutarate generates ATP and triggers the K_{ATP} channel-dependent pathway of insulin secretion. GDH is allosterically activated by leucine and inhibited by GTP and ATP. In addition to being highly expressed in the pancreas, GDH is expressed in liver, kidney, and brain (8).

Genetic defects in SUR1, KIR$_{6.2}$, GK, and GDH are responsible for congenital hyperinsulinism (9–23); other defects have also been identified: monocarboxylate transporter 1 (24) as well as 3-hydroxyacyl-CoA dehydrogenase (25).

HI/HA Syndrome

Dominant gain of function mutations in GDH cause a form of congenital hyperinsulinism associated with hyperammonemia (HI/HA, also known as GDH-HI) (16, 19, 26–29). De novo mutations are responsible

for nearly 80% of cases. These mutations impair normal inhibition of GDH by GTP.

GDH-Hyperinsulinism

As a result of impaired inhibition of GDH, unregulated allosteric activation of this enzyme by leucine arises (30) and manifests as excessive leucine-stimulated insulin secretion (Figure 16.2). Clinically, this "leucine sensitivity" is evidenced by protein-induced hypoglycemia (31) (Figure 16.3), a hallmark of HI/HA. Fasting hypoglycemia also occurs in HI/HA.

Unlike newborns with the more common K_{ATP} form of HI who are typically born large for gestational age and have severe hypoglycemia within the first few days of life, newborns with HI/HA have normal birth weight and their hypoglycemia is often not evident until later in infancy. Management of the hyperinsulinism is aimed at preventing both post-prandial and fasting hypoglycemia. Diazoxide, an agent which

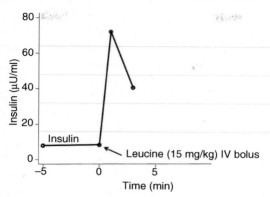

FIGURE 16.2   Acute insulin response to leucine in HI/HA. Shown is the insulin (solid line) response to an intravenous bolus of leucine (15 mg/kg) in the same child from Figure 16.1. Robust insulin secretion occurred in response to leucine (leu-AIR = 43 μU/mL) while hypoglycemia did not develop. The acute insulin responses to leucine in healthy controls are minimal (data not shown).

promotes opening of the K_{ATP} channel, works well in the treatment of the hyperinsulinism of HI/HA. Additionally, avoidance of pure protein meals is recommended to decrease the risk of protein-induced hypoglycemia.

Hyperammonemia

The other hallmark of GDH-HI is hyperammonemia. Plasma ammonium concentrations are usually in the range of 80–150 μmol/L (normal less than 35).

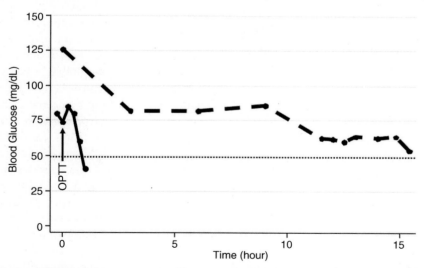

FIGURE 16.3   Fasting and protein-sensitive hypoglycemia in HI/HA. Shown are the blood glucose concentrations during fasting (dashed line) and following a protein meal in a 5-year-old female patient with HI/HA. This subject was able to fast for 15 hr before the blood glucose decreased to less than 60 mg/dL. Her fast was terminated at 16 hr for symptoms and blood glucose of 54 mg/dL. In contrast, the subject's blood glucose (solid line) decreased to 40 mg/dL within 1 hr of protein ingestion and continued to decrease over the next 30 min despite intravenous dextrose and oral carbohydrates (data not shown).

Despite plasma ammonium concentrations 2 to 5 times normal, individuals with HI/HA appear "asymptomatic" from their hyperammonemia, or at least, do not display symptoms typically associated with acute or chronic hyperammonemia. Plasma amino acids and urinary amino acids (used in the diagnosis of urea cycle defects) are normal. Protein intake, fasting, and blood glucose concentration do not impact plasma ammonium (20, 21, 27). Plasma ammonium is not improved with benzoate therapy (20, 28, 29) but is lowered by approximately 50% with *N*-carbamylglutamate, an *N*-acetyl glutamate analogue (21, 28). The clinical benefit of this decrease is not clear. The hyperammonemia is now thought to arise from upregulated GDH activity in kidney, although it was originally hypothesized to be of hepatic origin (32).

CENTRAL NERVOUS SYSTEM MANIFESTATIONS OF HI/HA

The CNS manifestations of HI/HA arise acutely from neuroglucopenia but may also arise in the absence of acute hypoglycemia. The occurrence of the latter issues in HI/HA has only recently been recognized, and the full spectrum of these neurodevelopmental conditions has yet to be determined. Neurologic issues related to seizures, learning disabilities, and behavior abnormalities may not be simple manifestations of hypoglycemic insults and have raised the possibility that either hyperammonemia or aberrant GDH activity in brain may be operative.

HYPOGLYCEMIC SEIZURES

A recent case report illustrates a typical presentation of HI/HA and how hypoglycemic episodes related to HI/HA may be misdiagnosed as intractable epilepsy. A 12-month-old female had two episodes of staring, drooling, and then generalized tonic–clonic seizures lasting 5–15 min. Subsequent sleep-deprived EEG and brain MRI were normal. A year later, she presented with a hypoglycemic episode (27 mg/dL). She was hospitalized for blood glucose monitoring and on the sixth day of hospitalization experienced a hypoglycemic episode (41 mg/dL). She was found to have a heterozygous activating mutation in *GLUD1*, the gene encoding for GDH. The patient's 32-year-old mother had "seizures" since infancy which involved episodes of lip movements, decreased consciousness, and improvement with food ingestion. Her seizures were intractable to several anticonvulsants. Mutational analysis of *GLUD1* revealed the mother had the same mutation as her daughter. In hindsight, the mother's seizures were likely manifestations of HI/HA-related hypoglycemia. Diazoxide treatment terminated the episodes in both child and mother (33).

Hypoglycemic seizures are usually focal with rapid secondary generalization. In neonates with hypoglycemia, seizures are associated with a higher risk of subsequent neuro-developmental abnormalities (34, 35). However, whether acute symptomatic seizures are indicative of more severe hypoglycemic brain injury is not clear, nor is it apparent whether these acute symptomatic seizures independently worsen outcome, perhaps by increasing energy (glucose) utilization. Hypoglycemia may result in cortical and deep gray structure injury. In neonates this injury may be most prominent in the occipital–parietal regions (36). Hypoglycemic brain injury may result in subsequent remote symptomatic epilepsy. These may appear as generalized convulsions, but since they arise from focal lesions, may have a focal mechanism of onset and be associated with focal or multifocal interictal epileptiform and nonspecific EEG abnormalities.

In young children with seizures, whether suspected or definite, evaluation for acute symptomatic seizure etiologies is pursued. This evaluation generally involves laboratory testing of glucose, electrolytes, blood count, and liver function tests. HI/HA commonly presents with hypoglycemic episodes, including seizures, during infancy and toddlerhood. Recognition of hypoglycemia as the inciting factor, however, may be delayed in HI/HA since affected individuals are asymptomatic between episodes and the pattern of hypoglycemia tends to be "atypical"—occurring after protein ingestion (ie, after meals) rather than with fasting, the much more common trigger of hypoglycemia. Importantly, testing of plasma ammonium in this setting may lead to the diagnosis of HI/HA. A slightly high ammonia value, while often attributed to slow blood flow during collection or delay in laboratory testing, should not be disregarded if HI/HA is considered.

Treatment of HI/HA-associated hypoglycemic seizures with valproate (before the diagnosis of HI/HA is made) may lead to further confusion regarding the underlying diagnosis. Recent studies demonstrate hyperammonemia is common in both children (37, 38) and adults (39) receiving valproate; the finding of hyperammonemia may be misinterpreted as representative of valproate rather than a clue to the HI/HA diagnosis. Several cases suggest that use of topiramate in addition to valproate may cause hyperammonemic encephalopathy (40, 41). Other anticonvulsants such as carbamazepine have more rarely been associated with hyperammonemia (42).

HI/HA AND EPILEPSY

Raizen et al questioned whether HI/HA is associated with epilepsy in the absence of acute hypoglycemia or remote symptomatic hypoglycemic brain injury (43). A 5-year-old boy with HI/HA successfully treated with diazoxide was noted to have paroxysmal eye blinking in the absence of hypoglycemia. His EEG revealed a high-voltage generalized spike pattern. Similar patients,

including a 7-year-old with electroclinical seizures characterized by unresponsive staring associated with several second bursts of irregularly generalized 3 Hz epileptiform activity (Figure 16.4), and a 4-year-old with bursts of irregular generalized, bifrontally predominant, epileptiform activity (Figure 16.5) have been followed at our Center. These abnormalities occurred during a scheduled admission for blood glucose monitoring and were identified at the time of documented normal blood glucose concentrations (>70 mg/dL).

Additional patients with HI/HA are reported to have seizures in the absence of hypoglycemic episodes (43–46). Further, the reported EEG features and seizure types are not typical of a symptomatic focal mechanism of onset and are more suggestive of a generalized mechanism of onset. These seizure phenotypes include atypical absence seizures and myoclonic seizures, often provoked by photic stimulation or hyperventilation, and generalized epileptiform features on

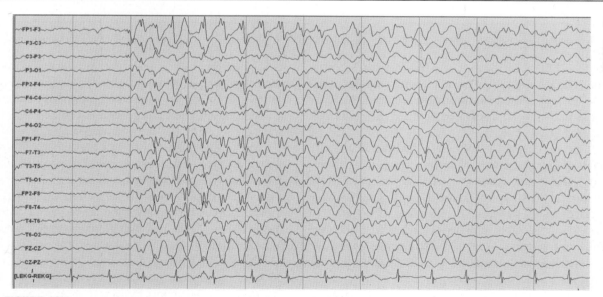

FIGURE 16.4 A 7-year-old with HI/HA treated with diazoxide presented with staring episodes lasting 2 to 10 sec without any associated abnormal movements. While in the hospital for routine monitoring of his home regimen and blood glucose "control," he underwent EEG monitoring. His EEG demonstrated a normal background (9 Hz occipital alpha activity with normal organization and normal sleep architecture). However, he had frequent irregular generalized bifrontally predominant sharp and wave discharges at about 3 Hz lasting for 3 to 10 sec. Some were associated with staring. These did not activate with sleep and did not change in duration or appearance during his fast.

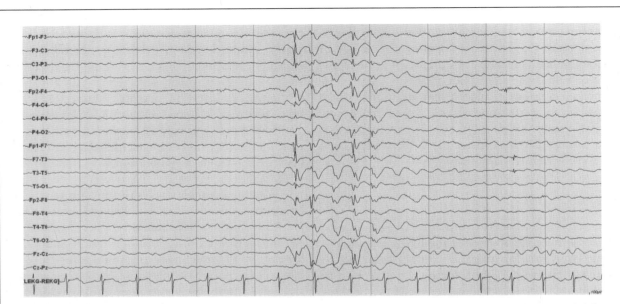

FIGURE 16.5   A 4-year-old patient with HI/HA treated with diazoxide presented with mild developmental delay. While in the hospital for a scheduled fasting test and frequent blood glucose monitoring to assess her home regimen, she underwent EEG monitoring. Her EEG demonstrated mild slowing (6 Hz activity with normal organization and normal sleep architecture). She had frequent irregular generalized and fragmented bifrontally predominant sharp and polyspike and wave discharges, sometimes in brief runs. None were associated with any clinical change. These did not activate with sleep and did not change in duration or appearance during her fast.

interictal EEG recordings. These findings indicate that while HI/HA may be associated with hypoglycemic episodes and related symptomatic seizures, this syndrome may also be associated with an increased risk for generalized epilepsy.

One retrospective study described the neurologic issues in 22 consecutive patients from 17 families with HI/HA. Subjects were a mean age of 12 years (18 months to 40 years). Hypoglycemic seizures were reported in 17 patients; 15 experienced generalized tonic–clonic seizures and two experienced prolonged hemiclonic seizures. Four of the five patients who did not have seizures presented with recurrent episodes of hypotonia, lethargy, and eye rolling leading to the diagnosis of hypoglycemia, and, ultimately HI/HA. At the time of evaluation, 14 subjects had epilepsy; the median age of recognition of nonhypoglycemic seizures was 6 years (range 2–12 years). Four of the 14 with epilepsy had never experienced hypoglycemic seizures. The most common seizure type was atypical absence (lasting longer than 30 sec, with or without eyelid myoclonias), myoclonic jerks of limbs, and

astatic seizures. Other seizure types included focal motor seizures and generalized tonic–clonic seizures. The inter-ictal EEG was abnormal in 12 of 14 patients with epilepsy and included generalized spike and wave discharges in eight and sleep activated photosensitive discharges in two. The EEG was normal in all eight without epilepsy. Seizures were well controlled with monotherapy in the majority of subjects, but were intractable in three. Ammonia levels were not different between patients with and without epilepsy (44). Most patients with epilepsy had mutations in exons 6 and 7 of *GLUD1* in this series (44), although the association with these GTP-binding domain mutations was not evident in the original Roizen et al series (43).

In the original report by Roizen et al responsiveness to seizure medications was present in 14 patients with HI/HA and nonhypoglycemic seizures (43). Two patients had seizures worsen with carbamazepine or oxcarbazepine and two patients had improvement on valproate. A 5-year-old patient developed drop attacks with euglycemia that improved on phenobarbital. However, when transitioned from phenobarbital to oxcarbazepine, he developed episodes of eyelid closure that correlated with high voltage, irregular generalized spike or polyspike and wave discharges of 3 to 5 Hz lasting 0.5 to 2 sec. His background EEG was normal without any evidence of encephalopathy. Ethosuximide reduced his seizures. He then had a generalized tonic seizure and was transitioned to zonisamide which reduced his seizures (43).

Also provocative regarding the role of GDH in the brain, developmental delay and cognitive impairment were present in 17 subjects. IQ testing demonstrated that learning disabilities were borderline in five, mild in nine, and moderate in three. Eleven patients required specialized education and the oldest four required protected employment due to cognitive disability. Patients with epilepsy were more likely to have cognitive problems. Mild behavioral problems occurred in four. Brain MRIs were normal in all except one patient (mild frontal atrophy). Ammonia levels were not different between individuals with and without learning disabilities (44).

Potential Mechanisms for Nonhypoglycemic Seizures in HI/HA

The mechanism of epilepsy in patients with HI/HA is unknown. While hypoglycemic brain injury could result in remote symptomatic seizures, evidence of insult on neuroimaging studies in HI/HA patients with such seizures is lacking (43–46).

Ammonia toxicity is also a possibility. The original descriptions of HI/HA characterize the hyperammonemia as being asymptomatic—lacking the usual symptoms of lethargy, headaches, coma, and encephalopathy despite serum ammonium levels as high as 300 μM. Moreover, EEG studies do not demonstrate evidence of metabolic encephalopathy, such as slowing, disorganization, or triphasic waves (43–45).

The mechanisms linking hyperammonemia to neurotoxicity are not fully understood. Ammonia "detoxification" occurs primarily in astrocytes via the amination of glutamate by glutamine synthetase. Glutamine can then be shuttled to neurons where it can be reconverted into glutamate or to GABA, an inhibitory neurotransmitter. Hyperammonemia may lead to enhanced glutamate amination in astrocytes, glutamate deficits, and alterations in intracellular compartmentalization of glutamate; these may be directly toxic to mitochondria and compromise energy

metabolism. For a complete review see (47). Accumulation of glutamine by astrocytes may also lead to cerebral edema.

Stanley originally proposed that the dearth of symptoms arises from enhanced glutamate oxidation by GDH which would prevent glutamine accumulation (48). Enhanced glutamate oxidation, however, would not necessarily prevent mitochondrial toxicity, glutamate deficits, and alterations in intracellular glutamate distributions.

The cases described above suggest hyperammonemia is not the source of seizures—plasma ammonium levels did not predict epilepsy and cerebral edema is not evident in individuals with HI/HA—although a contributing role of hyperammonemia cannot be excluded. Thus, HI/HA presents a unique model for understanding the mechanisms underlying neural ammonia toxicity.

A direct effect of enhanced GDH activity in the brain has also been proposed. GDH, highly expressed in the brain, is thought to have a larger presence in astrocytes than neurons. Oxidative deamination by GDH is the major route for the entrance of glutamate carbons in the form of alpha-ketoglutarate into the tricyclic acid cycle (49). Overactivity of GDH might decrease brain glutamine. Glutamine deficiency might compromise production of the major inhibitory neurotransmitter, GABA. GABA deficiency might lead to a hyperexcitable state as proposed by Olsen (50). The identification of mutations in the GABA receptor (51) in the setting of seizure disorders lends credence to a potential role for GABA deficiency in HI/HA.

A nerve-specific GDH, derived from the intronless *GLUD2* gene, is also present in brain (52). It is not under regulation like the GDH product of *GLUD1*. Its roles in HI/HA and its CNS manifestations have not been explored.

The finding of nonhypoglycemic seizures in the setting of HI/HA highlights the potential role of GDH in epilepsy and brain. Moreover, the prevalence of these seizures in HI/HA suggests a low clinical threshold for performing an EEG in an affected individual. Whether EEGs should be performed routinely at some specified interval in subjects with HI/HA has yet to be determined. As we learn more about HI/HA and its CNS manifestations, the clinical ramifications of enhanced GDH activity, the mechanisms by which ammonia insults brain, and the role of GDH in the CNS will hopefully be better delineated.

CLINICAL PEARLS

- Typical symptoms of acute and chronic hyperammonemia are absent in HI/HA.
- While most disorders of hypoglycemia arise in the setting of fasting, post-prandial hypoglycemia due to protein-sensitivity is the hallmark of HI/HA.
- Clinical manifestations of HI/HA vary, and some adults are only diagnosed after a child family member is diagnosed with HI/HA.

DIRECTIONS FOR FUTURE RESEARCH

The discovery that gain of function mutations in GDH cause hyperinsulinism has led to a greater understanding of insulin secretion. The association of these same mutations with hyperammonemia provides a framework for understanding how ammonia is normally metabolized by brain, how hyperammonemia insults brain activity, and the potential role of GDH in mitigating the toxic effect of hyperammonemia. Moreover, the finding of seizure disorders in the setting of GDH hyperactivity may provide a model for better understanding regulation of astrocytic and neuronal activity by brain.

KEY POINTS

- Hyperinsulinism suppresses generation of alternative brain fuels, ketones and lactate, rendering the brain particularly susceptible to insult due to hypoglycemia.
- Defects in the pathways of insulin secretion are responsible for congenital hyperinsulinism.
- Dominant mutations in *GLUD1*, encoding the mitochondrial enzyme GDH, cause a form of hyperinsulinism associated with hyperammonemia (HI/HA).
- Hypoglycemic seizures may be the first clue to the diagnosis of HI/HA.
- HI/HA may be associated with a seizure disorder with generalized clinical and electroencephalographic features that is unrelated acutely or remotely to hypoglycemia.
- The contributions of hyperammonemia and enhanced brain GDH activity to this seizure disorder have yet to be delineated.

REFERENCES

1. Sperling MA, Menon RK. Hyperinsulinemic hypoglycemia of infancy. *Endocrin Metab Clinics N America.* 1999;28:695–708.
2. Li CH, Matter A, Buettger C, Kwagh J, Collins HW, Stanley CA, Matschinsky FM, eds. A signaling role of glutamine in insulin secretion. ADA annual meeting; 2003; New Orleans.
3. Bryla J, Michalik M, Nelson J, Erecinska M. Regulation of the glutamate dehydrogenase activity in rat islets of langerhans and its consequence on insulin release. *Metabolism.* 1994;43:1187–95.
4. Colman RF. Glutamate dehydrogenase (bovine liver). In: SA Kuby, ed. A Study of Enzymes. NY: CRC Press; 1991:173–92.
5. Fahien LA, MacDonald MJ, Kmiotek EH, Mertz RJ, Fahien CM. Regulation of insulin release by factors that also modify glutamate dehydrogenase. *J Biol Chem.* 1988;263:13610–4.
6. Fajans SS, Floyd FC, Knopf RF, Guntshe EM, Rull JA, Thiffault CA, Conn JW. A difference in the mechanism by which leucine and other amino acids induce insulin release. *J Clin Endocr Metab.* 1967;27:1600–6.
7. Fajans SS, Quibrera R, Peck S, Floyd JC, Christensen HN, Conn JW. Stimulation of insulin release in the dog by a nonmetabolizable amino acid. Comparison with leucine and arginine. *J Clin Endocrin Metab.* 1971;33:35–41.
8. Hudson RC, Daniel RM. L-glutamate dehydrogenases: distribution, properties and mechanism. *Comp Biochem Physiol B.* 1993;106:767–92.
9. Dunne MJ, Kane C, Shepherd RM, Sanchez JA, James RF, Johnson PR, Aynsley-Green A, Lu S, Clement JPt, Lindley KJ, Seino S, Aguilar-Bryan L. Familial persistent hyperinsulinemic hypoglycemia of infancy and mutations in the sulfonylurea receptor. *New England Journal of Medicine.* 1997;336:703–6.
10. Glaser B, Chiu KC, Anker R, Nestorowicz A, Landau H, Ben-Bassat H, Shlomai Z, Kaiser N, Thornton PS, Stanley CA, et al. Familial hyperinsulinism maps to chromosome 11p14–15.1, 30 cM centromeric to the insulin gene. *Nat Genet.* 1994;7:185–8.
11. Glaser B, Chiu KC, Liu L, Anker R, Nestorowicz A, Cox NJ, Landau H, Kaiser N, Thornton PS, Stanley CA, et al. Recombinant mapping of the familial hyperinsulinism gene to an 0.8 cM region on chromosome 11p15.1 and demonstration of a founder effect in Ashkenazi Jews [published erratum appears in Hum Mol Genet 1995 Nov;4(11):2187–8]. *Hum Mol Genet.* 1995;4:879–86.
12. Glaser B, Ryan F, Donath M, Landau H, Stanley CA, Baker L, Barton DE, Thornton PS. Hyperinsulinism caused by paternal-specific inheritance of a recessive mutation in the sulfonylurea-receptor gene. *Diabetes.* 1999;48:1652–7.
13. Glaser B, Kesavan P, Heyman M, Davis E, Cuesta A, Buchs A, Stanley CA, Thornton PS, Permutt MA, Matschinsky FM, Herold KC. Familial hyperinsulinism caused by an activating glucokinase mutation. *N Engl J Med.* 1998;338:226–30.
14. Huopio H, Reimann F, Ashfield R, Komulainen J, Lenko HL, Rahier J, Vauhkonen I, Kere J, Laakso M, Ashcroft F, Otonkoski T. Dominantly inherited hyperinsulinism caused by a mutation in the sulfonylurea receptor type 1. *J Clin Invest.* 2000;106:897–906.

15. Kane C, Shepherd RM, Squires PE, Johnson PR, James RF, Milla PJ, Aynsley-Green A, Lindley KJ, Dunne MJ. Loss of functional KATP channels in pancreatic beta-cells causes persistent hyperinsulinemic hypoglycemia of infancy. *Nat Med.* 1996;2:1344-7.

16. MacMullen C, Fang J, Hsu BY, Kelly A, de Lonlay-Debeney P, Saudubray JM, Ganguly A, Smith TJ, Stanley CA. Hyperinsulinism/hyperammonemia syndrome in children with regulatory mutations in the inhibitory guanosine triphosphate-binding domain of glutamate dehydrogenase. *J Clin Endocrinol Metab.* 2001;86:1782-7.

17. Nestorowicz A, Inagaki N, Gonoi T, Schoor KP, Wilson BA, Glaser B, Landau H, Stanley CA, Thornton PS, Seino S, Permutt MA. A nonsense mutation in the inward rectifier potassium channel gene, Kir6.2, is associated with familial hyperinsulinism. *Diabetes.* 1997;46:1743-8.

18. Nestorowicz A, Wilson BA, Schoor KP, Inoue H, Glaser B, Landau H, Stanley CA, Thornton PS, Clement JPt, Bryan J, Aguilar-Bryan L, Permutt MA. Mutations in the sulonylurea receptor gene are associated with familial hyperinsulinism in Ashkenazi Jews. *Hum Mol Genet.* 1996;5:1813-22.

19. Stanley CA. The hyperinsulinism-hyperammonemia syndrome: gain-of-function mutations of glutamate dehydrogenase. In: S O'Rahilly, DB Dunger, eds. Genetic Insights in Paediatric Endocrinology and Metabolism. Bristol: BioScientifica, Ltd; 2000:23-30.

20. Weinzimer SA, Stanley CA, Berry GT, Yudkoff M, Tuchman M, Thornton PS. A syndrome of congenital hyperinsulinism and hyperammonemia. *Journal Of Pediatrics.* 1997;130:661-4.

21. Zammarchi E, Filippi L, Novembre E, Donati MA. Biochemical evaluation of a patient with a familial form of leucine-sensitive hypoglycemia and concomitant hyperammonemia. *Metabolism.* 1996;45:957-60.

22. Thomas PM, Cote GJ, Wohllk N, Haddad B, Mathew PM, Rabl W, Aguilar-Bryan L, Gage RF, Bryan J. Mutations in the sulfonylurea receptor gene in familial persistent hyperinsulinemic hypoglycemia of infancy. *Science.* 1995;268:426-9.

23. Thomas P, Ye YY, Lightner E. Mutations of the pancreatic islet inward rectifier Kir6.2 also leads to familial persistent hyperinsulinemic hypoglycemia of infancy. *Hum Mol Genet.* 1996;5: 1809-12.

24. Otonkoski T, Jiao H, Kaminen-Ahola N, Tapia-Paez I, Ullah MS, Parton LE, Schuit F, Quintens R, Sipila I, Mayatepek E, Meissner T, Halestrap AP, Rutter GA, Kere J. Physical exercise-induced hypoglycemia caused by failed silencing of monocarboxylate transporter 1 in pancreatic beta cells. *Am J Hum Genet.* 2007;81:467-74.

25. Clayton PT, Eaton S, Aynsley-Green A, Edginton M, Hussain K, Krywawych S, Datta V, Malingre HE, Berger R, van den Berg IE. Hyperinsulinism in short-chain L-3-hydroxyacyl-CoA dehydrogenase deficiency reveals the importance of beta-oxidation in insulin secretion. *J Clin Invest.* 2001;108:457-65.

26. Stanley CA, Fang J, Kutyna K, Hsu BY, Ming JE, Glaser B, Poncz M. Molecular basis and characterization of the hyperinsulinism/hyperammonemia syndrome: predominance of mutations in exons 11 and 12 of the glutamate dehydrogenase gene. HI/HA Contributing Investigators. *Diabetes.* 2000;49:667-73.

27. Miki Y, Tomohiko T, Obura T, Kato H, Yanagisawa M, Hayashi Y. Novel misense mutations in the glutamate dehydrogenase gene in the congenital hyperinsulinism-hyperammonemia syndrome. *J Pediatr.* 2000;136:69-72.

28. Huijmans JGM, Duran M, DeKlerk JBC, Rovers MJ, Scholte HR. Functional hyperactivity of hepatic glutamate dehydrogenase as a cause of the hyperinsulinism/hyperammonemia syndrome: Effect of treatment. *Pediatrics.* 2000;106:596-600.

29. Yorifuji T, Muroi J, Uematsu A, Hiramatsu H, Momoe T. Hyperinsulinism-hyperammonemia syndrome caused by mutant glutamate dehydrogenase accompanied by novel enzyme kinetics. *Hum Genet.* 1999;104:476-9.

30. Kelly A, Ng D, Ferry RJ, Jr., Grimberg A, Koo-McCoy S, Thornton PS, Stanley CA. Acute insulin responses to leucine in children with the hyperinsulinism/hyperammonemia syndrome. *J Clin Endocrinol Metab.* 2001;86:3724-8.

31. Hsu BY, Kelly A, Thornton PS, Greenberg CR, Dilling LA, Stanley CA. Protein-sensitive and fasting hypoglycemia in children with the hyperinsulinism/hyperammonemia syndrome. *Journal Of Pediatrics.* 2001;138:383-9.

32. Kelly A, Stanley CA. Disorders of glutamate metabolism. *Ment Retard Dev Disabil Res Rev.* 2001;7:287-95.

33. de las Heras J, Garin I, de Nanclares GP, Aguayo A, Rica I, Castano L, Vela A. Familial hyperinsulinism-hyperammonemia syndrome in a family with seizures: case report. *J Pediatr Endocrinol Metab.* 2010;23:827-30.

34. Pildes RS, Cornblath M, Warren I, Page-El E, Di Menza S, Merritt DM, Peeva A. A prospective controlled study of neonatal hypoglycemia. *Pediatrics.* 1974;54:5-14.

35. Koivisto M, Blanco-Sequeiros M, Krause U. Neonatal symptomatic and asymptomatic hypoglycaemia: a follow-up study of 151 children. *Dev Med Child Neurol.* 1972;14:603-14.

36. Volpe JJ. Hypoglycemia and Brain Injury. In: JJ Volpe ed. *Neurology of the Newborn.* Philadelphia: Saunders Elsevier; 2008:609-612.

37. Castro-Gago M, Gomez-Lado C, Eiris-Punal J, Diaz-Mayo I, Castineiras-Ramos DE. Serum biotinidase activity in children treated with valproic acid and carbamazepine. *J Child Neurol.* 2010;25:32-5.

38. Sharma S, Gulati S, Kabra M, Kalra V, Vasisht S, Gupta YK. Blood ammonia levels in epileptic children on 2 dose ranges of valproic acid monotherapy: a cross-sectional study. *J Child Neurol.* 2011;26:109-12.

39. Rousseau MC, Montana M, Villano P, Catala A, Blaya J, Valkov M, Allouard Y, Bugni E. Valproic acid-induced encephalopathy in very long course treated patients. *Brain Inj.* 2009;23:981-4.

40. Deutsch SI, Burket JA, Rosse RB. Valproate-induced hyperammonemic encephalopathy and normal liver functions: possible synergism with topiramate. *Clin Neuropharmacol.* 2009;32: 350-2.

41. Vivekanandan S, Nayak SD. Valproate-induced hyperammonemic encephalopathy enhanced by topiramate and phenobarbitone: a case report and an update. *Ann Indian Acad Neurol.* 2010;13:145-7.

42. Adams EN, Marks A, Lizer MH. Carbamazepine-induced hyperammonemia. *Am J Health Syst Pharm.* 2009;66:1468-70.

43. Raizen DM, Brooks-Kayal A, Steinkrauss L, Tennekoon GI, Stanley CA, Kelly A. Central nervous system hyperexcitability associated with glutamate dehydrogenase gain of function mutations. *Journal Of Pediatrics.* 2005;146:388-94.

44. Bahi-Buisson N, Roze E, Dionisi C, Escande F, Valayannopoulos V, Feillet F, Heinrichs C, Chadefaux-Vekemans B, Dan B, de Lonlay P. Neurological aspects of hyperinsulinism-hyperammonaemia syndrome. *Dev Med Child Neurol.* 2008; 50:945–9.

45. Bahi-Buisson N, El Sabbagh S, Soufflet C, Escande F, Boddaert N, Valayannopoulos V, Bellane-Chantelot C, Lascelles K, Dulac O, Plouin P, de Lonlay P. Myoclonic absence epilepsy with photosensitivity and a gain of function mutation in glutamate dehydrogenase. *Seizure.* 2008;17:658–64.

46. Perez Errazquin F, Sempere Fernandez J, Garcia Martin G, Chamorro Munoz MI, Romero Acebal M. Hyperinsulinism and hyperammonaemia syndrome and severe myoclonic epilepsy of infancy. *Neurologia.* 2011;26:248–52.

47. Hertz L, Kala G. Energy metabolism in brain cells: effects of elevated ammonia concentrations. *Metab Brain Dis.* 2007;22: 199–218.

48. Stanley CA. Hyperinsulinism/hyperammonemia syndrome: insights into the regulatory role of glutamate dehydrogenase in ammonia metabolism. *Mol Genet Metab.* 2004;81 Suppl 1:S45–51.

49. Sonnewald U, Westergaard N, Schousboe A. Glutamate transport and metabolism in astrocytes. *Glia.* 1997;21:56–63.

50. Olsen RW, DeLorey TM, Gordey M, Kang MH. GABA receptor function and epilepsy. *Adv Neurol.* 1999;79:499–510.

51. Wallace RH, Marini C, Petrou S, Harkin LA, Bowser DN, Panchal RG, Williams DA, Sutherland GR, Mulley JC, Scheffer IE, Berkovic SF. Mutant GABA(A) receptor gamma2-subunit in childhood absence epilepsy and febrile seizures. *Nat Genet.* 2001;28:49–52.

52. Plaitakis A, Metaxari M, Shashidharan P. Nerve tissue-specific (GLUD2) and housekeeping (GLUD1) human glutamate dehydrogenases are regulated by distinct allosteric mechanisms: implications for biologic function. *J Neurochem.* 2000;75:1862–9.

17

Glycine Encephalopathy and Epilepsy

Julia B. Hennermann

INTRODUCTION

Glycine encephalopathy (GE, OMIM 605899), or *non-ketotic hyperglycinemia*, is an autosomal recessive inborn error in the degradation of the amino acid glycine. This error results in an excessive accumulation of glycine in all tissues and body fluids, particularly in the central nervous system. The underlying defect is a deficiency in the glycine cleavage system (GCS), an intramitochondrial enzyme complex consisting of four different protein components [the P-protein (GLDC), the T-protein (AMT), the H-protein (GCSH), and the L-protein] (1). Most affected patients have a defect in the P-protein (80%), though some have a defect in the T-protein (20%) (1–4).

Glycine functions as both an excitatory and an inhibitory neurotransmitter. The excitatory effect is due to overstimulation of the *N*-methyl-D-aspartate (NMDA) receptor–channel complex, located in the cortex and the forebrain. Overstimulation of the glycine recognition site, located on the subunit NR1 of the NMDA receptor (5), causes an intracellular calcium accumulation. This accumulation produces neuronal injury, with subsequent cell death and intractable seizures (1, 6). Glycine has an inhibitory effect when the glycine receptors (GlyR) located in the spinal cord and the brain stem are stimulated. The stimulation of GlyR results in enhanced chloride permeability in the postsynaptic neurons, and is likely involved in the muscular hypotonia, neonatal apnea, and hiccupping found in children with GE (1, 5). The excitatory effect of these receptors on neural progenitor cells could be involved in the malformations sometimes observed in patients with GE (7).

CLINICAL PICTURE

The prevalence of GE is estimated to be 1 in 60,000 (1, 8). Depending on the age at manifestation and the outcome of the disease, different forms of GE may be discriminated: severe GE, attenuated GE, and late-onset GE. Most patients suffer from severe GE with presentation during the neonatal period. The existence of transient GE remains debatable.

SEVERE GE

Patients with severe GE present during the neonatal period, or, infrequently, during infancy, with poor outcomes ensuing. In patients with neonatal presentations, the first symptoms are hypotonia, seizures, coma, and/or apnea (9, 10). In the neonatal period, seizures often present as myoclonic epilepsy. It is not unusual for mothers to remark retrospectively on an in utero perception of fetal seizures. In some patients, seizures occur later than the neonatorum, although within the first 3 months of life. In patients with infantile presentations, hypotonia, and seizures predominate, whereas coma and apnea are less frequent. Some children show congenital malformations, including club feet, cleft lip/cleft palate, congenital hernias, cryptorchidism,

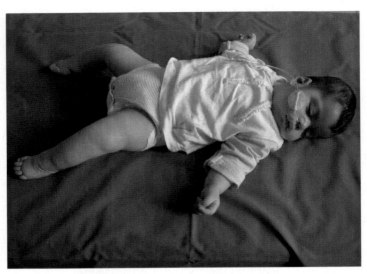

FIGURE 17.1   Infant (age $4\frac{1}{2}$ months) with a neonatal presentation of severe GE. Apart from club feet, the child had cerebral malformations including hypoplasia of the corpus callosum. The patient suffered from intractable seizures.

and, frequently, brain malformations (Figure 17.1). The occurrence of these malformations is always associated with a particularly poor outcome (10, 11). Patients develop spastic quadriparesis before the age of 6 months, truncal hypotonia, intractable seizures, severe neurodevelopmental impairment, frequent hiccupping, and microcephaly.

All children with severe GE show a poor outcome by a developmental age of approximately 6 weeks (11). At least 15% to 30% die during the neonatal period (9–11). In most patients with severe GE, seizures are intractable. Long-term problems in severe GE variably include feeding difficulties, gastroesophageal reflux, and esophagitis (10). Patients frequently require gastric tube feeding. Further problems involve the skeletal system, including hip dislocation, scoliosis, and osteoporosis (1).

ATTENUATED GE

Children with attenuated GE show a significantly better clinical outcome than children with severe GE (2). They may present during the neonatal or infantile period. In the neonatal period, the clinical picture resembles that of children with severe GE, showing hypotonia, seizures, myoclonic jerks, coma, and apnea, but with no congenital malformations. As the disease progresses,

they develop severe hyperactivity, choreiform movement disorders, behavioral problems, intellectual deficiency, and seizures (10, 11). Some children with attenuated GE present later, between the ages of 3 and 12 months. In these patients, hypotonia is the first symptom, followed by seizures and coma. In the majority of these cases, apnea is absent.

Intellectual deficiency is less pronounced in patients with attenuated GE than in those with severe GE (Figure 17.2). Children with attenuated GE often reach a DQ of 25–80. Although they learn to walk and show some motor skills, they predominantly manifest severe expressive language impairment. Unlike patients with severe GE, individuals with attenuated GE are very hyperactive and may develop choreiform movements. Seizures may occur, but they are less severe than those in patients with severe GE (10, 11).

LATE-ONSET GE

Late-onset GE seldom occurs. Patients present after the first 2 years of life with a clinical picture distinct from the earlier onset forms, showing cognitive decline and behavior problems. Hypotonia has not been reported in any of these patients, and seizures seldom occur. In some patients, leading symptoms include progressive spinocerebellar disease (12–14) or intermittent

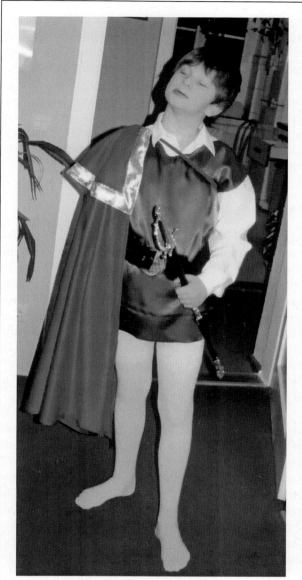

FIGURE 17.2 Boy (age $10\frac{1}{2}$ years) with neonatal presentation of attenuated GE and a good outcome. During the neonatal period and infancy, he suffered from myoclonic epilepsy, but his seizures stopped after infancy.

TRANSIENT GE

Rarely, children with transient GE have been reported. These children present during the neonatal period with the clinical features of GE and a transient increase of glycine in plasma and CSF levels. Patients usually progress to a good outcome with no or, in most cases, slight neurologic sequelae (17–24). None of the reported patients with transient GE had a proven enzymatic defect of the GCS, nor were they homozygous or compound heterozygous for mutations in the GCS genes. In contrast, in some patients, glycine elevation in the plasma and CSF has been shown to be secondary due to hypoxic ischemic encephalopathy, stroke, or central nervous infection (20, 25; own experiences).

DIAGNOSTIC APPROACHES

LABORATORY ANALYSIS

Glycine Determination

In term newborns presenting with myoclonic seizures, hypotonia, coma, and/or apnea, GE must be included in the differential diagnosis. The first diagnostic approach is to evaluate amino acid levels in the plasma and CSF. An increase in the plasma glycine concentration, CSF glycine concentration, and the CSF to plasma glycine ratio (greater than 0.08) is characteristic of GE. To discriminate GE from ketotic hyperglycinemia caused by other inborn errors of metabolism, urine organic acids also have to be analyzed. A secondary increase of glycine in plasma may be caused by medication (eg, treatment with valproate), starvation, encephalopathies of other origin (eg, hypoxic ischemic encephalopathy, leukencephalopathies) or blood-stained CSF (25–26). Recently, glycine elevations, associated with lactic acidosis and encephalopathy, have been reported in patients with mitochondrial dysfunction syndromes (27).

Children with neonatal-onset GE usually have higher concentrations of glycine in the CSF and a higher CSF to plasma ratio, regardless of their outcome, than children with onset in infancy. Plasma and CSF glycine concentrations decrease with age, especially CSF concentrations (28). However, it must be considered that, in a few patients with GE, glycine concentrations may be increased in CSF but not in plasma (2).

choreoathetosis (15). It has been suggested that genes other than GCS genes may be responsible for late onset GE (16), which would support the observation that late onset GE presents as a different variant of GE.

Enzymatic Analysis

To confirm a GE diagnosis, enzymatic analysis may be performed in liver tissue or in lymphoblasts. Enzymatic assays are generally more reliable in liver tissue than in lymphoblasts. For enzymatic analysis of the whole GCS complex, at least 20 mg of liver tissue, which may be obtained by needle biopsy, is required. To analyze the total GCS complex, including identifying the defective protein component, more than 150 mg of liver tissue is needed, which is obtained by an open liver biopsy (29).

Genetic Analysis

Mutation analysis in GE is challenging, as all four protein components of GCS map to different chromosomes, and mutations are predominantly private. Founder mutations have been described only in Finnish patients. *GLDC* on chromosome 9p24 codes for the P-protein. More than 100 *GLDC* mutations have been described; a few mutations occur more frequently, mainly in the Finish population. The missense mutation p.S564I, for example, has been identified in 70% of Finnish patients (30–32). Deletions of *GLDC* are very common, and may account for at least 20% of the mutations in patients with GE (33). *AMT*, on chromosome 3q21.1–21.2, codes for the T-protein. More than 25 *AMT* mutations have been identified, most of which are private mutations (16, 29, 32). *AMT* mutations have been speculated to be more frequent in attenuated forms of GE (29). Mutations in *GCSH*, which codes for the H-protein, are extremely rare (3, 16).

Prenatal Diagnosis

A prenatal diagnosis may be made after 11–12 wk of gestation by chorionic villus sampling (CVS). Molecular analysis may achieve reliable results in affected families with an index patient. False-negative results of prenatal diagnoses have been reported when performing enzymatic assay in chorionic villi and when determining glycine and serine concentrations in amniotic fluid (34–35).

EEG PATTERNS

Multifocal epilepsy and generalized slowing without epilepsy are common EEG patterns in patients with GE. During the neonatal period a typical burst-suppression pattern, which may be found in children with hypoxia and in other inborn errors of metabolism as well, may occur in GE. This pattern usually disappears after the neonatal period and then may change to hypsarrhythmia (1, 36). Burst suppression and hypsarrhythmia patterns are more frequent in patients with severe GE, and they predict a more severe outcome of the disease (10). Rarely, EEGs show focal epilepsy. Normal EEG patterns are uncommon in patients with GE, but may occur.

FINDINGS BY CEREBRAL MRI AND MRS

Various brain abnormalities and malformations have been described in GE. Hypoplasia or aplasia of the corpus callosum is the most common, occurring in up to 50% of patients. Further brain abnormalities include ventriculomegaly, hydrocephalus, brain atrophy, gyral malformations, cerebellar hypoplasia, delayed myelination, posterior fossa cysts, hypodensity of white matter, and intracranial hemorrhage (1, 37). All congenital brain malformations, especially hypoplasia of the corpus callosum, predict a poor outcome of the disease.

Long-echo time MR spectroscopy (MRS) may detect elevated glycine peaks in white and grey matter of affected patients (38). Cerebral glycine concentrations and ratios measured by MRS generally correlate well with the clinical course of GE (39). However, elevated cerebral glycine peaks are not detectable by MRS in patients with milder forms of GE (40). At the current state of knowledge, MRS is not established in day-to-day practice. Overall, MRS is a valuable but expensive tool in diagnosis and monitoring GE.

TREATMENT

Current therapy for GE is directed at decreasing glycine concentrations and blocking the effect of glycine at neurotransmitter receptors. Benzoate treatment and a low-protein diet can effectively reduce glycine plasma concentrations. There are a few NMDA receptor antagonists and GlyR blockers that may also be applied. Additionally, combined anticonvulsive treatment is necessary in most children, particularly in those with severe GE.

MEDICAL TREATMENT

Decrease of Glycine Concentrations

The therapeutic goal of treatment is to maintain plasma glycine levels ≤ 250 μmol/L. The most effective treatment is high-dose benzoate (250–750 mg/kg/d) (1). Benzoate is activated to benzoyl-CoA, which binds to glycine and is then excreted as hippurate in urine. Benzoate treatment does not ameliorate developmental delay, but it reduces seizure frequency and improves alertness in patients (41). The effect of benzoate is dose-dependent, and higher doses are required in more severely affected patients. Therapeutic plasma levels of benzoate are ≤ 3 μmol/L, and toxic levels are greater than 8 μmol/L (41). Benzoate toxicity is associated with a renal dysfunction syndrome (42). Further side effects of benzoate treatment are noncompliance due to unpalatability, esophagitis/gastritis, and carnitine deficiency (41). Compliance may be improved by application of coated benzoate granules, which are saliva resistant and neutral tasting (43, 44). Prophylaxis with an H_2-blocker is recommended for all children receiving benzoate treatment. Appropriate monitoring of benzoate treatment should include regular measurements of plasma glycine, carnitine, and benzoate (41, 42, 45).

NMDA Receptor Blockers

Dextromethorphan blocks the glutamate binding site of the NMDA receptor. It reduces seizures and improves alertness primarily in attenuated GE, but is less effective in severe GE (10, 46). Other NMDA receptor antagonists include tryptophan and ketamine, which target the glycine allosteric binding site (47).

GlyR Blockers

The inhibitory effect of glycine at GlyR is blocked by strychnine, which is effective in apneic infants. However, it may have deleterious side effects in long-term use (1). Diazepam also blocks the inhibitory effect of glycine at GlyR, but its effect is transient and tachyphylactic (48).

Anticonvulsant Treatment

To date no specific recommendations for anticonvulsant treatment in GE exist, and many patients require multiple medications. In early infancy, phenobarbital and benzodiazepines have been shown to be effective, particular for treatment of myoclonic seizures. A positive anticonvulsant effect has also been described in several patients receiving primidone, levetiracetam, phenytoin, vigabatrin, topiramate, carbamazepine, and clobazam (10). However, vigabatrin has also been shown to cause rapid, progressive deterioration in patients with severe GE (49). Felbamate, an NMDA-receptor-blocker (50), can be considered for the treatment of recalcitrant seizures, although potential toxicities mandate regular monitoring, for example, hematologic and hepatic functions. Lamotrigine and sulthiame are reported to be ineffective in the majority of patients with GE (10). Valproate treatment is not recommended, as it inhibits residual GCS enzyme activity and is associated with severe side effects in patients with GE (51, 52).

DIET

Decrease of Glycine Intake

Dietary glycine and serine restriction combined with benzoate therapy may be effective in patients with severe GE (1, 11, 45). Foods with a high content of glycine include those with a high content of natural protein, for example, meat, fish, dairy products, and gelatin (45). A glycine-free amino acid formula for nourishing infants with GE is available in some countries (eg, Gly-AM infant, Nutricia/SHS).

FUTURE DIRECTIONS

Certain clinical parameters, including cerebral MRI findings and a clinical scoring system, have been identified which may allow an early prediction of the outcome of the disease (10). At the moment, however, prediction of the outcome is not possible until after the neonatal period. As 20% of newborns with GE show a less severe outcome, this is an important issue concerning counselling and decision making in neonates with GE.

Further research needs to evaluate options for the treatment of patients with GE. Currently, no recommendations for an effective anticonvulsant treatment exist. Treatment may be optimized by introducing new anticonvulsants, possibly in combination with NMDA receptor antagonists blocking the glycine binding site of the NMDA receptor.

CLINICAL PEARLS

- Patients with GE present with hypotonia, seizures, coma, and/or apnea.
- Onset of clinical symptoms may be during neonatal period, infancy, or, rarely, after the age of 2 years. Fetal seizures may be reported.
- In the neonatal period seizures often present as myoclonic seizures.
- In the long-term, seizures are often intractable.
- Most patients have a poor outcome with a developmental age of maximal 6 weeks.
- However, developmental progress is made by 20% of the children with neonatal presentation and by 50% of the children with infantile presentation.
- A poor outcome may be predicted early in patients with malformations, including cerebral malformations.
- Treatment of GE includes benzoate and neurotransmitter receptor agonists.
- Combined anticonvulsive treatment is necessary in most children with GE.

Disclosures:
None.

Abbreviations:

CSF	cerebrospinal fluid
GlyR	glycine receptor
GCS	glycine cleavage system
GE	glycine encephalopathy
MRS	MR spectroscopy
NMDA	*N*-methyl-D-aspartate

REFERENCES

1. Hamosh A, Johnston MV. Nonketotic hyperglycinemia. In: CR Sciver, AL Beaudet, WS Sly, et al. eds. *The Metabolic and Molecular Bases of Inherited Disease*. 8th ed. New York: McGraw-Hill; 2001:2065–2078.
2. Applegarth DA, Toone JR. Nonketotic hyperglycinemia (Glycine encephalopathy): Laboratory diagnosis. *Mol Genet Metab*. 2001;74:139–146.
3. Applegarth DA, Toone JR. Workshop report. Glycine encephalopathy (nonketotic hyperglycinemia): review and update. *J Inherit Metab Dis*. 2004;27:417–422.
4. Tada K, Kure S. Non-ketotic hyperglycinemia: molecular lesion, diagnosis, and pathophysiology. *J Inherit Metab Dis*. 1993;16, 691–703.
5. Hernandes MS, Troncone LR. Glycine as a neurotransmitter in the forebrain: a short review. *J Neural Transm*. 2009;116: 1551–1560.
6. Lipton SA, Rosenberg PA. Excitatory amino acids as a final common pathway for neurological disorders. *N Engl J Med*. 1994;330:613–621.
7. Nguyen L, Rigo J-M, Rocher V, et al. Neurotransmitters as early signal for central nervous system development. *Cell Tissue Res*. 2001;305:187–202.
8. Applegarth DA, Toone JR, Lowry RB. Incidence of inborn errors of metabolism in British Columbia, 1969–1996. *Pediatrics*. 2000;105:e10.
9. Hoover-Fong JE, Shah S, van Hove JLK, et al. Natural history of nonketotic hyperglycinemia in 65 patients. *Neurology*. 2004;64:1847–1853.
10. Hennermann JB, Barufe J-M, Grieben U, et al. Prediction of long-term outcome in glycine encephalopathy: a clinical survey. *J Inherit Metab Dis*. 2012;35:253–261.
11. Van Hove JLK, Mahieu V, Schollen E, et al. Prognosis in nonketotic hyperglycinemia. *J. Inherit Metab Dis*. 2003; 26(Suppl. 2):71.
12. Bank WJ, Morrow G. Familial neuromuscular disease with nonketotic hyperglycinemia. *Trans Am Neurol Assoc*. 1971;96:21–23.
13. Hasegawa T, Shiga Y, Matsumoto A, et al. Late-onset nonketotic hyperglycinemia: a case report. *No To Shinkei*, 2002;54: 1068–1072.
14. Steiman GS, Yudkoff M, Berman PH, et al. Late-onset nonketotic hyperglycinemia and spinocerebellar degeneration. *J Pediatr*. 1979;94:907–911.
15. Brunel-Guitton C, Casey B, Coulter-Mackie M, et al. Late-onset nonketotic hyperglycinemia caused by a novel homozygous missense mutation in the *GLDC* gene. *Mol Genet Metab*. 2011;103:193–196.
16. Kure S, Kato K, Dinopoulos A, et al. Comprehensive mutation analysis of GLDC, AMT, and GCSH in nonketotic hyperglycinemia. *Hum Mutat*. 2006;27:343–352.
17. Aliefendioglu D, Aslan AT, Coskun T, et al. Transient nonketotic hyperglycinemia: two case reports and literature review. *Pediatr Neurol*. 2003;28:151–155.
18. Eyskens FJM, Van Doorn JWD, Marien P. Neurologic sequelae in transient nonketotic hyperglycinemia of the neonate. *J Pediatr*. 1992;121:620–621.
19. Korman SH, Boneh A, Ichinohe A, et al. Persistent NKH with transient or absent symptoms and a homozygous *GLDC* mutation. *Ann Neurol*. 2004;56:139–143.
20. Lang TF, Parr JB, Matthews EE, et al. Practical difficulties in the diagnosis of transient non-ketotic hyperglycinemia. *Dev Med Child Neurol*. 2008;50:157–159.
21. Luder AS, Davidson A, Goodman SI, et al. Transient nonketotic hyperglycinemia in Neonates. *J Pediatr*. 1989;114:1013–1015.
22. Maeda T, Inutsuka M, Goto K, et al. Transient nonketotic hyperglycinemia in an asphyxiated patient with pyridoxine-dependent seizures. *Pediatr Neurol*. 2000;22:225–227.
23. Schiffmann R, Kaye EM, Willis JK, et al. Transient neonatal hyperglycinemia. *Ann Neurol*. 1989;25:201–203.
24. Zammarchi E, Donati MA, Ciani F. Transient neonatal hyperglycinemia: a 13-year follow-up. *Neuropediatrics*. 1995;26: 328–330.

25. Aburahma S, Khassawneh M, Griebel M, et al. Pitfalls in measuring cerebrospinal fluid glycine levels in infants with encephalopathy. *J Child Neurol.* 2011;26:703–706.

26. Korman SH, Gutman A. Pitfalls in the diagnosis of glycine encephalopathy (non-ketotic hyperglycinemia). *Dev Med Child Neurol.* 2002;44:712–770.

27. Haack TB, Rolinski B, Haberberger B, et al. Homozygous missense mutation in BOLA3 causes mutliple mitochondrial dysfunctions syndrome in two siblings. *J Inherit Metab Dis.* 2012 May 5 [Epub ahead of print], PMID: 22562599.

28. Jones CM, Smith M, Henderson MJ. Reference data for cerebrospinal fluid and the utility of amino acid measurement for the diagnosis of inborn errors of metabolism. *Ann. Clin. Biochem.* 2006;43:63–66.

29. Toone JR, Applegarth DA, Levy HL, Coulter-Mackie MB, Lee G. Molecular genetic and biochemical characteristics of patients with T-protein deficiency as a cause of glycine encephalopathy. *Mol Genet Metab.* 2003;79:272–280.

30. Kure S, Takayanagi M, Narisawa K, et al. Identification of a common mutation in Finnish patients with nonketotic hyperglycinemia. *J Clin Invest.* 1992;90:160–164.

31. Toone JR, Applegarth DA, Coulter-Mackie MB, et al. Biochemical and molecular investigations of patients with nonketotic hyperglycinemia. *Mol Genet Metab.* 2000;70:116–121.

32. OMIM; http://www.ncbi.nlm.nih.gov

33. Kanno J, Hutchin T, Kamada F, et al. Genomic deletion with *GLDC* is a major cause of non-ketotic hyperglycinemia. *J Med Genet.* 2007;44:e69.

34. Applegarth DA, Toone JR, Rolland MO, et al. Non-concordance of CVS and liver glycine cleavage enzyme in three families with non-ketotic hyperglycinemia (NKH) leading to false negative prenatal diagnosis. *Prenat Diagn.* 2000;20:367–370.

35. Vianey-Saban C, Chevalier-Porst F, Froissart R, et al. Prenatal diagnosis of non ketotic hyperglycinemia: a 13-year experience, from enzymatic to molecular analysis. *J Inherit Metab Dis,* 2003;26(Suppl. 2):82.

36. Mises J, Moussali-Salefranques F, Laroque ML, et al. EEG findings as an aid to the diagnosis of neonatal nonketotic hyperglycinemia. *J Inherit Metab Dis.* 1982;5(Suppl. 2): 117–120.

37. Press GA, Barshop BA, Haas RH, et al. Abnormalities of the brain in nonketotic hyperglycinemia: MR manifestations. *AJNR.* 1989;10:315–321.

38. Heindel W, Kugel H, Roth B. Noninvasive detection of increased glycine content by proton MR spectroscopy in the brains of two infants with nonketotic hyperglycinemia. *AJNR.* 1993;14:629–635.

39. Choi C-G, Lee HK, Yoon J-H. Localized proton MR spectroscopic detection of nonketotic hyperglycinemia in an infant. *Korean J Radiol.* 2001;2:239–242.

40. Dinopoulos A, Kure S, Chuck G, et al. Glycine decarboxylase mutations: a distinctive phenotype of nonketotic hyperglycinemia in adults. *Neurology.* 2005;64:1255–1257.

41. Van Hove JLK, Kishnani P, Muenzer J, et al. Benzoate therapy and carnitine deficiency in non-ketotic hyperglycinemia. *Am J Med Genet.* 1995;59:444–453.

42. Wolff JA, Kulovich S, Yu AL, et al. The effectiveness of benzoate in the management of seizures in nonketotic hyperglycinemia. *AJDC.* 1986;140:596–660.

43. Breitkreutz J, Bornhöft M, Wöll F, et al. Pediatric drug formulations of sodium benzoate: I. Coated granules with a hydrophilic binder. *Eur J Pharm Biopharm.* 2003;56:247–253.

44. Breitkreutz J, El-Saleh F, Kiera C, et al. Pediatric drug formulations of sodium benzoate: II. Coated granules with a lipophilic binder. *Eur J Pharm Biopharm.* 2003;56:255–260.

45. Van Hove JLK, Vande Kerckhove K, Hennermann JB, et al. Benzoate treatment and the glycine index in nonketotic hyperglycinemia. *J Inherit Metab Dis.* 2005;28:651–663.

46. Hamosh A, Maher JF, Bellus GA, et al. Long-term use of high-dose benzoate and dextromethorphan for the treatment of nonketotic hyperglycinemia. *J Pediatr.* 1998;132:709–713.

47. Deutsch SI, Rosse RB, Mastropaolo J. Current status of NMDA antagonist interventions in the treatment of nonketotic hyperglycinemia. *Clin Neuropharmacol.* 1998;21:71–79.

48. Matalon R, Naidu S, Hughes JR, et al. Nonketotic hyperglycinemia: treatment with diazepam—a competitor for glycine receptors. *Pediatrics.* 1983;71:581–584.

49. Tekgul H, Serdaroglu G, Karapinar B, et al. Vigabatrin caused rapidly progressive deterioration in two cases with early moyclonic encephalopathy associated with nonketotic hyperglycinemia. *J Child Neurol.* 2006;21:82–84.

50. Harty TP, Rogawski MA. Felbamate block of recombinant N-methyl-D-aspartate receptors: selectivity for the NR2B subunit. *Epilepsy Res.* 2000;39:47–55.

51. Morrison PF, Sankar R, Shields WD. Valproate-induced chorea and encephalopathy in atypical nonketotic hyperglycinemia. *Pediatr Neurol.* 2006;35:356–358.

52. Hall DA, Ringel SP. Adult nonketotic hyperglycinemia crisis presenting as severe chorea and encephalopathy. *Movement Disord.* 2004;19:485–486.

Serine Synthesis Defects and Epilepsy

Tom J. de Koning

INTRODUCTION

Serine deficiency disorders are relatively new within the field of inborn errors of metabolism. In 1996, Jaeken and colleagues reported for the first time two siblings with a defect in the L-serine synthetic pathway (1). These patients suffered from severe neurological symptoms and were diagnosed because of low plasma and CSF serine concentrations upon routine amino acid analysis. The molecular defect in these patients affected the first step in the L-serine synthetic pathway, the enzyme 3-phosphoglycerate dehydrogenase (3-PGDH, Figure 18.1). In recent years, patients have been identified with defects in the two other enzymes of the L-serine pathway as well and invariably they presented with serious neurological symptoms.

To date only a limited number of patients have been reported with defects in the serine synthetic pathway and this might indicate that serine deficiency disorders are very rare disorders indeed. However, it might also be true that these patients are under- or mis-diagnosed. For historical reasons, most diagnostic procedures are aimed at the detection of elevated amino acid concentrations and not at detecting lowered amino acid values. Moreover, many diagnostic laboratories do not use age-related reference intervals for amino acids, representing another important factor applicable to diagnosing serine deficiency in particular in newborns and young infants.

FUNCTIONS OF L-SERINE IN THE CENTRAL NERVOUS SYSTEM

L-serine is a nonessential amino acid which means that it can be synthesized by body tissues and is not exclusively obtained from the diet. Although nonessential might suggest otherwise, L-serine is a key metabolite in many important cellular functions. For instance in cell proliferation L-serine is a starting point for the synthesis of nucleotides and the synthesis of other amino acids such as cysteine and glycine. With regard to the central nervous system (CNS), L-serine is predominantly related to neurotransmitter synthesis and the synthesis of phospholipids and glycolipids (2). Two neurotransmitters, glycine and D-serine, are directly synthesized from L-serine and these two neurotransmitters are functionally related since they are both ligands for N-methyl-D-aspartate (NMDA) receptors. In recent years it has become clear that D-serine, not glycine, is the natural ligand for the so-called "glycine site" in the majority of NMDA receptor subtypes (3). However, glycine is not only involved in excitatory neurotransmission through the activation of NMDA receptors, but also in inhibitory neurotransmission via glycine receptors in brain stem and spinal cord.

Besides being a precursor for neurotransmitters, L-serine is also the precursor for the synthesis of phosphoglycerides, glycerides, and complex macromolecules such as sphingolipids and glycolipids. These lipids are

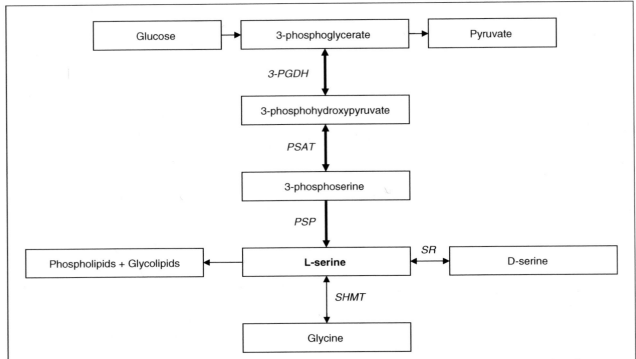

FIGURE 18.1   The synthesis pathway of L-serine. 3-PGDH, 3-phosphoglycerate dehydrogenase; PSAT, phosphoserine aminotransferase; PSP, phosphoserine phosphatase; SHMT, serine hydroxymethyltransferases; SR, serine racemase.

important membrane and myelin components and play a role in cellular differentiation, proliferation, migration, and cell survival ().

The transport of L-serine through the blood–brain barrier into the CNS appears to be rather limited and therefore the majority of L-serine is synthesized within the brain itself. In brain tissue L-serine is predominantly produced in astrocytes which supply neurons with the necessary amounts of L-serine for the functions listed above.

SERINE DEFICIENCY DISORDERS

The synthesis of L-serine takes place in three enzymatic steps (Figure 18.1) and genetic defects have been reported in all three enzymes. The majority of patients reported so far with serine deficiency suffered from a defect in the first step of the L-serine pathway; 3-phosphoglycerate dehydrogenase. Defects in the other two enzymes, phosphoserine aminotransferase and

phosphoserine phosphatase have been reported in single families only.

3-PHOSPHOGLYCERATE DEHYDROGENASE DEFICIENCY (3-PGDH)

Two clinical 3-PGDH deficiency phenotypes can be recognized, namely a severe infantile phenotype and a milder juvenile phenotype. In the severe infantile phenotype the majority of children presented with intrauterine growth retardation (IUGR) and congenital microcephaly, although both conditions do not necessarily need to be present in all patients. Intractable seizures develop within weeks to months after birth and the epileptiform discharges on EEG precede clinically manifest seizures. Once the children develop seizures, they demonstrate little to no psychomotor development and develop a severe spastic quadriplegia which becomes evident during the first years of life. The majority of children with infantile 3-PGDH deficiency were reported to be irritable and hypertonic, and appeared to be "unhappy" infants. In addition to the neurological symptoms listed above some children also had congenital cataracts, hypogonadism, adducted thumbs, inguinal and umbilical hernias, and megaloblastic anemia (2).

Several seizure types were observed in infants with infantile 3-PGDH deficiency, of which none appeared to be very specific. Infantile spasms, tonic–clonic seizures, tonic seizures, atonic seizures, gelastic seizures, and myoclonic seizures have all been reported at different ages in patients with infantile 3-PGDH deficiency (4, 5). In addition, EEG patterns appeared to be also nonspecific; both hypsarrhythmia and multifocal seizure activity evolving towards Lennox Gastaut syndrome are documented. On cranial MRI the brain has an atrophic appearance, which is due to a striking lack of white matter volume. Extensive hypomyelination and impaired and delayed myelination are evident (6).

Juvenile Phenotype

A juvenile onset and much milder phenotype of 3-PGDH deficiency has been reported by Tabatabaie et al. (7). In two siblings with normal early developmental milestones and subsequent mild-to-moderate developmental delay, absence seizures with the accompanying EEG abnormalities developed at school age. Neither microcephaly or pyramidal signs were present in either child. The patients were diagnosed at teenage, with one displaying severe behavior abnormalities and mood disturbance at the time of diagnosis. MRI of the brain in both siblings revealed no abnormalities and the striking hypomyelination seen in the infantile phenotype was not present. Until now only these siblings have been reported so it cannot be concluded whether the absence seizures present in these patients are specific for the juvenile phenotype. However, this is considered unlikely given the presence of multiple EEG patterns in the infantile phenotype.

With the description of this juvenile phenotype it is very likely that 3-PGDH deficiency can be accompanied by a wide spectrum of clinical symptoms varying from severe abnormalities at birth to mild intellectual deficiency with treatable seizures in childhood. This implies that not only infants with congenital microcephaly and seizures, but many more children with mild-to-moderate developmental delay and seizures, are potential candidates for amino acid analysis for serine deficiency.

Diagnosis: The diagnosis of both phenotypes of 3-PGHD deficiency can be suspected from amino acid analysis in plasma and CSF. Remarkably, no differences were present between the serine values of patients with the severe infantile form in comparison to the milder juvenile form. Therefore, the clinical phenotype cannot be predicted from amino acid analysis.

The deficiency of serine is much more pronounced in CSF and, in contrast to plasma, is not influenced by the absorption of amino acids from the diet. The latter is very important because plasma is typically used for diagnostic procedures and, thus, the diagnosis of 3-PGDH deficiency can be easily missed when plasma amino acids are not analysed in a fasting state. Therefore, CSF is preferred for diagnosing serine deficiency and plasma values can only be correctly interpreted when collected following an overnight fast. In addition, CSF amino acids have age-specific reference ranges (8). The values of serine are much higher in newborns and young infants than older children and adults. The use of age-specific reference ranges for diagnosing serine deficiency is important and diagnostic laboratories that have used pooled samples to determine their reference ranges are at risk to miss serine deficiency in newborns and infants (8 and personal observations).

Typical values for serine and glycine concentrations in 3-PGDH deficiency are depicted in Table 18.1. Analysis of urine amino acids to diagnose 3-PGDH deficiency is not helpful because, for poorly understood reasons, the urinary excretion of serine can be completely normal in serine deficiency.

The diagnosis of 3-PGDH deficiency can be confirmed by enzyme assay in cultured fibroblasts or mutation analysis (9). Mutation analysis may be preferred given the pitfalls in the interpretation of enzymatic assays of the serine synthetic pathway and the biochemical data from amino acid analysis (10).

Treatment

Patients with infantile 3-PGDH deficiency can be treated with oral supplementation of L-serine (500–700 mg/kg/d), which is associated with seizure control in the majority of children. In those children with an insufficient response on L-serine alone, glycine (200–300 mg/kg/d) can be added to the treatment (11, 12).

In general, treatment with amino acids has a very good effect on behavior, seizure control, and overall

TABLE 18.1 Clinical Disorders in Serine Synthesis Defects

Disorder	Clinical Features	Amino Acids[a]	Treatment	Response to Treatment
3-Phosphoglycerate dehydrogenase deficiency (3-PGDH)	*Infantile phenotype* (congenital) microcephaly, IUGR, intractable seizures, severe psychomotor retardation, spastic quadriplegia, cataracts, hypogonadism, hernia, megaloblastic anemia MRI: hypomyelination and delayed myelination *Juvenile phenotype* Mild–moderate intellectual deficiency, absence seizures, behavior problems MRI: no abnormalities	CSF serine 6–11 CSF glycine 1–normal Plasma serine 28–64 Plasma glycine 128–normal * CSF serine age 1 week: mean 59 μmol/L, reference interval 35–82 age 1 month: mean 52 μmol/L, reference interval 31–74 age 6 months: mean 44 μmol/L, reference interval 26–63 age 1 year: mean 41 μmol/L, reference interval 24–59 age 5 years: mean 34 μmol/L, reference interval 20–48 age 10 years: mean 31 μmol/L, reference interval 18–44 CSF serine 9 CSF glycine normal Plasma serine 58, 63 Plasma glycine normal	500–600 mg L-serine kg/day and glycine 200–300 mg/kg/d 100–150 mg L-serine/kg/d	Control of seizures or significantly lowered frequency, improvement of wellbeing. Increased white matter volume. No to limited effect on psychomotor development. *Antenatal treatment:* prevention of neurological abnormalities Control of seizures, improvement of behavior and school performance
3-Phosphoserine aminotransferase deficiency (PSAT)	*Symptomatic patient* secondary microcephaly, intractable seizures, early death MRI: generalized atrophy, including cerebellar vermis	CSF serine 5–18 CSF glycine less than 1 Plasma serine 30–51 Plasma glycine 110–121 * CSF serine age 1 week: mean 59 μmol/L, reference interval 35–82	500 mg/kg/d L-serine 200 mg/kg/d glycine	*Symptomatic patient* no clinical response to treatment *Presymptomatic patient* prevention of all neurological abnormalities

and pons, white matter abnormalities.
MRI *presymptomatic patient:* No abnormalities

age 1 month: mean 52 μmol/L, reference interval 31–74
age 6 months: mean 44 μmol/L, reference interval 26–63
age 1 year: mean 41 μmol/L, reference interval 24–59
age 5 years: mean 34 μmol/L, reference interval 20–48
age 10 years: mean 31 μmol/L, reference interval 18–44

3-Phosphoserine phosphatase deficiency (PSP)

Williams syndrome, IUGR, congenital microcephaly, slow psychomotor development, feeding difficulties.
MRI: not reported

CSF serine 18
CSF glycine normal
Plasma serine 55–80
Plasma glycine normal
* CSF serine age 1 week: mean 59 μmol/L, reference interval 35–82
age 1 month: mean 52 μmol/L, reference interval 31–74
age 6 months: mean 44 μmol/L, reference interval 26–63
age 1 year: mean 41 μmol/L, reference interval 24–59
age 5 years: mean 34 μmol/L, reference interval 20–48
age 10 years: mean 31 μmol/L, reference interval 18–44

200–300 mg/kg/d L-serine
Increase in head circumference
Lost to follow-up

aDifferent age-related reference ranges are shown for CSF serine.
IUGR, intrauterine growth retardation.

223

wellbeing. In the majority of patients the seizures will disappear and the EEG abnormalities will normalize, whereas in the remainder seizure frequency significantly improves. Unfortunately, amino acid therapy has only limited effects on psychomotor development in already symptomatic patients (13). We have shown that 3-PGDH deficiency is a treatable disorder, but treatment should optimally start before symptoms arise. In one case we applied intrauterine treatment to an affected fetus by giving the mother L-serine supplementation during pregnancy (5). Maternal treatment was initiated at 27 weeks of pregnancy and continued post-partum in the baby girl. In contrast to her severely affected siblings, the girl was born normocephalic and showed completely normal psychomotor development without any neurological symptoms until the current follow-up to the age of 11 years. Another case of presymptomatic treatment in serine deficiency will be discussed below (PSAT deficiency), and both cases emphasize the importance of early and prompt recognition and rapid intervention (5, 10).

Not surprisingly, treatment results were much better in the two affected patients with the milder juvenile phenotype, and much lower dosages of L-serine could be used to treat these patients effectively. Good treatment results were obtained with 100–150 mg/kg/d of L-serine and there was no need to add glycine. Both patients became seizure free and conventional antiepileptic drugs could be discontinued. Significant improvement in well-being, behavior, and school performance was documented during follow-up and all biochemical abnormalities normalized during treatment (7).

PHOSPHOSERINE AMINOTRANSFERASE (PSAT) DEFICIENCY

The second defect in the L-serine synthetic pathway is phosphoserine aminotransferase (PSAT) deficiency. This disorder was reported in 2007 by Hart et al., in two siblings. The symptoms were evident shortly after birth when the index patient, a boy, presented with feeding difficulties, jerky movements, and intractable seizures. Within weeks after symptom onset, microcephaly became evident. His seizures were therapy resistant to all drug regimens and vitamin supplements, and EEGs showed severe multifocal epileptiform activity. On MRI, generalized atrophy was present, but in contrast to 3-PGDH deficiency, there was also hypoplasia of the cerebellar vermis and pons, combined with multiple white matter abnormalities.

PSAT deficiency should be considered in the differential diagnosis of other causes of neonatal seizures such as the vitamin dependent seizures, glycine encephalopathy, and congenital disorders of glycosylation, with the latter group of disorders also often displaying cerebellar abnormalities.

Treatment

The index patient was treated with L-serine (500 mg/kg/d) and glycine (200 mg/kg/d) upon which the plasma and CSF serine and glycine levels normalized, although treatment had limited effect on seizure activity or any of his neurological symptoms. This child died at the age of 7 months. In contrast, his younger sister was diagnosed within hours after birth and immediate treatment prevented the onset of neurological symptoms up to 3 years of follow-up (10). Her height and head circumference showed some catch up growth upon amino acid treatment and imaging of her brain during follow-up revealed no abnormalities. The latter case is once again an important illustration that treatment in infantile serine deficiency should start before the onset of neurological symptoms and awareness among clinicians of this disorder is therefore important.

Diagnosis: The siblings published by Hart et al (10) also illustrated some pitfalls in confirmation of the diagnosis. Plasma serine and glycine in the index patient were only marginally below the reference range and were easily overlooked (Table 18.1), but in line with the other serine defects, the biochemical abnormalities were more pronounced in CSF than in plasma. Furthermore, the enzymatic assay of PSAT in the index patient was inconclusive and the defect could only be confirmed after mutation analysis and expression studies of the mutated protein. It is reasonable to assume that these diagnostic pitfalls are not specific for PSAT deficiency and that confirmation of the clinical and biochemical suspicion by mutation analysis is required in all serine deficiency disorders.

PHOSPHOSERINE PHOSPHATASE DEFICIENCY

Phosphoserine phosphatase (PSP) deficiency was reported only in a single case of a boy who suffered also from Williams syndrome (14). This boy had a proven microdeletion of 7q11.23 involving the elastin region, but in addition to the Williams syndrome phenotype he also had intrauterine growth retardation, feeding difficulties, hypospadias, and microcephaly. Biochemical analysis at the age of 1 year revealed low concentrations of serine in plasma and CSF, suspicious for a serine synthesis defect. In fact it turned out that the boy suffered from two disorders, Williams syndrome and PSP deficiency. The enzymatic defect in PSP was confirmed in cultured skin fibroblasts and by mutation analysis of the PSP gene (15).

The boy was treated with L-serine (300 mg/kg/d), which resulted in normalization of CSF serine concentration and catch-up in head circumference. However, the patient was lost to follow-up so unfortunately there is no documentation of long-term results of treatment. It appears that the PSP deficiency in this boy was rather mild given that there was not a history of severe psychomotor retardation or seizures.

Diagnosis: The values of serine and glycine in plasma and CSF of this patient are in Table 18.1. Serine was low to low normal in plasma, CSF serine was low, and glycine concentrations in CSF and plasma were normal. The diagnosis of PSP deficiency needs to be confirmed by enzymatic assay in cultured skin fibroblasts or mutation analysis, similar to the other serine deficiency disorders.

OVERLAPPING AND NONOVERLAPPING CLINICAL FINDINGS IN SERINE DEFICIENCY DISORDERS

From the patients reported to date with an infantile serine deficiency disorder, the overlapping symptoms were microcephaly, developmental delay and seizures. It is evident, however, that microcephaly may not be present at birth. The response to treatment with amino acids and the MRI findings were quite different in infantile 3-PGDH deficiency and PSAT deficiency. In 3-PGDH deficiency the seizures do respond to amino acid therapy, whereas in PSAT the response to amino acids was rather disappointing. The MRI in PSAT revealed generalized atrophy and abnormalities of the pons and cerebellum; this has not been reported in 3-PGDH deficiency. These differences could be important clues to aid diagnostic procedures. From the biochemical analysis no discrimination can be made between the three different forms of serine

deficiency disorders, nor is it possible to predict the severity of the clinical phenotype on the basis of the biochemical results.

CONCLUSIONS

Patients with serine deficiency present with neurological symptoms, varying from severe abnormalities at birth such as congenital microcephaly and neonatal seizures to milder phenotypes in childhood manifest as developmental delay and absence seizures. The laboratory diagnosis of serine deficiency disorders is straightforward by routine amino acid analysis in CSF and plasma. One should be aware that low values and even marginally low values of amino acids can be very informative and that age-related reference ranges should be used for interpreting serine concentrations. Serine deficiency disorders are treatable, warranting prompt diagnosis and treatment.

FUTURE DIRECTIONS

The symptoms observed in serine deficiency disorders provide a striking example of the importance of L-serine during development and postnatal functioning of the CNS. Serine deficiency disorders can serve as a model system to study, for instance, cellular proliferation (given the presence of microcephaly) or the synthesis and metabolism of D-serine and glycine in relation to NMDA coupled neurotransmission. In particular, the role of these L-serine derived metabolites in the etiology of seizures is most interesting. The fact that the patients' seizures disappear when sufficient L-serine is present underscores the link between serine metabolites and inhibition of excitation. It is hypothesized that D-serine is the principal agent responsible for this effect (3).

From a clinical viewpoint it is very relevant to identify the complete clinical spectrum associated with serine deficiency disorders and to know the prevalence of serine deficiency among different diagnostic categories such as neonatal seizures and mild cognitive deficiency. Finally, given the fact that serine deficiency disorders are treatable, the suitability of this group of disorders for newborn screening needs further consideration.

CLINICAL PEARLS

- Serine deficiency disorders are a treatable group of inherited metabolic epilepsies.
- Infantile and juvenile onset phenotypes are observed.
- Microcephaly (acquired or congenital), intractable seizures, and severe psychomotor retardation are key symptoms in infantile serine deficiency.
- For patients with infantile onset, treatment consists of L-serine (500–700 mg/kg/d) with glycine added (200–300 mg/kg/d) when the results are unsatisfactory with regard to the seizures.
- Children with the juvenile form present at school age with developmental delay and absence seizures.
- These children need 100–150 mg/kg/d L-serine therapy
- Beware of the pitfalls of amino acid analysis in diagnosing serine deficiency.

REFERENCES

1. Jaeken J, Detheux M, Van ML, et al. 3-Phosphoglycerate dehydrogenase deficiency: an inborn error of serine biosynthesis. *Arch Dis Child.* 1996;74:542–545.
2. Tabatabaie L, Klomp LW, Berger R, et al. L-Serine synthesis in the central nervous system: a review on serine deficiency disorders. *Mol Genet Metab.* 2010;99:256–262.
3. Fuchs SA, Berger R, de Koning TJ. D-Serine: the right or wrong isoform? *Brain Res.* 2011;1401:104–117.
4. Pineda M, Vilaseca MA, Artuch R, et al. 3-Phosphoglycerate dehydrogenase deficiency in a patient with West syndrome. *Dev Med Child Neurol.* 2000;42:629–633.
5. de Koning TJ, Klomp LW, van Oppen AC, et al. Prenatal and early postnatal treatment in 3-phosphoglycerate-dehydrogenase deficiency. *Lancet.* 2004;364:2221–2222.
6. de Koning TJ, Jaeken J, Pineda M, et al. Hypomyelination and reversible white matter attenuation in 3-phosphoglycerate dehydrogenase deficiency. *Neuropediatrics.* 2000;31:287–292.
7. Tabatabaie L, Klomp LW, Rubio-Gozalbo ME, et al. Expanding the clinical spectrum of 3-phosphoglycerate dehydrogenase deficiency. *J Inherit Metab Dis.* 2011;34:181–184.
8. Moat S, Carling R, Nix A, et al. Multicentre age-related reference intervals for cerebrospinal fluid serine concentrations: Implications for the diagnosis and follow-up of serine biosynthesis disorders. *Mol Genet Metab.* 2010;101:149–152.
9. Tabatabaie L, de Koning TJ, Geboers AJ, et al. Novel mutations in 3-phosphoglycerate dehydrogenase (PHGDH) are distributed throughout the protein and result in altered enzyme kinetics. *Hum Mutat.* 2009;30:749–756.
10. Hart CE, Race V, Achouri Y, et al. Phosphoserine aminotransferase deficiency: a novel disorder of the serine biosynthesis pathway. *Am J Hum Genet.* 2007;80:931–937.
11. de Koning TJ, Duran M, Dorland L, et al. Beneficial effects of L-serine and glycine in the management of seizures in 3-phosphoglycerate dehydrogenase deficiency. *Ann Neurol.* 1998;44:261–265.
12. de Koning TJ. Treatment with amino acids in serine deficiency disorders. *J Inherit Metab Dis.* 2006;29:347–351.
13. de Koning TJ, Duran M, Van ML, et al. Congenital microcephaly and seizures due to 3-phosphoglycerate dehydrogenase deficiency: outcome of treatment with amino acids. *J Inherit Metab Dis.* 2002;25:119–125.
14. Jaeken J, Detheux M, Fryns JP, et al. Phosphoserine phosphatase deficiency in a patient with Williams syndrome. *J Med Genet.* 1997;34:594–596.
15. Veiga-da-Cunha M, Collet JF, Prieur B, et al. Mutations responsible for 3-phosphoserine phosphatase deficiency. *Eur J Hum Genet.* 2004;12:163–166.

19

Lesch–Nyhan Disease and Epilepsy

Beth A. Markowski-Leeman and Hyder A. Jinnah

INTRODUCTION

Lesch–Nyhan disease is an X-linked recessive disorder characterized by a deficiency of the enzyme hypoxanthine-guanine phophoribosyltransferase (HPRT), resulting in the overproduction of uric acid. While the underlying mutations and phenotypes may differ between patients, a neurobehavioral syndrome that includes intellectual disability, self-injurious behavior, and motor dysfunction is characteristic. Variant forms may occur, in which there is a partial deficiency of the enzyme, milder symptoms, and a lack of overt self-injury.

Epilepsy occurs with greater prevalence in patients with Lesch-Nyhan disease (LND) and LND variants than in the general population. No studies, however, have addressed the relationship between LND and seizures. Hence, the precise frequency, risk factors, underlying mechanisms, semiology, and natural history of seizure disorders in LND are unclear. Furthermore, there are no guidelines for the appropriate evaluation and management of seizures in this population. The 28 cases of seizures in the setting of LND reported in the literature to date (Table 19.1) are reviewed below. The differential diagnoses, etiology, demographics, seizure types, electroencephalography (EEG) data, neuroimaging characteristics, pathological findings, and issues in evaluation and management of seizures specific to patients with LND are addressed.

DIFFERENTIAL DIAGNOSIS

To distinguish between seizures and the motor and behavioral manifestations of LND is important to ensure appropriate evaluation and treatment. The distinctions, however, can be difficult and may lead to an overestimation of the frequency of seizures in LND. The motor disorder in LND may include dystonic movements, characterized by involuntary, sustained, stereotypical, and at times repetitive muscle contractions, causing twisting or abnormal posturing. Opisthotonus, or arching of the back, is common (1, 2). When the posturing is sustained with whole-body dystonic tremors or myoclonic jerks, it may appear similar to a generalized tonic-clonic (GTC) seizure.

In "dystonic storm" or status dystonicus, the patient exhibits severe, potentially fatal, generalized dystonia and rigidity, often with a jerky tremor, refractory to standard medical management (3–5). Pain, exhaustion, and hyperpyrexia may be present. Similar to prolonged GTC seizures or status epilepticus, airway compromise, rhabdomyolysis leading to renal failure, and dehydration with metabolic derangements may be evident. Patients typically require intubation and sedation. The key distinguishing features between status dystonicus and status epilepticus, however, relate to level of consciousness, time course, semiology, and precipitating factors (Table 19.2). Loss of consciousness is a necessary feature of GTC seizures,

TABLE 19.1 Reports of LND and LND Variants With Seizures

Case	Age at sz Onset	Sz Type	Recurrence	Sz Frequency	Treatment	Other Meds	Treatment Outcome	EEG	Structural Lesions	Other Risk Factors
Berman (1969) Case 3	8 mos	NR	Yes	None after 13 mos	No AEDs listed	Allopurinol	NA	Diffuse background slowing	NR	Mother w/alcoholism, no prenatal care
Christie et al. (1982) Case LS	5 y	GTC	Yes	NR	NR	NR	NR	NR	NR	NR
Christie et al. (1982) Case SS	2 mos–3 y	NR	Yes	NR	NR	NR	NR	NR	NR	NR
Del Bigio et al. (2007)	9 y	GTC	Yes	2 szs in 1 y	NR	NR	NR	"Left occipital seizure focus"	Multifocal degeneration of internal granular layer of cerebellum, relative sparing of Purkinje cells, reactive astrogliosis of the molecular layer	NR
Ferrández et al. (1982)	<10 y	NR	Yes	NR	No AEDs listed	Allopurinol	NA	NR	NR	Anoxia at birth
Hoefnagel et al. (1965) Case III6	<2.8 y	GTC	Yes	Several last four mos of life	NR	NR	NR	NR	Two small areas of "softening" (left parietal lobe and brainstem) (Path)	NR
Hoefnagel et al. (1965) Case III8	6 y	GTC	Yes	1/yr	NR	NR	NR	NR	NR	NR
Jinnah (2006) Case 15	<10 y	GTC	Yes	NR	No AED	None	NA	NR	NR	NR
Jinnah (2006) Case 21	<12 y	GTC	Yes	NR	CBZ, clonazepam	Folate	NR	NR	NR	NR
Jinnah (2006) Case 41	<32 y	GTC	Yes	NR	Primidone, PB	Baclofen	NR	NR	NR	NR

Reference / Case	Age of onset	Seizure type		Seizure frequency	AED	Urate-lowering treatment	Seizure outcome	EEG	Imaging	Other
Jinnah (2010) Case 16 (V)	Childhood	NR	Yes	2 szs in 17 y	No AED	Allopurinol, baclofen, nifedipine	NA	NR	NR	NR
Kelley et al. (1969) Case AR (V)	13 y	GTC	Yes	NR	DPH, PB	Colchicine, probenecid	"Easily controlled"	NR	NR	NR
Kenney (1991)	<17 y	NR	Yes	NR	No AEDs listed	Allopurinol	NA	NR	NR	NR
Lohiya et al. (2003)	<30 y	GTC	Yes	NR	PB, VPA	Allopurinol	NR	NR	NR	NR
Lynch et al. (1991)	12 y	GTC	Yes	2/yr	CBZ, diazepam	Baclofen, allopurinol	Sz-free with CBZ	NR	Normal (CT, MRI)	NR
McCarthy et al. (2010)	<20 y	NR	Yes	"Minor epilepsy"	No AEDs listed	Allopurinol	NA	NR	NR	NR
Michener (1967) Case 1	5.5 mos*	GTC, focal (left UE/LE)	Yes	2 szs in 6.5 y	No AED	Probenecid, allopurinol	Sz-free with probenecid, allopurinol	Normal	Normal (PEG)	NR
Michener (1967) Case 4	22 mos**	GTC, "minor motor"	Yes	GTCs 1/year, several focal szs over 3 y	No AED	Probenecid	NA	Normal	NR	Febrile convulsion
Mitchell et al. (1984)	9 y	GTC	Yes	NR	NR	NR	NR	NR	Focal cerebellar gliosis (Path)	NR
Mizuno (1986) Case 5	<10 y	GTC, partial	Yes	NR	AEDs, type not specified	Benz-bromarone	Sz-free with AEDs	NR	NR	NR
Mizuno (1986) Case 9	neonatal	GTC	NR	NR	No AED	Benz-bromarone	"Healed naturally" as neonate	NR	No specific lesion (Path)	NR
Newcombe et al. (1966); Dreifuss et al. (1968)	16 mos	GTC	Yes	NR	AEDs, type not specified	Sodium bicarbonate, allopurinol	sz-free with AEDs	Right occipital slowing	Mild atrophy (PEG)	NR
Nyhan et al. (1967) Case DB	3 y	GTC	Yes	"Subsided" after 1 yr	NR	NR	NR	NR	NR	NR

(continued)

TABLE 19.1   Reports of LND and LND Variants With Seizures (*continued*)

Case	Age at sz Onset	Sz Type	Recurrence	Sz Frequency	Treatment	Other Meds	Treatment Outcome	EEG	Structural Lesions	Other Risk Factors
Nyhan et al. (1967) Case GW	<5 y	GTC	Yes	NR	NR	NR	NR	NR	NR	NR
Puliyel et al. (1984)	3 y	GTC, "tonic spasms"	Yes	3 szs in 7 y	PB, diazepam	NR	Two breakthrough szs in 7 y	NR	NR	NR
Riley (1960)	7.7 y	GTC	No	NA	No AED	Colchicine, benemid	NA	NR	NR	NR
Sass et al. (1965)	10.5 y	Tonic, w/left UE monoplegia	No	NA	No AEDs listed	Antibiotics	NA	NR	Cerebral atrophy or dysgenesis (PEG); "Slight size reduction," diffuse demyelinative, degenerative and vascular lesions, subarachnoid hemorrhage, urate granules (Path)	NR
Wada et al. (1968)	2 mos	GTC	Yes	NR	NR	NR	NR	Diffuse "dysrhythmia" w/spikes and sharp waves	Dilated lateral ventricles, frontal air accumulation (PEG); Hydrocephalus, medullary atrophy, diffuse degeneration, necrosis, demyelination and gliosis (Path)	Febrile convulsions

Seizures in the setting of LND and LND variants reported in the literature to date. NA = not applicable; NR = not reported; Sz = seizure, V = variant.

TABLE 19.2 **Differentiation of Status Dystonicus and Status Epilepticus**

	Status Dystonicus	Status Epilepticus
Onset/Offset	Sudden or gradual over days, weeks, or months	Sudden, within seconds to minutes
Consciousness	Preserved	Preserved with simple partial seizures Impaired with complex partial or generalized seizures
Focality	May be present at onset	May be present at onset
Tremor	May include tremor or flapping motions	May include tremor or large jerks; flapping often indicates nonepileptic etiology
Opisthotonus	Common	Rare; may be evident with frontal seizures
Myoclonus	Atypical in LND but common in status dystonicus	Evident with specific epilepsy syndromes (ie, JME)
Induced by stimulation or voluntary movement	Common	Rare
Other common precipitants	• Trauma or surgery • Excitement/anticipation • Stress • Infection, fever • Abrupt introduction, withdrawal or change of certain drugs (ie, initiation of clonazepam, zinc, D-penicilamine; discontinuation of lithium or tetrabenazine)	• Stress • Infection, fever • Sleep deprivation • Drug initiation (eg, buproprion, tramadol) or withdrawal (ie, anticonvulsants)
Hyperpyrexia	May be trigger or result from status dystonicus	May be trigger
Post-ictal state	None	Typically confusion, fatigue; frontal seizures associated with rapid return to baseline
Tongue-biting	• Conscious self-injury • Anterior tongue and lips	• During tonic phase, unconscious • Postero-lateral aspect of tongue
Airway compromise	Common	Common; often due to sedating medications
Metabolic derangements	Common	May be present
Rhabdomyolysis	Common	May be present
Management	May respond to anticonvulsants; most commonly treatments focus on benzodiazepines, dopamine agonists, anticholinergics, and/or propofol	Anticonvulsants, may require sedatives (eg, propofol, pentobarbital, midazolam)
Incidence	Rare	Common

Features differentiating status dystonicus from status epilepticus. JME = juvenile myoclonic epilepsy.

while consciousness is maintained in dystonia. Seizures are also of sudden onset and offset, over seconds to minutes, rather than the time course of weeks to months often seen with dystonic storm. Truncal twisting and arching is unusual in epilepsy, unless of frontal lobe onset. Finally, seizures, in contrast with dystonia, are rarely triggered by voluntary movement.

Other symptoms of LND must be distinguished from seizures, as well. These include tics or stereotypies due to tardive dyskinesia (1). Tongue biting may be a component of self-injurious behavior, and should be discriminated from the lacerations that may occur during a convulsion. The tongue bites sustained during convulsions occur during the tonic phase while consciousness is impaired, and lie along the postero-lateral aspect of the tongue. In contrast, patients with LND are aware during the biting behavior, with the lacerations typically located along the anterior portion of the tongue and lips (2). Patients with LND may have pronounced emotional lability with overt panic attacks, which must be differentiated from partial seizure activity (Table 19.3). Attention deficit hyperactivity disorder (ADHD), as well as other nonspecific attentional difficulties, may be

TABLE 19.3 Differentiation of Panic Attacks and Partial Seizures

	Panic Attacks	Partial Seizures
Duration of episode	Longer duration, last at least 5–15 min up to several hours	Brief, typically lasting 30 sec to 2 min
Variability of symptoms	Variable symptoms and sequence	More stereotyped
Consciousness	Preserved	May progress to alteration/loss of awareness
Postevent symptoms	No confusion/amnesia	May have confusion/amnesia
Symptom onset	Slow building of symptoms	Rapid shifts of symptoms
Déjà vu, olfactory or gustatory hallucinations	Rare Hallucinations in psychiatric disease perceived as internal to self, often with associated paranoia	Greater than 5% Hallucinations perceived as external to self, without paranoia
Smothering or choking sensation, tachypnea	Common	Rare
Anticipatory anxiety	Common	Uncommon
Associated symptoms (aphasia, gustatory hallucinations, behavioral arrest, automatisms)	Uncommon	May be associated as progress to CPS
Treatment	Response to benzodiazepines, antidepressants; other AEDs occasionally helpful	Response to AEDs, resection May rarely worsen with certain antidepressants (ie, tricyclics)
Recurrence	More associated with periods of emotional upset; occur in wakefulness	Sporadic; may occur during sleep
Agoraphobia	50%	No association
Family history	25.1% first-degree relatives with panic disorder	Uncommon
Palpitations	Tachycardia	Brady or tachycardia
Paresthesias	Peri-oral, distal extremities associated with hyperventilation	May be generalized although bilaterality rare; often focal, unilateral
EEG	Usually normal	Often abnormal
MRI	Usually normal	Lesions common
Age of onset	Most often 20–30 y	Any age

Features differentiating panic attacks from partial seizures. AEDs = antiepileptic drugs, CPS = complex partial seizures. Reprinted from *Wyllie's Treatment of Epilepsy*, 5th ed. Philadelphia: Lippincott Williams & Wilkins, 2011: 1043, with permission.

diagnosed in patients with LND variants and should be distinguished from the more discrete episodes of unresponsiveness characteristic of complex partial seizures. Hitting, biting, spitting, and vomiting on others may be evident in LND, with retained awareness of the aggressive behavior. This must be differentiated from the aggression seen during post-ictal confusion.

Less clearly differentiated from seizure activity, however, is episodic apnea with cyanosis of uncertain etiology infrequently seen in LND. Jinnah et al documented two such cases, and while "EEG studies provided no evidence for epilepsy," it was unclear whether EEGs were obtained during the spells (1). Three additional cases were observed in our center since that time. While these events resolved over time in some, others proved fatal. In addition, Lynch et al reported a case of LND with recurrent episodes of coma associated with acute illness (6). EEGs were not performed during these spells, as "there was nothing to suggest clinically nonconvulsive status epilepticus." It remains unclear what these events represent.

To definitively establish a diagnosis of seizures, the events in question must be captured on an EEG recording. To date, there have been no reports of continuous EEG monitoring in LND patients.

MECHANISMS OF SEIZURE GENERATION

The process by which HPRT deficiency leads to seizures is unknown. Evidence to support a direct role of uric acid in seizure generation is limited. A rat model suggests that generalized seizures induced by electroconvulsive shock or flurothyl are associated with increased levels of uric acid in the serum and striatal tissue, with levels reduced by systemic injection of allopurinol (7). Serum uric acid is also increased after status epilepticus or recurrent generalized convulsions (over 2–4 h) with cyanosis in humans (8). Nevertheless, the associations do not imply causation. The uric acid elevations may be a consequence of the seizure activity, resulting from impaired excretion or increased production due to muscle activity and breakdown.

While allopurinol may reduce seizure-associated uric acid elevations and decrease seizure frequency, these findings also fail to establish elevated uric acid as a causative factor (7, 9–11). Allopurinol inhibits the enzyme xanthine oxidase, which normally catalyzes

the conversion of hypoxanthine to xanthine and uric acid, thereby lowering uric acid levels. It has been suggested that the efficacy of allopurinol for seizure prevention correlates with the decrease in serum uric acid, with better results obtained with levels below 2 mg/dL (12). The present review, however, indicates no relationship between uric acid level and the occurrence of seizures, nor was there a difference in serum uric acid levels between responders and nonresponders to the use of allopurinol as an anticonvulsant (12). It may be that the efficacy of allopurinol relates to mechanisms of action other than alteration of uric acid levels. Allopurinol influences purine synthesis and degradation, specifically adenosine levels, which may have anticonvulsant properties. Its effect may also relate to structural similarities with traditional anticonvulsants.

Dreifuss et al was the first to propose that hyperuricemia was unlikely to cause the neurological symptoms of LND (13). Normal levels of CSF uric acid support this hypothesis. In addition, other disorders involving excessive production of uric acid do not include the neurobehavioral features of LND, that is, seizures are not a feature of gout. It is possible that the neurological complications of this hyperuricemic disorder arise in an indirect manner. The demands of excessive purine biosynthesis, toxic byproducts of purine synthesis, depletion of purine bases, or insufficiencies from diversion of substrates into the uric acid pathway may be responsible, and may be evident during critical periods for brain maturation.

Another mechanism that could increase the risk of epilepsy in LND involves adenosine. Adenosine is a neuroactive purine with the ability to reduce neuronal excitability and seizures. Several investigators have proposed that the enzyme defect in LND could lead to adenosine deficiency (14–19). While their studies focused primarily on abnormal interactions between adenosine and dopamine in the basal ganglia as a cause for the movement disorder and behavioral problems, adenosine deficiency also could lower seizure thresholds in the cerebral cortex. Clinically significant adenosine deficiency, however, has not been demonstrated in the LND brain to date.

Alternatively, other compounds in the pathway of HPRT may be responsible for seizure generation. Levels of xanthine, the precursor to uric acid, are also elevated in LND (20). Excessive xanthine may trigger a chain of events that produces increased endogenous convulsants (kynurenine and quinolinic acid) and diminished endogenous anticonvulsants (serotonin and gamma aminobutyric acid). While Gedye proposed that this pathway leads to self-injury, we posit that this pathway may explain, in part, the increased incidence of generalized convulsions in this population (21). Allopurinol may have anticonvulsant activity because it inhibits tryptophan pyrrolase, which reduces quinolinic acid production. While isolated reports of elevated CSF xanthine documented no associated CNS disorder, it may be that elevated xanthine is necessary but not sufficient for epileptogenesis. Perhaps the xanthine level must cross a certain threshold, the xanthine must be shunted down this particular metabolic pathway, or an underlying lowered seizure threshold by other mechanisms is also needed for epileptogenesis to occur. These hypotheses should be further explored in LND.

DEMOGRAPHICS

PREVALENCE

While uncommon, and perhaps not characteristic of LND, the prevalence of epilepsy in LND is likely increased relative to the general population. In the United States, 1% of the population under age 20 years will be diagnosed with epilepsy, with a worldwide prevalence of 0.5% to 1%. Jinnah et al. reviewed 254 LND cases in the literature, in which 1.3% had seizures as the presenting feature of the disorder (1). Estimates of the prevalence of seizures during the course of the disease ranged from 7% to 10.5% to approximately 35% to 50% as suggested by older literature (1, 2, 13). Seizures may also be evident in patients with partial HPRT deficiencies. In the review by Jinnah et al. 3.1% of patients with LND variants presented with seizures, with lifetime prevalence estimated at 2.2% to 14.9% (22).

AGE OF ONSET

Although seizures may be the presenting feature of LND in a small number of patients, the first signs more commonly relate to delayed motor development. Seizures typically occurred in later stages of the disorder, in early childhood (23). Of the 28 individual cases of seizures described in the literature to date, only 16 listed a clear age of onset, ranging from the neonatal period to 13 years.

RISK FACTORS

The classic risk factors for epilepsy in the general population do not appear to play a significant role in LND, suggesting that seizures are a consequence of the disease itself. Birth injuries, febrile seizures, family histories of epilepsy, head trauma, and CNS infections were not commonly noted. In one case, seizures were preceded by anoxia at birth, and another patient was born to a mother with alcoholism and no prenatal care (24, 25). Typically, however, the prenatal, birth, and neonatal histories were unremarkable (23, 26–31). In one patient, the initial seizure occurred in the setting of a fever secondary to an upper respiratory infection, and in one infant, seizures occurred repeatedly in association with fever of unknown origin (26, 30). In the remaining 26 cases, however, seizures occurred without known fevers or infections. Nor does family history of seizures necessarily suggest an increased risk in a given patient. Seizures may be evident in a patient with LND, but not present in a sibling with the disorder (23, 26, 32). Furthermore, two brothers were born of parents with febrile seizures, yet neither of the children with LND had epilepsy (33). Finally, no cases of serious head trauma with loss of consciousness or CNS infections were noted in patients with LND and epilepsy.

Although Michener described a case in which a seizure occurred when the serum uric acid level peaked, the level of uric acid in serum or urine does not typically correlate with the risk for seizures (26). Nor does the underlying HPRT genetic mutation appear to be predictive, although limited genetic data are available. Seizures have been reported in patients with IVS7 + 5G > A, G209A, and G212T mutations, as well as an E2-3 deletion (1, 22). Further studies are needed to evaluate the relationship between mutation type and risk of epilepsy.

Learning and intellectual disabilities are often associated with seizures in the general population, and patients with LND typically have static encephalopathy. IQ estimates in LND patients with seizures ranged from 32 to 110, with the majority demonstrating significant impairments. It is difficult to establish accurate IQs in this patient population, however, as many cannot participate in standard testing due to motor or behavioral issues. Hence, it has not been possible to obtain a reliable or valid assessment of the relationship between seizures and cognitive function.

SEIZURE CLASSIFICATION

The vast majority of seizures reported are GTC. Semiologies provided in reports on 22 patients include GTCs alone ($n = 17$), tonic seizures alone ($n = 1$), GTCs and partial seizures ($n = 3$), and GTCs and tonic seizures ($n = 1$). Although descriptions of generalized convulsions were consistent with GTCs, the possibility of prolonged opisthotonic posturing with superimposed dystonic tremors could not be excluded. Whether the GTCs were of primary generalization at onset is also uncertain. A focal onset followed by secondary generalization, missed by observers or not otherwise reported, is possible. In many cases, seizures were reported by caregivers but not directly observed by investigators. Evidence for focality was suggested by the co-occurrence of GTC or tonic seizures with "minor motor" seizures, partial seizures, a focal seizure of the left arm and leg, and a likely Todd's paralysis of the left upper extremity (26, 31, 34). Right occipital slowing evident in the EEG of one patient and a left occipital abnormality in another were also suggestive of focal epileptogenic processes (13, 27, 35). Insufficient data exists, however, to suggest a common focus of epileptogenesis across patients. In metabolic epilepsies, it is also possible for the focus to shift, or for a focal process to become generalized over time. To document that these events are in fact epileptic, establish whether convulsions are of primary or secondary generalization, and determine the site of onset would require capturing seizures during video-EEG monitoring.

EEG CHARACTERISTICS

No specific EEG signature of LND has been identified. EEG is considered to be of limited value in establishing the diagnosis of LND, and is not often obtained or reported. When reported, findings are often normal, abnormalities are nonspecific, or findings are not clearly described. Nor are there consistent associations to suggest normalization by medications or relationships to uric acid levels.

Of the 28 individual reports of seizures, six had documented EEGs, only one with a clear epileptiform abnormality, consisting of a "diffuse dysrhythmia with spikes and sharp waves" (30). The remaining studies were normal ($n = 2$), showed diffuse slowing ($n = 1$), demonstrated focal right occipital slowing ($n = 1$), or revealed a "left occipital seizure focus" not further described ($n = 1$) (Table 19.1). Several EEG reports of patients with LND but no history of seizures are shown in Table 19.4, many of which were abnormal. When present, abnormalities typically consisted of generalized slowing and "dysrhythmias." One patient was noted to have epileptiform abnormalities, consisting of "some paroxysmal, rather sharp 7–12 sec activity" in the "frontotemporal area, predominantly on the right" (36). Whether this subject later developed seizures is unknown, and the predictive value of EEG is this population is unclear.

An "intermittent ill-localized slow wave abnormality from the right temporal region" was also evident in one patient; however, data are insufficient to suggest a particular focus of EEG abnormality in patients with LND (37). As previously noted, in metabolic disorders, apparent generalized changes may evolve from focal abnormalities ("secondarily" generalized), and focal discharges may change in location over time.

STRUCTURAL ABNORMALITIES

In the majority of LND patients with epilepsy, neuroimaging findings were not reported, as they are not considered to be useful in establishing the diagnosis. No lesions specific to LND have been identified, and in general, the majority of imaging studies in LND and LND variants are normal (6, 20, 38). It is possible that lesions were overlooked in older studies, however, as imaging was limited to less detailed pneumoencephalography or CT scans. Atrophy was the most common abnormality noted, often suggested by pneumoencephalography (13, 26, 27, 31, 33). Atrophy was evident in 12% to 18% of patients on CT or MRI, which may be subtle and require volumetric techniques in order to detect (1, 22).

Nor have there been any consistent neuropathological changes noted on autopsy in LND patients. In some cases, no lesions are identified (37). When lesions are found, it is unclear whether they are related to the disease process, and whether uric acid plays any role in their generation. The most common abnormality is mild to moderate microcephaly (39, 40). In addition to low brain weight, Bassermann et al. noted slight cerebral edema (40). Wada et al. found severe hydrocephalus with thinning of the

TABLE 19.4   Electroencephalography in LND and LND Variants

Case	EEG	Structural Lesions	Treatment
Andrés et al. (1987) (V)	Normal	Normal (CT)	Allopurinol, sodium bicarbonate
Bassermann et al. (1979)	"No signs of seizures"	No lesions (Path)	NR
Bunn et al. (1975) Case MB	"Irregular slow activity from all areas"	NR	NR
Gasperini et al. (2010)	Normal	Normal (US); WM atrophy of bilateral temporal/insular regions (MRI)	NR
Geerdink et al. (1973) Case 1	Normal background, fronto-temporal (primarily right) "paroxysmal, rather sharp 7–12 sec activity"	NR	Probenecid, sodium bicarbonate, colchicine as needed, allopurinol, benzofuran
Hatanaka et al. (1990)	"Dysrhythmia"	Normal (CT)	Allopurinol
Kelley et al. (1969) Case FL (V)	"Diffuse dysrhythmia"; repeat EEG normal	NR	Allopurinol (prior to EEG), colchicine as needed; trials of probenecid, phenylbutazone, alkalinizing agents (eg, Shohl's solution, sodium bicarbonate), folic acid
Kelley et al. (1969) Case ML (V)	Normal	NR	Allopurinol (prior to EEG)
Lesch et al. (1964) Case EW	"Disorganized," no "seizure discharges"	Minimal cerebral atrophy bilaterally (PEG)	NR
Mahnovski et al.	"Diffuse moderate cortical damage"	Brain weight slightly low, "focal degenerative changes" (Path)	NR
Michener (1967) Case 2	Normal	Possible "mild degree cortical atrophy," with follow-up imaging normal (PEG)	Probenecid (after EEG)
Michener (1967) Case 3	"Immature cortical discharge, diffusely with no evidence of focal defect or gross asymmetry"	NR	Probenecid (after EEG)
Michener (1967) Case 5	"Diffuse cerebral dysrhythmia, possible of subcortical origin"	NR	Probenecid (after EEG)
Michener (1967) Case 6	Normal	NR	Probenecid (after EEG)

(continued)

TABLE 19.4 **Electroencephalography in LND and LND Variants** (*continued*)

Case	EEG	Structural Lesions	Treatment
Partington et al. (1967) Case 1, A	"Marked dysrhythmia," slow background, "intermittent ill-localized slow wave abnormality from the right temporal region"	NR	Allopurinol, sodium citrate/citric acid (after EEG)
Partington et al. (1967) Case 2, S	Normal	No lesions (Path)	NR
Reed et al. (1966)	Normal	NR	Diazepam, phenobarbital, probenecid, sodium bicarbonate (after EEG)*
Rijksen et al. (1981) (V)	"Very irregular without marked abnormalities"	NR	Allopurinol (prior to EEG)
Schulman et al. (1971)	Normal	NR	Adenine, allopurinol (after EEG)
Shnier et al. (1972) Case 1	"General dysrhythmia suggesting a generalized cerebral abnormality"	NR	Allopurinol (after EEG)
Shnier et al. (1972) Case 2	"Generalized dysrhythmia"	NR	Allopurinol (after EEG)
Watts et al. (1974)	Normal	NR	Trials of blood transfusion, adenine, allopurinol, tetrabenazine, thiopropazate, chlorpromazine

EEG features of patients with LND and LND variants, but no reported seizures. Path = pathology; PEG = pneumoencephalogram; US = ultrasound; V = variant; WM = white matter; *Unclear whether AEDs were initiated after the EEG; uric acid lowering agents were given after the EEG was obtained.

cortex, neocortical, and cerebellar degenerative and necrotic changes, and diffuse demyelination and gliosis (30). Sass et al. documented widespread demyelinating and vascular lesions in the central white matter of the cortex and cerebellum, some containing urate granules, similar to the changes seen with uremia (31). Rare foci of recent subarachnoid hemorrhage were also noted. Hoefnagel et al. reported a patient with two small areas of "softening" in the left parietal lobe and brainstem, without further description (23). Crome et al. found cortical neuronal loss, superficial gliosis, and in one case, multiple foci of cerebellar cortical necrosis (41). Del Bigio described two cases of multifocal internal granular layer atrophy with relative sparing of Purkinje cells, and suggested that common cerebellar abnormalities could underlie some features of LND (35). In the four brains examined at autopsy in our center, however, none exhibited cerebellar lesions. While it is possible that differences between studies are due to severity of disease, this is unlikely. Due to these variable findings, we presume that seizures in LND are not due to a common structural lesion.

EVALUATION AND MANAGEMENT

AFEBRILE SEIZURES

The American Academy of Neurology established practice parameters for the evaluation and treatment of the first nonfebrile seizure in children (42, 43). Routine EEG was recommended as a standard of care to predict the risk of recurrence and classify the seizure type or syndrome. Toxicology and other laboratory studies, lumbar puncture, and neuroimaging were suggested in individual cases based upon age and clinical presentation. MRI was the preferred imaging modality, to be considered in the event of a prolonged post-ictal focal deficit or a failure to return to baseline after several hours. Furthermore, imaging "should be seriously considered in any child with a significant cognitive or motor impairment of unknown etiology, unexplained abnormalities on neurologic examination, a seizure of partial (focal) onset with or without secondary generalization, an EEG that does not represent a benign partial epilepsy of childhood or primary generalized epilepsy, or in children under 1 year of age." Many patients with seizures in the setting of LND will fall into these latter categories.

The decision to treat an otherwise healthy child with anticonvulsants after the first seizure should be individualized, weighing the risk of side effects against the benefits of preventing recurrence. The determination largely depends upon the risk of repeated seizures. An abnormal neurological examination, epileptiform discharges on EEG, and a "remote symptomatic" etiology may carry an increased risk of recurrence. A remote symptomatic etiology refers to seizures "without immediate cause but with a prior identifiable major brain insult such as severe trauma or accompanying a condition such as cerebral palsy or mental retardation," as in LND. In the setting of a remote symptomatic etiology, recurrence rates exceed 50%. In our review of the literature, 25 of the 28 LND patients with seizures were clearly documented to have had repeated events. Hence, in the LND population, one may consider chronic treatment after the first unprovoked seizure. Further studies are needed, however, to establish a standard of care in this patient group.

FEBRILE SEIZURES

In neurologically healthy children, simple febrile seizures confer a minimally heightened risk of epilepsy compared to the general population, and are considered to be benign events with good prognoses. Recent guidelines from the American Academy of Pediatrics for the evaluation of children with simple febrile seizures suggest that clinicians focus on identifying the cause of the fever, with lumbar puncture performed when there is concern for meningitis (44).

EEG, bloodwork, and neuroimaging are generally not indicated, nor is treatment with antiepileptic drugs (AEDs). Although treatment with anticonvulsants may reduce the probability of additional febrile seizures, the risk of side effects typically outweighs the benefit. Furthermore, chronic AED use will not prevent later afebrile seizures. Antipyretics may reduce the risk of febrile seizures if administered early, however, and should be considered.

Nevertheless, these guidelines do not apply to children with known neurologic abnormalities or complex febrile seizures, which are focal, last $\geq$15 min, and/or recur within 24 hours. Such patients are at a higher risk for development of epilepsy, with risks increased in the setting of a complex febrile seizure, a family history of epilepsy, and neurodevelopmental abnormalities such as cerebral palsy (45). Consistent with this data, the two LND patients described with febrile seizures both had recurrent events. The AAP guidelines do not pertain to patients with LND, and there are no specific treatment recommendations for this patient group. It is suggested, however, that imaging be obtained in a child with a febrile seizure and possible structural defect, as in cases of microcephaly or spasticity, with MRI the preferred modality.

ANTICONVULSANT MEDICATIONS: OPTIONS, SIDE EFFECTS AND DRUG–DRUG INTERACTIONS

Data regarding anticonvulsant therapy in this population are insufficient to establish guidelines for the choice of AED. In many cases, seizures appeared to be easily controlled by older generation anticonvulsants, including phenytoin, phenobarbital, and carbamazepine (6, 13, 27, 32, 34, 46). These patients were treated prior to the availability of the newer generation of anticonvulsants (rufinamide, lacosamide, vigabatrin, pregabalin, oxcarbazepine, zonisamide, levetiracetam, tiagabine, topiramate, lamotrigine, gabapentin, and felbamate), and it is unclear whether these agents would be effective. In addition, it is impossible to determine in an individual case whether seizures were controlled by the traditional anticonvulsants, responded to the treatments for LND (ie, allopurinol), or would have abated regardless of treatment.

Given this limited information, the choice of AED should be individualized and guided by the side effect profile. Certain potential adverse effects of anticonvulsants are of particular concern in patients with

LND. Although data are conflicting, and declines may be minimal, cognitive impairments have been demonstrated with use of valproic acid (VPA), phenobarbital, primidone, carbamazepine, and phenytoin. Barbiturates are particularly concerning in this regard, and use should be carefully considered in children who may already have baseline cognitive deficits. Effects of newer agents on cognition in children have not been adequately studied. Phenobarbital, lamotrigine, and gabapentin may cause irritability or aggression, particularly in children and patients with learning disabilities. Levetiracetam can exacerbate irritability, and despite mood stabilizing properties, carbamazepine and VPA may cause paradoxical irritability. Topiramate and zonisamide may cause nephrolithiasis, and should be avoided in patients with a history of kidney stones. Since kidney stones are common in LND even during allopurinol treatment, it may be wise to discourage use. Topiramate and zonisamide can also lead to significant weight loss, which may be problematic in the underweight LND population. The majority of AEDs may also cause nausea or vomiting, most commonly associated with oxcarbazepine and VPA. Lamotrigine may produce insomnia, of concern in patients with poor sleep at baseline. Resting or intention tremors are classically associated with VPA, but tremor may also be evident with pregabalin, oxcarbazepine, rufinamide, lacosamide, and tiagabine. Tremors may be alleviated by primidone or topiramate.

Possible interactions between anticonvulsants and the medications used to treat the symptoms of LND should also be considered. Allopurinol, used to reduce uric acid levels in nearly all patients with LND, may cause a drug hypersensitivity syndrome including a rash. A similar syndrome may be evident with certain anticonvulsants (eg, lamotrigine, carbamazepine, phenytoin, phenobarbital, and primidone, as well as sulfa-based drugs such as topiramate and zonisamide), and it is important to distinguish which agent caused the adverse reaction in a given patient. Significant interactions between allopurinol and anticonvulsants, however, are rare. Zagnoni et al. and Coppola et al. found no significant changes in plasma AED levels with use of allopurinol in subjects taking concomitant VPA or phenobarbital (11, 12). Two patients, however, did have an increase in phenytoin levels with allopurinol, which led to phenytoin dosage reduction in one and withdrawal from the study due to phenytoin intoxication in the other (11). Although results for

carbamazepine have been more variable, Coppola et al. found a small but statistically significant increase in carbamazepine levels with allopurinol use (7 and 9 µg/mL during placebo and allopurinal phases, respectively) (12).

Of note, uric acid levels may be altered by AEDs, with decreases induced by carbamazepine and phenytoin. The effects of VPA and barbiturates have been variable. Uric acid levels typically become progressively lower with longer duration of AED therapy. Effects on uric acid levels were independent of AED levels, however, and did not correlate with seizure frequency (11, 12, 47, 48).

No interactions between AEDs and sodium bicarbonate, used to increase urinary alkalinization and promote uric acid solubility, have been reported. Metoclopramide, often used to improve gastric motility in LND, has no known interactions with AEDs. Nor have interactions been noted with baclofen or trihexyphenidyl, medications used to reduce muscle tone. Dantrolene, however, has theoretical interactions with barbiturates and benzodiazepines in that they may cause additive respiratory depression. When these drugs are used in combination, the patient should be monitored for decreased respiratory drive, with reduction in the dose of one or more drugs when necessary.

ALLOPURINOL IN THE TREATMENT OF SEIZURES

Traditionally, allopurinol is believed to have no effect on the neurological manifestations of LND. Although data are conflicting, some results indicate that allopurinol may be an effective anticonvulsant, reducing seizures in an estimated 30% to 75% of patients. The drug may be most effective when seizures are of recent onset, and are complex partial or secondarily generalized. The efficacy of allopurinol may also correlate with the decrease in serum uric acid, with better results obtained with levels below 2 mg/dL, as previously noted.

Much of the available data, however, derive from isolated case reports or uncontrolled studies. Coleman et al. described a 22-month-old with hyperuricosuria and complex partial and GTC seizures in the setting of tyronsinemia (9). The EEG was initially normal, but at 4 years of age, the child developed focal EEG abnormalities. The EEGs gradually evolved to a severely abnormal generalized pattern. By 8 years of age, the EEG demonstrated a disorganized background with nearly constant high voltage spikes and 3 to 5 seconds spike-wave discharges bilaterally. The seizures could not be controlled by more traditional AEDs, including phenobarbital, phenytoin, primidone, mephobarbital, acetazolamide, carbamazepine, and diazepam. Allopurinol, however, controlled the seizures within 3 days, leading to reduction of the other AEDs, normalization of the EEG, and cognitive improvement. Although he had several breakthroughs, they typically occurred in association with elevated uric acid levels, alterations in the dosage of allopurinol, or consumption of foods containing large amounts of purines.

The authors published a series including two similar patients, with hyperuricosuria and seizures beginning at age 22 months which were refractory to traditional AEDs (10). Although uric acid levels were elevated, they were not definitively diagnosed with LND. One patient had GTC seizures occurring every 2 to 3 months, despite treatment with phenobarbital, primidone, and carbamazepine. After treatment with allopurinol, seizures occurred less than once per year. The other patient had a febrile GTC, followed by the onset of afebrile convulsions. Phenobarbital and carbamazepine did not control the GTCs, occurring every 2 months. With allopurinol, the patient attained seizure freedom with improved behavior. While there were two breakthrough seizures, they were associated with a lowered allopurinol dose or ingestion of purine-containing foods.

An uncontrolled study suggesting responder rates (percentage of patients with less than or equal to 50% reduction in seizure frequency) of nearly 75% led to a double blind, randomized, placebo-controlled, add-on crossover trial of allopurinol in patients with medically refractory seizures and normal uric acid (11, 49). Allopurinol significantly reduced total seizure counts by 10.5%, and secondary generalized seizures by 27.9%. While results are conflicting, allopurinol may also be effective for simple partial, complex partial, atonic, myoclonic, tonic, absence, and atypical absence seizures (12, 49). The responder rates to allopurinol in these controlled studies ranged from 14% to 23.5% (11, 12). While long-term efficacy has been questioned, when breakthrough seizures occurred, they were often in the setting of allopurinol dosage reduction.

Of the 28 patients with LND and seizures described in the literature, one had possible resolution of seizure activity with allopurinol. It is not clear whether the seizures would have resolved regardless of treatment, and events were rare. It is also unknown whether seizures would be more frequent, or of greater prevalence, if the majority of LND patients were not taking allopurinol. Further studies regarding the anticonvulsant effects of allopurinol in this population are needed.

OTHER MANAGEMENT ISSUES: TREATMENT OF SLEEP AND BEHAVIORAL DISORDERS IN LND

Clinicians should also address factors that may reduce seizure thresholds in these patients. Sleep difficulties are common in LND, including sleep apnea. The resulting sleep deprivation may lower seizure thresholds. Sleep apnea may be alleviated by proper positioning at night to prevent hyperextension and blockage of the airway. Improved sleep quality may then reduce seizure frequency.

Antidepressant and antipsychotic medications are used to manage behavioral disorders (ie, self-injury) in LND, but may risk exacerbation of seizures. While the likelihood of seizures associated with these agents has not been studied specifically in LND, data from the general population suggests that the risks are minimal. The misconception that all antidepressants significantly lower seizure threshold and should be avoided is largely based upon data from overdoses, which have little predictive value when levels are within therapeutic range (50, 51). Lower doses of antidepressants may in fact have anticonvulsant properties (52). While the medications with substantial risk are few, it is prudent to avoid bupropion, particularly the immediate-release formulation, and maprotiline, which induce seizures in 0.36% to 5.8% and 12.2% to 15.6% of patients, respectively (52). In addition, the tricyclic antidepressants (TCAs; amitriptyline, amoxapine, clomipramine, desipramine, doxepin, imipramine, nortriptyline, protriptyline, trimipramine) are relatively contraindicated in children with epilepsy due to the lowering of seizure thresholds. These medications increase the risk of seizures in the general population up to 0.1% to 4% at therapeutic levels and 8.4% to 22% in the setting of overdose (levels greater than 1000 mg/mL). The risk of clomipramine also increases with concomitant VPA, with status epilepticus occurring in some cases. Status epilepticus has also been reported with amoxapine (52).

In contrast, selective serotonin reuptake inhibitors (SSRIs; citalopram, escitalopram, fluoxetine, fluvoxamine, paroxetine, sertraline) are unlikely to worsen seizure frequency or severity (Table 19.5). Weight gain is of concern when used in combination with

TABLE 19.5 Antidepressants Commonly Used in Patients With Epilepsy

Medication	Hepatic Enzyme Effects	Interactions With AEDs/ Antidepressants	Seizure Risk (Percent Incidence in General Population)	Notes
SSRI				
Citalopram	Little effect	Levels decreased by: DPH CBZ PB Primidone	0.1–0.3 18.0 at 600–1,900 mg	
Escitalopram	Little effect		0–0.04%	• Myoclonus reported with concurrent LMT
Fluoxetine	Inhibitor	↑ DPH levels ↑ CBZ levels ↑ TCA levels ↑ VPA levels (rare)	0–0.3	• Possible anticonvulsant effects • Serotonin syndrome, isolated case of Parkinsonian syndrome with concurrent CBZ • Long half life, less withdrawal
Fluvoxamine	Inhibitor	↑ DPH levels Levels decreased by: DPH CBZ PB Primidone	0.05–0.2	
Paroxetine	Little effect		0.07–0.1%	• May cause weight gain • Short half life, withdrawal syndrome
Sertraline	Little effect	↑ TCA levels Levels decreased by: DPH CBZ PB Primidone OXC (minimal) TPX (minimal)	0-0.3	• May cause weight gain
SNRI				
Venlafaxine			0.1–0.3% 0 with XR formulation 5.0 with overdose	• Not for use in young children; may use in older adolescents • More complicated titration • Significant withdrawal • Use extended release • May cause lethargy, irritability, hypertension
Tetracyclic				
Mirtazapine			0.04	• Not for use in young children; may use in older adolescents • May cause sedation, weight gain • Lacks SE of nausea, • May cause agranulocytosis; do not use with CBZ

AED = antiepileptic drug; CBZ = carbamazepine; DPH = phenytoin; LMT = lamotrigine; OXC = oxcarbazepine; PB = phenobarbital; SE = side effects; SNRI = selective serotonin-norepinephrine reuptake inhibitor; SSRI = selective serotonin reuptake inhibitor; TCA = tricyclic antidepressant; TPX = topiramate; VPA = valproic acid. Reprinted from *Wyllie's Treatment of Epilepsy*, 5th ed. Philadelphia: Lippincott Williams & Wilkins, 2011: 1039, with permission.

AEDs that cause the same effect, including gabapentin, VPA, CBZ, and pregabalin, although this may be beneficial in underweight patients with LND. Among the SSRIs, sertraline has been best studied in the setting of epilepsy; however, clinicians often favor the use of the newer citalopram and escitalopram due to their lack of hepatic enzyme effects.

The typical antipsychotics carry a greater risk of seizure exacerbation, with seizure induction rates in the general population of 0.5% to 1.2%. Risk is increased by a history of seizures or abnormal EEGs, CNS disorders, rapid titration, and high doses (53). Among the typical antipsychotics, haloperidol appears to be the safest (Table 19.6). Other typical

TABLE 19.6 Atypical Antipsychotics

Drug	Levels Decreased by	Levels Increased by	Seizure Risk	Notes
Clozapine	DPH CBZ PB Primidone OXC* TPX*	VPA	Avoid use; black box warning for higher seizure risk 4.4% at >600 mg/day** <1% at <300 mg/day** Patients with epilepsy had increased seizure frequency on <300 mg/day	• Concomitant CBZ increases risk of leucopenia and neuroleptic malignant syndrome
Olanzapine	DPH CBZ PB Primidone	VPA	Higher seizure risk 0.9	
Ziprasidone	DPH CBZ PB Primidone OXC* TPX*		0.4–0.5	• Affective and anxiolytic properties • May cause akathisia
Risperidone	DPH CBZ PB Primidone OXC* TPX*		Lower seizure risk 0.3	• More likely to cause extrapyramidal side effects
Quetiapine	DPH CBZ PB Primidone OXC* TPX*		0.8	• Affective and anxiolytic properties • Only neuroleptic that did not cause EEG changes
Aripiprazole	CBZ	Fluoxetine*** Paroxetine***	0.4	• May cause akathisia

*Moderate, dose-dependent effects, **Studies in patients without epilepsy, ***May be minimal effects; CBZ = carbamazepine; DPH = phenytoin; OXC = oxcarbazepine; PB = phenobarbital; TPX = topiramate; VPA = valproic acid. Reprinted from *Wyllie's Treatment of Epilepsy*, 5th ed. Philadelphia: Lippincott Williams & Wilkins, 2011: 1046, with permission.

agents with lower seizure-inducing potential include molindone, fluphenazine, perfenzine, and trifluoperazine (53). The atypical antipsychotics, however, have lower epileptogenic potential and are preferred in patients with epilepsy. Ziprasidone, quetiapine, aripiprazole, risperidone, and olanzapine have relatively low rates of seizure induction (54, 55). Blood glucose and lipid profiles must be followed with these agents, however, particularly in those taking AEDs associated with weight gain (eg, VPA, gabapentin, pregabalin, and CBZ). Agents to avoid include clozapine, chlorpromazine, and loxapine, as they are associated with a high incidence of seizures in nonepileptic patients.

SUDDEN DEATH

Approximately 1 in 1000 people with epilepsy, and 1 in 150 people with medically refractory seizures, will die suddenly of unknown cause each year (56, 57). Sudden unexpected death in epilepsy (SUDEP) is defined as "sudden, unexpected, witnessed or unwitnessed, non-traumatic, and non-drowning death in patients with epilepsy, with or without evidence of a seizure and excluding documented status epilepticus where necropsy examination does not reveal a toxicological or anatomical cause for death" (56, 57). Evidence often suggests that seizures, which may lead to apnea, and less commonly cardiac arrhythmias, may have occurred near the time of death. Autopsy commonly reveals pulmonary edema. Risk factors include young adulthood, male sex, GTC seizures, poor medication adherence, remote symptomatic epilepsy, use of psychotropic medications, alcohol abuse, and unwitnessed seizures. Fortunately, SUDEP in childhood is rare.

A similar phenomenon, however, occurs in LND. It has been suggested that sudden death in LND relates to neurological dysfunction or aspiration associated with hiatal hernias or GERD. We raise the concern, however, that sudden death in LND could be related to SUDEP, given the increased incidence of epilepsy and abnormal EEG activity in this population. Furthermore, only 8 of the 28 patients with a history of seizures were known to be taking AEDs, with lack of treatment potentially leading to added risk. Mizuno provided an example of SUDEP in a patient with LND and seizures, in which the patient woke, was playing in his bed, was told to go back to sleep, and within 2 hours was found dead (34). An autopsy

suspected "suffocation," but no CNS, respiratory, or cardiovascular changes were noted. Two other children with LND had died in relation to witnessed seizure activity (23). All were in a high-risk category: male, with a history of GTC seizures, and not taking AEDs. Such events underscore the importance of treating recurrent seizures in LND with anticonvulsants, and avoiding abrupt AED withdrawal. No data exists, however, to suggest that treatment after a single unprovoked seizure will prevent sudden death.

KEY POINTS

Seizures occur with greater frequency in LND than in the general population. The mechanisms underlying seizure generation are unknown, but are unlikely to be a direct consequence of elevated uric acid. Seizures must be distinguished, however, from the motor disorder of LND, in which dystonic spasms with superimposed tremor or myoclonus may have a similar appearance. The majority of seizures in LND are GTC, but whether they are of primary or secondary generalization is unclear. No specific EEG, neuroimaging or neuropathological signatures have been identified, and findings are often normal. Nor are there specific guidelines regarding treatment. As seizures tend to be recurrent in this population, we suggest consideration of treatment after the first unprovoked seizure. The choice of medication should be individualized, however, and based upon side effect profiles. In many cases seizures have been easily controlled by the older generation of anticonvulsants (eg, phenytoin, phenobarbital, and carbamazepine), but no data have been published regarding use of newer agents.

CLINICAL PEARLS

- Seizures must be differentiated from dystonia with superimposed tremors or myoclonus. Status dystonicus or "dystonic storm" may closely resemble convulsive status epilepticus.
- The majority of seizures in LND are GTC. Partial and tonic seizures are reported less commonly.
- Consider treatment after the first afebrile convulsion, as seizures tend to be recurrent in this population.
- Phenobarbital, lamotrigine, and gabapentin may cause irritability or aggression in children and patients with learning disabilities. Carbamazepine and valproic acid may also cause paradoxical irritability.

- Topiramate and zonisamide should be avoided in LND due to the risk of nephrolithiasis.
- Allopurinol may significantly increase phenytoin levels, and cause a hypersensitivity syndrome similar to that seen with anticonvulsants (ie, lamotrigine). It may also have an anticonvulsant effect.
- Carbamazepine and phenytoin may decrease uric acid levels.

REFERENCES

1. Jinnah HA, Visser JE, Harris JC, et al. Delineation of the motor disorder of Lesch-Nyhan disease. *Brain.* 2006;129(Pt 5):1201–1217.
2. Christie R, Bay C, Kaufman IA, et al. Lesch-Nyhan disease: clinical experience with nineteen patients. *Dev Med Child Neurol.* 1982;24:293–306.
3. Mishra D, Singhal S, Juneja M. Status dystonicus a rare complication of dystonia. *Indian Pediatr.* 2010;47(10):883–885.
4. Teive HA, Munhoz RP, Souza MM, et al. Status dystonicus: study of five cases. *Arq Neuropsiquiatr.* 2005;63(1):26–29.
5. Manji H, Howard RS, Miller DH, et al. Status dystonicus: the syndrome and its management. *Brain.* 1998;121(Pt 2):243–252.
6. Lynch BJ, Noetzel MJ. Recurrent coma and Lesch-Nyhan syndrome. *Pediatr Neurol.* 1991;7:389–391.
7. Nomikos GG, Zis AP, Damsma G, et al. Electroconvulsive shock increases interstitial concentrations of uric acid in the rat brain. *Brain Res.* 1994;660(1):50–56.
8. Warren DJ, Leitch AG, Leggett RJ. Hyperuricaemic acute renal failure after epileptic seizures. *Lancet.* 1975;2(7931):385–387.
9. Coleman M, Landgrebe M, Landgrebe A. Progressive seizures with hyperuricosuria reversed by allopurinol. *Arch Neurol.* 1974;31(4):238–242.
10. Coleman M, Landgrebe M, Landgrebe A. Purine seizure disorders. *Epilepsia.* 1986;27(3):263–269.
11. Zagnoni PG, Bianchi A, Zolo P, et al. Allopurinol as add-on therapy in refractory epilepsy: a double-blind placebo-controlled randomized study. *Epilepsia.* 1994;35(1):107–112.
12. Coppola G, Pascotto A. Double-blind, placebo-controlled, cross-over trial of allopurinol as add-on therapy in childhood refractory epilepsy. *Brain Dev.* 1996;18(1):50–52.
13. Dreifuss FE, Newcombe DS, Shapiro SL, et al. X-linked primary hyperuricemia (hypoxanthine-guanine phosphoribosyltransferase deficiency encephalopathy). *J Ment Defic Res.* 1968;12:100–107.
14. Kopin IJ. Neurotransmitters and the Lesch-Nyhan syndrome. *N Engl J Med.* 1981;305:1148–1150.
15. Stone TW. Physiological roles for adenosine and adenosine 5′-triphosphate in the nervous system. *Neurosci.* 1981;6:523–555.
16. Green RD, Proudfit JK, Yeung SH. Modulation of striatal dopaminergic function by local injection of 5′-N-ethylcarboxamide adenosine. *Science.* 1982;218:58–61.
17. Baumeister AA, Frye GD. The biochemical basis of the behavioral disorder in the Lesch-Nyhan syndrome. *Neurosci Biobehav Rev.* 1985;9:169–178.
18. Torres RJ, DeAntonio I, Prior C, et al. Adenosine transport in peripheral blood lymphocytes from Lesch-Nyhan patients. *Biochem J.* 2004;377:733–739.
19. Jinnah HA, Hess EJ, Wilson MC, et al. Localization of hypoxanthine-guanine phosphoribosyltransferase mRNA in the mouse brain by in situ hybridization. *Mol Cell Neurosci.* 1992;3:64–78.
20. Andres A, Praga M, Ruilope LM, et al. Partial deficit of hypoxanthine guanine phosphoribosyl transferase presenting as acute renal failure. *Nephron.* 1987;46:179–181.
21. Gedye A. Serotonin-GABA treatment is hypothesized for self-injury in Lesch-Nyhan syndrome. *Med Hypoth.* 1992;38:325–328.
22. Jinnah HA, Ceballos-Picot I, Torres RJ, et al. Attenuated variants of Lesch-Nyhan disease. *Brain.* 2010;133:671–689.
23. Hoefnagel D, Andrew ED, Mireault NG, et al. Hereditary choreoathetosis, self-mutilation, and hyperuricemia in young males. *N Engl J Med.* 1965;273:130–135.
24. Ferrandez A, Mayayo E, Nyhan WL, et al. Report of a patient with Lesch-Nyhan syndrome caused by total deficiency of HGPRT and with normal activity in female family members. *An Esp Pediatr.* 1982;17(1):60–64.
25. Berman PH, Balis ME, Dancis J. Congenital hyperuricemia: an inborn error of purine metabolism associated with psychomotor retardation athetosis, self-mutilation. *Arch Neurol.* 1969;20:44–53.
26. Michener WM. Hyperuricemia and mental retardation. *Am J Dis Child.* 1967;113:195–206.
27. Newcombe DS, Shapiro SL, Sheppard GL, et al. Treatment of x-linked primary hyperuricemia with allopurinol. *JAMA.* 1966;198(3):315–317.
28. Riley ID. Gout and cerebral palsy in a three-year-old boy. *Arch Dis Child.* 1960;35:293–295.
29. Mitchell G, McInnes RR. Differential diagnosis of cerebral palsy: Lesch-Nyhan syndrome without self-mutilation. *Can Med Assoc J.* 1984;130:1323–1324.
30. Wada Y, Arakawa T, Loizumi K. Lesch-Nyhan syndrome: autopsy findings, in vitro study of incorporation of 14C-8-inosine into uric acid, guanosine-monophosphate, adenosine-monophosphate in the liver. *Tohoku J Exp Med.* 1968;95:253–260.
31. Sass JK, Itabashi HH, Dexter RA. Juvenile gout with brain involvement. *Arch Neurol.* 1965;13:639–655.
32. Puliyel JM, Kumar M. Lesch Nyhan syndrome. *Indian Pediatr.* 1984;21:251–252.
33. Lesch M, Nyhan WL. A familial disorder of uric acid metabolism and central nervous system function. *Am J Med.* 1964;36:561–570.
34. Mizuno T. Long-term follow-up of ten patients with Lesch-Nyhan syndrome. *Neuropediatrics.* 1986;17: 158–161.
35. Del Bigio MR, Halliday WC. Multifocal atrophy of cerebellar internal granular neurons in Lesch-Nyhan disease: case reports and review. *J Neuropathol Exp Neurol.* 2007;66(5):346–353.
36. Geerdink RA, De Vries WHM, Willemse J, et al. An atypical case of hypoxanthine-guanine phosphoribosyltransferase deficiency (Lesch-Nyhan syndrome). I. clinical studies. *Clin Genet.* 1973;4:348–352.

37. Partington MW, Hennen BKE. The Lesch-Nyhan syndrome: self-destructive biting, mental retardation, neurological disorder and hyperuricemia. *Dev Med Child Neurol.* 1967;9: 563–572.

38. Hatanaka T, Higashino H, Woo M, et al. Lesch-Nyhan syndrome with delayed onset of self-mutilation: hyperactivity of interneurons at the brainstem and blink reflex. *Acta Neurol Scand.* 1990;81:184–187.

39. Crussi FG, Robertson DM, Hiscox JL. The pathological condition of the Lesch-Nyhan syndrome. *Am J Dis Child.* 1969;118:501–506.

40. Bassermann R, Gutensohn W, Jahn H, et al. Pathological and immunological observations in a case of Lesch-Nyhan syndrome. *Eur J Pediatr.* 1979;132: 93–98.

41. Crome L, Stern J. *The Pathology of Mental Retardation.* London: J. & A. Churchill Ltd.; 1967.

42. Hirtz D, Ashwal S, Berg A, et al. Practice parameter: evaluating a first nonfebrile seizure in children: report of the quality standards subcommittee of the American Academy of Neurology, The Child Neurology Society, and The American Epilepsy Society. *Neurology.* 2000;55(5):616–623.

43. Hirtz D, Berg A, Bettis D, et al. Practice parameter: treatment of the child with a first unprovoked seizure: Report of the Quality Standards Subcommittee of the American Academy of Neurology and the Practice Committee of the Child Neurology Society. *Neurology.* 2003;60(2):166–175.

44. Neurodiagnostic evaluation of the child with a simple febrile seizure. *Pediatrics.* 2011;127(2):389–394.

45. Millar JS. Evaluation and treatment of the child with febrile seizure. *Am Fam Physician.* 2006;73(10);1761–1764.

46. Kelley WN, Greene ML, Rosenbloom FM, et al. Hypoxanthine-guanine phosphoribosyltransferase deficiency in gout. *Ann Int Med.* 1969;70:155–206.

47. Krause KH, Berlit P, Schmidt-Gayk H, et al. Antiepileptic drugs reduce serum uric acid. *Epilepsy Res.* 1987;1(5):306–307.

48. Ring HA, Heller AJ, Marshall WJ, et al. Plasma uric acid in patients receiving anticonvulsant monotherapy. *Epilepsy Res.* 1991;8(3):241–244.

49. DeMarco P, Zagnoni P. Allopurinol and severe epilepsy. *Neurology.* 1986;36(11):1538–1539.

50. Balit CR, Lynch CN, Isbister GK. Bupropion poisoning: a case series. *Med J Aust.* 2003;178(2):61–63.

51. Cuenca PJ, Holt KR, Hoefle JD. Seizure secondary to citalopram overdose. *J Emerg Med.* 2004;26(2):177–181.

52. Pisani F, Spina E, Oteri G. Antidepressant drugs and seizure susceptibility: from in vitro data to clinical practice. *Epilepsia.* 1999;40(Suppl 10):S48–S56.

53. Kanner AM. The use of psychotropic drugs in epilepsy: what every neurologist should know. *Semin Neurol.* 2008;28(3): 379–388.

54. Nadkarni S, Arnedo V, Devinsky O. Psychosis in epilepsy patients. *Epilepsia.* 2007;48(Suppl 9):17–19.

55. Mahgoub NA. A report of successful treatment of psychosis in epilepsy with risperidone. *J Neuropsychiatry Clin Neurosci.* 2007;19(3):347–348.

56. Nashef L, Brown S. Epilepsy and sudden death. *Lancet.* 1996;348(9038):1324–1325.

57. Hirsch LJ, Donner EJ, So EL, et al. Abbreviated report of the NIH/NINDS workshop on sudden unexpected death in epilepsy. *Neurology.* 2011;76(22):1932–1938.

20

Sulfite Oxidase Deficiency/Molybdenum Cofactor Deficiency and Epilepsy

Jörn Oliver Sass and Barbara Plecko-Startinig

INTRODUCTION

First reported in 1967 and 1978, respectively, isolated sulfite oxidase deficiency (ISOD) and sulfite oxidase deficiency due to molybdenum cofactor deficiency (MOCOD) are neurometabolic diseases which have attracted increasing attention in the last few years (1, 2). They are panethnic conditions of autosomal recessive inheritance (3). Although therapeutic attempts are usually of limited success, animal data and a recent human pilot study have opened a perspective for treatment of the most frequent type of MOCOD (4–6).

CLINICAL PRESENTATIONS OF MOCO DEFICIENCY AND ISOLATED SULFITE OXIDASE DEFICIENCY

NEONATAL MANIFESTATION

The typical presentation of MOCOD as well as of ISOD is that of a child born after uneventful pregnancy and delivery who presents with poor feeding within days after birth. This nonspecific period is followed by the onset of seizures within days or a few weeks. Seizures are mainly myoclonic or tonic-clonic, are often therapy-resistant and may develop into status epilepticus (7–9). Though seizures may be intractable in the beginning, some patients become seizure free or are finally controlled under monotherapy with one anticonvulsant (10).

Along the evolution of seizures many patients exhibit signs of encephalopathy with periods of prolonged crying, apneic spells, opisthotonic postures, and erratic eye movements or myoclonias provoked by stimulation (3, 8, 11, 12). Few patients may need early resuscitation and ventilation, leading to a false diagnosis of hypoxic ischemic encephalopathy (8, 10, 13).

In all patients onset of seizures is accompanied by rapid neurologic deterioration with truncal hypotonia but brisk reflexes and hypertonicity of all extremities and profound intellectual deficiency. EEG reveals multi-focal spike-wave activity or burst-suppression patterns (7, 9) but may show unilateral predominance of epileptic discharges (8, 14). Amplitude-integrated EEG, a tool for cerebral function monitoring in modern ICUs, was applied in one child with MOCOD and showed rapid evolution from a normal pattern with sleep–wake cycling during the very early phase of seizure onset to a burst suppression pattern over the following 3 days (9).

Subtle dysmorphic features have been described in about 75% of patients, consisting of a somewhat coarse and elongated face with long philtrum, small nose, puffy cheeks, and widely spaced eyes (2, 3, 15). Asymmetry of the skull, frontal bossing, and enophthalmus have been described in single patients (10, 15). Head circumference is normal at birth, but most patients will acquire microcephaly during infancy (3). A few cases with MOCOD have been described with macrocephaly associated with hydrocephalus (10). Due to impaired function of xanthine dehydrogenase, patients with MOCOD may excrete smooth brownish xanthine stones (7).

Beyond the neonatal period subluxation of the lense may occur in MOCOD as well as in ISOD (1, 16, 17). Other ocular abnormalities seen in ISOD are nystagmus, myopia, areactive pupils, and optic atrophy (18).

In contrast to nonspecific MRI changes seen in many other epilepsies caused by inborn errors of metabolism, cranial imaging may be especially helpful in diagnosing MOCOD. In the typical case MRI shows evolution from cytotoxic brain edema with loss of gray–white matter differentiation to cystic white matter changes and global brain atrophy (9, 19). Following the recognition of the severe neonatal phenotype, milder forms have been diagnosed and seem to be more prevalent among patients with ISOD.

LATE ONSET FORMS

Aside from the typical manifestation, ISOD and MOCOD can manifest with later onset forms, which are much more nonspecific. In many of these cases onset of illness is triggered by a febrile illness. Children with late onset forms may have a completely uneventful neonatal period and normal early psychomotor development over several months. Some patients have nonspecific motor or speech delay with varying degrees of muscular hypotonia prior to the onset of clear neurologic illness (20, 21). Neurological manifestations comprise nonspecific agitation with encephalopathy (22), chorea, dystonia (20), or hemiplegia of acute or subacute onset (20, 23). Seizures may occur (10) but in contrast to neonatal onset cases are not a constant or prominent feature. While many patients with late onset forms show recovery and developmental progress following the onset of neurologic symptoms (10, 21), some develop progressive neurodegeneration with complete loss of acquired skills (10). Single patients have been described with isolated visual impairment due to lens subluxation (10) or a marfanoid habitus, with their neurologic illness and lens subluxation occurring as late as the 8th year of life (23). Interestingly, in late onset MOCOD as well as ISOD dysmorphic features seem to be infrequent and at least two patients were described with macrocephaly (21, 22) at the time of neurologic presentation.

In all late onset patients it was the family history, radiologic features or, less reliably, decreased plasma uric acid that prompted investigations for MOCOD or ISOD.

MRI IN TYPICAL AND LATE ONSET MOCOD AND ISOD

In the typical case of neonatal onset, imaging is always strikingly abnormal and can be suggestive of the underlying disorder. It is now well known that imaging in MOCOD as well as in ISOD reflects different stages of brain damage. Thus, changes observed depend on the time when imaging is performed. During the first days of life, brain magnetic resonance imaging (MRI) reveals diffuse brain edema and swelling of white as well as of gray matter, involving the globus pallidus and midbrain (9,1024). These changes are also visible on cranial ultrasound (9), but are nonspecific per se and sometimes misinterpreted as acute sequelea of a perinatal hypoxic brain insult (13, 25, 26). Diffusion-weighted imaging demonstrates widespread diffusion restriction in a child with ISOD, along with elevated lactate and decreased *N*-acetylaspartate on proton magnetic resonance spectroscopy, suggesting energy failure associated with neuronal dysfunction and myelin disintegration (27). Abnormal shape of the frontal horns may be caused by marked atrophy of the basal ganglia (28). Some patients have associated primary malformations including a hypoplastic pons and cerebellar vermis with posterior fossa cysts or Dandy–Walker malformation (10, 14, 29, 30). In a single patient, hypoplasia of the right hemisphere with a thickened cortex of the contralateral side was found at autopsy (11). One patient with neonatal onset MOCOD had hydrocephalus with macrocephaly at birth and needed ventriculo-peritoneal shunting (10).

Within several days to weeks the initial pattern of brain edema gives way to extended cystic changes mainly within white matter with variable frontal or occipital preponderance, thinning of the corpus callosum and marked brain atrophy (10, 19). This process is reflected by arrest of head growth and rapidly developing postpartum microcephaly. CT scans at that stage may show calcifications of the basal ganglia. In one case of neonatal onset MOCOD imaging at the age of 8 days revealed intraventricular as well as intraparenchymal hemorrhage in addition to diffuse encephalomalacia (30).

Though in the typical case cystic lesions do not occur until several days or weeks of seizure onset, single patients may show cystic changes in late pregnancy or at birth, pointing toward an intrauterine onset of brain damage in most severely affected cases (10, 31).

In late onset cases cranial imaging is much more nonspecific but revealed some abnormalities in all patients reported so far. Bilateral signal changes of the globus pallidi associated with some degree of mild cortical atrophy were described in several patients with mild MOCOD (20, 21, 23) while one patient with late onset global developmental delay and bilateral lense subluxation had symmetric signal abnormality within the cerebellar deep nuclei. Bilateral hypodensity of frontal white matter was found in one case of late onset ISOD (22). Interestingly, one late onset patient with MOCOD had cortical malformation, which was not associated with seizures (21). In all cases symmetric involvement of the deep gray or white matter was suggestive of a metabolic disorder.

BIOCHEMICAL BASIS AND LABORATORY DIAGNOSTICS

Both sulfite oxidase deficiency due to MOCOD and ISOD can be identified via elevated urine sulfite levels in fresh, neutralized urine examined using test sticks based on Ellman's reagent. However, such dipstick tests have yielded both false-negative (32, 33) and false-positive results (34).

Increased concentrations of urinary thiosulfate can also point to sulfite oxidase deficiency, but this is not a routine parameter in clinical chemistry and has been reported with both false-positive (35) and false-negative results (36).

One may expect a decrease in sulfate excretion in individuals with sulfite oxidase deficiency, but this strongly depends on the diet and there are no reliable reference values for pediatric patients, thus the use of this parameter in the detection of sulfite oxidase deficiency appears not feasible (32). Lack of (rarely assessed) urinary urothione can serve as a marker of MoCo deficiency, but not of isolated sulfite oxidase deficiency (37).

High taurine levels are frequently found in newborns (38), thus, such a finding is a low-specificity marker of sulfite oxidase deficiency only. Sulfocysteine (especially in urine) is a frequently used parameter, which often requires shipment on dry ice, which is not easy to accomplish in some clinical settings. In conventional amino acid analysis (which provides taurine

and other amino acid data in the same run) early eluting sulfocysteine may well be affected by interfering signals. Thus, a specialized method should be used.

A rather stable parameter is the peak height ratio of S-sulfonated transthyretin and other oxidized transthyretin isoforms in electrospray ionisation (ESI) mass spectrometry (39). However, this test is not routinely available. As in antiquitin deficiency, individuals with sulfite oxidase deficiency may present with elevated urinary levels of alpha-aminoadipic semialdehyde (40). This is probably due to a reaction of accumulated sulfite with the semialdehyde.

A widely available test, which has been shown to be useful in the diagnosis of sulfite oxidase deficiency, is the determination of total homocysteine (41). It requires less than 100 μL of plasma or serum. Patients with sulfite oxidase deficiency are characterized by pronounced hypohomocysteinemia, usually undetectable plasma total homocysteine values, if appropriate preanalytical conditions are ensured. Low concentrations of plasma cystine are also in agreement with a diagnosis of sulfite oxidase deficiency, but represent a rather nonspecific finding.

Patients with sulfite oxidase deficiency due to MOCOD present with additional deficiency of xanthine dehydrogenase. Consequently, they are sometimes diagnosed via hypouricemia recognized in the routine clinical chemistry laboratory. This may contribute to the fact that the prevalence of MOCOD appears to be higher than that of ISOD. Normal serum values of uric acid (which can also be ingested with the food) do not exclude MOCOD, but low uric acid concentrations in serum and urine in combination with elevated urinary levels of hypoxanthine/xanthine strongly indicate this disease or xanthine dehydrogenase deficiency. The latter is usually well distinguished from MoCo deficiency because of its much milder phenotype, usually limited to the development of xanthine stones in some of the patients (42). Notably, MOCOD leads also to deficiency of aldehyde oxidase (which catalyzes the hydroxylation of various compounds) (43), and of mitochondrial amidoxime reducing component, which has been identified as a general detoxifying and pro-drug metabolizing enzyme with yet unknown physiological substrates (44).

Confirmation of sulfite oxidase deficiency can be accomplished by a specific enzyme activity test in cultivated fibroblasts (45). Mutation analysis is also available. In isolated sulfite oxidase deficiency, the *SUOX* gene can be sequenced. Three types of MoCo deficiency can be distinguished based on the genetic defect. Two-thirds of the patients have mutations in the *MOCS1* gene (46). They lack the first precursor in the biosynthetic pathway of MoCo, cyclic pyranopterin monophosphate (cPMP) (47), and are designated type A patients. Type B patients have mutations in the *MOCS2* gene, which encodes the molybdopterin synthase, and accumulate cPMP (48). Only a single patient with MoCo deficiency type 3 has been identified. That girl presented with the deletion of two exons of *GEPH* gene (49).

PATHOPHYSIOLOGY

While the congruency of the clinical presentations in ISOD and MOCOD strongly points to sulfite oxidase deficiency as the underlying cause of most symptoms, details of the pathomechanisms are not yet known. Whereas lack of sulfate is unlikely to contribute to clinical features in ISOD and MOCOD, direct effects of sulfite may affect formation of disulfide bridges and may thus explain ectopia lentis reported for some patients (1, 16, 50) and may cause a decrease of antioxidant levels in the brain (20). High sulfite levels can also result in degradation of thiamine (vitamin B$_1$) and of unsaturated fatty acids (50, 51). Inhibition of glutamate dehydrogenase by sulfite may affect the energy supply of the brain (52). Whereas contributions of multiple factors to the pathology of sulfite oxidase deficiency are well possible, the most convincing approach is based on the fact that the structure of accumulating sulfocysteine very much resembles that of glutamate and may thus result in activation of neuroreceptors such as the NMDA (*N*-methyl-D-aspartate) receptors (53). This could also explain fatal consequences of cysteine loading in the first patient diagnosed with ISOD (3).

TREATMENT

For many years treatment in MOCOD and ISOD was purely symptomatic. In neonatal onset forms, seizures were reported to be resistant against conventional anticonvulsants. Due to structural similarity of the accumulating compound *S*-sulfocysteine and glutamic acid overstimulation of the NMDA receptor (NMDAR) was assumed (53) and lead to treatment of one patient with dextromethorphan, an NMDAR antagonist. In

this patient, seizures stopped and EEG improved markedly (54). Recently, a favorable effect of vigabatrin, a GABA-ergic drug, has been reported in combination therapy with other anticonvulsants (55).

In 1993, a first short-term trial of dietary restriction was undertaken in a 3-month-old girl with MOCOD (56). A combination of methionine restriction with supplementation of cysteine led to moderate improvement of clinical symptoms and head growth during a 2 month observational period. In 2000, a first attempt of long-term dietary treatment was described in two unrelated patients with late onset ISOD (22). To decrease the overall sulfur load, natural protein (and thus the intake of the sulfur-containing amino acids methionine and cystine) was restricted and adequate protein intake provided by an amino acid supplement free of methionine and cystine. This treatment resulted in marked reduction of urinary levels of metabolites such as *S*-sulfocysteine. This was accompanied by a stable clinical course and continuous developmental progress. Unfortunately, other authors could not prove efficacy of this concept in single patients with ISOD (24, 57, 58).

Increase of plasma cysteine and consecutive sulfite excess during catabolic events can trigger neurometabolic crises and a cysteine loading test was fatal in the first patient described with ISOD (3).

Administration of L-cysteamine as a chelating agent of sulfites had no effect in lowering levels of relevant metabolites (22), as was the case for D-penicillamine (59) and for 2-mercaptoethanesulfonic acid (60). Supplementation of molybdenum may be beneficial in the small patient group with MoCo type C deficiency and mutations of the gephyrin gene.

FUTURE DIRECTIONS

Using a mouse model (61), a treatment approach based on substitution therapy with cPMP has been established for MoCo deficiency type A (62). Recently, results from intravenous cPMP replacement in humans with MoCo deficiency type A have been purported to result not only in remarkable normalization of biomarkers for this disease, but also in clinical improvement and prevention of ongoing sulfite neurotoxicity (5, 6). Currently available information suggests that early diagnosis and treatment of MoCo deficiency type A may be crucial to suppress brain damage.

CLINICAL PEARLS

- Every newborn with epileptic encephalopathy of unclear etiology should undergo testing for sulfite oxidase deficiency (ISOD, MOCOD).
- As treatment becomes available for the group of MOCOD type A patients, early diagnosis may become crucial to prevent irreversible brain damage.
- The detection of hypouricemia should result in testing for molybdenum cofactor deficiency, especially in an encephalopathic newborn.
- While more specialized investigations are important for confirmation, assessment of total homocysteine in plasma or serum is a widely available routine test which may help with the diagnosis of molybdenum cofactor deficiency and isolated sulfite oxidase deficiency because of their association with hypohomocysteinemia.

REFERENCES

1. Mudd SH, Irreverre F, Laster L. Sulfite oxidase deficiency in man: demonstration of the enzymatic defect. *Science.* 1967;156:1599–1602.
2. Duran M, Beemer FA, van de Heiden C, et al. Combined deficiency of xanthine oxidase and sulphite oxidase: a defect of molybdenum metabolism or transport? *J Inherit Metab Dis.* 1978;1:175–178.
3. Johnson JL, Duran M. Molybdenum cofactor deficiency and isolated sulfite oxidase deficiency. In: CR Scriver, AL Beaudet, WS Sly, et al., eds. *The Metabolic and Molecular Bases of Inherited Disease.* New York: McGraw-Hill: 2001: 3163–3177.
4. Schwarz G, Santamaria-Araujo JA, Wolf S, et al. Rescue of lethal molybdenum cofactor deficiency by a biosynthetic precursor from *Escherichia coli. Hum Mol Genet.* 2004:13:1249–1255.
5. Veldman A, Santamaria-Araujo JA, Sollazzo S, et al. Successful treatment of molybdenum cofactor deficiency type A with cPMP. *Pediatrics.* 2010;125:e1249–e1254.
6. Veldman A, Hennermann JB, Schwarz G, et al. Timing of cerebral developmental disruption in molybdenum cofactor deficiency. *J Child Neurol.* 2011;26:1059–1060.
7. Bonioli E, DiStefano A, Palmieri A, et al. Combined deficiency of xanthine oxidase and sulphite oxidase due to a deficiency of molybdenum cofactor. *J Inherit Metab Dis.* 1996;19:700–701.
8. Schiaffino MC, Fantasia AR, Minniti G, et al. Isolated sulphite oxidase deficiency: clinical and biochemical features in an Italian patient. *J Inherit Metab Dis.* 2004;27:101–102.
9. Sie SD, de Jonge RC, Blom HJ, et al. Chronological changes of the amplitude-integrated EEG in a neonate with molybdenum cofactor deficiency. *J Inherit Metab Dis.* 2010; DOI: 10.1007/s10545-010-9198-z.

10. Vijayakumar K, Gunny R, Grunewald S, et al. Clinical neuroimaging features and outcome in molybdenum cofactor deficiency. *Pediatr Neurol.* 2011;45:246–252.
11. Roesel RA, Bowyer F, Blankenship PR, et al. Combined xanthine and sulphite oxidase defect due to a deficiency of molybdenum cofactor. *J Inherit Metab Dis.* 1986;9:343–347.
12. van Gennip AH, Abeling NG, Stroomer AE, et al. The detection of molybdenum cofactor deficiency: clinical symptomatology and urinary metabolite profile. *J Inherit Metab Dis.* 1994;17:142–145.
13. Hobson EE, Thomas S, Crofton PM, et al. Isolated sulphite oxidase deficiency mimics the features of hypoxic ischaemic encephalopathy. *Eur J Pediatr.* 2005;164:655–659.
14. Topcu M, Coskun T, Haliloglu G, et al. Molybdenum cofactor deficiency: report of three cases presenting as hypoxic-ischemic encephalopathy. *J Child Neurol.* 2001;16:264–270.
15. Munnich A, Saudubray JM, Charpentier C, et al. Multiple molybdoenzyme deficiencies due to an inborn error of molybdenum cofactor metabolism: two additional cases in a new family. *J Inherit Metab Dis.* 1983;6(Suppl 2):95–96.
16. Edwards MC, Johnson JL, Marriage B, et al. Isolated sulfite oxidase deficiency: review of two cases in one family. *Ophthalmology.* 1999;106:1957–1961.
17. Hughes EF, Fairbanks L, Simmonds HA, et al. Molybdenum cofactor deficiency-phenotypic variability in a family with a late-onset variant. *Dev Med Child Neurol.* 1998;40:57–61.
18. Shih VE, Abroms IF, Johnson JL, et al. Sulfite oxidase deficiency. Biochemical and clinical investigations of a hereditary metabolic disorder in sulfur metabolism. *N Engl J Med.* 1977;10(297):1022–1028.
19. Appignani BA, Kaye EM, Wolpert SM. CT and MR appearance of the brain in two children with molybdenum cofactor deficiency. *AJNR Am J Neuroradiol.* 1996;17:317–320.
20. Graf WD, Oleinik OE, Jack RM, et al. Ahomocysteinemia in molybdenum cofactor deficiency. *Neurology.* 1998;51:860–862.
21. Johnson JL, Coyne KE, Rajagopalan KV . Molybdopterin synthase mutations in a mild case of molybdenum cofactor deficiency. *Am J Med Genet.* 2001;104:169–173.
22. Touati G, Rusthoven E, Depondt E, et al. Dietary therapy in two patients with a mild form of sulphite oxidase deficiency. Evidence for clinical and biological improvement. *J Inherit Metab Dis.* 2000;23:45–53.
23. Mize C, Johnson JL, Rajagopalan KV . Defective molybdopterin biosynthesis: clinical heterogeneity associated with molybdenum cofactor deficiency. *J Inherit Metab Dis.* 1995;18:283–290.
24. Sass JO, Gunduz A, Araujo Rodrigues, et al. Functional deficiencies of sulfite oxidase: differential diagnoses in neonates presenting with intractable seizures and cystic encephalomalacia. *Brain Dev.* 2010;32:544–549.
25. Bakker HD, Abeling NG, ten Houten R, et al. Molybdenum cofactor deficiency can mimic postanoxic encephalopathy. *J Inherit Metab Dis.* 1993;16:900–901.
26. Eyaid WM, Al-Nouri DM, Rashed MS, et al. An inborn error of metabolism presenting as hypoxic-ischemic insult. *Pediatr Neurol.* 2005;32:134–136.
27. Eichler F, Tan WH, Shih VE, et al. Proton magnetic resonance spectroscopy and diffusion-weighted imaging in isolated sulfite oxidase deficiency. *J Child Neurol.* 2006;21:801–805.

28. Schuierer G, Kurlemann G, Bick U, et al. Molybdenum-cofactor deficiency: CT and MR findings. *Neuropediatrics*. 1995;26:51–54.

29. Pintos-Morell G, Naranjo MA, Artigas M, et al. Molybdenum cofactor deficiency associated with Dandy-Walker malformation. *J Inherit Metab Dis*. 1995;18: 86–87.

30. Teksam O, Yurdakok M, Coskun T. Molybdenum cofactor deficiency presenting with severe metabolic acidosis and intracranial hemorrhage. *J Child Neurol*. 2005;20:155–157.

31. Carmi-Nawi N, Malinger G, Mandel H, et al. Prenatal brain disruption in molybdenum cofactor deficiency. *J Child Neurol*. 2011;26:460–404. Epub 2011 Jan 31.

32. van der Klei-van Moorsel JM, Smit LM, et al. Infantile isolated sulphite oxidase deficiency: report of a case with negative sulphite test and normal sulphate excretion. *Eur J Pediatr*. 1991;150:196–197.

33. Simmonds HA, Hofmann GF, Pérignon JL, et al. Diagnosis of molybdenum cofactor deficiency. *Lancet*. 1999;353:675.

34. Duran M, Aarsen G, Fokkens RH, et al. 2-Mercaptoethanesulfonate-cysteine disulfide excretion following the administration of 2-mercaptoethanesulfonate—a pitfall in the diagnosis of sulfite oxidase deficiency. *Clin Chim Acta*. 1981;111:47–53.

35. Mann G, Kirk JM. Antibiotic interference in urinary thiosulphate measurements. *J Inherit Metab Dis*. 1994;17:120–121.

36. Carragher FM, Kirk JM, Steer C, et al. False negative thiosulphate screening test in a case of molybdenum cofactor deficiency. *J Inherit Metab Dis*. 1999;22:842–843.

37. Johnson JL, Rajagopalan KV. Structural and metabolic relationship between the molybdenum cofactor and urothione. *Proc Nat Acad Sci*. 1982;79:6856–6860.

38. Bremer HJ, Duran M, Kamerling JP, et al. *Disturbances of Amino Acid Metabolism: Clinical Chemistry and Diagnosis*. Baltimore-Munich: Urban & Schwarzenberg; 1981.

39. Kishikawa M, Sass JO, Sakura N, et al. The peak height of S-sulfonated transthyretin and other oxidized isoforms as a marker for molybdenum cofactor deficiency, measured by electrospray ionization mass spectrometry. *Biochim Biophys Acta*. 2002;1588:135–138.

40. Footitt EJ, Mills PB, Clubley C, et al. Alpha-aminoadipic semialdehyde is elevated in molybdenum cofactor deficiency. *J Inherit Metab Dis*. 2011;34(Suppl 3):S84.

41. Sass JO, Nakanishi T, Sato T, et al. New approaches towards laboratory diagnosis of isolated sulphite oxidase deficiency. *Ann Clin Biochem*. 2004;41:157.

42. Raivio KO, Saksela M, Lapatto R. Xanthine oxidoreductase—role in human pathophysiology and in hereditary xanthinuria In: CR Scriver, AL Beaudet, WS Sly, et al., eds. *The Metabolic and Molecular Bases of Inherited Disease*. New York: McGraw-Hill; 2001:2639–2652.

43. Garattini E, Fratelli M, Terao M. The mammalian aldehyde oxidase gene family. *Hum Genomics*. 2009;4:119–130.

44. Wahl B, Reichmann D, Niks D, et al. Biochemical and spectroscopic characterization of the human mitochondrial amidoxime reducing components hmARC-1 and hmARC-2 suggests the existence of a new molybdenum enzyme family in eukaryotes. *J Biol Chem*. 2010;285:37847–37859.

45. Johnson JL, Wuebbens MM, Mandell R, et al. Molybdenum cofactor biosynthesis in humans. Identification of two complementation groups of cofactor-deficient patients and preliminary characterization of a diffusible molybdopterin precursor. *J Clin Invest*. 1989;83:897–903.

46. Reiss J, Johnson JL. Mutations in the molybdenum cofactor biosynthetic genes MOCS1, MOCS2, and GEPH. *Hum Mutat*. 2003;21:569–576.

47. Santamaria-Araujo JA, Fischer B, Otte T, et al. The tetrahydropyranopterin structure of the sulfur-free and metal-free molybdenum cofactor precursor. *J Biol Chem*. 2004;279: 15994–15999.

48. Reiss J, Dorche C, Stallmeyer B, et al. Human molybdopterin synthase gene: genomic structure and mutations in molybdenum cofactor deficiency type B. *Am J Hum Genet*. 1999;64:706–711.

49. Reiss J, Gross-Hardt S, Christensen E, et al. A mutation in the gene for the neurotransmitter receptor-clustering protein gephyrin causes a novel form of molybdenum cofactor deficiency. *Am J Hum Genet*. 2001;68:208–213.

50. Til HP, Feron VJ, De Groot AP. The toxicity of sulphite. I. Long-term feeding and multigeneration studies in rats. *Food Cosmet Toxicol*. 1972;10:291–310.

51. Southerland WM, Akogyeram CO, Toghrol F, et al. Interaction of bisulfite with unsaturated fatty acids. *J Toxicol Environ Health*. 1982;10:479–491.

52. Zhang X, Vincent AS, Halliwell B, et al. A mechanism of sulfite neurotoxicity: direct inhibition of glutamate dehydrogenase. *J Biol Chem*. 2004;279:43035–43045.

53. Olney JW, Misra CH, de Gubareff T. Cysteine-S-sulfate: brain damaging metabolite in sulfite oxidase deficiency. *J Neuropathol Exp Neurol*. 1975;34:167–177.

54. Kurlemann G, Debus O, Schuierer G. Dextromethorphan in molybdenum cofactor deficiency. *Eur J Pediatr*. 1996;155:422–423.

55. Gümüş H, Ghesquiere S, Per H, et al. Maternal uniparental isodisomy is responsible for serious molybdenum cofactor deficiency. *Dev Med Child Neurol*. 2010;52:868–872. Epub 2010 June 22.

56. Boles RG, Ment LR, Meyn MS, et al. Short-term response to dietary therapy in molybdenum cofactor deficiency. *Ann Neurol*. 1993;34:742–744.

57. Lee HF, Mak BS, Chi CS, et al. A novel mutation in neonatal isolated sulphite oxidase deficiency. *Neuropediatrics*. 2002;33: 174–179.

58. Chan KY, Li CK, Lai CK, et al. Infantile isolated sulphite oxidase deficiency in a Chinese family: a rare neurodegenerative disorder. *Hong Kong Med J*. 2002;8:279–282.

59. Tardy P, Parvy P, Charpentier C, et al. Attempt at therapy in sulphite oxidase deficiency. *J Inherit Metab Dis*. 1989;12:94–95.

60. Endres W, Shin YS, Günther R, et al. Report on a new patient with combined deficiencies of sulphite oxidase and xanthine dehydrogenase due to molybdenum cofactor deficiency. *Eur J Pediatr*. 1988;148:246–249.

61. Lee HJ, Adham IM, Schwarz G, et al. Molybdenum cofactor-deficient mice resemble the phenotype of human patients. *Hum Mol Genet*. 2002;11:3309–3317.

62. Schwarz G, Santamaria-Araujo JA, Wolf S, et al. Rescue of lethal molybdenum cofactor deficiency by a biosynthetic precursor from Escherichia coli. *Hum Mol Genet*. 2004;13:1249–1255.

Creatine Disorders and Epilepsy

Ton de Grauw

CREATINE DEFICIENCY SYNDROMES

In 1994, the first inborn error of creatine metabolism was reported in a 22-month-old boy with developmental delay, a movement disorder, and low creatinine excretion in the urine (1). MRI of the brain showed bilateral globus pallidus abnormalities and H-MRS showed absence of the creatine peak. EEG showed a low voltage pattern with multifocal spikes. Creatine and creatinine were decreased, but guanidinoacetate/creatinine (GAA/Crn) was elevated in the urine as expected. Subsequently, it was found that this patient and an additional patient, a 4-year-old female, had mutations in the guanidino acetate methyl transferase (GAMT) gene (2). Since then, two more creatine deficiency syndromes have been recognized. Both creatine transporter (CrT) deficiency and arginine glycine amidino transferase (AGAT) deficiency were first reported in 2001 (3, 4).

CREATINE PHYSIOLOGY

About 50% of the daily creatine requirement is met through the diet. In addition, the body produces creatine in the kidney (AGAT), liver (GAMT) (Figure 21.1), and possibly in the pancreas (5). Because the intracellular creatine concentration is higher than the concentration in the blood by a factor of 1,000, an active transporter (CrT) is required for creatine uptake into tissues. SLC6A8, a gene on the X-chromosome, was found to be the CrT gene (6). Although a second gene was found on chromosome 16 (SLC1A10), this was labeled a pseudogene (7). Muscle, heart, brain, retina, and the GI tract all require active uptake of creatine. Creatine is also reabsorbed in the kidney through this active uptake process.

Through the creatine kinase (CK) reaction, creatine is phosphorylated and stored for energy-requiring processes in the cell. Four distinct types of CK subunits exist, and they are each expressed in different tissues. The cytosolic M-CK (M for muscle) and B-CK (B for brain) form dimeric molecules and combine into three isoenzymes: MM-CK, MB-CK, and BB-CK. Two mitochondrial isoenzymes have been recognized: ubiquitous Mi-CK and sarcomeric Mi-CK. Both are located in the mitochondrial intermembrane space.

Adult humans contain approximately 120 g of creatine. Creatine is metabolized intracellularly to creatinine by a nonenzymatic process at a rate of 1.7% of the total creatine pool per day, which equals about 2 g/day of creatinine production.

Creatine physiology continues to be evaluated. Recently, after the recognition that creatine deficiency affects the CNS, one study showed that creatine may occasionally function as a neurotransmitter (8). Additionally, it has been shown in rat brains that AGAT and GAMT are present in the CNS, although mostly in separate cells (9). These authors also showed that GAA requires CrT for uptake in the GAMT-containing cells to produce creatine.

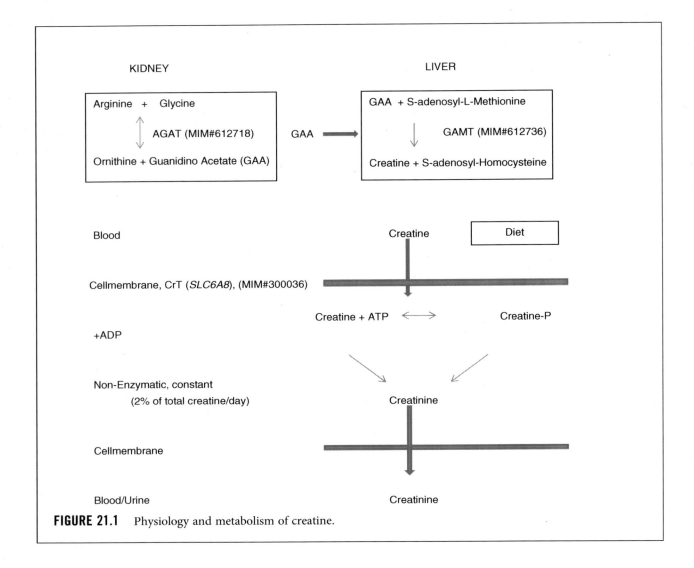

FIGURE 21.1   Physiology and metabolism of creatine.

AGAT DEFICIENCY

Only eight patients with AGAT deficiency have been reported (4, 10–12). All of them presented with developmental delay and intellectual deficiency without any specific neurological problems or deficits on physical or neurological examination. Laboratory tests showed low creatine (Cr) and low guanidino acetic acid (GAA) levels in the blood and urine. All had low or absent creatine in the brain as measured by proton MR spectroscopy. Creatine supplementation improved cognitive function dramatically in young patients, but less so in the adults. One subject was diagnosed in the neonatal period, started on creatine supplementation in the first few months, and is reported to be developing normally (12).

Although one of the patients had febrile seizures, none of the patients developed epilepsy, including two subjects who were not diagnosed until their twenties (11). Some of the patients had EEGs done, all of which were normal.

GAMT DEFICIENCY

GAMT deficiency, which was first described in 1994, was the first creatine deficiency syndrome to be reported. Initially, patients reported with severe developmental delay and severe neurological problems, such as movement disorders and epilepsy (1). The neurological symptoms of seizures and abnormal movements (eg, tremors, chorea) responded dramatically to creatine supplementation, but developmental progress was limited (13). Abnormal neurological function was primarily attributed to GAA levels in the blood, which remained elevated. Later, patients were reported with milder phenotypes (14).

All GAMT deficiency patients present with developmental delay and approximately 50% develop seizures. A recent report on eight patients showed developmental delay in all of them, and seizures in four patients (one developed myoclonic seizures, the others were not described) (15). Three of these patients had an EEG, two of which showed slow background activity; one showed generalized epileptiform activity.

Currently, the standard treatment for GAMT deficiency consists of creatine monohydrate and dietary restrictions. The therapeutic dose of creatine monohydrate is unknown, but patients are usually treated with 5 to 20 g/day. Although treatment with creatine monohydrate has proven effective in restoring normal creatine concentration in tissues, it does not correct the high level of GAA, which is neurotoxic. Thus, patients are treated with a low-protein diet to limit arginine intake and decrease GAA production. So far, this treatment has resulted in lower GAA levels, but the reported patients continue to have substantially increased GAA blood concentrations. Additionally, patients are treated with ornithine supplementation to avoid ornithine deficiency secondary to arginine restriction. Table 21.1 shows GAA concentrations in the blood and urine remain high in two of our patients

TABLE 21.1   Creatine Treatment (With Protein Restriction) in GAMT Patients

	Patient 3			
DATE	**GAA/CRN (U)** (NL: 8–150)	**CR/CRN (U)** (NL: 28–1350)	**GAA (B, μmol/L)** (NL: 0.3–2.8)	**CR (B, μmol/L)** (NL: 20–110)
05/27/08	1986	49		
START TREATMENT	15 g creatine/day			
08/11/08	349	11,781		
02/02/09	427	18,233		
05/18/09	530	39,555		
01/11/10	456	10,302	8.7	950
12/08/10	465	5,950	13.4	677
	Patient 4			
DATE	**GAA/CRN (U)** (NL: 8–150)	**CR/CRN (U)** (NL: 28–1350)	**GAA (B, μmol/L)** (NL: 0.3–2.8)	**CR (B, μmol/L)** (NL: 20–110)
05/27/08	1083	33		
START TREATMENT	10 g creatine/day			
08/11/08	310	29,649		
02/02/09	285	22,881		
05/18/09	526	46,307		
01/11/10			10.8	433
12/08/10	728	26,004	34.6	2457

who were put on creatine supplements and protein restriction.

Four patients currently being followed for GAMT deficiency are described here. Two brothers (Patients 1 and 2) with intellectual deficiency and partial epilepsy were diagnosed at the ages of 16 and 20 years, respectively. Seizures were well controlled, and they remained seizure-free for a 10-year period after antiepileptic drugs were discontinued. The family refused treatment with creatine.

A 4-year-old girl (Pt 3) was diagnosed after she presented with staring spells and developmental delay. MRI of the brain was normal, but h-MRS showed absence of the creatine peak (Figure 21.2). Prior to the diagnosis of GAMT deficiency, she was diagnosed with autism at our developmental pediatrics clinic. Her EEG showed a moderately slow background and runs of generalized spike-and-slow wave discharges at 2 to 3 Hz; some of these discharges were associated with clinical symptoms of absence seizures. She was started on creatine monohydrate, a low-protein diet, and ornithine supplementation. The absence seizures were quickly controlled, and a 24-hour EEG 3 months

later was completely normal. Another 3 months later, her MRI was normal and h-MRS showed a normal creatine concentration (Figure 21.3). Her cognitive function started to improve after 6 to 9 months.

Currently, she is 7 years old and in regular first grade with some assistance. Her IQ has increased from 59 at age 4 to 79 at present. Unfortunately, her absence seizures returned and she was started on lamotrigine, which controlled her seizures quickly. The EEG showed normal background and two electroclinical seizures with generalized $2\frac{1}{2}$ Hz spike and slow wave discharges. This finding is comparable to the absence seizures and EEG abnormalities that have been found in patients with glucose transporter (GLUT1) deficiency (16), a pattern that raises the question of whether or not disorders of energy metabolism could be associated with early-onset absence epilepsy.

A younger sister of patient 3 (Pt 4) with more severe developmental delay was diagnosed with GAMT deficiency at 18 months of age. MRI of the brain showed increased signal of the globus pallidus bilaterally on T2 and FLAIR images (Figure 21.4). She never had seizures, and EEG showed mild generalized

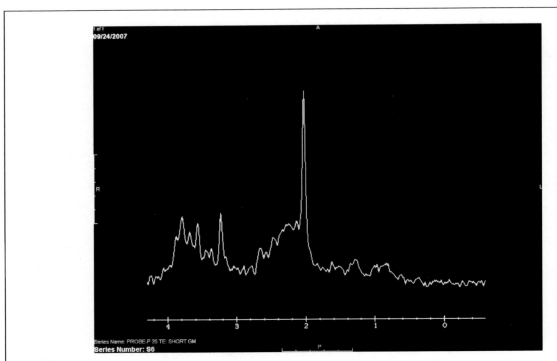

FIGURE 21.2   h-MRS of patient 3 showing absent creatine peak at 3.03 ppm before treatment.

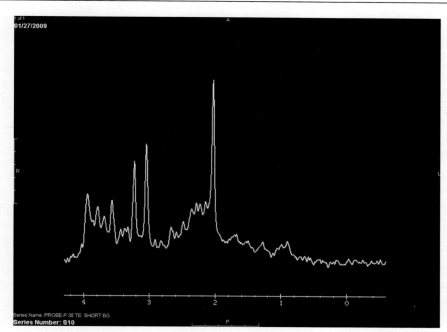

FIGURE 21.3 h-MRS of patient 3 showing normal creatine peak at 3.03 ppm after treatment with 15 g of creatine monohydrate.

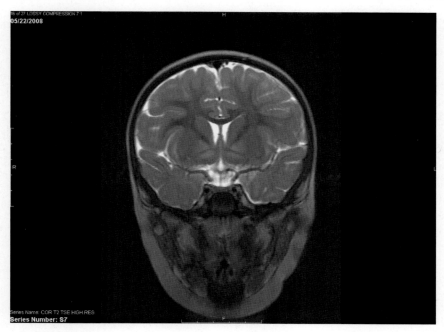

FIGURE 21.4 MRI of the brain, coronal view showing increased signal in globus pallidus bilaterally.

slowing. Treatment normalized her development as well as her brain MRI. The abnormal signal in the globus pallidus has been reported in some of the aforementioned case reports; however, it has not been reported in the other creatine deficiency syndromes.

CRT DEFICIENCY

The creatine transporter gene, SLC6A8, was found in 1995. It is located on the X-chromosome at Xq28 (6). Since our first report of a patient with CrT deficiency in 2001, we have identified several others with the disease. A phenotype of males with intellectual deficiency with predominantly language involvement has now been described. Carrier females may present with learning disabilities (17). Many other cases have been published, and it has been suggested that CrT deficiency is the second most common cause of X-linked mental retardation (XLMR) after Fragile X syndrome (18). Over the past 10 years, patients have been described with phenotypes ranging in severity (19, 20).

Most of the patients develop epilepsy that is controlled with antiepileptic medication. Fons et al reported on epilepsy in six patients. They did not find any specific seizure type or EEG abnormality except for generalized slow background (21). Nonlesional partial epilepsy appears to be the most common epilepsy type, but generalized convulsions and other generalized epilepsies have been reported. Although no long-term outcome studies have been done, it is our experience that seizures decrease in adolescence and adulthood. Five of our patients had EEG's done for seizures. Two of the EEGs were completely normal. One EEG showed mild background slowing, and another showed mild background slowing with bilateral occipital intermittent polymorphic delta activity. One patient had an EEG done showing generalized bursts of polyspikes without clinical changes. A 24-hour EEG in one of the patients showed multifocal epileptiform discharges without seizures, and sleep did not activate the epileptiform activity.

CONCLUSION

Although patients with creatine deficiency syndromes often present with seizures, preliminary studies have failed to identify a specific seizure type or specific EEG abnormality. Variation in seizure severity is common. Seizures in patients with creatine synthesis defects may respond to creatine supplementation, but treatment may require antiepileptic drugs. The creatine transporter deficiency syndrome remains untreatable, but many patients' seizures can be treated successfully with medication.

CLINICAL PEARLS

1. Three creatine deficiency disorders: all have identical phenotype
2. Phenotype includes: developmental delay, seizures, autistic features, movement disorders
3. Urinary screening for Cr and GAA is most appropriate: AGAT: ↓ CR, ↓ GAA; GAMT: ↓ CR, ↑ GAA; CRT: ↑ CR
4. AGAT and GAMT deficiency are (partially) treatable
5. CRT deficiency appears to be relatively common

REFERENCES

1. Stockler S, Holzbach U, Hanefeld F, et al. Creatine deficiency in the brain: a new, treatable inborn error of metabolism. *Pediatr Res.* 1994;36(3):409–413.
2. Stockler S, Hanefeld F. Guanidinoacetate methyltransferase deficiency: a newly recognized inborn error of creatine biosynthesis. *Wien Klin Wochenschr.* 1997;109(3):86–88.
3. Salomons GS, vanDooren SJ, Verhoeven NM, et al. X-linked creatine-transporter gene (SLC6A8) defect: a new creatine-deficiency syndrome. *Am J Hum Genet.* 2001;68(6):1497–1500.
4. Item CB, Stockler-Ipsiroglu S, Stromberger C, et al. Arginine glycine amidinotransferase deficiency: the third inborn error of creatine metabolism in humans. *Am J Hum Genet.* 2001;69(5):1127–1133.
5. Wyss M, Kaddurah-Daouk R. Creatine and creatinine metabolism. *Physiol Rev.* 2000;80(3):1107–1213.
6. Gregor P, Nash SR, Caron MG, et al. Assignment of the creatine transporter gene (SLC6A8) to human chromosome Xq28 telomeric to G6PD. *Genomics.* 1995;25(1):332–333.
7. Hoglund PJ, Adzic D, Scicluna SJ, et al. The repertoire of solute carriers of family 6: Identification of new human and rodent genes. *Biochem Biophys Res Commun.* 2005;336(1):175–189.
8. Almeida LS, Salomons GS, Hogenboom F, et al. Exocytotic release of creatine in rat brain. *Synapse.* 2006;60(2):118–123.
9. Braissant O, Beard E, Torrent C, et al. Dissociation of AGAT, GAMT and SLC6A8 in CNS: relevance to creatine deficiency syndromes. *Neurobiol Dis.* 2010;37(2):423–433.

10. Battini R, Leuzzi V, Carducci C, et al. Creatine depletion in a new case with AGAT deficiency: clinical and genetic study in a large pedigree. *Mol Genet Metab.* 2002:77(4):326–331.

11. Edvardson S, Korman SH, Livine A, et al. L-arginine: glycine amidinotransferase (AGAT) deficiency: clinical presentation response to treatment in two patients with a novel mutation. *Mol Genet Metab.* 2010;101(2–3):228–232.

12. Schulze A, Battini R. Pre-symptomatic treatment of creatine biosynthesis defects. *Subcell Biochem.* 2007;46:167–181.

13. Stockler S, Hanefeld F, Frahm J. Creatine replacement therapy in guanidinoacetate methyltransferase deficiency, a novel inborn error of metabolism. *Lancet.* 1996;348(9030):789–790.

14. O'Rourke DJ, Ryan S, Salomons G, et al. Guanidinoacetate methyltransferase (GAMT) deficiency: late onset of movement disorder and preserved expressive language. *Dev Med Child Neurol.* 2009;51(5):404–407.

15. Dhar SU, Scaglia F, Li FY, et al. Expanded clinical and molecular spectrum of guanidinoacetate methyltransferase (GAMT) deficiency. *Mol Genet Metab.* 2009;96(1):38–43.

16. Mullen SA, Suls A, DeJonghe P, et al. Absence epilepsies with widely variable onset are a key feature of familial GLUT1 deficiency. *Neurology.* 2010;75(5):432–440.

17. deGrauw TJ, Cecil KM, Byars AW, et al. The clinical syndrome of creatine transporter deficiency. *Mol Cell Biochem.* 2003;244(1–2):45–48.

18. Rosenberg EH, Almeida LS, Kleefstra T, et al. High prevalence of SLC6A8 deficiency in X-linked mental retardation. *Am J Hum Genet.* 2004;75(1):97–105.

19. Mancardi MM, Caruso U, Schiaffino MC, et al. Severe epilepsy in X-linked creatine transporter defect (CRTR-D). *Epilepsia.* 2007;48(6):1211–1213.

20. Alcaide P, Rodriguez-Pombo P, Ruiz-Sala P, et al. A new case of creatine transporter deficiency associated with mild clinical phenotype and a novel mutation in the SLC6A8 gene. *Dev Med Child Neurol.* 2010;52(2):215–217.

21. Fons C, Sempere A, Sanmarti FX, et al. Epilepsy spectrum in cerebral creatine transporter deficiency. *Epilepsia.* 2009;50(9):2168–2170.

22

Cerebral Folate Deficiency and Epilepsy

Fernando Scaglia

INTRODUCTION

Folates are required cofactors for one-carbon methyl transfer reactions and are involved in several biological processes including DNA synthesis, regulation of gene expression through methylation reactions, determination of embryonic central nervous system development, and synthesis of amino acids and neurotransmitters (1–5). Folate must be obtained from an exogenous source in mammals as the liver stores folate for only a few months. Dietary folate is absorbed in the intestine, metabolized in the liver to 5-methyltetrahydrofolate (5-MTHF), and then distributed in the bloodstream. The uptake of 5-MTHF in cells is carried out by different transport systems including the proton-coupled folate transporter (PCFT), the reduced folate carrier (RFC), and two GPI-anchored receptors, folate receptor alpha (FRα), and beta (FRβ) (6). The physiological form of folate, 5MTHF, is actively transported from the plasma to the central nervous system by an FRα-mediated endocytotic process in choroid epithelial cells and reaches a two- to fourfold higher concentration in the cerebrospinal fluid compared to the serum. FRα is a high-affinity receptor that functions at the physiological nanomolar range of extracellular folate concentrations (7). Thus far, five different inherited disorders of folate metabolism are known which lead to generalized folate deficiency (8–10).

CEREBRAL FOLATE DEFICIENCY IS ASSOCIATED WITH DIVERSE NEUROLOGICAL CONDITIONS

Initially, low cerebrospinal fluid (CSF) levels of 5-methyltetrahydrofolate (5-MTHF) were observed in an 18-year-old teenager with progressive sensorineural hearing loss, cerebellar ataxia, and pyramidal tract dysfunction (11). Low CSF levels of 5-MTHF were also documented in five children who presented at 6 months of age with irritability, deceleration of head growth, disturbed sleep, psychomotor delay, cerebellar ataxia, epilepsy, pyramidal signs, and cerebral atrophy (12). These clinical findings were corroborated in a larger series of 20 subjects (13).

Moreover, CFD was documented in a child who presented with a progressive neurological syndrome consisting of epilepsy, intellectual disability, and autistic features in the presence of normal peripheral folate levels (14). Folinic acid supplementation corrected the CSF abnormalities and the patient exhibited remarkable motor improvement with restoration of independent gait, hand use, and oral feeding. A follow-up EEG showed no epileptiform activity, although background slowing persisted. The fact that autistic features are salient in CFD was demonstrated in another report of seven children with CFD (15). Five subjects met criteria for autism spectrum disorder and six had epilepsy. The epilepsy improved with folinic acid treatment in only one subject, whereas in the other five, there was no response to this treatment. In another report, one patient with hypomyelination with atrophy of the basal ganglia and cerebellum syndrome was found to have CFD (16).

Other neurogenetic conditions that have been associated with CFD include isolated Rett syndrome (17) and atypical Aicardi–Goutières syndrome associated with microcephaly, severe developmental delay, dyskinesia, epilepsy, and CNS calcifications (18). On the basis of these reports, developmental delay, regression, dyskinesia, epilepsy, and autistic features could be considered core clinical features of this neurometabolic condition.

CEREBRAL FOLATE DEFICIENCY ASSOCIATED WITH INBORN ERRORS OF METABOLISM

CFD has been recognized as a neurobiochemical feature associated with an inborn error of serine biosynthesis, 3-phosphoglycerate dehydrogenase deficiency (19). This is a condition that is associated with epilepsy, congenital microcephaly, and psychomotor retardation. In this syndrome, the epilepsy can be successfully treated with serine supplementation. CFD may also be associated with a number of metabolic disorders involving folate metabolism: 5,10-methylene-tetrahydrofolate reductase deficiency (20), dihydropteridine reductase deficiency (21); hereditary folate malabsorption (10), dihydrofolate reductase deficiency (22), and glutamate formiminotransferase deficiency (23). However, in all of these conditions the folate deficiency is systemic and not confined to the central nervous system.

CEREBRAL FOLATE DEFICIENCY ASSOCIATED WITH THE PRESENCE OF BLOCKING AUTOANTIBODIES

The underlying etiology for CFD has remained elusive for a long time, although in some cases may be associated with the presence of blocking autoantibodies to folate receptors (24). These patients may present in early childhood with generalized tonic–clonic seizures and develop intractable epilepsy that is refractory to treatment with folinic acid (25). However, these patients may present in adolescence with schizophrenic symptoms and worsening catatonia (26).

CEREBRAL FOLATE DEFICIENCY IS ASSOCIATED WITH MITOCHONDRIAL ENCEPHALOMYOPATHIES

Among mitochondrial syndromes, Kearns–Sayre syndrome has been reported to be associated with low levels of CSF 5-MTHF (27–30). It is thought that the low CSF 5-MTHF could be caused by the ensuing lack of ATP production required for the active ATP-dependent folate transport across the blood–brain barrier. Moreover, one additional publication reported low plasma folate in addition to low CSF 5-MTHF (31). Autopsy studies in deceased patients with Kearns–Sayre syndrome have demonstrated oncocytic transformation of epithelial cells in the choroid plexus accompanied by the presence of mtDNA deletions and decreased expression of mitochondrial DNA encoded proteins (30). This factor could also contribute to the observed low levels of CSF 5-MTHF as the uptake of 5-MTHF occurs primarily in the choroid plexus (32). Beneficial effects with folinic acid supplementation such as reversal of white matter demyelination have been reported in these patients (29).

A patient with a severe mitochondrial complex I encephalomyopathy associated with psychomotor retardation, weakness, hypotonia, ataxia, refractory epilepsy, spastic diplegia, leukoencephalopathy with demyelination, and low CSF 5-MTHF has been reported (33). The patient had onset of generalized and focal epileptic seizures at 1 year of age. Seizures could not be controlled with conventional antiepileptic therapy. At age 1 year and 2 months, the use of ubiquinone, vitamin C, and vitamin E decreased the frequency of akinetic and adverse motor seizures with persistence of other clinical signs and symptoms. At age 1 year and 10 months, folinic acid and riboflavin were added and after 1 year, the seizures were fully controlled and the electroencephalogram normalized. The ataxia and hypotonia improved and this patient was then able to sit after 4 years of treatment. Follow-up brain MRI revealed reversal of signs of hypomyelination and absence of lactate peak on MR spectroscopy. Reduced folate transport across the choroid plexus has been observed in other mitochondrial encephalomyopathies.

Another mitochondrial syndrome where CFD has been described is Alpers disease (34). Patients present with psychomotor retardation followed by regression, intractable epilepsy, abnormal breathing pattern, cortical atrophy, and liver dysfunction (35). The syndrome is caused by mutations in the *POLG* gene encoding the mitochondrial DNA polymerase gamma (36). A $3\frac{1}{2}$-year-old girl with Alpers disease and two pathogenic POLG mutations (p.A467T/p.G848S) was found to have CFD (34). EEG activity was suppressed with the presence of focal spike waves over the temporal region. Laboratory investigations demonstrated elevated CSF neopterin, IL-6, IL-8, IFN-gamma, reduced CSF 5-MTHF, and increased serum and CSF folate receptor blocking autoantibodies. Treatment with oral leucovorin was initiated. Over a period of 17 months, levels of folate receptor blocking autoantibodies continued to increase. Combined therapy with phenobarbital and vigabatrin led to suppression of the status epilepticus and marked reduction of focal seizures. During the time the child received folinic acid therapy, the high-amplitude slow waves on EEG decreased and the epileptiform activity was less pronounced. The low 5-MTHF CSF levels in this patient could be caused by interference of transport across the blood–brain barrier due to the action of autoantibodies as well as defective transport due to ATP depletion in the choroid plexus. Moreover, increased utilization and catabolism of 5-MTHF due to oxidative stress has been postulated (33). Currently, it is not known whether the production of folate receptor autoantibodies in Alpers syndrome may represent a constant finding or be associated with a cerebral inflammatory response.

OTHER SECONDARY CAUSES OF CFD

One secondary cause of CFD may be associated with the use of valproic acid that may impair the uptake of folate that occurs primarily in the choroid plexus (32). This hypothesis may be linked to the observation that the use of antiepileptic drugs known to have antifolate effects during pregnancy increases the risk of neural tube defects and other birth defects in the offspring of women suffering from epilepsy (37–38).

MUTATIONS IN THE *FOLR1* GENE CAUSE CFD ASSOCIATED WITH NEURODEGENERATION AND DISTURBED MYELIN METABOLISM

Recently, patients with impaired transport of folate to the CNS caused by loss of function mutations in the *FOLR1* gene encoding the folate receptor alpha have

been reported. The patients exhibited psychomotor decline, progressive movement disturbances, white matter disease, and epilepsy (39–40). Patients typically exhibit null mutations as in the report by Steinfeld et al where two siblings were compound heterozygous for two nonsense mutations, p.Q118X and p.C175X (40). These patients had an initial period of normal development. Myoclonic–astatic seizures have been described in the most affected patients (39). MR-based *in vivo* metabolite analysis indicated depletion of white matter choline and inositol. *FOLR1* mutations cause severe CFD in these patients. These patients have almost undetectable levels of CSF 5MTHF with a decrease in CSF 5MTHF concentrations greater than 80% below the lower limit of reference values. Glial choline and inositol depletion and CSF 5-MTHF were restored by folinic acid therapy. However, the epilepsy in these patients has been described as drug refractory (40).

Furthermore, progressive myoclonic epilepsy was described in an additional patient with a homozygous p.C105R mutation in the *FOLR1* gene (41). The epilepsy in this patient was treated successfully with high-dose folinic acid supplementation. CFD caused by a homozygous mutation (p.R204X) in the *FOLR1* gene was described in a patient with congenital deafness, labyrinthine aplasia, microtia, and microdontia syndrome (LAMM) (42). This report stressed the importance of CSF folate evaluation in patients with unexplained neurological presentation in the setting of a malformation syndrome. Folinic acid treatment helped to regain consciousness in this child but the epilepsy was only managed successfully with pyridoxal-5-phosphate.

TREATMENT

The mainstay of treatment of CFD is the use of folinic acid with a starting dose of 0.5 mg/kg body weight that would be increased to 1 mg/kg of body weight. This treatment has led to normalization of CSF 5-methyltetrahydrofolate and improvement in clinical symptoms (14, 43, 15). In cases of CFD caused by FOLR1 mutations, the increase in CSF 5-MTHF requires considerable doses of folinic acid of up to 5 mg/kg per day. Folinic acid is a more stable and metabolic active form of folate when compared to folic acid which is an oxidized, metabolically inactive form of folate. It has been thought that folic acid may have adverse effects such as the induction of epileptic seizures (13). Neurological dysfunction and epilepsy can be reversed by folate therapy (14, 44).

CONCLUSIONS

The CNS folate deficiency with normal content of folate in the peripheral tissues is compatible with defective folate transfer across the choroid plexus. Although the responsible mechanism in most of the CFD cases remains elusive, mutations in the *FOLR1* gene have been described in few cases. In some patients, the presence of folate receptor auto-antibodies suggests that CFD may be caused by blocking folate transport into the CSF. It has been postulated that the antibodies would bind to the folate receptors on the choroid plexus. However, in the majority of cases CFD may represent a common final pathway of different pathological mechanisms leading to neuronal dysfunction and perturbed CNS metabolism. Since there is some evidence that some aspects of cerebral dysfunction including epileptic manifestations can be reversed by therapy with folinic acid, a case could be made to screen the CSF of subjects with unknown neurological disorders for the presence of CFD.

CLINICAL PEARLS

1. CFD is a condition associated with decreased levels of 5-methyltetrahydrofolate in the cerebrospinal fluid with normal plasma and red blood cell folate levels.
2. In the majority of cases, CFD may represent a common final pathway of different pathological mechanisms leading to neuronal dysfunction and perturbed CNS metabolism.
3. In a minority of patients, mutations in *FOLR1* that impair folate transport to the central nervous system, have been reported.
4. Epilepsy, intellectual disability, developmental regression, dyskinesias, and autism are salient features of this condition.
5. Some features of cerebral dysfunction including epileptic manifestations can be reversed or ameliorated by folinic acid supplementation.

SUMMARY

Cerebral folate deficiency (CFD) is a neurometabolic condition associated with low levels of 5-methyltetrahydrofolate in the cerebrospinal fluid with normal folate levels in plasma and red blood cells. CFD has been found in diverse neurological conditions and for the majority of patients does not represent a defined neurogenetic syndrome but the common result of different genetic and metabolic disorders. There seems to be a role for blocking autoantibodies against membrane-associated folate receptors of the choroid plexus in certain cases. Successful treatment of CFD with high doses of folinic acid has been reported in some subjects with CFD.

REFERENCES

1. Blount BC, Mack MM, Wehr CM, et al. Folate deficiency causes uracil misincorporation into human DNA and chromosome breakage: implications for cancer and neuronal damage. *Proc Natl Acad Sci USA.* 1997;94(7):3290–3295.
2. Linhart HG, Troen A, Bell GW, et al. Folate deficiency induces genomic uracil misincorporation and hypomethylation but does not increase DNA point mutations. *Gastroenterology.* 2009;136(1):227–235.
3. Ghoshal K, Li X, Datta J, et al. A folate- and methyl-deficient diet alters the expression of DNA methyltransferases and methyl CpG binding proteins involved in epigenetic gene silencing in livers of F344 rats. *J Nutr.* 2006;136(6):1522–1527.
4. Pogribny IP, Karpf AR, James SR, et al. Epigenetic alterations in the brains of Fisher 344 rats induced by long-term administration of folate/methyl-deficient diet. *Brain Res.* 2008;1237: 25–34.
5. Fournier I, Ploye F, Cottet-Emard JM, et al. Folate deficiency alters melatonin secretion in rats. *J Nutr.* 2002;132(9): 2781–2784.
6. Matherly LH, Goldman DI. Membrane transport of folates. *Vitam Horm.* 2003;66:403–456.
7. Weitman SD, Weinberg AG, Coney LR, et al. Cellular localization of the folate receptor: Potential role in drug toxicity and folate homeostasis. *Cancer Res.* 1992;52:6708–6711.
8. Rosenblatt DS, Fenton WA. Inherited disorders of folate and cobalamin transport and metabolism. In: CR Scriver, AL Beaudet, WS Sly , et al. eds. *The Metabolic and Molecular Bases of Inherited Disease.* 8th ed. New York: McGraw-Hill; 2001:3897.
9. Hilton JF, Christensen KE, Watkins D, et al. The molecular basis of glutamate formiminotransferase-cyclodeaminase deficiency. *Hum Mut.* 2003;22:67–73.
10. Qiu A, Jansen M, Sakaris A, et al. Identification of an intestinal folate transporter and the molecular basis for hereditary folate malabsorption. *Cell.* 2006;127(5):917–928.

11. Wevers RA, Hansen SI, van Hellenberg Hubar JL, et al. Folate deficiency in cerebrospinal fluid associated with a defect in folate binding protein in the central nervous system. *J Neurol Neurosurg Psychiatry*. 1994;57(2):223–226.
12. Ramaekers VT, Häusler M, Opladen T, et al. Psychomotor retardation, spastic paraplegia, cerebellar ataxia and dyskinesia associated with low 5-methyltetrahydrofolate in cerebrospinal fluid: a novel neurometabolic condition responding to folinic acid substitution. *Neuropediatrics*. 2002;33(6):301–308.
13. Ramaekers VT, Blau N. Cerebral folate deficiency. *Dev Med Child Neurol*. 2004;46(12):843–851.
14. Moretti P, Sahoo T, Hyland K, et al. Cerebral folate deficiency with developmental delay, autism, and response to folinic acid. *Neurology*. 2005;64(6):1088–1090.
15. Moretti P, Peters SU, Del Gaudio D, et al. Brief report: autistic symptoms, developmental regression, mental retardation, epilepsy, and dyskinesias in CNS folate deficiency. *J Autism Dev Disord*. 2008;38(6):1170–1177.
16. Mercimek-Mahmutoglu S, Stockler-Ipsiroglu S. Cerebral folate deficiency and folinic acid treatment in hypomyelination with atrophy of the basal ganglia and cerebellum (H-ABC) syndrome. *Tohoku J Exp Med*. 2007;211(1):95–96.
17. Ramaekers VT, Hansen SI, Holm J, et al. Reduced folate transport to the CNS in female Rett patients. *Neurology*. 2003;61(4):506–515.
18. Blau N, Bonafé L, Krägeloh-Mann I, et al. Cerebrospinal fluid pterins and folates in Aicardi–Goutières syndrome: a new phenotype. *Neurology*. 2003;61(5):642–647.
19. de Koning TJ, Duran M, Dorland L, et al. Beneficial effects of L-serine and glycine in the management of seizures in 3-phosphoglycerate dehydrogenase deficiency. *Ann Neurol*. 1998;44(2):261–265.
20. Rozen R. Molecular genetics of methylenetetrahydrofolate reductase deficiency. *J Inherit Metab Dis*. 1996;19(5):589–594.
21. Ponzone A, Spada M, Ferraris S, et al. Dihydropteridine reductase deficiency in man: from biology to treatment. *Med Res Rev*. 2004;24(2):127–150.
22. Banka S, Blom HJ, Walter J, et al. Identification and characterization of an inborn error of metabolism caused by dihydrofolate reductase deficiency. *Am J Hum Genet*. 2011;88(2):216–225.
23. Arakawa T, Tamura T, Higashi O, et al. Formiminotransferase deficiency syndrome associated with megaloblastic anemia responsive to pyridoxine or folic acid. *Tohoku J Exp Med*. 1968;94:3–16.
24. Ramaekers VT, Rothenberg SP, Sequeira JM, et al. Autoantibodies to folate receptors in the cerebral folate deficiency syndrome. *N Engl J Med*. 2005;352(19):1985–1991.
25. Bonkowsky JL, Ramaekers VT, Quadros EV, et al. Progressive encephalopathy in a child with cerebral folate deficiency syndrome. *J Child Neurol*. 2008;23(12):1460–1463.
26. Ho A, Michelson D, Aaen G, et al. Cerebral folate deficiency presenting as adolescent catatonic schizophrenia: a case report. *J Child Neurol*. 2010;25(7):898–900.
27. Dougados M, Zittoun J, Laplane D, et al. Folate metabolism disorder in Kearns–Sayre syndrome. *Ann Neurol*. 1983;13(6):687.
28. Macron JM, Mizon JP, Rosa A. Disorders of folate metabolism in the Kearns–Sayre syndrome. *Rev Neurol (Paris)*. 1983;139(11):673–677.
29. Pineda M, Ormazabal A, López-Gallardo E, et al. Cerebral folate deficiency and leukoencephalopathy caused by a mitochondrial DNA deletion. *Ann Neurol*. 2006;59(2):394–398.
30. Tanji K, Schon EA, DiMauro S, et al. Kearns–Sayre syndrome: oncocytic transformation of choroid plexus epithelium. *J Neurol Sci*. 20001;178(1):29–36.
31. Allen RJ, DiMauro S, Coulter DL, et al. Kearns–Sayre syndrome with reduced plasma and cerebrospinal fluid folate. *Ann Neurol*. 1983;13(6):679–682. http://www.ncbi.nlm.nih.gov/pubmed?term=%22Papadimitriou%20A%22%5BAuthor%5D
32. Hyland K, Shoffner J, Heales SJ. Cerebral folate deficiency. *J Inherit Metab Dis*. 2010;33(5):563–570.
33. Ramaekers VT, Weis J, Sequeira JM, et al. Mitochondrial complex I encephalomyopathy and cerebral 5-methyltetrahydrofolate deficiency. *Neuropediatrics*. 2007;38(4):184–187.
34. Hasselmann O, Blau N, Ramaekers VT, et al. Cerebral folate deficiency and CNS inflammatory markers in Alpers disease. *Mol Genet Metab*. 2010;99(1):58–61.
35. Gordon N. Alpers syndrome: Progressive neuronal degeneration of children with liver disease. *Dev Med Child Neurol*. 2006;48(12):1001–1003.
36. Nguyen KV, Sharief FS, Chan SS, et al. Molecular diagnosis of Alpers syndrome. *J Hepatol*. 2006;45(1):108–116.
37. Wolff T, Witkop CT, Miller T, et al. Folic acid supplementation for the prevention of neural tube defects: An update of the evidence for the U.S. preventive services task force. *Ann Intern Med*. 2009;150(9):632–629.
38. Dansky LV, Rosenblatt DS, Andermann E Mechanisms of teratogenesis: folic acid and antiepileptic therapy. *Neurology*. 1992;42(4 Suppl 5):32–42.
39. Cario H, Bode H, Debatin KM, et al. Congenital null mutations of the FOLR1 gene: a progressive neurologic disease and its treatment. *Neurology*. 2009;73(24):2127–2129.
40. Steinfeld R, Grapp M, Kraetzner R, et al. Folate receptor alpha defect causes cerebral folate transport deficiency: a treatable neurodegenerative disorder associated with disturbed myelin metabolism. *Am J Hum Genet*. 2009;85(3):354–363.
41. Pérez-Dueñas B, Toma C, Ormazábal A, et al. Progressive ataxia and myoclonic epilepsy in a patient with a homozygous mutation in the FOLR1 gene. *J Inherit Metab Dis*. 2010;33(6):795–802.
42. Dill P, Schneider J, Weber P, et al. Pyridoxal phosphate-responsive seizures in a patient with cerebral folate deficiency (CFD) and congenital deafness with labyrinthine aplasia, microtia and microdontia (LAMM). *Mol Genet Metab*. 2011;104(3):362–368.
43. Hansen FJ, Blau N. Cerebral folate deficiency: life-changing supplementation with folinic acid. *Mol Genet Metab*. 2005;84(4):371–373.
44. Botez MI, Peyronnard JM, Bérubé L, et al. Relapsing neuropathy, cerebral atrophy and folate deficiency. A close association. *Appl Neurophysiol*. 1979;42(3):171–83.

23

Homocysteinemias and Epilepsy

William M. McClintock

A group of disorders of the metabolism of homocysteine and folate lie at the central juncture of the transsulfuration and remethylation reactions whereby homocysteine is converted into methionine and cystathionine. These disorders have in common increased levels of homocysteine in the serum and urine.

METABOLISM OF HOMOCYSTEINE

Homocysteine is at a critical juncture of the metabolism of sulfur containing amino acids, acting as an intermediate in the metabolism of methionine through the cycle of transmethylation. This cycle uses methyltetrahydrofolate and the cofactors of vitamins B2 and B12. The other important pathway is the irreversible degradation by transsulfuration to cysteine using vitamin B6 as a cofactor. These processes are in equilibrium, and serve as an important feedback to the various pathways that allow for proper biosynthesis.

The transmethylation pathway is a cycle that allows the reformation of methionine from homocysteine using methyltetrahydrofolate as a catalyst, with cobalamin (B12) as a cofactor. The central enzyme is methionine synthase (MTR) which uses 5-methyltetrahydrofolate (5-methyl THF) as a methyl group donor forming methionine from homocysteine. Betaine can also be used as a methyl donor, which is the rationale of its therapeutic use. Methionine is then further metabolized by the enzyme methionine adenosyltransferase to S-adenosylmethionine (AdoMet) requiring

ATP. AdoMet is then used through the action of several methyltransferases in the processes of biosynthesis in the production of DNA, RNA, proteins, and neurotransmitters. A by-product is S-adenosylhomocysteine (AdoHcy) which is a strong inhibitor of most methyltransferases. AdoHcy is further metabolized through the enzyme S-adenosylhomocysteine hydrolase (SAHH) back to homocysteine with adenosines as by-products. MTR uses vitamin B12 as a cofactor, and a genetic defect of MTR is one of the major forms of homocystinuria.

The methyl donor 5-methyl THF is also metabolized within an important cycle, with the most important metabolic step the conversion of 5,10-methylenetetrahydrofolate (5,10-methylene THF) to 5-methyl THF. This metabolic step is catalyzed by the critical enzyme 5,10-methylenetetrahydrofolate reductase (MTHFR), using riboflavin (vitamin B2) as a cofactor. Through several pathways these tetrahydrofolate products are converted into 10-formyltetrahydrofolate which is used in purine biosynthesis. Disorders of MTHFR can thereby lead to abnormalities of homocysteine metabolism and megaloblastic anemia. There are several genetic variations leading to dysfunction of the MTHFR enzyme.

The alternative metabolism of homocysteine is the irreversible transsulfuration to cysteine with cystathionine beta-synthase (CBS) as the main enzyme catalyzing this metabolic pathway. CBS is a pyridoxine (vitamin B6)-dependent enzyme. Cystathionine gamma-lyase (CTH) catalyzes the breakdown of cystathionine to cysteine and alpha-ketobutyrate, and is also a vitamin B6-dependent enzyme. Cysteine is important as a precursor to protein synthesis and the formation of glutathione, used by the body for reactions of antioxidation and detoxification. In most tissues homocysteine is remethylated or transported out of the cell, and degradation is done mainly in the liver.

The disorders within this pathway can lead to a variety of neurological manifestations by several mechanisms. Neurons can be affected directly. An important mechanism is the effect on vascular endothelial cells that may cause injury to the brain due to stroke. Disruption of structural proteins may also have neurological consequences. As mentioned above, there may be an effect on the formation of neurotransmitters. The major disorders are enzymatic deficits of the metabolism of homocysteine or the metabolism of folate impairing MTHFR which is an important cofactor in the homocysteine metabolic pathway. This group of disorder leads to a wide range of clinical and neurological presentations. These disorders may present anywhere from the newborn period to adult life. The unifying finding of all these disorders is the increased serum or urine levels of homocysteine. The disorders of homocysteine metabolism and MTHFR deficiency will be discussed. Parenthetically, deficiency of folic acid has similar effects.

HOMOCYSTEINURIA

There are three main enzymes in the pathway of conversion of homocysteine into methionine and their metabolism that have been found to cause neurological disorders associated with homocysteinuria. These are: CBS, MTR, and MTHFR. Homocysteinuria can also occur with the methylmalonic acidurias. The overall incidence of homocysteinuria is 1:335,000 persons, but is as high as 1:65,000 in Ireland.

CBS DEFICIENCY

CBS deficiency is the most common cause of homocysteinuria. There have been over 150 mutations found in the CBS gene, most of which are missense mutations. The location of the gene is on chromosome 21 located at 21q22.3. The CBS enzyme is responsible for the transsulfuration leading to the conversion of homocysteine into cystathionine. Some of the patients with CBS deficiency respond to pyridoxine therapy and modest restriction of methionine in their diet. The pathophysiology of the neurologic deficits are thought to be secondary to the lack of an essential amino acid, methionine, and toxic effects of homocysteine and methionine, as well as possibly other metabolic by-products. The brain is also affected because of the effect on blood vessels leading to thrombosis and strokes. Homocysteine elevations have been shown to independently raise the risk of atherosclerosis and thereby the risk of stroke and heart disease. Connective tissue involvement leads to disorders of eyes and bones.

The major clinical manifestations of this enzyme defect involve the brain, eye, blood vessels, and bones. Intellectual deficiency is the most frequent central nervous system symptom. The first clinical signs may be nonspecific developmental delay in early infancy. The ultimate IQ varies greatly, anywhere from profound impairment to normal intelligence. Pyridoxine responsive patients tend to fare better than the nonresponders, and early treatment can lead to normal intelligence. Psychiatric disorders have been reported and include psychosis and other behavioral disorders. Stroke and focal seizures are also occasionally seen. The skeletal manifestations lead to a Marfanoid appearance. The bones are longer with osteoporosis and defects in the vertebrae, arachnodactyly, pes planus, scoliosis, and genu valgum. Eye involvement is the result of abnormalities of the collagen of the fibers holding the lens in place leading to displacement of the lens. The lens is displaced downward as opposed to upward in Marfan syndrome, which can help with the differential diagnosis. The resulting abnormality of the lens leads to glaucoma, myopia, cataracts, and corneal changes. Vasculopathy produced by the effect on the endothelial cell leads to both arterial and venous thrombosis. The brain, kidney, and lungs can be involved with infarctions. There is an increased risk of cardiac infarction. A controversy has developed because although it is clear that there is an increased risk in adults with mildly elevated homocysteine levels for stroke and myocardial infarction, treatment trials thus far have not shown a benefit from treatments that lower homocysteine levels. This is opposed to those with genetic homocystinuria where treatment to lower levels has been shown to be a benefit.

The diagnosis is made by finding increased homocysteine in the urine or serum. On most standard testing for quantitative plasma amino acids it is important to be aware that increased levels of homocysteine may be missed for technical reasons. If one of the disorders of hyperhomocysteinemia is suspected, it would be prudent to check homocysteine itself in the plasma or urine. Serum amino acids will also reveal low levels of cysteine and elevated methionine. Direct testing for the enzyme defect on fibroblasts or leukocytes is required to confirm the diagnosis. For patients that are responsive to pyridoxine, treatment includes treatment with pyridoxine in combination with B12 and folate, along with modest restriction of methionine in the diet. For nonresponders treatment is with a methionine restricted, cysteine-supplemented diet. B2, B12, and folate are often added. Betaine is also given. This compound is a methyl donor that promotes the remethylation of homocysteine to methionine (1).

MTR DEFICIENCY

This disorder is differentiated from CBS deficiency by the finding of increased levels of homocysteine and low or normal levels of methionine. This enzyme uses cobalamin (vitamin B12) as a cofactor, and vitamin B6 is a cofactor in the pathway of the formation of 5-methylene THF. In humans, methionine is an essential amino acid. There can be deficits in the MTR enzyme itself or in enzymes involved in the synthesis of methylcobalamin. MTR is an autosomal recessive disorder caused by mutation of the MTR gene on chromosome 1 located at 1q43. There have been over 20 mutations of this gene found.

The clinical presentation of MTR deficiency is often in early infancy with encephalopathic features. Poor feeding, lethargy, hypotonia, and seizures are most frequently seen. There are milder affected patients presenting later with developmental delay, gait abnormalities or white matter lesions. Because of the defect of cobalamin, megaloblastic anemia is often seen. Diagnostic studies show high homocysteine found in urine and serum. B12 and folate levels are normal or high and methylmalonic aciduria is usually not seen. When the diagnosis is made treatment is begun with hydroxycobalamin in high doses. This often leads to rapid biochemical normalization. Prenatal therapy has been used.

METHYLENE TETRAHYDROFOLATE REDUCTASE DEFICIENCY

There are recessively inherited disorders of the MTHFR enzyme which lead to hyperhomocysteinemia. The biochemical profile is high serum homocysteine and low methionine. There are widespread changes in the brain and blood vessels. There are genotype and phenotype correlations that are related to the severity of enzyme deficiency. Phenotypes have been divided into infantile, late infantile, and juvenile/late onset forms. More severe deficiency leads to earlier presentation and more severe CNS manifestations. There is good correlation between the severity of the phenotype and severity of loss of enzyme activity. The most severe deficiencies can present as the early infantile type with severe epileptic encephalopathy (2). These children present with hypotonia, lethargy, feeding difficulties, and recurrent apnea. There may be a rapid progression to coma and death. They can present with early infantile encephalopathy and infantile spasms within the first year of life. Seizures tend to then evolve into a picture of multiple seizure types. These have included myoclonic, generalized tonic clonic, atypical absence, partial complex, and tonic seizures. Status epilepticus and nonconvulsive status epilepticus have been seen. Seizures are often intractable to multiple antiepileptic drugs and other interventions such as the ketogenic diet and vagus nerve stimulator. A picture similar to Lennox Gastaut syndrome has developed in a number of patients. EEGs most often demonstrate generalized spike wave, fast spike discharges, and polyspike discharges. Progressive microcephaly and global encephalopathy ensue as seizures continue. MRI reveals generalized atrophy and decreased white matter volume, with a picture of demyelination. MR spectroscopy has revealed a decreased choline peak. Treatment late with metabolic supplements (see below) has not been helpful. There is evidence that treatment begun very early can preserve brain growth and development.

The late infantile onset (1–10 years) is associated with a milder phenotype. Developmental delay is seen. Ataxia and pyramidal tract signs are present. Tone abnormalities with extrapyramidal movements may appear. A speech disorder is common. Occasional thrombotic events and lens dislocation may be seen. Various seizure types are usually present. Juvenile or later onset (older than 10 years) is similar to the late

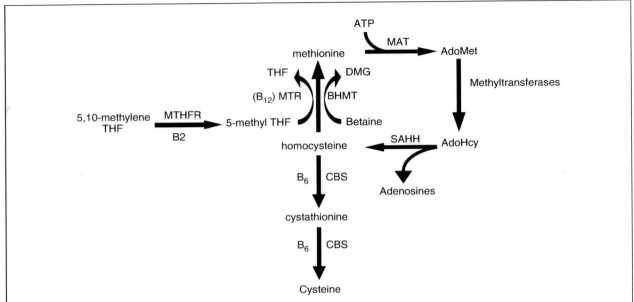

FIGURE 23.1 Schematic representation of the pathways for homocysteine metabolism. AdoHcy, *S*-adenosylhomocysteine; AdoMet, *S*-adenosylmethionine; BHMT, betaine-homocysteine methyltransferase; CBS, cystathionine beta-synthase; CTH, cystathionine gamma-lyase; MAT, methionine-adenosyltransferase; MTHFR, methylenetetrahydrofolate reductase; MTR, methionine synthase; SAHH, *S*-adenosylhomocysteine hydrolase.

infantile form, but with a milder phenotype. These patients present in late teenage or adult life with mild mental slowing, strokes, or psychiatric features. There was an early case report of schizophrenia responsive to folic acid secondary to MTHFR deficiency. Psychiatric disorders have been reported and responsive to treatment to lower the homocysteine levels (3). Communicating hydrocephalus has also been seen.

In the later onset patients who present from late infancy to early childhood, the picture can be one of a progressive encephalopathy. Episodic neurological signs may be present as well as peripheral neuropathy. A progressive myelopathy or neuropathy may be seen. Arterial or venous thrombosis may lead to stroke or infarction in other organs (4). These patients have many characteristics in common with Angelman syndrome and it is thought that a disorder of methylation may link these disorders together.

This is an autosomal recessive disorder with localization to chromosome 1p36.3. There is the milder thermolabile enzyme form which is common and is a proposed genetic risk factor for atherothrombotic vascular disease and neural tube defects. It is estimated that up to 20% of the population is homozygous for this mutated form of MTHFR with mild homocysteinemia (5). The most common mutations are 677C to T and 1298A to T. Treatment of the milder, later onset forms of MTHFR deficiency utilizing vitamins to lower homocysteine levels has not led to a reduced incidence of cardiovascular or atherosclerotic events (6). The severe forms discussed above lead to much less enzyme activity and are rarer.

Treatment of the early onset, more severe, forms of MTHFR deficiency includes the use of high doses of betaine, starting at 100 mg/kg/d, and then titrating slowly to a maximum of 20 g/d until there is normalization of the homocysteine levels (6–8). This treatment can lead to improved behavior and stabilization of neurological deterioration (9). Reversal of long-term neurological abnormalities has not been achieved. The use of pyridoxine, folic acid, folinic acid, and vitamin B12 has been tried with limited success. Supplementation with methionine is also used, and has led to improvement in at least a few reports.

KEY POINTS

1. This group of disorders is characterized biochemically by increased homocysteine levels. Some also have low methionine levels.
2. There is a very wide spectrum of phenotypic expression including epilepsy, encephalopathy, microcephaly, ataxia, psychiatric disorders, and peripheral neuropathy.
3. Early treatment may improve outcome.
4. Clinicians may miss one of these disorders by just checking serum amino acids. Assay of serum homocysteine or urine amino acids may be required to ensure proper diagnosis.

REFERENCES

1. Castro R, Rivera I, Ravasco P, et al. 5,10-methylenetetrahydrofolate reductase (MTHFR) 677C–>T and 1298A–>C mutations are associated with DNA hypomethylation. *J Med Genet.* 2004; 41:454–458.
2. Prasad AN, Rupar CA, Prasad C. Methylenetetrahydrofolate reductase (MTHFR) deficiency and infantile epilepsy. *Brain Dev.* 2011;33:758–769.
3. Freeman JM, Finkelstein JD, Mudd SH. Folate-responsive homocystinuria and "schizophrenia". A defect in methylation due to deficient 5, 10-methylenetetrahydrofolate reductase activity. *N Engl J Med.* 1975;292:491–496.
4. Blom HJ, Smulders Y. Overview of homocysteine and folate metabolism. With special references to cardiovascular disease and neural tube defects. *J Inherit Metab Dis.* 2011;34: 75–81.
5. Yap S, Boers GH, Wilcken B, et al. (2001). Vascular outcome in patients with homocystinuria due to cystathionine betasynthase deficiency treated chronically: A multicenter observational study. *Arterioscler Thromb Vasc Biol.* 21:2080–2085.
6. Marti-Carvajal AJ, Sola I, Lathyris D, Salanti G. Homocysteine lowering interventions for preventing cardiovascular events. *Cochrane Database Syst Rev.* 2009;CD006612.
7. Craig SA. Betaine in human nutrition. *Am J Clin Nutr.* 2004;80:539–549.
8. Schwahn BC, Hafner D, Hohlfeld T, et al. Pharmacokinetics of oral betaine in healthy subjects and patients with homocystinuria. *Br J Clin Pharmacol.* 2003;55:6–13.
9. Ueland PM, Holm PI, Steiner H. Betaine: A key modulator of one-carbon metabolism and homocysteine status. *Clin Chem Lab Med.* 2005;43(10):1069–1075.

24

Congenital Disorders of Glycosylation and Epilepsy

Susan Sparks

INTRODUCTION

When evaluating seizures in the context of multisystem involvement, failure to thrive, or muscle weakness, defects in protein glycosylation must be included in the differential. The diagnosis should also be explored in patients with cerebellar atrophy, stroke-like episodes, muscle weakness and hypotonia in conjunction with eye and brain abnormalities, and nonregressive early onset encephalopathy (1).

Glycosylation defects encompass abnormalities in the synthesis of N-linked glycoproteins, O-linked glycoproteins, or both. Since the characterization of N-linked defects in the 1980s, the field of clinical glycobiology has rapidly progressed and now includes defects in glycosyltransferases for some forms of congenital muscular dystrophies. By far the most abundant and well studied of the glycosylation defects are the group of disorders known as Congenital Disorders of Glycosylation (CDG) (formerly known as carbohydrate-deficient glycoprotein syndrome—CDGS).

Congenital disorders of glycosylation (CDG) are a group of disorders of abnormal glycosylation of N-linked oligosaccharides caused by deficiency in 29 different enzymes in the N-linked oligosaccharide synthetic pathway. Type I CDG comprises those disorders in which there are defects that affect the biosynthesis of oligo-linked oligosaccharides in the cytosol or the endoplasmic reticulum (ER), as well as defects involving the transfer of oligosaccharides

onto nascent glycoproteins. Type II CDG comprises all defects of further trimming and elongation of N-linked oligosaccharides in the ER and Golgi. Most commonly, the disorders begin in infancy; manifestations range from severe developmental delay and hypotonia with multiple organ system involvement to hypoglycemia and protein-losing enteropathy with normal development. However, most types have been described in only a few individuals, and thus understanding of the phenotypes is limited. In PMM2-CDG (*CDG-Ia*), the most common type reported, the clinical presentation and course are highly variable, ranging from death in infancy to mild involvement in adults.

DIAGNOSIS/TESTING

The diagnostic test for all types of CDG is transferrin isoform analysis to determine the number of sialylated N-linked oligosaccharide residues linked to serum transferrin. Such testing is clinically available. Additional analysis of serum N-glycans, serum O-glycans, and glycosylation of muscle proteins on muscle biopsy may help with the diagnosis of other defects of glycosylation. While the enzyme is known in most CDG types, the enzymatic assays have been developed for only a couple of types. Thus, clarification of type requires molecular genetic testing, which is available clinically for many of the types.

PMM2-CDG (*CDG-Ia*)

With over 800 patients described worldwide, PMM2-CDG (*CDG-Ia*) is the most common and best understood of this rare group of disorders. PMM2-CDG (*CDG-Ia*) is caused by a deficiency of phosphomannose mutase (PMM), the enzyme responsible for converting mannose 6-phosphate to mannose 1-phosphate in the activation of mannose necessary for attaching the mannose saccharides to the protein. The typical clinical course of PMM2-CDG (*CDG-Ia*) has been divided into an infantile multisystem stage, late-infantile and childhood ataxia-intellectual disability stage, and adult stable disability stage. Recent reports have widened the phenotypic spectrum to include hydrops fetalis at the severe end (2) and a mild neurologic phenotype in adults with multisystemic involvement at the mild end (3, 4). The infantile multisystem stage, the most commonly seen stage, is characterized by inverted nipples, abnormal subcutaneous fat distribution, and cerebellar hypoplasia, in combination with facial dysmorphism and psychomotor retardation.

SEIZURES

Studies have indicated that seizures occur in 20% to 60% of patients with PMM2-CDG (*CDG-Ia*) (5–9). These tend to be intermittent and easily controlled with standard antiepileptic therapy. Seizures range from febrile seizures, or those only associated with mild infections, to generalized (tonic-clonic, atonic, and absence) and focal seizures (simple and complex partial). In one study of 23 patients with PMM2-CDG (*CDG-Ia*) who had seizures, the mean age of the first seizure was 17 months with a range of 3 to 53 months (6).

STROKE-LIKE EPISODES

In the infantile and adult stages of PMM2-CDG (*CDG-Ia*), affected individuals may have stroke-like episodes or transient unilateral loss of function sometimes associated with fever, seizure, dehydration, or trauma. These episodes are typically accompanied by altered mental status. Recovery may occur over a few weeks to several months. Persistent neurologic deficits after a stroke-like episode occasionally occur but are rare. Studies have indicated that stroke-like episodes

occur in 15% to 50% of individuals with PMM2-CDG (*CDG-Ia*) (5–8). In one large study (23 patients with PMM2-CDG (*CDG-Ia*)), the mean age of first event was 3.6 years (range 0.6–8.8 years) with half of those having recurrent episodes with recovery in between (6). The etiology of these stroke-like episodes has not been fully elucidated.

Imaging studies done on patients at the time of the event were either normal or showed nonspecific edema. Ishikawa et al. (2009) (10) described one patient who had serial imaging during two separate stroke-like episodes. The first episode occurred at 5.2 years of age associated with high fever and presentation with right hemiplegia, conjugate eye deviation to the left, and vomiting leading to subsequent intermittent clonic convulsions of the right extremities resolving with midazolam infusion. This episode was associated with diminished responsiveness lasting an hour and an EEG demonstrating right hemispheric high-voltage slow waves superimposed on intermittent low-voltage fast waves, and a moderately low-voltage pattern in the left hemisphere. There were several days of irritability following the initial presentation. A head CT on the first day revealed a hypodense lesion in the left temporo-parietal watershed area, and laboratory studies suggested disseminated intravascular coagulation (DIC) which resolved with therapy. Seria imaging identified a subdural hematoma on the right side and acute-phase diffusion-weighted imaging revealed a hyperintense lesion in the left temporo-occipital area with left cerebral atrophy. Occlusion of the distal left middle cerebral artery was demonstrated on magnetic resonance angiography. These findings suggested that this initial episode was an ischemic stroke, complicated by a subdural hematoma. His hemiplegia persisted for several months, and subsequently improved gradually. He subsequently had several episodes of hemiplegia resolving within 12 hours without any imaging evidence of ischemia or infarction. There were also episodes of seizures without accompanying hemiparesis. He had a second stroke-like episode at the age of 6.8 years, described clinically as a clonic seizure followed by subsequent hemiplegia of the left extremities, vomiting, and deviation of the eyes to the right. Initially unconscious, he regained alertness within an hour. He had persistent hemiplegia with intermittent partial motor seizures of the left extremities requiring continuous midazolam and phenytoin infusions. Imaging of this event demonstrated marked edema throughout the right hemisphere, followed by a focal lesion in the right temporo-occipital white matter, and MRA showed no vascular changes. His symptoms resolved after 5 weeks and a follow-up MRI 1 year later demonstrated reduced hyperintensity in the corresponding lesion on T2-weighted and FLAIR images. This second stroke-like episode did not show vascular changes like the first; however, the edema on imaging suggested hypoxia. Therefore the pathophysiology of the stroke-like episodes may be due to ischemia.

Dinopolos et al. (11) evaluated three patients with PMM2-CDG (*CDG-Ia*) during stroke-like episodes with continuous EEG monitoring and brain imaging. All three patients presented with hemiparesis, irritability, and altered mental status in the presence of a febrile illness. Evidence of neuronal hyperexcitability was demonstrated on the electrographic recordings of all three patients, although there was no evidence of ischemia or vascular changes on imaging studies. All three were treated with intravenouslorazepam which resolved the epileptic discharges on EEG and improved their level of consciousness. The hemiparesis resolved within 2 to 4 days of treatment. They were all sent home with medication (carbamazepine, oxcarbazepine, or topiramate) with no subsequent episodes in the time studied (2.5–4 years).

Both of these studies highlight the uncertainty of the underlying pathophysiology and specific mechanism of stroke-like episodes in CDG. Ischemia has been proposed as a possible etiology of these events because both procoagulant (factor XI) and anticoagulant (protein C, antithrombin III, and protein V) proteins are reported to be deficient in most patients with PMM2-CDG (*CDG-Ia*) (12, 13). Many of the coagulation proteins undergo significant posttranslational modification with glycosylation and abnormal coagulation factor activity is seen in patients with CDG which could contribute to the etiology of stroke-like episodes. However, the role of coagulant and anticoagulant deficiencies in relation to the clinical events is unclear. Of 24 patients with PMM2-CDG (CDG-Ia) and uniform deficiencies of factor XI, protein C and antithrombin III and variable deficiencies of Factors II, V, VII, IX, X, antifibrinolytic enzyme, and alpha-2 plasminogen inhibitor, six had hemorrhage, three had deep vein thromboses, four had stroke-like episodes, and one developed DIC (12–17). Other factors that support ischemia as the cause of the events include

platelet hyperaggregability and transient decrease of endogenous anticoagulants during catabolic stress (14).

Epileptic seizures are not uncommon in patients with PMM2-CDG (CDG-Ia) and often are observed in association with stroke-like events. Todd's paralysis is a transient focal neurologic deficit known as postictal paralysis which can follow a convulsive motor seizure. However, in many patients with stroke-like episodes, paralysis occurs without seizure activity and persists longer than 24 hours (18). The pathogenesis of the observed neuronal hyperexcitability in patients with PMM2-CDG (CDG-Ia) is unclear, but is presumably related to a deficient glycosylation at the neuronal level (19). Focal neuronal hyperexcitability has also been documented in patients with the mitochondrial encephalopathy lactic acidosis and stroke (MELAS) syndrome and has been proposed as the triggering mechanism of stroke-like events (20).

Another etiology that has been proposed is transient disease-related noncytotoxic, that is, vasogenic, edema (5). Both Pearl and Krasnewich (5) and Ishikawa et al. (10) described patients with PMM2-CDG (*CDG-Ia*) who demonstrated neuroradiologic evidence of transient edema during stroke-like events. Transient cortical hypoperfusion, induced by the coagulation defects, that was severe enough to cause neuronal dysfunction but mild enough to be undetected by MRI modalities cannot, however, be excluded.

OTHER NEUROLOGIC FINDINGS IN PMM2-CDG (*CDG-Ia*)

Hypotonia, ataxia, developmental delay/intellectual disability, and absent deep tendon reflexes have been observed in up to 100% of the individuals with PMM2-CDG (*CDG-Ia*) (6). Progressive peripheral neuropathy occurs in adults with PMM2-CDG (*CDG-Ia*) (21). A 42-year-old man was eventually diagnosed with PMM2-CDG (*CDG-Ia*) after years of progressive cerebellar ataxia and a peripheral neuropathy (22).

NEURODEVELOPMENT

Miossec-Chauvet et al. (8) evaluated nine patients with PMM2-CDG (*CDG-Ia*), eight who had severe delay and one with moderate delay. The ability to control the head was acquired between 6 and 12 months, sit between 16 and 30 months, and stand with assistance between 2.5 and 10 years. A single patient in this series could walk without help. Development of fine motor skills was also delayed, with control of palm grasp around 12 to 18 months of age. Eight of the nine patients acquired precision grasp with impairments related to dysmetria and tremor. Speech ability varied the most with one child aged 3 years not speaking at all, another aged 12.5 years only saying a few words, and six patients who learned to combine a few words at 4 years of age. Only two patients acquired more elaborate speech with the rudiments of reading. Two patients in this study were adults, both with cognitive impairment (one severe and one moderate). There were severe deficiencies in attention, concentration, and reasoning ability; reduced spontaneous speech and verbal fluency; and intellectual and behavioral disorders. Additional findings in one patient included memory impairments, dyspraxia, and deficits in visuospatial organization. In a larger study of 20 patients with PMM2-CDG (*CDG-Ia*), 19 had developmental delay (one was only 3 months at evaluation). Of the older individuals, two could walk unaided (2 years and 7 years), but two others could not walk (ages 6 years and 9 years) (9).

Detailed developmental and neuropsychological assessment were performed on four patients (ages 14–26 years) with PMM2-CDG (*CDG-Ia*) (23). All four had marked delay in all areas of psychomotor development and gained to walk with aid, perform manipulative abilities and develop communicative language after the seventh year. Acquired abilities remained stable, while self-help skills gradually improved over time. On neuropsychological assessment, there was cognitive impairment of variable degree with particular impairment of visuoperceptual skills, visuospatial organization, eye–hand coordination, verbal memory, and language.

Interestingly, there can be significant variability between siblings with PMM2-CDG (*CDG-Ia*). Drouin-Garraud et al. (1) describes three siblings with mild neurologic involvement but varying presentation of clinical symptoms. The first patient presented as a neonate with hypotonia and alternating convergent strabismus. He started to walk at 21 months, and delayed speech became obvious. At the age of 7 years, he had moderate cerebellar ataxia, intention tremor, dysmetria, and dysarthria, and an IQ tested at 66. At 13 years, there was moderate instability and tremor and he attended a special school. The second sibling presented in the first year of life with global hypotonia,

and convergent strabismus. She walked at 30 months. Her expressive speech was limited; however, she had good receptive language. From the age of 4 years, she experienced generalized seizures. The third sibling did not present with neurologic signs until 18 months when moderate ataxia was noted. She walked at 23 months. MRI was normal at 6 weeks, but at 20 months a follow-up study demonstrated vermis and hemispheric cerebellar atrophy.

In older individuals and adults, independence for daily life is limited. In the study by Miossec-Chauvet (8), six of the nine patients could dress and feed themselves and had bowel and bladder control, at least during the day. The older patients were entirely dependent on another person for their daily activities and lived either in institutions or with their families. In another study of four adults with PMM2-CDG (*CDG-Ia*), one patient lives independently with help during the day and is employed in an assisted work setting. The other three require variable levels of assistance with daily care, but lead full active lives (21). In another study of three adult patients with PMM2-CDG (*CDG-Ia*) (7), the cognitive deficits and motor impairment were stable. They all finished special school and have sheltered employment. While none are able to walk unassisted due to their walking pattern being impaired by ataxia and weakness in the lower limbs, short distances are possible with walkers, but wheelchair is necessary for outdoor mobility and longer distances.

NEUROIMAGING IN PMM2-CDG (*CDG-Ia*)

There have been multiple series published demonstrating varying degrees of cerebellar hypoplasia on brain imaging of patients with PMM2-CDG (CDG-Ia). In a total of 58 patients, 53 had evidence of cerebellar hypoplasia (5, 6, 8, 9). In one study in which 10 patients had subsequent imaging (1 month to 7 years later), eight patients demonstrated progression of the cerebellar atrophy (6). Cerebellar hypoplasia is not always apparent in the younger individuals, but seen almost universally in patients after infancy (6). Additional features on MRI include both infratentorial and supratentorial changes compatible with atrophy, enlarged cisterna magna and superior cerebellar cistern, Dandy–Walter malformations, white matter cysts, and delayed or insufficient myelination (24, 25). Serial CTs performed on three children with PMM2-CDG (*CDG-Ia*) revealed that enlargement of the spaces between the folia of the cerebellar hemispheres, especially from the anterior to the posterior aspect, as well as atrophy of the anterior vermis, seemed to progress until around age 5 years (26). Progression of cerebellar atrophy on MRI after age 5 years is variable. After age 9 years, progression of the cerebellar atrophy was not evident. Development of the supratentorial structures was normal.

RARE CDG SUBTYPES

For many types of CDG, the phenotype is not completely known because only a few affected individuals have been described and reported (Table 24.1). Neurodevelopment varies between the types, with PMI-CDG (CDG-Ib) having normal cognition. Seizures range from rarely or never seen to intractable infantile spasms that are refractory to treatment. Imaging findings range from normal to cerebral hemispheric anomalies.

DYSTROGLYCANOPATHIES (DEFECTS OF GLYCOSYLATION OF ALPHA-DYSTROGLYCAN)

There is a group of muscular dystrophies with abnormal glycosylation of alpha-dystroglycan, an important component of the dystrophin–glycoprotein complex necessary for muscle integrity and function. The glycosylation of alpha-dystroglycan is important for binding the ligands in the extracellular matrix, such as laminin, perlecan, and neurexin (27, 28). As a group, they are known as the dystroglycanopathies and clinically range from adult-onset limb-girdle muscular dystrophy to severe, congenital weakness with CNS and eye involvement. The CNS pattern varies, but typically demonstrates abnormal migration and at the severe end of the spectrum has type II, or "cobblestone" lissencephaly. Eye involvement ranges from myopia to microophthalmia. At the milder end of the spectrum, limb-girdle muscular dystrophy may be the only manifestation, without brain or eye involvement. Diagnosis of this group of disorders relies on the demonstration of absent glycosylation of alpha-dystroglycan on muscle or nerve biopsy using monoclonal antibodies to the glycosylated epitopes of alpha-dystroglycan followed by specific molecular analysis (29, 30).

CLINICAL SYNDROMES

DYSTROGLYCANOPATHIES–WALKER–WARBURG SYNDROME (WWS)

Walker–Warburg syndrome (WWS) was initially described in 1942 (31), and further characterized by Warburg (32). WWS is an extremely severe condition, with a life expectancy of less than 3 years. Signs of WWS are already present at birth, and imaging techniques can detect features such as encephaloceles and severe hydrocephalus prenatally. There is profound weakness and generalized hypotonia at birth. Muscle bulk is reduced and contractures develop soon after birth, although it may take a few months to develop. Seizures have been described.

Brain abnormalities include migration defects with type II lissencephaly/agyria ("cobblestone type"), combined with pontocerebellar hypoplasia. Obstructive hydrocephalus may complicate the clinical picture. White matter shows hypomyelination. There are hindbrain malformations with atrophy of the cerebellar vermis and hemispheres and a flattened aspect of the pons and brainstem. Arachnoid cysts are common especially in the posterior fossa. Additional structural abnormalities include hypoplasia/agenesis of the corpus callosum, encephalocele, and Dandy–Walker malformations (33).

Eye abnormalities can include microcornea and/or microphthalmia, either unilateral or bilateral, hypoplastic or absent optic nerves, and colobomas which may involve the retina. Retinal dysplasia or detachment may be present. Other anterior chamber malformations include cataracts, iris hypoplasia or malformation, and abnormal or shallow anterior chamber angle which can result in glaucoma.

Additional features include male genital anomalies such as small penis and undescended testes and severe feeding difficulties that likely require tube or grastrostomy feeding. Rarely there can be mild facial dysmorphism such as low set or prominent ears and cleft lip or palate (33). Mild renal dysplasia and imperforate anus have been reported (34).

WWS–MOLECULAR PATHOGENESIS/GENETICS

There is genetic heterogeneity in WWS. Mutations have been demonstrated in the *O*-mannosyltransferase 1 (*POMT1*) gene (29, 35, 36), the *O*-mannosyltransferase

TABLE 24.1   Subtypes of CDG and Their Neurologic Findings

Type/Gene	Microcephaly	Hypotonia	Developmental Delay/Intellectual Disability	Seizures	Stroke-Like Episodes	MRI Findings	Other Findings
PMM2-CDG (CDG-Ia)	±	+++	+ → +++	- → ++	+	Cerebellar hypoplasia	Peripheral neuropathy, ataxia, coagulopathy, plus multisystemic features
MPI-CDG (CDG-Ib)	-	±	-	±	-	normal	Cyclic vomiting, PLE, FTT, hypoglycemia
ALG6-CDG (CDG-Ic)	-	++/+++	+/++	- → +++	-	normal	Retinal degeneration, endocrine abnormalities
ALG3-CDG (CDG-Id)	+	+++	+++	+++	-	Cerebral atrophy; hypoplastic corpus callosum	Optic nerve atrophy, distinctive features
DPM-CDG (CDG-Ie)	+	+++	+++	- → +++	-	Normal or delayed myelination	Distinctive features, knee contractures
MPDU1-CDG (CDG-If)	-	+++	+++	+++	-	Cerebral atrophy	Generalized scaly, erythematous skin
ALG12-CDG (CDG-Ig)	+ (progressive)	+++	++/+++	±	-		Immunodeficiency, feeding difficulties
ALG8-CDG (CDG-Ih)	-	±	- → ? (most with early death)	- → +++	-	Cortical atrophy	Coagulopathy, PLE, anemia, thrombocytopenia
ALG2-CDG (CDG-Ii)	+	+	+++	+++	-	Delayed myelination	Iris colobomas, visual impairment
DPAGT1-CDG (CDG-Ij)	+	+	+++	+++	-	Normal (PET scan demonstrated multifocal areas of decreased activity)	
ALG1-CDG (CDG-Ik)	+	+++	+++	+++	-	Normal to cerebral atrophy	Severe presentation, coagulopathy, immunodeficiency, cardiomyopathy, nephrotic syndrome
ALG9-CDG (CDG-IL)	+	+++	+++	+ → +++	-	Cerebral and cerebellar atrophy	Hepatomegaly, FTT, pericardial effusion, renal cysts
DOLK-CDG (CDG-Im)	+	+++	? (early death)	++	-		Ichthyosis, dilated cardiomyopathy

CDG type						MRI	Clinical features
RFT1-CDG (CDG-In)	+	+++	+++	++	–		Feeding issues, FTT, visual impairment, SNHL
DPM3-CDG (CDGIo)	–	–	±	–	+		Muscle weakness, cardiomyopathy
ALG11-CDG (CDG-Ip)	+	+++	+++	+++	–		Distinctive features, FTT, persistent vomiting and gastric bleeding
SRD5A3-CDG (CDG-Iq)	–	++	+/++		–		Congenital eye malformations
MAGT1-CDG		++	+ → +++	+++	–		
MAGT2-CDG (CDG-IIa)	–	++	– → +++	+++	–	Normal	Distinctive features, Diminished platelet aggregation
MOGS-CDG (CDG-IIb)	–	++	? (early death)	+++	–		Distinctive features, generalized edema
SLC35C1-CDG (CDG-IIc)	+	+++	+++	–	–		Distinctive features, leukocytosis
B4GALT1-CDG (CDG-IId)	–		+	–	–	Dandy-Walker malformation; progressive hydrocephalus	Coagulopathy, elevated serum creatine kinase
COG7-CDG (CDG-IIe)	+	+++	? (early death)	+++	–	Cortical and/or cerebellar atrophy; hypoplasia of corpus callosum	Distinctive features with wrinkled and loose skin; multi-systemic involvement
SLC35A1-CDG (CDG-IIf)							Macrothrombocytopenia, neutropenia, immunodeficiency
COG1-CDG (CDG-IIg)	+ (progressive)	++	+	–	–	Slight cerebellar and cerebral atrophy	FTT, rhizomelic short stature, mild hepatosplenomegaly
COG8-CDG (CDG-IIh)	+ (progressive)	++	+	++	–	Brainstem and cerebellar atrophy	FTT, polyneuropathy, strabismus, ataxia
COG5-CDG (CDG-IIi)	–	+	+	–	–	Brainstem and cerebellar atrophy	ataxia
COG4-CDG (CDG-IIj)	+	++	++	+	–		Ataxia, absent speech, recurrent infections
COG6-CDG (CDG-IIL)	+	+	? (early death)	+++	–	Cerebral atrophy; intracranial hemorrhage	Vomiting, intracranial hemorrhage with altered mental status, early death

Involvement of features ranges from absent (–) to severe (+++). FTT: failure to thrive; MRI: Magnetic resonance imaging; PET: Positron emission tomography; PLE: Protein-losing enteropathy; SNHL is sensorineural hearing loss.

2 (*POMT2*) gene (37), the *fukutin* gene (38), the fukutin-related protein (*FKRP*) gene, and most recently in *LARGE* (39). These genes are discussed in detail below. Abnormal alpha-dystroglycan expression has been documented in patients with WWS with up to 70% of cases having no molecular diagnosis (33, 40).

DYSTROGLYCANOPATHIES—MUSCLE EYE BRAIN DISEASE

Muscle eye brain disease (MEB) was initially described in patients in Finland (41), with the combination of congenital muscular dystrophy, mental retardation, eye, and structural brain involvement. While there is an increased prevalence in Finland, MEB has been demonstrated in all ethnic backgrounds (42). The severity of MEB varies from a typical neonatal presentation to a milder presentation with seizures and autism (43). The typical presentation of MEB is neonatal onset of profound muscle hypotonia and poor visual alertness. The muscle weakness is generalized and includes the facial and neck muscles. Patients at this severe end never achieve sitting and may die during the first years of life. Moderately affected patients usually show high myopia, but have some preserved vision enabling them to establish eye contact. Their maximum motor ability is to sit unsupported, and occasionally speak a few words. Patients at the milder end of the spectrum may acquire ambulation for a number of years. Often their functional abilities are more impaired by the coexistence of spasticity and ataxia than muscle weakness.

Typical eye features include high myopia, optic disc pallor, retinal dysplasia, persistent hyperplastic primary vitreous, glaucoma, and cataracts. Later on, the progressive high myopia may lead to retinal detachment. Visual evoked potentials demonstrate high amplitudes and delayed latencies. Electroretinograms are abnormal and progressive (44).

CNS findings include structural brain abnormalities on brain MRI, including neuronal migration defects and type II "cobblestone" lissencephaly similar to WWS (45). Other features include partial absence of the corpus callosum, hypoplasia of the pyramidal tracts and obstructive hydrocephalus requiring a shunt. Patients with milder MEB may only have flattening of the brainstem, hypoplasia of the cerebellar vermis, or cerebellar cysts (46). Mental retardation is present in the typical and moderated patients

with MEB. Seizures and myoclonic jerks may also be present.

MEB—MOLECULAR PATHOGENESIS/GENETICS

Linkage analysis was used to localize the gene responsible for MEB to chromosome 1p32-34 (47) and subsequently mutations in the glycosyltransferase O-mannose beta-1,2-N-acetylglucosaminyltransferase (*POMGnT1*) were shown to cause MEB (48). See below for more details on *POMGnT1*.

DYSTROGLYCANOPATHIES—FUKUYAMA CONGENITAL MUSCULAR DYSTROPHY

Fukuyama congenital muscular dystrophy (FCMD) was initially described in Japan in 1960 (49). It is the second most common form of muscular dystrophy in Japan after Duchenne muscular dystrophy. Clinically, there is a spectrum of severity ranging from severe, to typical presentation, to mild (50). Classically, patients with FCMD present with neonatal onset of generalized muscle weakness, severe brain involvement, frequent seizures, mental retardation, and abnormal eye function. Symptoms may begin in utero with poor fetal movement. Asphyxia at birth is not uncommon. There may be functional improvement, and most patients achieve standing with support and occasional ambulation with support. There is progressive involvement of respiratory muscles, and respiratory failure in the middle-late teens is an invariable complication. Cardiac involvement is almost invariable and typically develops in the second decade of life (51). There are progressive contractures of the hips, ankles, and knees. There is loss of independent sitting after 9 years of age, and scoliosis commonly develops. At the mild end of the spectrum, patients can walk or stand with support, and at the severe end of the spectrum, neither head control nor ability to sit without support is ever achieved (50).

Brain abnormalities are similar to WWS and MEB, with migration defects, cobblestone lissencephaly, and hindbrain malformations. Brain MRI also demonstrates increased white matter signal on T2-weighted images due to delayed myelination (52). There can be hypoplasia of the pons and cerebellar cysts (53).

Cognitive ability ranges from profound intellectual disability to mild-moderate, where patients learn to speak in short sentences and may even be able to read and write a few characters. Most patients develop seizures before 3 years of age.

About 50% of the classical FCMD cases show signs of ocular involvement ranging from abnormal eye movements, poor visual pursuit, and strabismus to severe myopia, hyperopia, or cataracts. At the more severe end of the spectrum, however, there can be retinal detachment and microophthalmos.

FCMD–MOLECULAR PATHOGENESIS/GENETICS

FCMD is caused by mutations of the *FKTN* gene on chromosome 9q31 (54).

DYSTROGLYCANOPATHIES–CONGENITAL MUSCULAR DYSTROPHY WITH MUSCLE HYPERTROPHY (MDC1C)

The typical form of MDC1C presents with weakness and hypotonia at birth, or in the first few months of life, followed by marked delay of motor milestones. The maximum motor achievement is to sit or to take a few steps with support in the first decade of life. Progressive respiratory muscle weakness leads to ventilatory insufficiency in the first or second decade of life. Other characteristic features include marked enlargement of the leg muscles, sometimes followed by striking tongue hypertrophy. Wasting and weakness of the shoulder muscles and facial weakness are common. Cardiac involvement is present in the form of a dilated cardiomyopathy (55).

Brain MRI findings in MDC1C range from normal, to isolated cerebellar cysts, to cerebellar cysts associated with structural brain changes. These changes involve the posterior fossa and the cortex. In one patient there was focal nodular heterotopia and in another cerebellar dysplasia and pontine hypoplasia (56). Signs of cortical or subcortical atrophy and focal and diffuse white matter changes have been observed in some patients with MDC1C (57).

MDC1C–MOLECULAR PATHOGENESIS/GENETICS

MDC1C is caused by mutations in the *fukutin-related protein*, or *FKRP*, gene (see below).

DYSTROGLYCANOPATHIES–CONGENITAL MUSCULAR DYSTROPHY WITH SEVERE MENTAL RETARDATION AND ABNORMAL GLYCOSYLATION (MDC1D)

To date, only a single patient with MDC1D has been reported. She is a 17-year-old girl who presented at 5 months of age with congenital onset of muscular dystrophy, profound intellectual disability, white matter changes, and subtle structural abnormalities on brain MRI. Her maximal motor ability was walking 200 yards and jumping at 9 years of age, but thereafter a gradual decline in function was observed, and at 17 years, she was only able to walk a few steps independently. There was muscle hypertrophy of the quadriceps, calf and arm muscles. Contractures at the ankles and elbows were mild. Hearing and vision were normal, and there was no cardiac involvement (58).

The brain MRI at 14 years of age demonstrated abnormal white matter changes mostly in the periventricular region to the arcuate fibers, particularly anteriorly and in the temporal regions. The brainstem was hypoplastic. There was mild pachygyria with the cortex in the frontal lobes being moderately thick and dysplastic, and in the posterior frontal, temporal and parietal regions, the gyri were mildly simplified with shallow sulci (58).

MDC1D–MOLECULAR PATHOGENESIS/GENETICS

MDC1D is caused by a mutation in LARGE (see below; (58)).

GENES INVOLVED IN THE DYSTROGLYCANOPATHIES (TABLE 24.2)

A. *POMT1* and *POMT2*

POMT1 catalyses the first step in O-mannosyl glycan synthesis, with the attachment of a mannose via an O-glycosyl linkage to the Ser/Thr of the protein (59). POMT2 is a second O-mannosyltransferase, which complexes with POMT1 for the O-mannosyltransferase activity (60, 61). Mutations in *POMT1* and *POMT2* cause WWS. Mutations in *POMT1* have also been described in patients with a milder phenotype consisting of congenital muscular dystrophy, calf hypertrophy, microcephaly and mental retardation (36) and in Limb-girdle muscular dystrophy

TABLE 24.2   Genes Causing Secondary Alpha-Dystroglycanopathies

Gene	Chromosome location	Protein	Phenotype
POMT1	9q34	Protein-O-mannosyltransferase 1	WWS, LGMD2K
POMT2	14q24	Protein-O-mannosyltransferase 2	WWS
POMGnT1	1p32-p34	O-linked mannose β1,2-N-acetylglucosaminyltransferase	MEB
FKTN	9q31-q33	Fukutin	WWS, FCMD, LGMD2L
FKRP	19q13.3	Fukutin-related protein	MDC1C, LGMD2I
LARGE	22q12.3-q13.1	Large	WWS, MDC1D

FCMD: Fukuyama congenital muscular dystrophy; LGMD: Limb-girdle muscular dystrophy; MDC: Congenital muscular dystrophy type 1C or 1D; MEB: muscle-eye-brain disease; WWS: Walker-Warburg syndrome.

type 2K (LGMD2K; (62)). Mutations in *POMT2* have been shown to cause a milder phenotype, more consistent with MEB, as well as in patients with congenital muscular dystrophy, microcephaly, and severe intellectual disability, with or without ocular involvement (63).

B. *POMGnT1*

Linkage analysis was used to localize the gene responsible for MEB to chromosome 1p32–34 (47) and subsequently mutations in the glycosyltransferase O-mannose beta-1,2-N-acetylglucosaminyltransferase (*POMGnT1*) were shown to cause MEB (48). *POMGnT1* has 22 exons, with the coding region beginning in exon 2 (48). Mutations are located throughout the gene and include a combination of missense, nonsense and frameshift mutations (42, 48, 64). There has been some genotype-phenotype correlation with a more severe CNS phenotype in the patients carrying mutations towards the 5′ of the gene compared to those located towards the 3′ (42). However, in one family with 2 siblings carrying the same mutation, one had typical features of MEB, but her sibling was much more severe, with some features suggestive of WWS (65). POMGnT1 catalyzes the transfer of *N*-acetylglucosamine to O-linked mannose of glycoproteins including dystroglycan. Reduction of POMGnT1 activity in skeletal muscle of MEB patients has been demonstrated (48, 66, 67).

C. FCMD

FCMD is caused by mutations of the *FKTN* gene on chromosome 9q31 (54, 68). The *FKTN* gene spans more than 100 kb of genomic DNA and is composed of 10 exons (68). Its protein product, fukutin, is a 461 amino acid, 53.7 kD, transmembrane protein with sequence homology to a bacterial glycosyltransferase, but its precise function is unknown (69). A recent report has shown there is co-localization and molecular interaction of fukutin and POMGnT1 suggesting that fukutin may form a complex with POMGnT1 and modulate its enzymatic activity (70).

A retrotransposal insertion into the 3′ UTR of fukutin mRNA accounts for 87% of FCMD chromosomes and is considered to be a relatively mild mutation as it only partially reduces the stability of the full length mRNA. Carrier frequency in Japan is 1:90 (71). Compound heterozygotes between this mutation and deletions or non-sense mutations have a more severe phenotype than individuals homozygous for the retrotransposal insertion (50). While targeted inactivating mutations of both alleles in the mouse are not compatible with life, recently two patients with functional null mutations in a homozygous state were identified. Interestingly, they both had a more severe WWS-like phenotype indicating that complete loss of fukutin function is compatible with life in the human (38, 72). *FKTN* mutations have also been reported in patients with a limb girdle muscular dystrophy phenotype (LGMD2L; (73)). Some of these patients have presented in the first months of life with a CMD phenotype.

A study in Japan noted that patients who were heterozygous for the founder mutation had seizures earlier than those who were homozygous for the founder mutation. In addition, some patients with compound heterozygous mutations demonstrated intractable seizures (74).

D. FKRP

MDC1C is caused by mutations in the *fukutin-related protein*, or *FKRP*, gene. The *FKRP* gene consists of four exons, one of which encodes for a 495 amino acid protein which, like fukutin, is targeted to the medial-Golgi apparatus (75). Sequence homology suggests *FKRP* is a member of the glycosyltransferase family (76). Mutation analysis in patients with MDC1C revealed either two missense mutations or a missense mutation combined with a null mutation (77). So far no patient has been reported with two null *FKRP* alleles and perhaps this would not be compatible with life. Mutations in *FKRP* also cause the milder allelic condition of LGMD2I (78). The most common mutation in *FKRP* is the 826C > A (Leu276Ile) mutation which is associated with LGMD2I and has not been seen in MDC1C (77). This common mutation has been calculated to occur at a heterozygous frequency of 1:400 in the UK (77). The second allelic mutation in patients with the Leu276Ile change determines the severity of the LGMD2I phenotype although the degree of intra-familial clinical variability suggests that additional factors may also play a significant role (79).

One patient with MEB has been described with a mutation in the *FKRP* gene (80). This patient had congenital muscular dystrophy, anterior chamber abnormalities, and characteristic brain abnormalities including cobblestone lissencephaly.

There are two surprising features associated with *FKRP* gene alterations. The first is that *FKRP* mutations are very common especially among Caucasians with a heterozygous frequency of 1:400 (77). The second is the large range of severity of phenotype associated with mutations in a single gene, *FKRP*. This ranges from an in utero-onset of muscular dystrophy with a WWS phenotype to mild LGMD variants with muscular dystrophy onset in adulthood.

LARGE and LARGE2

The *LARGE* gene is the 5th largest gene in the human genome, spanning 664 kb of genomic DNA on chromosome 22q12.3-q13.1, and has homology to the glycosyltransferase gene family (81). The predicted protein contains an N-terminal cytoplasmic domain, a transmebrane region, and two putative catalytic domains (82). The proximal catalytic domain has close homology to Waaj, a bacterial family GT8 glycosyltransferase (83) involved in lipo-oligosaccharide synthesis (84). The distal catalytic domain demonstrates homology with the human UDP-GlcNAc:Gal-beta1,3-*N*-acetylglucosaminyltransferase (83). There is a second gene, *LARGE2* with close homology to *LARGE* (85, 86). Mutations in LARGE were originally described in MDC1D. More recently, a large intragenic deletion was demonstrated in the LARGE gene in a patient with severe CMD, more consistent with WWS (39).

CLINICAL PEARLS

- Defects in protein glycosylation should be considered in the differential diagnosis of seizures, especially in the context of multisystemic disease, hypotonia, or failure to thrive.
- Protein glycosylation defects encompass N-linked, O-linked, or combined defects.
- Over 35 different defects have been described in the group of protein glycosylation defects.
- PMM2-CDG (CDG-Ia) is the prototype and most prevalent form of CDG, presenting with hypotonia, developmental delay, inverted nipples, abnormal fat pads, and cerebellar hypoplasia along with various other multisystemic issues.
- Defects in glycosylation should also be on the differential diagnosis of muscular dystrophy, especially if there are ophthalmologic and CNS findings.

REFERENCES

1. Drouin-Garraud V, et al. Neurological presentation of a congenital disorder of glycosylation CDG-Ia: implications for diagnosis and genetic counseling. *Am J Med Genet.* 2001; 101(1):46–49.
2. Van de Kamp JM, et al. Congenital disorder of glycosylation type Ia presenting with hydrops fetalis. *J Med Genet.* 2007; 44(4):277–280.

3. Barone R, et al. Borderline mental development in a congenital disorder of glycosylation (CDG) type Ia patient with multisystemic involvement (intermediate phenotype). *J Inherit Metab Dis.* 2007;30(1):107.

4. Coman D, et al. Congenital disorder of glycosylation type 1a: three siblings with a mild neurological phenotype. *J Clin Neurosci.* 2007;14(7):668–672.

5. Pearl PL, Krasnewich D. Neurologic course of congenital disorders of glycosylation. *J Child Neurol.* 2001;16(6):409–413.

6. Kjaergaard S, Schwartz M, Skovby F. Congenital disorder of glycosylation type Ia (CDG-Ia): phenotypic spectrum of the R141H/F119L genotype. *Arch Dis Child.* 2001;85(3): 236–239.

7. Perez-Duenas B, et al. Long-term evolution of eight Spanish patients with CDG type Ia: typical and atypical manifestations. *Eur J Paediatr Neurol.* 2009;13(5):444–451.

8. Miossec-Chauvet E, et al. Neurological presentation in pediatric patients with congenital disorders of glycosylation type Ia. *Neuropediatrics.* 2003;34(1):1–6.

9. De Lonlay P, et al. A broad spectrum of clinical presentations in congenital disorders of glycosylation I: a series of 26 cases. *J Med Genet.* 2001;38(1):14–19.

10. Ishikawa N, et al. Different neuroradiological findings during two stroke-like episodes in a patient with a congenital disorder of glycosylation type Ia. *Brain Dev.* 2009;31(3):240–243.

11. Dinopoulos A, et al. Radiologic and neurophysiologic aspects of stroke-like episodes in children with congenital disorder of glycosylation type Ia. *Pediatrics.* 2007;119(3):e768–e772.

12. Young G, Driscoll MC. Coagulation abnormalities in the carbohydrate-deficient glycoprotein syndrome: case report and review of the literature. *Am J Hematol.* 1999;60(1):66–69.

13. Fiumara A, et al. Haemostatic studies in carbohydrate-deficient glycoprotein syndrome type I. *Thromb Haemost.* 1996;76(4): 502–504.

14. Van Geet C, Jaeken J. A unique pattern of coagulation abnormalities in carbohydrate-deficient glycoprotein syndrome. *Pediatr Res.* 1993;33(5):540–531.

15. Okamoto N, et al. Decreased blood coagulation activities in carbohydrate-deficient glycoprotein syndrome. *J Inherit Metab Dis.* 1993;16(2):435–440.

16. Iijima K, et al. Hemostatic studies in patients with carbohydrate-deficient glycoprotein syndrome. *Thromb Res.* 1994;76(2): 193–198.

17. Stibler H, et al. Complex functional and structural coagulation abnormalities in the carbohydrate-deficient glycoprotein syndrome type I. *Blood Coagul Fibrinolysis.* 1996;7(2):118–126.

18. Gallmetzer P, et al. Postictal paresis in focal epilepsies—incidence, duration, and causes: a video-EEG monitoring study. *Neurology.* 2004;62(12):2160–2164.

19. Marx J. Getting it together at the synapse. *Science.* 1992; 258(5086):1304–1306.

20. Iizuka T, Sakai F. Pathogenesis of stroke-like episodes in MELAS: analysis of neurovascular cellular mechanisms. *Curr Neurovasc Res.* 2005;2(1):29–45.

21. Krasnewich D, O'Brien K, Sparks S. Clinical features in adults with congenital disorders of glycosylation type Ia (CDG-Ia). *Am J Med Genet C Semin Med Genet.* 2007;145C(3):302–306.

22. Schoffer KL, O'Sullivan JD, McGill J. Congenital disorder of glycosylation type Ia presenting as early-onset cerebellar ataxia in an adult. *Mov Disord.* 2006;21(6):869–872.

23. Barone R, et al. Developmental patterns and neuropsychological assessment in patients with carbohydrate-deficient glycoconjugate syndrome type IA (phosphomannomutase deficiency). *Brain Dev.* 1999;21(4):260–263.

24. Peters V, et al. Congenital disorder of glycosylation IId (CDG-IId)—a new entity: clinical presentation with Dandy-Walker malformation and myopathy. *Neuropediatrics.* 2002;33(1):27–32.

25. Holzbach U, et al. Localized proton magnetic resonance spectroscopy of cerebral abnormalities in children with carbohydrate-deficient glycoprotein syndrome. *Acta Paediatr.* 1995;84(7):781–786.

26. Akaboshi S, Ohno K, Takeshita K. Neuroradiological findings in the carbohydrate-deficient glycoprotein syndrome. *Neuroradiology.* 1995;37(6):491–495.

27. Ibraghimov-Beskrovnaya O, et al. Primary structure of dystrophin-associated glycoproteins linking dystrophin to the extracellular matrix. *Nature.* 1992;355(6362):696–702.

28. Kanagawa M, et al. Disruption of perlecan binding and matrix assembly by post-translational or genetic disruption of dystroglycan function. *FEBS Lett.* 2005;579(21):4792–4796.

29. Beltran-Valero de Bernabe D, et al. Mutations in the O-mannosyltransferase gene POMT1 give rise to the severe neuronal migration disorder Walker-Warburg syndrome. *Am J Hum Genet.* 2002;71(5):1033–1043.

30. Muntoni F, et al. 114th ENMC International Workshop on congenital muscular dystrophy (CMD), 8th Workshop of the International Consortium on CMD, 3rd Workshop of the MYO-Cluster project Genre. *Neuromuscul Disord.* 2003; 13(7–8):579–588.

31. Walker A Lissencephaly. *Arch Neurol Psychol.* 1942;48:13–29.

32. Warburg M. Hydrocephaly, congenital retinal nonattachment, and congenital falciform fold. *Am J Ophthalmol.* 1978;85(1): 88–94.

33. Vajsar J, Schachter H. Walker-Warburg syndrome. *Orphanet J Rare Dis.* 2006;1:29.

34. Dobyns WB, et al. Diagnostic criteria for Walker-Warburg syndrome. *Am J Med Genet.* 1989;32(2):195–210.

35. Kim DS, et al. POMT1 mutation results in defective glycosylation and loss of laminin-binding activity in alpha-DG. *Neurology.* 2004;62(6):1009–1011.

36. Van Reeuwijk J, et al. The expanding phenotype of POMT1 mutations: from Walker-Warburg syndrome to congenital muscular dystrophy, microcephaly, and mental retardation. *Hum Mutat.* 2006;27(5):453–459.

37. Van Reeuwijk J, et al. POMT2 mutations cause alpha-dystroglycan hypoglycosylation and Walker-Warburg syndrome. *J Med Genet.* 2005;42(12):907–912.

38. De Bernabe DB, et al. A homozygous nonsense mutation in the fukutin gene causes a Walker-Warburg syndrome phenotype. *J Med Genet.* 2003;40(11):845–848.

39. Van Reeuwijk J, et al. Intragenic deletion in the LARGE gene causes Walker-Warburg syndrome. *Hum Genet.* 2007;121(6): 685–690.

40. Jimenez-Mallebrera C, et al. Profound skeletal muscle depletion of alpha-dystroglycan in Walker-Warburg syndrome. *Eur J Paediatr Neurol.* 2003;7(3):129–137.

41. Santavuori P, et al. Muscle-eye-brain disease (MEB). *Brain Dev.* 1989;11(3):147–153.

42. Taniguchi K, et al. Worldwide distribution and broader clinical spectrum of muscle-eye-brain disease. *Hum Mol Genet.* 2003;12(5):527–534.

43. Haliloglu G, et al. Clinical spectrum of muscle-eye-brain disease: from the typical presentation to severe autistic features. *Acta Myol.* 2004;23(3):137–9.

44. Pihko H, et al. Ocular findings in muscle-eye-brain (MEB) disease: a follow-up study. *Brain Dev.* 1995;17(1):57–61.

45. Haltia M, et al. Muscle-eye-brain disease: a neuropathological study. *Ann Neurol.* 1997;41(2):173–180.

46. Muntoni F, Voit T. The congenital muscular dystrophies in 2004: a century of exciting progress. *Neuromuscul Disord.* 2004;14(10):635–649.

47. Cormand B, et al. Assignment of the muscle-eye-brain disease gene to 1p32-p34 by linkage analysis and homozygosity mapping. *Am J Hum Genet.* 1999;64(1):126–135.

48. Yoshida A, et al. Muscular dystrophy and neuronal migration disorder caused by mutations in a glycosyltransferase, POMGnT1. *Dev Cell.* 2001;1(5):717–724.

49. Fukuyama Y, Kwazura M, Haruna H. A peculiar form of congenital muscular dystrophy. *Paediatr Univ Tokyo.* 1960;4:5–8.

50. Saito K, et al. Haplotype-phenotype correlation in Fukuyama congenital muscular dystrophy. *Am J Med Genet.* 2000;92(3):184–190.

51. Nakanishi T, et al. Cardiac involvement in Fukuyama-type congenital muscular dystrophy. *Pediatrics.* 2006;117(6):e1187–e1192.

52. Fukuyama Y, Osawa M, Suzuki H. Congenital progressive muscular dystrophy of the Fukuyama type—clinical, genetic and pathological considerations. *Brain Dev.* 1981;3(1):1–29.

53. Aida N, et al. Cerebellar MR in Fukuyama congenital muscular dystrophy: polymicrogyria with cystic lesions. *AJNR Am J Neuroradiol.* 1994;15(9):1755–1759.

54. Toda T, et al. Localization of a gene for Fukuyama type congenital muscular dystrophy to chromosome 9q31-33. *Nat Genet.* 1993;5(3):283–286.

55. Mercuri E, et al. Congenital muscular dystrophy with secondary merosin deficiency and normal brain MRI: a novel entity? *Neuropediatrics.* 2000;31(4):186–189.

56. Mercuri E, et al. Spectrum of brain changes in patients with congenital muscular dystrophy and FKRP gene mutations. *Arch Neurol.* 2006;63(2):251–257.

57. Quijano-Roy S, et al. Brain MRI abnormalities in muscular dystrophy due to FKRP mutations. *Brain Dev.* 2006;28(4):232–242.

58. Longman C, et al. Mutations in the human LARGE gene cause MDC1D, a novel form of congenital muscular dystrophy with severe mental retardation and abnormal glycosylation of alpha-dystroglycan. *Hum Mol Genet.* 2003;12(21):2853–28561.

59. Willer T, et al. O-Mannosyl glycans: from yeast to novel associations with human disease. *Curr Opin Struct Biol.* 2003;13(5):621–630.

60. Manya H, Endo T. Defective O-mannosyl glycosylation causes congenital muscular dystrophies. *Tanpakushitsu Kakusan Koso.* 2004;49(15 Suppl):2451–2456.

61. Akasaka-Manya K, et al. Physical and functional association of human protein O-mannosyltransferases 1 and 2. *J Biol Chem.* 2006;281(28):19339–19345.

62. Balci B, et al. An autosomal recessive limb girdle muscular dystrophy (LGMD2) with mild mental retardation is allelic to Walker-Warburg syndrome (WWS) caused by a mutation in the POMT1 gene. *Neuromuscul Disord.* 2005;15(4):271–275.

63. Yanagisawa A, et al. New POMT2 mutations causing congenital muscular dystrophy: identification of a founder mutation. *Neurology.* 2007;69(12):1254–1260.

64. Vervoort VS, et al. POMGnT1 gene alterations in a family with neurological abnormalities. *Ann Neurol.* 2004;56(1):143–148.

65. Teber S, et al. Severe muscle-eye-brain disease is associated with a homozygous mutation in the POMGnT1 gene. *Eur J Paediatr Neurol.* 2008;12(2):133–136.

66. Manya H, et al. Loss-of-function of an N-acetylglucosaminyl-transferase, POMGnT1, in muscle-eye-brain disease. *Biochem Biophys Res Commun.* 2003;306(1):93–97.

67. Zhang W, et al. Enzymatic diagnostic test for muscle-eye-brain type congenital muscular dystrophy using commercially available reagents. *Clin Biochem.* 2003;36(5):339–344.

68. Kobayashi K, et al. Structural organization, complete genomic sequences and mutational analyses of the Fukuyama-type congenital muscular dystrophy gene, fukutin. *FEBS Lett.* 2001;489(2–3):192–196.

69. Toda T, et al. Fukuyama-type congenital muscular dystrophy (FCMD) and alpha-dystroglycanopathy. *Congenit Anom (Kyoto).* 2003;43(2):97–104.

70. Xiong H, et al. Molecular interaction between fukutin and POMGnT1 in the glycosylation pathway of alpha-dystroglycan. *Biochem Biophys Res Commun.* 2006;350(4):935–941.

71. Toda T, et al. The Fukuyama congenital muscular dystrophy story. *Neuromuscul Disord.* 2000;10(3):153–159.

72. Silan F, et al. A new mutation of the fukutin gene in a non-Japanese patient. *Ann Neurol.* 2003;53(3):392–396.

73. Godfrey C, et al. Fukutin gene mutations in steroid-responsive limb girdle muscular dystrophy. *Ann Neurol.* 2006;60(5):603–610.

74. Yoshioka M, et al. Seizure-genotype relationship in Fukuyama-type congenital muscular dystrophy. *Brain Dev.* 2008;30(1):59–67.

75. Torelli S, et al. Sub-cellular localisation of fukutin related protein in different cell lines and in the muscle of patients with MDC1C and LGMD2I. *Neuromuscul Disord.* 2005;15(12):836–843.

76. Brockington M, et al. Mutations in the fukutin-related protein gene (FKRP) cause a form of congenital muscular dystrophy with secondary laminin alpha2 deficiency and abnormal glycosylation of alpha-dystroglycan. *Am J Hum Genet.* 2001;69(6):1198–1209.

77. Poppe M, et al. The phenotype of limb-girdle muscular dystrophy type 2I. *Neurology.* 2003;60(8):1246–1251.

78. Brockington M, et al. Mutations in the fukutin-related protein gene (FKRP) to identify limb girdle muscular dystrophy 2I as a milder allelic variant of congenital muscular dystrophy MDC1C. *Hum Mol Genet.* 2001;10(25):2851–2859.

79. Mercuri E, et al. Phenotypic spectrum associated with mutations in the fukutin-related protein gene. *Ann Neurol.* 2003;53(4): 537–542.

80. Beltran-Valero de Bernabe, D, et al. Mutations in the FKRP gene can cause muscle-eye-brain disease and Walker-Warburg syndrome. *J Med Genet.* 2004;41(5):e61.

81. Peyrard M, et al. The human LARGE gene from 22q12.3–q13.1 is a new, distinct member of the glycosyltransferase gene family. *Proc Natl Acad Sci USA.* 1999;96(2):598–603.

82. Grewal PK, et al. Mutant glycosyltransferase and altered glycosylation of alpha-dystroglycan in the myodystrophy mouse. *Nat Genet.* 2001;28(2):151–154.

83. Coutinho PM, et al. An evolving hierarchical family classification for glycosyltransferases. *J Mol Biol.* 2003;328(2):307–317.

84. Heinrichs DE, Yethon JA, Whitfield C. Molecular basis for structural diversity in the core regions of the lipopolysaccharides of Escherichia coli and Salmonella enterica. *Mol Microbiol.* 1998;30(2):221–232.

85. Brockington M, et al. Localization and functional analysis of the LARGE family of glycosyltransferases: significance for muscular dystrophy. *Hum Mol Genet.* 2005;14(5):657–665.

86. Fujimura K, et al. LARGE2 facilitates the maturation of alpha-dystroglycan more effectively than LARGE. *Biochem Biophys Res Commun.* 2005;329(3):1162–1171.

Lysosomal Storage Diseases and Epilepsy

Pranoot Tanpaiboon and Grisel Lopez

INTRODUCTION

Lysosomes are cytoplasmic organelles surrounded by a single layer lipoprotein membrane. They are components of all plant and animal eukaryotic cells, except red blood cells (1). Lysosomes contain a variety of acid hydrolases required for degrading macromolecules such as polysaccharides, proteins, lipids, and nucleic acids. The products of digestion, such as sugars (glucose, galactose) and lipids (ceramide, sphingosine), are released to the cytoplasm and are then recycled for biosynthetic purposes. The process of degradation and reusing breakdown products for biosynthesis is called metabolic salvage (2, 3).

Therefore, lysosomes are important for maintaining cell homeostasis involving metabolic salvage. Homeostasis helps cells adapt to a changing environment and maintain normal function (4).

Furthermore, lysosomes are involved in a number of cellular processes, such as cholesterol homeostasis, autophagy, phagocytosis, membrane repair, bone and tissue remodeling, immunity, neurotransmission, intracellular signaling, and cell apoptosis. Lysosomes, thus, not only function as "end point degradative compartments," but also play important roles in complex cellular regulation and recycling mechanisms (5, 6).

PHYSIOLOGY OF LYSOSOME AND LYSOSOMAL ENZYME TRAFFICKING

The production of the majority of lysosomal enzymes starts in the rough endoplasmic reticulum (RER). Consequently, the precursors of enzymes are modified as well as attached with mannose-6-phosphate (M6P) in the Golgi apparatus as a part of posttranslational modification and targeting processes. The lysosomal enzymes containing M6P move to the trans-Golgi network, where N-acetylglucosamine residues of M6P are removed by an uncovering enzyme (N-acetylglucosamine-1-phospho-diester or α-N-acetylglucosaminidase), causing the enzymes containing M6P to expose their receptors (M6P receptor). The interaction between the lysosomal enzymes and the M6P receptors facilitates enzyme traffic to the late endosomes (prelysosomal compartment) and the lysosomes (endosome–lysosome system or E/L system).

Ultimately, the receptor–ligand complexes are transported to the late endosomes and then to the lysosomes. The process of enzyme transferring from the late endosomes to the lysosomes is not fully understood. Several hypotheses have been proposed including:

• The late endosome matures to become the lysosome.

- The enzymes are transported via vesicles to the lysosome.
- The endosome and lysosome fuse to form a hybrid organelle.

The M6P receptor is salvaged from the late endosome to the trans-Golgi network; therefore, the acid hydrolases in lysosomes lack the M6P receptors.

A small portion of the enzyme precursors do not bind to the receptors and are secreted with secretory proteins from the trans-Golgi network. These enzyme precursors are recaptured into clathrin-coated pits (CCP) by cation-independent M6P receptors. They are respectively transported to the early endosomes, the late endosomes, and the lysosomes (5, 7, 8). Lysosomal degradation pathways (or endosome–lysosome (E/L) function) require the ubiquitin–proteasome pathway and autophagy (9).

After autophagic (intracellular macromolecules) and phagocytic (extracellular macromolecules) vacuoles combine with the E/L system, macromolecules in vacuoles are delivered and broken down by the lysosome (5). Some lysosomal enzymes, especially lipid hydrolases, require special proteins, sphingolipid activator proteins (Saps), to present the lipid substrates to the lysosomal enzymes.

Autophagy (auto phagos: self eating) is a catabolic process involving the degradation of a cell's own components. The autophagosomes deliver cytoplasmic materials, including soluble macromolecules and organelles, to the lysosomes for degradation. The role of autophagy is essential during cell starvation because the recycling of cell material by cytoplasmic component degradation processes provides the elements necessary for cell survival and energy production. Autophagy also is a cellular housekeeping function eliminating redundant or unused substances from cells.

There are at least three different types of autophagy, including:

- Macroautophagy, which is the most studied type
- Chaperone-mediated autophagy (CMA), which requires a specific peptide motif and lysosomal-associated membrane protein 2 (LAMP-2a)
- Microautophagy, which originates from small portions of the cytoplasm.

Impairment or alteration of autophagy function may be related to the pathophysiology of cancer, neurodegenerative diseases, lysosomal storage diseases, aging, immunity, and inflammation (4, 10, 11).

It is hypothesized that impairment of autophagy secondary to the lysosomal storage disorders plays an important role in the pathophysiology of the lysosomal storage disorders, especially the neuropathic type.

LYSOSOMAL STORAGE DISORDERS

Lysosomal storage disorders (LSDs) are a large group of inherited inborn errors of metabolism (IEM), currently including approximately 50 diseases. Each group is characterized by specific accumulated intralysosomal substrates. There are many steps engaging enzyme synthesis. The interruption in any synthesis step leads to lysosomal enzyme dysfunction and/or impaired macromolecule degradation. The majority of diseases in this group are caused by a deficiency of lysosomal acid hydrolases. Some LSDs are caused by other mechanisms such as deficiency of activator proteins, trafficking defects, defects in biogenesis of lysosomes, or lysosomal membrane transporter defects (12, 13).

Although the overall incidence of each disease is rare, the cumulative incidence is common, with one in 7,700 live births (14). Certain ethnic groups have high carrier frequency for specific diseases. For example, Gaucher disease type I, Niemann–Pick type A, mucolipidosis type IV, gangliosidosis type II (GM2), and Tay–Sachs disease have a high prevalence in the Ashkenazi Jewish population.

Most LSDs are inherited in an autosomal recessive pattern. Exceptions include Fabry disease, mucopolysaccharidosis II (MPS II or Hunter syndrome), and Danon disease (a defect in lysosomal membrane associated protein 2 or LAMP2), which are inherited in an x-linked pattern. Autosomal dominant inheritance has been reported in adult-onset neuronal ceroid lipofuscinosis (ANCL). More than two-thirds of LSDs are neuropathic LSDs in which the main clinical symptom is neurodegeneration (3, 11, 15).

PATHOPHYSIOLOGY OF LYSOSOMAL STORAGE DISORDERS

The original hypothesis for the pathological mechanism of LSDs was the cytotoxic effect of a specific storage substance. It was believed that the storage of a single major substrate, normally degraded by a specific lysosomal enzyme, disturbed cell function, caused cell and organ enlargement, and ultimately led to cell death (16). Although accumulation of macromolecules in the lysosomes is ordinarily confined to cells, tissues, and organs in which substrate turnover is high, the current concept of LSD pathophysiology has been expanded beyond the "one enzyme–one substrate relationship." It is widely accepted that LSDs are not "pure storage diseases," but the consequence of dysfunction of complex cellular signaling mechanisms (9, 17).

The primary storage material can cause a series of secondary impairment of other biochemical pathways, as well as dysfunction in a variety of cells. The interruption of other biochemical pathways leads to build up of secondary co-accumulated substances, which may disturb normal cellular function, disrupt lysosomal biogenesis, and cause cell death. Settembre et al proposed that the accumulated substances interrupt autophagosome–lysosome fusion, which ultimately leads to progressive accumulation of poly-ubiquitinated protein and dysfunctional mitochondria (17). Defects of fusion between autophagosomes and lysosomes also cause accumulation of autophagosomes, as demonstrated in mouse embryonic fibroblasts (MEFs) and macrophages (18).

Considering autophagy has a housekeeping function, impairment of autophagy leads to multiple consequences associated with cellular homeostasis destruction (3, 9, 17), such as:

- Cell damage and inflammation because of accumulation of protein and toxic substances
- Dysfunctional mitochondria and increased susceptibility to mitochondrial-mediated cell apoptosis because of mitochondrial turnover impairment
- Defect in clearance of oxidized organelles produced by oxidative stress and inflammatory processes

Alteration of macrophage and microglial cell function, possibly secondary to primary storage, impairs the innate immune system, which consequently increases levels of proinflammatory response, including chemokines and cytokines (9, 13, 19). An inflammatory component plays an important role in the pathophysiology of neurodegeneration of many neuropathic LSDs including GM1-gangliosidosis, GM2-gangliosidosis, Mucopolysaccharidosis III B (Sanfilippo type B), Niemann–Pick type C (NPC) and neuronal ceroid lipofucinosis (NCL). Inflammation has been described as part of the pathophysiology of hepatosplenomegaly in Gaucher disease as well (13, 19–22).

Aggregation of protein and inflammatory response in the nervous system are characteristic of adult neurodegenerative disorders such as Alzheimer's and Parkinson's disease; therefore, neuropathic LSDs likely share similar pathophysiology with common adult onset neurodegenerative conditions.

In addition to the cytotoxic effects of accumulating substances, enzyme blockage also decreases the products of digestion. These products are precursors of metabolic biosynthesis and are sources of energy for cells. Insufficiency of metabolic products results in energy deprivation and affects other metabolic pathways.

Other possible pathophysiologic mechanisms include defect of neuronal growth factor transportation and alteration of vesicular trafficking (9).

CLASSIFICATION

Lysosomal storage disorders can be classified according to the major accumulated substrate, underlying mechanism, or defective enzyme. Subgroups are usually divided by age of onset. The commonly used classification is type of major accumulated substrate (12, 23, 24).

Glycogen
Pompe
Dannon disease (defect of LAMP2)

Lipid
NPC
Cholesterol ester storage disease (CESD)/Wolman disease

Monosaccharide/Amino Acid Monomer
Infantile free sialic acid storage disease (ISSD)
Intermediate and mild form (Salla)

Mucolipidoses (ML)
Mucolipidosis type II (I cell disease)
Mucolipidosis type III (pseudo Hurler polydystrophy)
Mucolipidosis type IV

Mucopolysaccharidoses (MPS)
MPS type I   type I H (Hurler or severe form); type I HS (Hurler–Schie or intermediate form) and type I S (Schie or attenuated form)

MPS type II (Hunter)
MPS type III (Sanfilippo) A, B, C, and D
MPS type IV (Morquio) A and B
MPS type VI (Maroteaux–Lamy)
MPS VII (Sly)
MPS IX (Natowicz)

Multiple Enzyme Defects

Multiple sulfatase deficiency
Galactosialidosis   early infantile, late infantile, juvenile/adult form

Neuronal Ceroid Lipofuscinosis (NCLS)

Congenital NCL
Infantile (INCL, Santavuori–Haltia)
Late infantile (LINCL, Jansky–Bielschowsky)
Juvenile (JNCL, Batten disease)
Adult (ANCL, Kuf's disease)
Northern epilepsy (NE) or progressive epilepsy with mental retardation (EPMR)

Oligosaccharidoses

Alpha-Mannosidosis
Beta-Mannosidosis
Fucosidosis
Schindler disease
Aspartylglucosaminuria (AGU)
Sialidosis type I (Cherry-red spot myoclonus syndrome)
Sialidosis type II (Mucolipidosis type I)

Peptide

Pycnodysostosis
Cystinosis

Sphingolipidoses

GM1 gangliosidosis   infantile, late infantile, and adult form

GM2 gangliosidosis   Tay–Sachs, Sandhoff and GM2 activator deficiency (AB variant)

Gaucher disease (GD)   type I, II, and III
                        Saposin C deficiency

Niemann–Pick   types A and B

Fabry

Faber

Krabbe (globoid cell leukodystrophy)   early infantile, late infantile, adult
                                        Saposin A deficiency

Metachromatic leuko-dystrophy (MLD)   late infantile, juvenile, and adult
                                        Saposin B deficiency

Multiple Sphingolipids

Prosaposin deficiency (pSap)

CLINICAL MANIFESTATIONS

Clinical manifestations vary and can involve multiple organs, including neurological (both central and peripheral nervous systems), cardiovascular, ophthalmological, gastrointestinal, and respiratory systems. Some features are disease-specific, while others are observed in several diseases. Additionally, there is significant overlap between the clinical presentations of different disease groups. For example, several oligosaccharidoses and the majority of mucopolysaccharidoses present with delayed development, coarse facial features, hepatosplenomegaly, and corneal clouding.

The clinical spectrum and severity are variable within the same enzyme defect, although related. The clinical presentation of subtypes of each disease may be a continuum of overlapping features. Age of onset is broad, encompassing both prenatal, including a very rare manifestation with hydrops fetalis, and adult presentation.

The common signs and symptoms are described as follows:

(I) **Neurological manifestations**
   (a) Mental retardation, macro- or micro-cephaly, epilepsy, myoclonus, peripheral neuropathy, spasticity, hypotonia, dysphagia, stridor, cerebellar ataxia, extrapyramidal signs, aggressive behavior, psychiatric problems
   (b) Characteristic abnormal eye movements are noted in some neuropathic LSDs
      (i) Abnormal saccades are seen in late-onset GM2 gangliosidosis and Gaucher disease type III

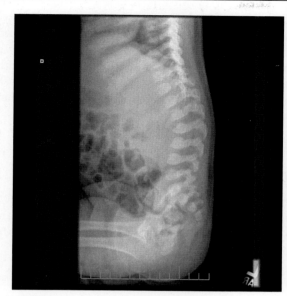

FIGURE 25.1 Lateral spine x-ray of a 7-month-old boy with mucopolysaccharidosis type I (Hurler) shows anterior beaking of spines and platyspondyly.

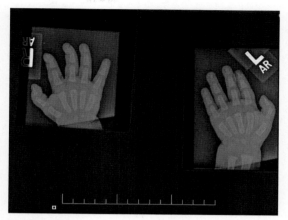

FIGURE 25.2 Hand x-ray of a 7-month-old boy with mucopolysaccharidosis type I (Hurler) shows bullet shape metacarpals with widened distal portion.

  (ii) Vertical supranuclear gaze palsies are seen in Niemann Pick C (NPC) disease

  (iii) Horizontal supranuclear gaze palsies are seen in Gaucher disease types II and III

(II) **Extraneurological manifestations**

 (a) Coarse facial features: prominent forehead, bushy eyebrows, puffiness of eyelids, flattening of nasal bridge, thick lips, and macroglossia

 (b) Bone and joints

  (i) Dysostosis multiplex: thickened skull, enlarged J-shaped sella, broad ribs, spinal beaking, and platyspondyly (Figure 25.1), odontoid hypoplasia, pointing of proximal part and broad distal part of metacarpal (bullet-shaped appearance) (Figure 25.2), underdeveloped pelvis

  (ii) Limitation of joint mobility

 (c) Ophthalmologic

  (i) Cherry-red spot

  (ii) Retinitis pigmentosa

  (iii) Optic atrophy

  (iv) Cataracts

  (v) Corneal clouding

 (d) Ears and hearing

  (i) Hearing impairment

  (ii) Recurrent otitis media

 (e) Cardiovascular

  (i) Valvular disease

  (ii) Cardiomyopathy

 (f) Pulmonary

  (i) Pulmonary infiltration

 (g) Gastrointestinal

  (i) Hepatosplenomegaly

  (ii) Neonatal cholestatic liver disease

  (iii) Reflux

 (h) Hematology

  (i) Pancytopenia, anemia, or thrombocytopenia

 (i) Skin

  (i) Angiokeratoma (Figure 25.3)

  (ii) Multiple mongolian spots

  (iii) Hirsutism

  (iv) Hypopigmented to skin-colored papules/nodules (pebbling skin)

  (v) Xanthomata

DIAGNOSIS

A complete physical examination, including full ophthalmologic, hearing, and cardiac assessments, is important for individuals with possible LSDs. Family history, ethnic background, and ascertainment of consanguinity can provide useful information resulting in a correct diagnosis.

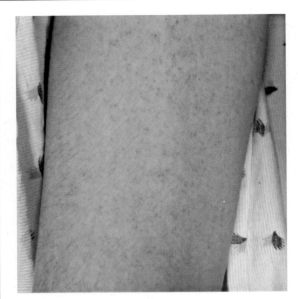

FIGURE 25.3   Angiokeratoma, cluster of small raised red spots on thigh, of a 13-year-old boy with fucosidosis.

ROUTINE INVESTIGATIONS

Basic investigations, such as complete blood count (CBC), comprehensive metabolic panel, ferritin, and bone x-ray, among others, can provide information about the baseline health status, convey evidence of possible coexisting diseases, and narrow the differential diagnosis. For example, pancytopenia and hyperferritinemia suggest Gaucher disease. Severe liver disease is seen in Niemann-Pick C. Neurological deficits can result in undernutrition, iron deficiency, anemia, and low albumin. Low levels of high-density lipoprotein (HDL) are occasionally observed in untreated Gaucher disease and Niemann Pick C.

Elevation of biochemical markers suggests active disease activity, an indication that is used for monitoring treatment response. Chitotriosidase (CHITO), angiotensin-converting enzyme (ACE), and tartrate-resistant acid phosphatase (TRAP) are recommended biochemical markers for monitoring response to therapy in patients with Gaucher disease. However, these markers should not be used and interpreted in isolation. CHITO is produced by activated macrophages and is the most sensitive biomarker for changing disease activity. Approximately 6% of the population has chitotriosidase deficiency; therefore, monitoring CHITO in these individuals is not useful.

Skeletal surveys are used to detect dysostosis multiplex, seen in many LSDs such as MPS, some oligosaccharidoses, ML, ISSD, GM1 gangliosidosis, and galactosialidosis. Cervical spine x-ray is necessary to evaluate instability and subluxation in patients with dysostosis multiplex. Characteristic Erlenmeyer flask deformity of the femur may be seen in Gaucher disease with bone involvement (25–28).

BIOCHEMICAL TESTS

Screening Test

Urine oligosaccharide and glycosaminoglycan (GAG) screening tests are useful initial methods. There are no specific precautions regarding diet or timing when obtaining the specimen.

Urine Glycosaminoglycan Analysis

Both quantitative and qualitative analysis for urine GAGs are available. A quantitative test can be analyzed by a colorimetric method using dimethylene blue (DMB) or by spectrophotometry (SP). Quantitative analysis is applied as an initial investigation for MPS, to monitor the amount of GAGs after bone marrow transplantation, or during treatment with enzyme therapy. Qualitative urine GAG analysis is performed by thin-layer chromatography (TLC) or electrophoresis. Pattern recognition can be used to indicate a possible diagnosis, as excretion patterns are generally disease-specific. However, quantitative and qualitative urine GAG analysis should be interpreted together for a complete evaluation. A urine specimen with slightly elevated or normal total GAG may contain an abnormal excretion profile of GAGs.

Increased total GAG excretion has been observed in diseases affecting connective tissue metabolism such as Lowe syndrome (oculocerebrorenal syndrome), osteopetrosis, and pycnodysostosis. Caution in the execution and interpretation of these tests is important to avoid false-positive results. For example, adhesive from a urine bag can cause artificial elevation of total GAGs and an abnormal electrophoresis pattern.

Urine Oligosaccharides Analysis

Urine oligosaccharide screening tests are analyzed by TLC or matrix-assisted laser desorption and time of flight mass spectrometry (MALDI-TOF). The interpretation is similar to TLC or electrophoresis for

GAGs. Excretion profiles of oligosaccharides are usually specific to the enzyme defect. However, TLC is less sensitive than MALDI-TOF in identifying excretion products of mucolipidosis II or III and sialidosis. The MALDI-TOF method can also detect large organic molecules up to several kiloDaltons and has been used for detection and characterization of peptides, proteins, oligosaccharides, and nucleotides (29). A recently developed MALDI-TOF technique can also identify glycosylated and small glycopeptides (30).

Urine oligosaccharide screening tests may show an abnormal pattern of oligosaccharide excretion in individuals suffering from the oligosaccharidoses group, Pompe disease, sphingolipidoses (including GM1 and GM2), mucolipidosis, and galactosialidosis.

Other Urine Screening Tests

Quantitative urine free and bound sialic acid assays can be performed by chromatographic technique, either through spectrophotometric or fluorimetric thiobarbituric acid assays. Free sialic acid storage disease, sialidosis, galactosialidosis, and sialuria (an increase of sialic acid in the cytoplasm) can all cause elevated urine sialic acid (31–33).

Abnormal screening results must be confirmed by the appropriate enzyme assay for a final diagnosis. If LSDs are still strongly suspected but urine screening tests are negative, enzyme analysis of various diseases suggested by clinical findings should be considered.

Enzyme Analysis

Enzyme analysis is a definitive diagnostic test and is commercially available for the majority of LSDs. The level of the enzyme residual activity may or may not be associated with disease severity. Specific enzyme assays should be performed in the appropriate material. The type of specimen required for each disease is shown in Table 25.1. Pseudodeficiency can occasionally be shown in GM2 gangliosidosis and MLD. An individual that carries the pseudodeficiency gene will have low normal enzymatic activity; however, one will not have symptoms of the disease or pathologic storage of a specific substance.

The limitations of enzyme testing are:

• Determination of carrier status and differentiation between normal individuals and carriers of the

disease are limited since the level of activity in carriers may overlap with the level of activity seen in normal controls.
• Normal results in symptomatic patients can be a finding of activator-deficient LSDs such as GM2 activator deficiency. This result is contrary to pseudodeficiency, in which deficiency of enzyme activity is noted but the accumulation of pathologic metabolites and symptoms identical to those associated with enzyme deficiency are not detected. Substrate loading tests on cultured fibroblasts can also be used to diagnose these conditions.

Other Biochemical Tests

Intracellular cholesterol transport assay provides a definite diagnosis for Niemann–Pick C (NPC). The assay is analyzed by assessing the ability of cultured fibroblasts to esterify cholesterol after loading with low-density lipoprotein cholesterol (LDL). The filipin staining test is also a sensitive and specific tool to diagnose NPC. This test requires fibroblasts cultured in LDL-enriched medium. The stain detects cholesterol-filled perinuclear vesicles (26).

Molecular Analysis

Molecular tests are beneficial in the following situations:

• To distinguish between carrier and normal individuals
• To confirm a diagnosis when a biochemical test is inconclusive
• To detect an individual with pseudodeficiency
• To diagnose diseases for which enzyme tests are not available
• To provide information for genetic counseling and prenatal diagnosis for at-risk pregnancies if a family mutation is known. Biochemical testing for prenatal diagnosis is possible only in very few centers and requires many precautions; therefore, molecular testing on the proband (affected individual), and/or parents is necessary.

Histology–Pathology

Bone marrow aspiration/biopsy may show typical storage cells indicating some LSDs. Gaucher cells, macrophages containing storage materials, can be detected in the bone marrow and most other tissues and

TABLE 25.1   Lysosomal Storage Diseases (LSDs) With Primary Neurological Involvement, Primary Defect and Diagnostic Method

Storage materials	Diseases	Primary defect	Diagnosis
Lipid	Niemann–Pick C	Intracellular cholesterol transport	Impair intracellular cholesterol transport, positive filipin test
Monosaccharide	Free sialic acid storage disease	Lysosomal transport protein sialin	All forms: High free sialic acid in urine, tissue, and FB, especially lysosomal localization
	• Infantile free sialic acid storage disease (ISSD)		
	• Intermediate salla disease		All forms: Molecular test (SLC17A5 gene)
	• Mild form (salla disease)		
Mucolipidoses	Mucolipidoses		
	• Type II (I cell disease)	*N*-acetylglucosamine-1-phosphotransferease	High urine oligosaccharide, normal urine GAGs, 5–20 times higher than normal of nearly all lysosomal enzymes in blood and tissue
	• Type III (pseudo Hurler polydystrophy)	*N*-acetylglucosamine-1-phosphotransferease	
	• Type IV	Receptor-stimulated cation channel (mucolipidin)	
Mucopolysaccharidoses (MPS)	MPS		All types: high and abnormal pattern of urine GAGs, deficiency of a specific enzyme analysis,[a] molecular test
Dermatan, heparan sulfate	• Type IH (Hurler)	l-Iduronidase	Low enzyme activity in WBC, FB
Dermatan, heparan sulfate	• Type II (Hunter)	Iduronate-sulfatase	Low enzyme activity in WBC, FB, P, S
Heparan sulfate	• Type III A (Sanfilippo type A)	Heparan-*N*-sulfatase	Low enzyme activity in WBC, FB
	• Type III B (Sanfilippo type B)	*N*-acetyl-α-glucosaminidase	Low enzyme activity in WBC, FB, P, S
	• Type III C (Sanfilippo type C)	α-Glucosaminide-acetyl-CoA transferase	
	• Type III D (Sanfilippo type D)	*N*-Acetylglucosamine-6-sulfatase	Low enzyme activity in FB
Dermatan, heparan, chondroitin sulfate	• Type VII (Sly)	β-Glucoronidase	Low enzyme activity in WBC, FB, P, S

(continued)

TABLE 25.1   Lysosomal Storage Diseases (LSDs) With Primary Neurological Involvement, Primary Defect and Diagnostic Method   (*continued*)

Storage materials	Diseases	Primary defect	Diagnosis
Multiple enzyme defects	Multiple sulfatase deficiency	Sulfatase-modifying factor-1 (SUMF1)	Low enzyme activity of several sulfatase in WBC, FB; high urine GAGs and high urine sulfatides
	Galactosialidosis	β-Galactosidase and neuraminidase secondary to defect of protective protein, cathepsin A	Low enzyme activity in FB, WBC
Neuronal ceroid lipofuscinosis (NCL)	NCL		All types: Electron microscopy of biopsied tissues, or buffy coat; molecular test; enzyme analysis in FB, WBC can be performed in CTSD, PPT1, and TPP1
	• Congenital	Cathepsin D (CTSD)	
	• Infantile (INCL)	Palmitoyl-protein thioesterase-1 (PPT1)	
	• Late infantile (LNCL)	Tripeptidyl peptidase 1 (TPP1)	
	• Juvenile (JNCL)	A transmembrane protein	
	• Adult (ANCL)	Ceroid lipofuscinosis neuronal protein 3 (CNT3)	
	• Northern epilepsy (NE)	Ceroid lipofuscinosis neuronal protein 8 (CLN8)	
Oligosaccharidoses (glycoproteinoses)			All types: high and abnormal pattern of urine oligosaccharides, deficiency of specific enzyme analysis,[a] molecular test
	Alpha-mannosidosis	A-Mannosidase	Low enzyme activity in WBC, FB
	Beta-mannosidosis	B-Mannosidase	Low enzyme activity in WBC, FB
	Fucosidosis	α-Fucosidase	Low enzyme activity in WBC, FB
	Schindler disease	α-N-acetylgalactosaminidase	Low enzyme activity in WBC, FB
	Aspartylglucosaminuria (AGU)	Aspartylglucosaminidase	Low enzyme activity in WBC, FB
	Sialidosis		Low enzyme activity in FB
	• Severe infantile	α-Neuraminidase	
	• Mild infantile (mucolipidosis I)	α-Neuraminidase	
	• Adult	α-Neuraminidase	
Sphingolipidoses			Deficiency of a specific enzyme analysis,[a] molecular test

(continued)

TABLE 25.1 Lysosomal Storage Diseases (LSDs) With Primary Neurological Involvement, Primary Defect and Diagnostic Method *(continued)*

Storage materials	Diseases	Primary defect	Diagnosis
Ceramide	Farber disease	Ceramidase	Low enzyme activity in FB
Galactocerebroside	Globoid cell leukody-strophy (GLD or Krabbe disease)	β-Galactocerebrosidase	Low enzyme activity in WBC, FB
	• Infanitle		
	• Late infantile		
	• Adult		
	• Saposin A deficiency	Sphingolipid activator protein A (SAPA)	
Gangliosidoses	GM1 gangliosidoses	β-Galactosidase	High urine oligosaccharides, deficiency of specific enzyme analysis,[a] molecular test
	• Infantile		
	• Late infantile		
	• Adult		
	GM2 gangliosidoses	β-Hexosaminidase	High urine oligosaccharide
	• Sandhoff disease	β-Hexosaminidase A and B (α-subunit)	Low enzyme activity in WBC, FB, P
	• Tay–Sachs	β-Hexosaminidase A (β-subunit)	Low enzyme activity[b] in S, WBC, FB
	• GM2 activator deficiency (AB variant GM2)	β-Hexosaminidase activator	Abnormal urine oligosaccharide but normal enzyme activity, requires molecular test
Glucocerebroside	Gaucher disease	β-Glucocerebrosidase	Deficiency of a specific enzyme analysis[a]
	• Type II		Low enzyme activity in WBC, FB, DBS
	• Type III		Low enzyme activity in WBC, FB, DBS
	• Saposin C deficiency	Sphingolipid activator protein C (SAPC)	Nearly normal glucosylcerami-dase activity, imunochemical analysis, molecular test
Sphingomyelin	Niemann–Pick	Sphingomyelinase	Deficiency of a specific enzyme analysis[a]
	• Type A		Low enzyme activity in WBC, FB
	• Type B		Low enzyme activity in WBC, FB
Sulfatide	Metachromatic leuko-dystrophy (MLD)	Arylsulfatase A	Deficiency of a specific enzyme analysis,[a] high urine sulfatides

(continued)

TABLE 25.1 **Lysosomal Storage Diseases (LSDs) With Primary Neurological Involvement, Primary Defect and Diagnostic Method** (*continued*)

Storage materials	Diseases	Primary defect	Diagnosis
	Late infantile		Low enzyme activity in WBC, FB
	Juvenile		Low enzyme activity in WBC, FB
	Adult		Low enzyme activity in WBC, FB
	• Saposin B deficiency	Sphingolipid activator protein B (SAPB)	High urine sulfatides, SapB level in urine and FB
Multiple sphingolipids	Prosaposin deficiency (pSap)	Precursor of sphingolipid activator protein	Combined deficiency of galactosylceramidase and ceramidase in WBC, FB; elevation free ceramide in FB

FB, fibroblast, DBS, dry blood spot; GAGs, glycosaminoglycans; P, plasma, S, serum, WBC, white blood cell.
[a]Demonstration of low specific enzyme activity upon analysis in the appropriate material.
[b]Serum is used for all genders, but for women who are pregnant or on birth control, WBC is recommended.
Source: Adapted from Refs. 24, 34, 35, 36, 37–39.

demonstrate a characteristic "wrinkled tissue paper" or "crumpled silk" appearances. Pseudo-Gaucher cells have been reported in non-LSDs such as lymphomas, acute lymphocytic leukemia, and thalassemia. Foam cells containing white or empty-appearing lipid inclusions (lipid-laden macrophages) and/or sea-blue histiocytes are another typical LSD storage cell. These cells are found in Niemann–Pick disease (40).

Tissue and skin fibroblast histology, pathology, and electron microscope studies could be helpful in the determination of several diseases. Furthermore, these methods are important in the diagnosis of NCLs. Some types of NCLs have pathologic inclusions that may be identified in lymphocytes (41).

Newborn Screening

Because of therapeutic advances in LSDs, some diseases have been included in newborn screening panels in several U.S. states and in some other countries. These diseases include Pompe, Fabry, and the neuropathic LSDs (Krabbe, Niemann-Pick, and Gaucher diseases). The benefits, complications, ethical concerns, and financial issues associated with the early diagnosis of these diseases have been debated (42).

TREATMENT

Currently, specific treatment is available for some LSDs. Furthermore, several new treatments are under clinical trials and development. Although the cytotoxic effect of accumulated substrates is not the only pathophysiology of LSDs, the main purpose of treatment is to decrease storage materials with the expectation that lowering accumulation may reverse pathology.

To reduce accumulated substrates, the treatment can be achieved by:

• Increasing enzyme activity and improving residual enzyme activity
• Reducing accumulated substrates by inhibiting biosynthesis of substrates

Increasing enzyme activity and improving residual enzyme activity can be accomplished by:

• Exogenous enzyme replacement therapy (ERT)
• Hematopoietic stem cell transplantation (HSCT) and bone marrow transplantation (BMT)
• Enzyme enhancement by pharmacological chaperones
• Gene therapy

In normal circumstances, a small portion of the newly synthesized lysosomal enzyme is secreted into the cytoplasm without binding to the mannose-6-phosphate (M6P) receptor on the lysosome. Later, these enzymes can be taken back into the cells and consequently delivered to lysosomes through M6P receptors. This concept is important for cross-correction by enzymes produced from hematopoietic stem cell derivatives and exogenous ERT (43).

1. *Enzyme Replacement Therapy (ERT)*

Exogenous enzyme supplementation is administered through intravenous injection. This is a lifelong treatment. Gaucher disease type I is a prototype for exogenous enzyme therapy, which has become a standard of care. The treatment improves quality of life, hematological parameters, bone problems, and visceromegaly. It also reduces the risk of clinically significant long-term sequelae. Patient response to treatment in each parameter is highly variable (28, 44). Currently, ERT for Fabry disease, MPS type I, II, and VI, and Pompe disease have been approved by the US Food and Drug Administration (FDA). The benefits, safety, and tolerability of ERT have been studied, and the treatment is well-tolerated overall. Clinical trials for ERT for Niemann Pick A and B, as well as MPS IV are underway. Although enzyme therapy is successful in treatment of nonneuropathic-type Gaucher disease, ERT is noncurative. Additionally, there are limitations to ERT, which can be summarized as follows:

○ Irreversible pathology may not respond to ERT
○ Some clinical symptoms of LSDs are not caused by cytotoxic effects of the accumulated substrates, but by other mechanisms such as autophagy and inflammation. Therefore, ERT may not affect symptoms resulting from these pathogenic factors.
○ ERT is not beneficial for neuropathic LSDs because the exogenous enzyme is unable to cross the blood–brain barrier. The M6P receptors involved in enzyme uptake and transporting the enzyme to the lysosome are not expressed in the adult blood–brain barrier, although they are present in newborns (45–48).

Intrathecal enzyme replacement therapy for MPS I, II, and IIIA is currently being studied (see www.clinicaltrial.gov). Intrathecal enzyme infusion was shown to improve symptoms of meningitis in a patient with MPS VI (49).

2. *Hematopoietic stem cell transplantation (HSCT) and bone marrow transplantation (BMT)*

HSCT/BMT provides donor-derived cells, which can cross the blood–brain barrier and enter the brain. After migration into the brain, the donor-derived cells differentiate into microglia. In somatic organs, donor-derived cells can differentiate into other cells such as macrophages and Kupffer cells. Subsequent to engraftment, donor-derived cells become a permanent normal source of the enzyme and may ultimately restore biochemical function through cross-correction. HSCT/BMT can also modify the CNS inflammatory response, an important pathophysiology of neuropathic GM1 gangliosidosis, GM2 gangliosidosis, NCL, and NPC. The efficacy of HSCT in reducing inflammation has been demonstrated in mouse models (50–52). HSCT/BMT has been used in cases where ERT is not effective or available, especially for neuropathic LSDs. Cell sources for these transplants include bone marrow and unrelated donor-umbilical cord blood transplantation (UCBT) (53).

Improvement of neurologic symptoms after HSCT has been demonstrated in MPS IH (Hurler), early-stage-infantile onset Krabbe disease, late-onset Krabbe disease, and early-stage juvenile/adult MLD. In MPS I, successful HSCT/BMT has been shown to preserve neurocognitive function. These treatments could also decrease liver and spleen sizes, improve pulmonary and cardiac function, and enhance the quality of life in patients with MPS I. If the transplant is performed during the first 2 years of life, improvements are significant. However, benefits to cornea, heart valves, and bone are limited. During the first year posttransplantation, deterioration in development may be observed due to the slow process of donor-derived microglia replacement in the CNS. As mentioned earlier, microglia are a source of enzymes in the CNS.

In general, neurologic outcomes for HSCT/BMTs performed in presymptomatic, early-stage or mild phenotype individuals are better than those in symptomatic individuals or those with severe phenotypes. Unsatisfactory outcomes of symptomatic stage transplantations may be related to the process of engraftment and cross-correction, which might not occur quickly enough to counteract the rapid progression of disease (48, 52, 54–57).

The advantages of HSCT/BMT in other diseases have been reported with a small number of patients. These diseases include Alpha mannosidosis (58, 59), Fucosidosis (60), Farber disease (61), Aspartylglucosaminuria (56, 62, 63), Sialidosis (mucolipidosis type I), I cell disease (64), and Wolman disease (65, 66).

Combinations of HSCT and ERT have been conducted. ERT that is commenced prior to transplantation (with or without ERT after transplantation) and continued until full engraftment has been shown to be well tolerated and beneficial. It has been demonstrated that this combination of treatments does not disturb engraftment or increase morbidity (57, 67, 68).

3. *Pharmacological chaperones*

A pharmacological chaperone is a small molecule with good biodistribution to a number of organs, and includes molecules that can cross the blood–brain barrier. Pharmacological chaperones are useful for treating LSDs caused by enzyme misfolding. Some types of mutations, including missense mutations, in-frame deletions, and splice site mutations, cause enzyme misfolding but do not impair an active site of the enzyme. Misfolded enzymes are degraded prematurely by cell control mechanisms and do not become functionally active enzymes. Chaperones promote enzyme activity by enhancing refolding and promoting enzyme delivery to the lysosomes. This concept has been studied in Gaucher disease type I, Fabry, Pompe, and GM1/GM2 gangliosidosis (43, 45, 47).

4. *Gene therapy*

The goal of gene therapy is to provide a permanent and continuous source of enzyme at the therapeutic level. This treatment may also reach the end organs, including the bones and brain, better than other methods. Gene therapy can be achieved by ex vivo and in vivo gene therapy. For ex vivo therapy, human stem cells are transfected with the gene using a viral vector and subsequently transplanted to patients. On the other hand, in vivo gene therapy uses the liver or brain as a depot organ for viral vectors. Gene therapy studies have been conducted in animal models for several neuropathic LSDs, including INCL, LINCL, MPS II, MPS VII, MLD, and Krabbe. Benefits have been demonstrated in some studies; for example, one study showed a significantly slower rate of neurological decline in

10 children with LINCL after adeno-associated virus serotype 2 vector was injected in several locations in the CNS (43).

(I) **Substrate reduction therapy**

The objective of substrate reduction therapy (SRT) is to inhibit synthesis of accumulated substrates and accordingly reduce the amount of substrate of the deficient lysosomal enzyme.

(i) The imino sugar *N*-butyl-deoxynojirimycin (NB-DNJ or miglustat) is a chaperone that blocks sphingolipid synthesis by inhibiting glucosylceramide synthase. NB-DNJ was first approved in patients with Gaucher disease type I. Because glycosylceramide is a precursor of many sphingolipids, NB-DNJ has been studied in a few neuropathic LSDs, including GM1 gangliosidosis, GM2 gangliosidoses (Tay–Sachs and Sandhoff), and Niemann Pick C (45, 69).

In Niemann–Pick C, NB-DNJ stabilized symptoms in juvenile/adult patients and delayed regression rate of neurological symptoms in children. In addition, horizontal saccadic eye movement velocity and swallowing function were improved (70, 71). Significant improvement in extra pyramidal symptoms and seizures was reported in a child with NPC after 40 days of treatment with NB-DNJ (72). Currently, the drug has been approved for use in NPC in Europe.

(ii) Isoflavones, particularly genistein, inhibit synthesis of glycosaminoglycans (GAGs). It was demonstrated that isoflavones could reduce GAGs in cultured human fibroblasts obtained from MPS IIIA (Sanfilippo) and MPS VII (Sly) patients. A pilot study conducted in children with MPS IIIA and B demonstrated decline of GAGs concentration as well as improvement of hair morphology and cognitive function after treatment with isoflavones. A 2-years follow-up of eight patients with Sanfilippo treated with isoflavone extract showed a variety of responses, including improvement, stability, and decline in cognitive function. More studies need to be conducted to determine the efficacy, dosage and safety of isoflavones to treat MPS IIIA (73, 74).

In addition to specific and supportive treatment, genetic counseling is also important. Appropriate genetic counseling informs families making personal medical decisions and helps them to prepare for any subsequent pregnancies. Counseling also helps to identify other affected family members and facilitates early treatment of these patients.

EPILEPSY IN LYSOSOMAL STORAGE DISORDERS

Epilepsy is a condition characterized by recurrent unprovoked seizures. A seizure is considered to be a manifestation of abnormal discharges of a set of neurons in the brain. Seizures can be provoked (secondary to a known brain insult such as an infection, fever, or tumor) or unprovoked (without an identifiable precipitant). There are specific classifications used for the diagnosis of seizures and epileptic syndromes proposed by the International League against Epilepsy (75). The timing of seizure presentation can aid in the differential diagnosis of patients with LSDs. For example, seizures tend to occur after other symptoms are present in Gaucher disease type III, GM2 gangliosidoses, JNCL, MLD, and Niemann–Pick type C. In contrast, the lipofuscinoses LINCL and Northern Epilepsy have seizure onset usually before other symptoms are present. In INCL, ANCL type A and sialidosis type I, seizures usually occur early in the disease presentation. The recognition of seizure timing is vital in order to manage and improve the patient's quality of life. LSDs should be included in the differential diagnosis of patients with epilepsy and unexplained intellectual deficiency, organomegaly, familial history suggestive of genetic diseases, and clinical presentations that do not match any classical epilepsy syndrome. The recognition of the relationship between LSDs and epilepsy is vital and further research is warranted.

Epilepsy is observed in almost all neuropathic LSDs. Age of seizure onset is variable. There is no specific seizure type or electroencephalography (EEG) signature that is pathognomonic for any given LSD diagnosis. Thus, it is difficult to diagnose LSDs based on the type of epilepsy attack. However, myoclonic epilepsy occurs frequently in some of these diseases, especially the late-onset group. A diagnostic flow chart for LSDs and myoclonus is shown in Flowchart

1. Neuropathic LSDs with myoclonus as a part of their clinical manifestation include (12, 24, 35, 76–79):

Lipid storage	Niemann–Pick type C
Neuronal ceroid lipofuscinosis	Infantile, late infantile, juvenile, adult and Northern epilepsy form
Oligosaccharidoses	Aspartylglucosaminuria
	Fucosidosis type II
	Schindler disease
	Sialidosis type I (Macular cherry-red spot/myoclonus syndrome)
	Sialidosis type II (mucolipidosis type I)
Sphingolipidoses	Gaucher type II
	Gaucher type III
	Late-onset Krabbe
	Late-onset Tay–Sachs disease
	Niemann–Pick type A, B
Multiple enzyme defect	Late infantile and juvenile-onset galactosialidosis
	Multiple sulfatase deficiency
Activator protein deficiency	Prosaposin

Symptomatic treatment with AEDs seems to be effective in most cases; however, careful attention and close monitoring of seizure frequency and/or severity needs to be followed because, in rare occasions, AEDs may worsen epilepsy. Although LSDs are rare diseases among patients with epilepsy, accurate diagnosis is vital in terms of management, treatment, counseling, and prognosis. When managing LSD patients, the possibility of epilepsy should always be considered.

Because LSDs are rare disorders, limited literature exists concerning epilepsy. Moreover, seizures can and often occur due to metabolic or infectious processes that complicate the clinical presentation of these patients and are not necessarily due to the disease process itself. However, we will discuss some examples of LSDs that are associated with epilepsy as part of their clinical presentation.

NEUROIMAGING IN CHILDREN WITH LSDs AND EPILEPSY

Gaillard et al (80) proposed guidelines for imaging children with newly diagnosed epilepsy not secondary to febrile illness, acute symptomatic causes, or neonatal seizures. In general, neuroimaging was indicated if there is evidence of focal epilepsy (focal findings on neurological exam, focal onset by history, or focal abnormalities on EEG), evidence of stigmata on examination of neurocutaneous or cerebral malformation syndromes, in children younger than 2 years of age once simple febrile seizures are excluded, and in children with characteristics of generalized epilepsy syndromes (such as Lennox–Gaustaut). Changes in seizure pattern, worsening of seizures (frequency or severity), and developmental regression also merit neuroimaging evaluation if not previously done. Finally, new-onset seizures in the context of a medical emergency, such as status epilepticus or increased intracranial pressure, merit radiological evaluation. Because structural abnormalities are commonly the cause of seizures, MRI is the modality of choice. CT should be considered if the presence of blood or calcifications is suggested by the clinical presentation (80).

NEUROPATHIC LSDs

Neuropathic LSDs comprise two-thirds of all LSDs. The common characteristic features of neuropathic LSDs are neurodegeneration, developmental regression, and mental retardation. Secondary neurological complications are noted in some LSDs. For example, cerebrovascular accidents and carpal tunnel syndrome occur in Fabry disease, and hypoplastic cervical spine causing cord compression appears in MPS. In addition, cataplexy (sudden loss of muscle tone evoked by strong emotions such as laughter or anger) has been reported in approximately 20% of children with Niemann–Pick type C, although less commonly in adults (4%) (81). A summary of lysosomal storage disorders with primary neurological involvement classified by major storage material is shown in Table 25.1.

NIEMANN–PICK DISEASE TYPE C

Niemann–Pick disease type C (NPC) is a panethnic autosomal recessive lipidosis characterized by accumulation of unesterified cholesterol and glycolipids in the endosomal/lysosomal system (81, 82). Resembling other LSDs, the clinical course and presenting symptoms diverge. Age of onset ranges from perinatal to adult onset. Classic NPC (late infantile and juvenile) involves the majority of cases (~60–70%). Clinical manifestations are hydrop fetalis, neonatal cholestatic jaundice, hepatosplenomegaly, and hearing loss. Isolated hepatosplenomegaly is usually an initial symptom of late infantile (2- to 6-year-old). Prominent clinical features of adult onset are cerebellar ataxia, vertical supranuclear opthalmoplegia, dysarthria, dysphagia, and splenomegaly. Psychiatric symptoms are more commonly seen than in classic NPC (81).

Patients with NPC do not show neurological manifestations during the neonatal period (83). However, in the early infantile form (age of onset from 2 months to 2 years), some patients can present with severe symptoms, including delay of developmental motor milestones from 8 to 9 months and central hypotonia. The late infantile form age of onset ranges from 2 to 6 years, and death generally occurs between 7 and 12 years of age (83). Neurological symptoms including hypotonia, ataxia, dystonia, myoclonus, cataplexy, cognitive deterioration, and vertical supranuclear ophthalmoplegia are commonly seen. Partial or generalized seizures alone or in combination may occur. The seizures generally respond to standard antiepileptic drug treatment, but refractory cases may occur. Severe epilepsy has a bad prognosis and is associated with a shortened life span. Canafoglia et al described a patient with late infantile NPC with a clinical presentation of worsening myoclonus, generalized seizures, cerebellar symptoms, mild mental impairment, and gaze palsy (84). The seizures were treated with antiepileptic drugs, including benzodiazepines. EEG showed abnormally high and diffuse background alpha-activity, enhanced by intermittent photic stimulation, but did not show any clear epileptic abnormalities. Approximately half of the patients with juvenile NPC (onset from 6 to 15 years) show variable types of seizures. The lifespan is quite variable, with some patients surviving up to 30 years of age or later (83).

Iturriaga et al reported an analysis of symptom presentation in patients with biochemically confirmed NPC that included age at onset of disease, age at diagnosis, and neurological involvement, among other parameters. The study included 30 patients with ages ranging from 4 days to 35 years. Epilepsy appeared in 33% of patients with early infantile NPC, 67% of patients with late infantile NPC, and 55% of patients with juvenile NPC. No epilepsy appeared in subjects with adult-onset NPC. Seizures were well controlled with only one antiepileptic drug (85).

Uc Ergun Y. et al reported two cases of the juvenile form with seizure disorders. The first case was a 45-year-old man with a history of complex partial seizures since adolescence with rare generalization. EEG was described as showing diffuse slowing of the background activity with generalized brain dysfunction. Brain MRI showed mild posterior periventricular white matter hyperintensity on T2-weighted images. The second case described a 14-year-old girl with progressive dystonia, ophthalmoparesis, dysarthria, ataxia, cognitive deterioration, and seizure disorder. Her seizures were partial with secondarily generalized tonic–clonic seizures (86).

Diagnosis

• Biochemical test demonstrating impaired intracellular cholesterol transport is a definite diagnosis.
• Filipin stain on fibroblast or bone marrow cells shows fluorescent positive intracellular compartments indicating cholesterol storage.
• Identifying disease-causing mutations in NPC1 and/or NPC2 gene can also confirm the diagnosis.

Treatment

Disease-Specific Treatment

Several medications have been studied, such as Cucumin, steroid binding agents, and steroid-lowering agents. Only NB-DNJ (miglustat) has been approved for NPC as a disease-specific treatment in Canada, the European Union, South Korea, Brazil, Russia, and Australia. The mechanism of NB-DNJ is not well known. It is believed that the elevation of ceramide, as a result of glucosylceramide synthase inhibition, leads to alteration of the chemical coefficient of cholesterol in the membrane, consequently assisting cholesterol efflux from the lysosome. NB-DNJ may reduce the production of gangliosides (GM2 and GM3); therefore, it reduces an accumulation of gangliosides that are toxic to the CNS. Improving intracellular calcium homeostasis, which plays an important role in pathogenesis, has also been postulated to be the action of NB-DNJ.

Supportive Treatment

• Medications for cataplexy, medications for extrapyramidal symptoms, antipsychotic drugs, and AEDs.

• Instruction to prevent aspiration, nutritional treatment.

Neuronal Ceroid Lipofuscinoses

Neuronal ceroid lipofuscinoses (NCLs) are a group of rare, inherited, neurodegenerative LSDs with characteristic accumulation of autofluoroscent lipopigments and proteins in the lysosomes. Defects in a transmembrane protein and an enzyme deficiency underlie the pathogenesis of NCLs.

Patients with NCLs are considered genetically heterogenous as more than 160 mutations have been identified in eight reported NCL genes to date (CLN1, CLN2, CLN3, CLN5, CLN 6, CLN7, CLN8, and CLN10) (87). Mutations in each gene lead to a distinct phenotype, making NCLs more heterogeneous in nature.

The CLN1 gene located on chromosome 1p32 encodes the soluble lysosomal enzyme pamitoylprotein thioesterase1 (PPT1). The CLN2 gene located on chromosome 11p15 encodes another soluble lysosomal enzyme, tripeptidyl-peptidase1 (TPP1). The CLN3 and CLN5 genes encode lysosomal membrane proteins. Deficiency of PPT1 typically causes INCL and deficiency of TPP1 causes classic LINCL. A minority of patients with JNCL have PPT1 or TPP1 deficiency. Mutations in CLN3 cause JNCL (87). The Finnish variant form of late infantile neuronal ceroid lipofuscinosis (vLINCLfin) is caused by mutations in the CLN5. The CLN6 is located on chromosome 15p23. Mutations in the CLN6 cause a variant late infantile neuronal ceroid lipofuscinosis (vLINCL). The CLN7 is located on chromosome 4q28.1–q28.2. Mutations in the CLN7 cause the Turkish variant late infantile neuronal ceroid lipofuscinosis (vLINCL).

The CLN8 gene is located on chromosome 8p23 and is mutated in Finnish families with the variant Northern epilepsy (NE) (progressive epilepsy with mental retardation, PEMR) and in Turkish, Italian, and Israeli patients with a more severe variant late infantile NCL. The CLN8 protein is a nonglycosylated membrane protein whose function is unknown (87). The CLN10 is located on chromosome 11p15.5 and mutations have been described in three patients with both congenital NCL and with a severe course of neurodegeneration beginning at early school age (88).

Clinical features can be categorized by age of onset including congenital (onset before or around birth), infantile (onset 6–12 months), late infantile (onset

2–4 years old), juvenile (onset 4–9 years old), adult (30 years old), and Northern epilepsy (NE or progressive myoclonic epilepsy and mental retardation in Finland). Common symptoms of NCLs are cognitive decline, motor function impairment, vision loss, and seizures. Myoclonus is a frequent feature of INCL, LINCL, JNCL, ANCL, and NE. NCLs with progressive myoclonus should be differentiated from other causes of progressive myoclonic epilepsies such as sialidosis type I, Lafora progressive myoclonus epilepsy, Unverricht–Lundborg disease, mitochondrial diseases including MERRF, and Dentatorubral-pallidoluysian atrophy (15, 41).

Children with INCL are normal at birth. The symptoms usually start after 6 months of age and include seizures, microcephaly, and visual loss. Mental and motor deterioration occurs, leading to a vegetative state and eventual death by 10 years of age (87). Myoclonus, atonic, and tonic–clonic seizures manifest at the end of the first year in patients with the infantile form of NCL, in whom EEG shows early and severe depression. MRI of the brain usually shows deterioration of cortical, cerebellar, and white matter areas. Seizures are followed by rapid dementia and motor dysfunction (89).

LINCL has a later clinical onset. Classic LINCL or Jansky–Bielschowsky has an onset between 2 and 4 years of age. The clinical course of LINCL is characterized by dementia, seizures, visual impairment, and delayed and/or loss of developmental milestones, especially after seizure manifestation (35, 87, 90). The seizures vary in type and include generalized tonic–clonic, atonic, astatic, myoclonic, absence, and partial-onset seizures. Action myoclonus can become prominent after the onset of seizures, which could be a clinical clue for early diagnosis (41, 89). The EEG pattern in patients with LINCL may show spikes with slowing in the occipital region with photic stimulation (6). MRI of the brain shows progressive cerebral and cerebellar atrophy with normal basal ganglia and thalami (6, 41).

JNCL is the most common form of NCL worldwide. Onset is usually between the ages of 4 and 8 years (mean age 5 years) with a highly variable clinical course and a life expectancy of 20 to 30 years (87). Progressive visual failure due to retinitis pigmentosa and optic atrophy may be the only sign for 2–5 years (41, 87). Seizures may manifest between the ages of 5 and 18 years and can be generalized tonic–clonic, complex partial, and/or myoclonic seizures (77). EEG tracing can show

disorganization, spikes, and slow wave complexes (77). CT and MRI may reveal cerebral and, to a lesser degree, cerebellar atrophy in the later stages (age greater than 15 years) (41).

The adult form of NCL (ANCL, Kuf's disease) represents 10% of all cases of NCLs (91). It usually manifests around 30 years of age, although in some cases symptoms may appear as early as 11 years of age (41). Unlike other types of NCLs, ophthalmologic studies in patients with ANCL are normal and no ocular symptoms are observed (41). Family studies have shown both recessive (Kuf's disease) and dominant modes (Parry disease) of inheritance (92). However, the genetic locus of the gene responsible for ANCL (CLN4) is yet to be determined.

On the basis of clinical phenotypes, ANCL has been classified into two major subgroups. Type A is characterized by the presence of progressive myoclonus epilepsy (PME) as well as dementia, ataxia, and both pyramidal and extrapyramidal signs (41). Seizures are often hard to control and can be tonic–clonic with a long tonic phase with photosensitivity (77). Type B is marked by behavioral changes, dementia, and a peculiar facial dyskinesia (41). EEG shows photosensitivity at low frequencies, a feature not commonly encountered in other adult epilepsy syndromes (41, 77, 92).

Onset of symptoms of Northern epilepsy occurs between the ages of 5 and 10 and includes slow and progressive mental deterioration, generalized tonic–clonic seizures, and, in some cases, complex partial seizures (90). Vision problems are uncommon in patients with NE. Seizures tend to be resistant to common AEDs and become more frequent as patients approach puberty; however, clonazepam has been somewhat effective (90). After puberty, seizures become less frequent but mental deterioration continues to progress (41). Brain imaging may demonstrate cortical atrophy in patients over 40 years of age, but this is rare before the age of 30. EEG tracing shows slowing of background activity. Rhythmic delta activity is abundant, while more specific patterns can be missing. Epileptiform activity on EEG can be frequently observed, but is not predominant (93).

Neuroimaging in NCLs

D'Incerti et al reported that magnetic resonance imaging in all the different forms of NCLs demonstrate cerebral and cerebellar atrophy, mild hyperintensity of cerebral white matter on T2-weighted images, thinning of the cortex, and hypointensity of the thalami on T2-weight images (94). The author suggested that cerebral atrophy is one of the cardinal manifestations of NCLs and that when interpreting MRI studies of young patients with progressive encephalopathy, if severe atrophy or rapid enlargement of the ventricles and sulci is observed, NCL must be considered. Rapid progression of atrophy is often observed in both the INCL and LINCL. In contrast, cerebral atrophy associated with JNCL and ANCL is often subtle early in the course of disease, or may remain completely absent.

Diagnosis

- Enzyme analysis is available only for Palmitoyl-protein thioesterase1 (PTT1), tripeptidyl-peptidase 1 (TPP1), and cathepsin D (CTSD). The test can be performed in white blood cells, fibroblasts, or chorionic villi.
- Histology demonstrates characteristic pathologic inclusions in tissues and sometimes in lymphocytes. The specific morphology of inclusions may indicate specific type of NCLs; granular osmiophilic deposits (GROD) in INCL, curvilinear in LINCL, and fingerprint in JNCL and ANCL. Mixed inclusion patterns are also seen in almost every type (36).
- Molecular testing

Stockler-Ipsiroglu et al suggested a diagnostic work-up for young children with epilepsy and mental retardation. Initial determination of PPT1 and TPP1 would include or exclude a diagnosis of CLN1 and CLN2. If *both* tests are negative, a tissue biopsy (skin or rectal) for demonstration of lipofuscin inclusion bodies by electron microscopy should follow if there is a high clinical index of suspicion. If this study demonstrates positive lipofuscin inclusions, the *CLN6, 7,* and *8* genes should be investigated for a final molecular diagnosis. Older children with retinopathy and mental regression should undergo vacuolated lymphocyte demonstration and mutation analysis of the *CLN 3* gene. If these are negative, other CLNs or mild variants of CLN1 and CLN2 should be considered and respective testing initiated (95).

Treatment

There is no effective therapy for NCLs. The therapy that exists is mainly supportive. Common problems such as malnutrition, sleep problems, behavioral-psychiatric problems, and spasticity require palliative care.

Seizures are often not responsive to antiepileptic therapy; therefore, AEDs should be selected with caution. Antiepileptic drugs (AEDs) such as valproate (VPA), clonazepam, and lamotrigine (LTG) have been studied in patients with JNCL by Aberg LE et al. In this study, LTG and VPA appeared equally effective. In addition, LTG in monotherapy or LTG in combination with clonazepam (CZP) was superior to other AEDs or combinations. Other new AEDs such as levetiracetam and topiramate may provide some benefit. Certain antiepileptic drugs such as carbamazepine and phenytoin have been associated with exacerbation of seizure activity and could also cause clinical deterioration (41). LTG may aggravate seizures and myoclonus in LINCL (41).

Other supportive medical treatment includes melatonin for sleep problems, baclofen for spasticity, anti-Parkinson drugs, and antipsychotics drugs such as respiridone, clonazepam, and sulpiride. Prior to initiating these medications, drug interaction should be considered and each drug should be selected with proper precautions. The safest and most commonly used drugs in the lowest possible doses are recommended (41, 96, 97).

A combination of vitamin E and sodium selenite, acting as antioxidants, has been used in JNCL. Gene therapy in LINCL has been investigated (36). Several clinical trials have been conducted to determine the most effective treatments, which can be summarized as follows:

- Cystaemine trial for PPT1 deficiency INCL
- Stem cell therapy for PPT1 deficiency INCL
- Gene therapy for INCL, LINCL, and JNCL
- Combination between intracranial gene therapy with either neonatal BMT or cysteamine demonstrated satisfactory results in animal models (98, 99).

Mucopolysaccharidoses

Mucopolysaccharidoses (MPSs) are a group of LSDs characterized mainly by accumulation of GAGs or mucopolysaccharides. Each type of MPS shares many clinical features. The degree of severity is a continuum within each type. Cognitive impairment and mental retardation are characteristic of MPS IH, severe form MPS II and all subtype of MPS III. Skeletal manifestations are noted in all types with variable severity. Coarse facial features are shown in all types, especially early onset, but are less prominent in MPS IV. In mild cases such as MPS IS (Scheie), patients may present with only joint contractures and mild skeletal abnormalities without intellectual deficiency. MPS III has severe behavioral disturbances. Seizures have been reported in neurological involvement in the MPSs. The incidence of seizures in MPS II is 13% according to one large cohort study. Other neurological symptoms are hydrocephalus, spinal cord compression, cervical myelopathy, optic nerve compression, and carpal tunnel syndrome. These features may be associated with accumulated GAGs in tissue surrounding nerves or in choroid plexus (100).

Diagnosis

- Brain imaging study: Described in MPS II, brain MRI reveals ventriculomegaly as well as widely distributed white-matter lesions, predominantly peri and supraventricularly, but also in the basal ganglia and corpus callosum. Imaging also demonstrates enlargement of the perivascular spaces (100, 101). A skeletal survey shows dysostosis multiplex.
- Quantitative and qualitative urine GAGs studies are appropriate initial screening tests.
- Enzyme analysis and molecular testing are used to make a definite diagnosis.

Treatment

ERT is available for MPS I, II, and VI. ERT has limited ability to cross the blood–brain barrier, which consequently reduces the benefits of the treatment in the CNS. Improvements in neurological symptoms have been documented in some patients under high-dose ERT. However, the overall benefit of using high-dose ERT to overcome neurodegeneration is controversial. ERT generally improves hepatomegaly, respiratory function, walking ability, joint movement, left ventricular hypertrophy, and growth. Intrathecal ERT treatment for MPS I, II, and IIIA is under clinical trials.

The advantage of hematopoietic stem cell transplantation (HSCT) has only been displayed in MPS I. Successful HSCT preserves neurocognition and alleviates some somatic symptoms, including inhibiting changing of facial features, improvement of joint stiffness and heart function, and reducing liver–spleen size.

Valvular heart diseases and corneal cloudiness are not improved significantly after HSCT.

Improvement of cognitive function in MPS IIIA and B patients treated with a genistein-rich isoflavone extract was demonstrated in one pilot study. A large clinical trial of genistein on MPS IIIA has been conducted, but the efficacy of the treatment is still being evaluated (74).

Oligosaccharidoses

Oligosaccharidoses or glycoproteinoses are a group of LSDs caused by defects of glycoprotein degradation. A stepwise removal of terminal monosaccharides from polypeptide chains requires several enzymes. The deficiency of an enzyme in each step leads to accumulation of glycoproteins (oligosaccharide chains attached to a side chain of polypeptides). Many clinical features of oligosaccharidoses overlap with MPS. Somatic phenotypes including coarse facies, hepatosplenomegaly, deafness, and corneal clouding range from mild to severe. Cataracts and cloudy corneas are noted in alpha-mannosidosis. Cherry-red spots are seen in sialidoses types I and II. Angiokeratoma has been reported in most types of oligosaccharidoses, except Schindler disease and sialidosis. Neurological manifestations are demonstrated in every disease in this group; however, the severity varies broadly. Intellectual disability, pyramidal tract signs, cerebellar problems, and seizures are commonly seen as well. Myoclonus is noted in some diseases including aspartylglucosaminuria (AGU), Fucosidosis type II, Schindler disease, sialidosis type I (Macular cherry-red spot/myoclonus syndrome), and sialidosis type II (mucolipidosis type I). Sialidosis type I is a prototype of LSDs presenting with polymyoclonus and progressive visual loss.

Sialidosis

Sialidosis is an autosomal recessive lysosomal storage disorder caused by mutations in the *NEU 1* gene, resulting in deficiency of the enzyme sialidase (alpha neuraminidase). There is subsequent accumulation and urinary excretion of neuraminidase substrates, mainly sialylated glycoproteins and oligosaccharides (102). Lai et al recommended that the *NEU1* mutations be screened in patients presenting with action myoclonus, ataxia, and seizures, even without macular cherry-red spots. Laboratory findings show high levels of sialylated oligosaccharides in the urine and low activity of neuraminidase in skin fibroblasts (103). Urinary oligosaccharide analysis has been used as a rapid diagnostic screening method (104). Death usually occurs in the third decade (76).

Sialidosis has been classically divided into two clinical types, types I and II. Type I sialidosis, also known as cherry-red spot myoclonus syndrome, is the milder form that presents in the second decade of life (103). The clinical phenotype is characterized by the presence of the macular cherry-red spot, cerebellar ataxia, seizures, myoclonus, and a decrease in visual acuity secondary to retinal degeneration (102). Progressive debilitating action-like myoclonus is often the first symptom and gradually leads to motor deterioration that is often unresponsive to medications (76). Tonic–clonic seizures are present in 50% of cases and are usually controlled with AEDs (77). Some patients show minimal or no signs of intellectual impairment (105).

EEG tracings in patients with sialidosis type I have been reported as normal, although typically show a low-voltage background of fast activity with disease progression, and minimal or no photosensitivity, which contrasts with ANCL (76, 77).

Type II sialidosis, or mucolipidosis type I, is the more severe form of the disease and is subdivided into congenital, infantile, and juvenile forms based on the age of onset. Phenotypes of sialidosis type II are similar to MPS, such as coarse facies, dysostosis multiple, hepatosplenomegaly, cornea clouding, developmental delay, myoclonus, and visual and hearing impairment (102). Sialidosis type II is much more common than sialidosis type I. However, type I seems to be more frequent in Italians, and type II has a higher frequency in Japan (102, 105).

Louboutin et al reported a 21-year-old French male individual with sialidosis type I. Visual deterioration at 16 year of age was the initial presentation. By age 19, he was unsteady on his feet and had developed abnormal speech. At 20 year of age, he developed myoclonic jerks with mild response to clonazepam. He did not have cognitive deficits. The CT scan and cerebral MRI were normal. The EEG was abnormal with diffuse paroxymal features described as generalized spikes and spike and wave complexes. After treatment with antiepileptic drugs, the rest EEG abnormalities disappeared (106). Lai et al reported 17 Taiwanese patients with sialidosis type I. Three of them had seizures as part of their clinical presentation. The seizure types were generalized tonic–clonic and myoclonic. The seizures were

managed with AEDs and EEGs showed abnormalities described as diffuse paroxysmal features, such as spike-wave complexes, in only two patients. Brain MRIs showed mild-to-moderate diffuse brain atrophy in five patients (102).

In summary, myoclonic seizures are well documented in type I sialidosis. However, epileptic seizures and myoclonus can also be seen in patients with sialidosis type II (107).

Diagnosis

- Urine oligosaccharide screening shows excretion pattern consistent with each disease.
- The diagnosis is confirmed by enzyme analysis and/ or molecular testing.

Treatment

Only symptomatic treatment is available. HSCT has been attempted in alpha-mannosidosis, fucosidosis, AGU, and sialidosis type II and the success of HSCT was reported in several patients. To date, there are no specific AEDs recommended. For sialidosis type I, dantrolene, 5-hydroxytryptophan (5HTP), and clonazepam were successful medications reducing myoclonus in a few case reports (76).

Sphingolipidosis

Sphingolipidoses are a group of LSDs caused by a defect in sphingolipid degradation. Ceramide is a basic structure of almost all sphingolipids. Examples of more complex forms include shingomyelin, cerebroside (ceramide and glucose), and gangliosides. Sphingolipids are essential components of myelin sheaths and neuronal tissue. Progressive neurological problems, cognitive deficiency, peripheral neuropathy, extra pyramidal symptoms, epilepsy, and cherry-red spots are typical features of sphingolipidoses. Coarse facies, dysostosis multiplex, and visceromegaly are noted in some diseases. Early-onset GM1 gangliosidosis has symptoms similar to severe MPS. Myoclonus has been reported in Gaucher type II, Gaucher type III, Late-onset Krabbe, Late-onset Tay–Sachs disease, and Niemann–Pick types A and B.

MLD and Krabbe, which are also categorized as leukodystrophies, involve the central and peripheral nervous systems. The early-onset group presents with irritability, spasticity, developmental delay, and, ultimately, deafness, and blindness. Behavioral problems are seen in juvenile onset. In MLD adult forms, psychiatric symptoms, especially schizophrenia, can be an initial symptom, ultimately followed by regression of cognitive function. Adult Krabbe shows central and peripheral nervous system symptoms, including eventual cognitive decline, blindness, and seizures (108, 109).

Gaucher Disease

Gaucher disease (GD) is an autosomal recessive disorder. The disease results from the inherited deficiency of the enzyme glucocerebrosidase (EC 3.2.1.45), which cleaves the glycolipid glucocerebroside into glucose and ceramide (110). The gene for beta-glucocerebrosidase was mapped to 1q21 (GenBank No. J03059). The most common mutations are N370S (c.1226 A > G), 84GG, L444P (c.1448 T > C), and IVS2(+1) (111). L444P/L444P and D409H/D409H (c.1342G > C) mutations are associated with the development of neurological manifestations. Although the diagnosis of GD can be established by finding deficient glucocerebrosidase activity in leukocytes or cell lines, the identification of a mutation in the glucocerebrosidase (*GBA*) gene confirms the diagnosis and facilitates genetic counseling.

The disorder has been classically divided into three types based upon the presence or absence and rate of progression of neurological manifestations (110). Type I, nonneuronopathic GD, is by far the most common type. It is associated with the N370S mutation, which is thought to protect against neurological symptoms except for Parkinson-like syndromes. Patients with GD type I have variable clinical presentations and disease progression. In some patients, the disease manifestations are significant and commonly include organomegaly, anemia, thrombocytopenia, and bone involvement. Type II, acute neuronopathic GD, is more stereotypic, with early onset between birth and 3 to 4 months of age of rapidly progressive and devastating neurological deterioration. Most affected children succumb to the disease within the first year or two of life. Type III or chronic neuronopathic GD encompasses multiple different phenotypes, although homozygosity for the L444P mutation predominates, with a mean age at diagnosis of 2.3 years (111). Patients can not only have primarily visceral involvement with slowed horizontal saccadic eye movements, but also myoclonus, ataxia, seizures, and dementia.

A subgroup of individuals with GD type III may manifest with uncontrollable myoclonic epilepsy and rapid CNS deterioration with death occurring over a very short period of time (112). In general, myoclonic epilepsy occurs after the development of other symptoms such as abnormal eye movements, ataxia, and dementia (110). In addition, reports in the literature have described some GD type III patients with generalized tonic–clonic epilepsy as part of the clinical presentation (113).

Electroencephalography in patients with GD and epilepsy may show several abnormal patterns such as poly spikes with occipital predominance increased by photic stimulation, diffuse slowing with presence of high-voltage sharp waves during sleep, multifocal spike and wave paroxysms, or normal background including absence of a correlation with EEG spikes and clinical myoclonus. Some patients manifest abnormal EEGs without convulsive disorders (77, 114–117) Neuroimaging studies in patients with GD are usually normal.

Gangliosidosis

A ganglioside is a molecule found predominately in neuronal membranes, although there is evidence that intracellular pools of gangliosides are involved in important signaling, transport, and regulatory functions (118). GM1 gangliosidosis is a lysosomal storage disorder due to a deficiency of the enzyme β-galactosidase. This enzyme hydrolyzes the terminal β-galactosyl residues from GM1 gangliosides, glycoproteins, and GAGs. GM2 gangliosidosis is due to an inherited deficiency of β-hexosaminidase A, β-hexosaminidase B, or GM2 activator in the lysosomes, which results in accumulation of GM2 ganglioside in the lysosomes.

GM1 Gangliosidosis

The clinical manifestation of GM1 gangliosidosis results from massive storage of GM1 ganglioside and related glycoconjugates in tissues, especially the CNS. The precise molecular mechanism leading to pathogenesis is not completely understood. However, observation of neuronal vacuolation accompanied by astrogliosis and microgliosis has been associated with neuronal cell death (119).

Three clinical forms are identified depending on age of onset of symptoms: type I (infantile), type II (late-infantile), and type III (adult) (120). Type I is the most severe form, with psychomotor retardation by 6 months of age. In addition, the diagnosis is suspected in infants with visceromegaly, cherry-red spot, and facial and skeletal abnormalities. Type II patients usually develop symptoms between 7 months and 3 years of age. The symptoms include slow progressive neurological deterioration and seizures. Type III is the mildest form, with onset of symptoms between 3 and 30 years of age. Patients tend to show symptoms consistent with cerebellar dysfunction, speech problems, short stature, and vertebral deformities (120). Magnetic resonance imaging of infantile onset shows diffuse hypomyelination, T2 hyperintensity of bilateral caudate and putamen, and a normal T2 signal intensity of the corpus callosum (Figures 25.4 and 25.5). Similar to MRI of infantile onset, CT of the brain demonstrates bilateral thalamic hyperdensity. Hypomyelination is not detected in late onset (121, 122).

GM2 gangliosidoses (Tay–Sachs Disease, Sandhoff Disease, AB Variant)

The GM2 ganglioside is degraded by beta-hexosaminidase A and/or beta-hexosaminidase B along with GM2 activator in the lysosome. Defects in these enzymes or this enzyme activator lead to GM2 ganglioside storage in the lysosomes, especially the lysosomes of CNS neurons (123).

Tay–Sachs disease, Sandhoff disease, and the GM2 gangliosodosis AB variant are clinically indistinguishable. Type I GM2 gangliosidosis is the infantile acute-onset form where clinical symptoms are present by the age of 6 months. In type I patients, seizures are common by the end of the first year of life and are highly variable in type. Subtle complex partial seizures or absence attacks typically become more frequent and more severe with time (124). Complete seizure control is difficult, but partial seizure control can be achieved by using conventional anticonvulsant medications. EEG abnormalities are relatively mild initially, but then show rapid progressive deterioration until death (124). Sakuraba et al reported a 1.5-year-old Japanese male patient with the infantile acute onset form of GM2 gangliosidosis AB variant who had myoclonic seizures at the age of 1 year. EEG revealed hypsarrhythmia. Anticonvulsants and vitamin B6 were effective in preventing myoclonus, despite the rapid progression of psychomotor disease (125).

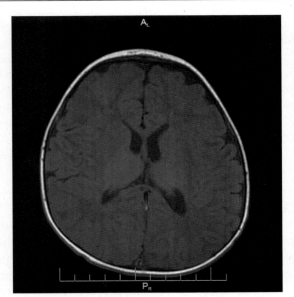

FIGURE 25.4 Axial T1 weight and Figure 25.5. Axial T2 weight MRI of 8-month-old with GM1 gangliosidosis shows increase intensity of both thalamus and delayed myelination.

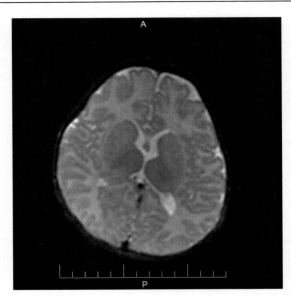

FIGURE 25.5 Axial T1 weight and Figure 25.5. Axial T2 weight MRI of 8-month-old with GM1 gangliosidosis shows increase intensity of both thalamus and delayed myelination.

Type II GM2 gangliosidosis, the subacute or juvenile form, has a variable age of onset between 2 and 18 years (126). It is characterized by progressive spasticity with seizures and dementia, leading to a vegetative state by late childhood or mid-adolescence (126). Maegawa et al studied a cohort of 21 patients with subacute GM2 gangliosidosis. In that cohort, seizures started between 1.5 and 32.0 years of age. Brain imaging studies showed cerebellar atrophy followed by generalized cerebral atrophy (127). Other reports in the literature described seizures in this group of patients as poorly controlled generalized tonic–clonic seizures (128, 129).

Type III GM2 gangliosidosis, the late-onset form, develops in late childhood and adulthood. It has a slower progression compared to the other forms (126). Type III affected individuals present with neurological and psychiatric symptoms including ataxia, weakness, spasticity, dysarthria, dysphagia, dystonia, psychosis, mania, depression, and cognitive decline (130). Motor symptoms and cerebellar ataxia are predominant manifestations in this form (123). Seizures in type III GM2 gangliosidosis are extremely rare.

MRI of infantile onset GM2 gangliosidosis is identical from those of GM1. T2 hyperintensity of bilateral caudate and putamen is observed in infantile onset GM2. Thalamic hyperdensity is observed in CT of the brain (Figure 25.6). Hypomyelination is not noted in late-onset GM2 gangliosidosis (122, 131).

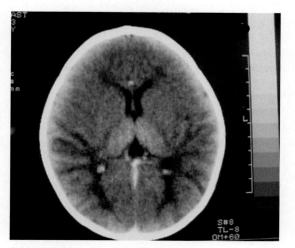

FIGURE 25.6 Axial CT brain of a 19-month-old boy with GM2 gangliosidosis shows symmetrically increased density within the thalamus (bright thalamus).

Metachromatic Leukodystrophy

Epileptic seizures are observed at a relatively late stage of metachromatic leukodystrophy (MLD). Approximately 25% of patients with the late infantile form, 50% to 60% of those with the juvenile form, and a few percent of patients with the adult form develop seizures (132). Different types of seizures have been reported, including generalized seizures, petit mal, petit mal variant, astatic seizures, and simple partial or complex partial seizures in the late infantile and juvenile forms (132, 133). EEGs may show nonspecific background abnormalities having diffuse and focal features (133). Bostantjopoulou et al reported two cases of adult form MLD with epilepsy. EEG findings were bilateral high-voltage delta frequency slow activity with variable frontal dominance and at times asymmetry (132).

Brain MRI in MLD may show periventricular leukodystrophy with symmetric confluent high signal density regions on T2-weighted images developing first in periventricular regions and further spreading into the hemispheres (77). Demyelination can also be seen in the posterior limbs of the internal capsule, descending pyramidal tracts, and the cerebellar white matter. Subcortical fibers are spared until late-stage MLD. Low-density tigroid stripes extending radially within abnormal white matter are typical but not specific. Brain atrophy is a late sign. There is no contrast enhancement of the abnormal white matter (Figures 25.7 and 25.8) (109).

Diagnosis

- Elevation of CSF protein and delayed nerve conduction velocity (NCV) are demonstrated in MLD and Krabbe.
- Urine oligosaccharide screening is abnormal in Gaucher disease, GM1, and GM2 gangliosidoses.
- Increase urine sulfatide excretion is noted in MLD and multiple sulfatase deficiency. Multiple sulfatase deficiency may present with similar clinical features seen in MLD, such as central and peripheral nervous system involvement. Unlike MLD, multiple sulfatase deficiency can have abnormal urine GAG excretion. Enzyme assay for several sulfatides, including iduronate sulfatase, heparin sulfatase, aryl-sufatase A & B, and steroid sulfatase, is helpful for differentiation (12).

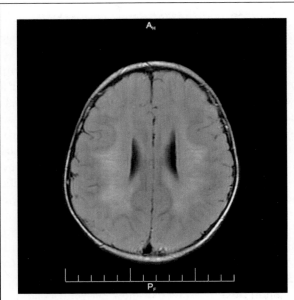

FIGURE 25.7   Axial FLAIR MRI of a 29-month-old with MLD shows symmetric, increased T2 signal within the deep cerebral white matter.

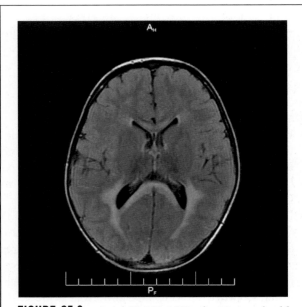

FIGURE 25.8   Axial FLAIR MRI of a 29-month-old with MLD shows symmetric, increased T2 signal within the deep cerebral white matter.

- The diagnosis is confirmed by enzyme analysis and/or molecular testing.

Treatment

There is presently no curative therapy for MLD. Seizures should be treated with antiepileptic drugs (134). ERT has been approved in nonneuropathic Gaucher and Fabry diseases. As mentioned earlier, the limitation of ERT is neurologic restoration. High-dose ERT may stabilize cognitive function. SRT is applied for mild–moderate Gaucher disease. Other treatment options such as chaperones and gene therapy are still under investigation. HSCT has provided promising results in the presymptomatic and early stages of disease in Krabbe and MLD.

Multiple Enzyme Defects

Galactosialidase

Deficiency of combined beta galactosidase and sialidase (neuraminidase) resulting from the defect of a protective protein (cathepsin A) causes galactosialidosis. Cathepsin A, a lysosomal protein, is encoded by the *PCCA* gene and functions to protect both beta galactosidase and sialidase from intralysosomal proteolysis. Age of onset varies from early, late infantile, and juvenile/adult. Similar to the majority of sphingolipidoses, cherry-red spots are usually detected. Other phenotypes also noted in GM1 gangliosidosis and MPS are seen in galactosialidosis, including dysostosis multiplex, coarse facial features, hepatosplenomegaly, cardiac involvement, corneal clouding and sometimes angiokeratoma. Neurological symptoms including developmental delay are usually seen in children, whereas progressive intellectual disability, seizures, and myoclonus are usually found in the juvenile/adult form.

Diagnosis (12, 135)

- Vacuolated lymphocytes may be identified. This finding may be seen in other LSDs such as NCL, mucolipidoses, oligosaccharidoses, and lipid storage LSDs.
- Urine oligosaccharide screening detects sialyloligosaccharides, similar to patients with sialidosis.
- Enzyme analysis demonstrating deficiency of both beta galactosidase and sialidase provides a definite diagnosis.

Treatment

No definitive treatment exists, although stem cell therapy has been studied in animal models.

Multiple Sulfatase Deficiency (MSD or Austin Disease)

A defect in sulfatase-modifying factor1 (SUMF1) causes deficiency of 12 sulfatases. SUMF1 functions to activate all sulfatases. Impairment of SUMF1 leads to defects of posttranslational modification and enzyme activation. The function of some sulfatases is known, and isolated enzyme deficiencies have been linked to specific diseases including MPS II, MPS IIIA, MPS IIID, MPS VI, MLD, X-linked ichthyosis, and chondrodysplasia punctata. Therefore, clinical features of MSD are a combination of symptoms of isolated sulfatase deficiency, such as organomegaly, developmental delay, coarse facies, corneal clouding, and ichthyosis.

Diagnosis
- Abnormal urine GAGs, abnormal oligosaccharide screening results, and elevation of urine sulfatides may be identified.
- Enzyme analysis shows decreased activity of sulfatases, including iduronate sulfatase, heparin sulfatase, arylsufatase A & B, and steroid sulfatase.

Treatment
No definitive treatment is available; however, enzyme therapy is currently being studied (74, 136).

CONCLUSION

LSDs comprise a group of disorders causing defects at the organelle and sub-organelle level. As might be expected, this results in a wide range of pathophysiologies and clinical consequences. The complex pathophysiology of LSDs bears similarity to those of common adult neurodegenerative diseases. This similarity can often complicate and delay diagnosis, as more common conditions might be considered initially. However, with new therapeutic options available or under development, it is more important than ever to consider an LSD diagnosis in a patient with unexplained neurologic symptoms. The molecular and genetic heterogeneity of these disorders further complicate the clinical diagnosis of these conditions; however, a structured workup based on metabolites, enzyme activity, genetics, presentation, and symptoms is the most likely way to yield the correct diagnosis.

Neurologic manifestations are the most debilitating clinical impacts of LSDs. Epilepsy is a common part of these neurological manifestations and can be the initial symptom. Epilepsy is usually present along with other specific signs and symptoms of each disease. A small portion of LSDs have characteristic seizure types, and the age of onset of epilepsy varies from neonate to adult. Therefore, LSDs should be included in the differential diagnosis of epilepsy, especially when accompanied by declining cognitive function.

Specific treatment is only available for some diseases. None of the currently available therapies successfully alleviates neurological manifestations. In addition, there are no specific antiepileptic drugs recommended for this group of patients. Currently, a variety of new treatments specifically for CNS manifestations are under investigation. These include direct introduction of recombinant enzyme into the cerebrospinal fluid.

In summary, LSDs are serious debilitating illnesses that can have significant impact on the CNS. Although current therapies are limited in effective treatment of the CNS manifestations, new strategies are constantly being explored to address this. Any patient with unexplained neurologic symptoms accompanied by cognitive changes should result in consideration of a diagnosis of an LSD. Early diagnosis is important for genetic counseling of other family members and to determine whether enzymatic or other interventional therapies will be useful.

CLINICAL PEARLS

- Lysosomes are organelles which contain a variety of enzymes used for large molecule degradation.
- Their functions are essential for maintaining cell homeostasis.
- Lysosomal storage disorders (LSDs) are a large group of inborn errors of metabolism; each group is characterized by specific accumulated intralysosomal substrates.
- Functional impairment or insufficient lysosomal enzymes are the most common etiology of LSDs.
- Cytotoxic effects of a specific storage substance are not the only pathophysiologic mechanism of LSDs; other complex mechanisms include dysfunction of cell signaling and disturbance of cell homeostasis.
- Most LSDs are inherited in an autosomal recessive pattern; there is a 25% chance of having another child with the same disease.

- Clinical manifestations are broad, usually involve multiple organs, and have overlap between different disease groups.
- Neurological manifestations are the most common presentation.
- Epilepsy is a common part of the neurological manifestations.
- Epilepsy may develop anytime during the course of disease.
- A small number of LSDs have characteristic seizure types, for example, myoclonus in sialidosis type I.
- Urine oligosaccharide and glycosaminoglycan (GAG) screening are useful to identify LSDs.
- Definitive diagnosis can be made by enzyme and molecular analysis.
- Specific treatment is available for some diseases although none of the current therapies successfully alleviate neurological symptoms.
- LSDs should be considered in the differential diagnosis of seizures with regression of development or multisystem involvement.

REFERENCES

1. de Duve C. Lysosomes revisited. *Eur J Biochem.* 1983;137(3): 391–397.
2. Tettamanti G, Bassi R, Viani P, et al. Salvage pathways in glycosphingolipid metabolism. *Biochimie.* 2003;85(3–4):423–437.
3. Walkley SU. Pathogenic cascades in lysosomal disease—Why so complex? *J Inherit Metab Dis.* 2009;32(2):181–189.
4. Todde V, Veenhuis M, van der Klei IJ. Autophagy: Principles and significance in health and disease. *Biochim Biophys Acta.* 2009;1792(1):3–13.
5. Saftig P. Physiology of the lysosome. In: A Mehta, M Beck, G Sunder-Plassmann. eds. *Fabry Disease: Perspectives from 5 Years of FOS.* Oxford: Oxford PharmaGenesis; 2006, Chapter 3.
6. Wolf NI, Garcia-Cazorla A, Hoffmann GF. Epilepsy and inborn errors of metabolism in children. *J Inherit Metab Dis.* 2009;32(5):609–617.
7. Stuart K. Trafficking of lysosomal enzymes in normal and disease states. *J Clin Invest.* 1986;77:1–6.
8. Barranger JA, Cabrena-Salazarr MA. Lysosomal biogenesis and disease. In: D Brooks, E Pakinson-Lawrence. eds. *Lysosomal Storage Disorders.* New York: Springer; 2007:7–43.
9. Bellettato CM, Scarpa M. Pathophysiology of neuropathic lysosomal storage disorders. *J Inherit Metab Dis.* 2010; 33(4):347–362.
10. Levine B, Mizushima N, Virgin HW. Autophagy in immunity and inflammation. *Nature.* 2011;469(7330):323–335.
11. Underwood BR, Massey DCO, Rubinsztein DC. Autography and human genetic disease. In: D Valle, AL Beaudet,
B Volgelstein. eds. *The Online Metabolic and Molecular Bases of Inherited Disease (OMMBID).* Available at www.ommbid. com. 2011. Accessed May 25, 2011.
12. Zschocke J, Hoffmann GF. Lysosomal metabolism. In: J Zschocke, GF Hoffmann. eds. *Vademecum Metabolicum: Manual of Metabolic Paediatrics.* 2nd ed. Stuttgart: Schattauer; 2004:111–123.
13. Parkinson-Lawrence EJ, Shandala T, Prodoehl M, et al. Lysosomal storage disease: Revealing lysosomal function and physiology. *Physiology (Bethesda).* 2010;25(2):102–115.
14. Meikle PJ, Hopwood JJ, Clague AE, et al. Prevalence of lysosomal storage disorders. *JAMA.* 1999;281(3):249–254.
15. Shahwan A, Farrell M, Delanty N. Progressive myoclonic epilepsies: A review of genetic and therapeutic aspects. *Lancet Neurol.* 2005;4(4):239–248.
16. Her HG. Inborn lysosomal diseases. *Gastroenterology.* 1965;48:625–633.
17. Settembre C, Fraldi A, Rubinsztein DC, et al. Lysosomal storage diseases as disorders of autophagy. *Autophagy.* 2008;4(1):113–114.
18. Settembre C, Fraldi A, Jahreiss L, et al. A block of autophagy in lysosomal storage disorders. *Hum Mol Genet.* 2008;17(1): 119–129.
19. Jeyakumar M, Thomas R, Elliot-Smith E, et al. Central nervous system inflammation is a hallmark of pathogenesis in mouse models of GM1 and GM2 gangliosidosis. *Brain.* 2003;126(Pt 4):974–987.
20. Smith D, Wallom KL, Williams IM, et al. Beneficial effects of anti-inflammatory therapy in a mouse model of Niemann–Pick disease type C1. *Neurobiol Dis.* 2009;36(2):242–251.
21. Sano R, Tessitore A, Ingrassia A, et al. Chemokine-induced recruitment of genetically modified bone marrow cells into the CNS of GM1-gangliosidosis mice corrects neuronal pathology. *Blood.* 2005;106(7):2259–2268.
22. Li HH, Zhao HZ, Neufeld EF, et al. Attenuated plasticity in neurons and astrocytes in the mouse model of Sanfilippo syndrome type B. *J Neurosci Res.* 2002;69(1):30–38.
23. Pastores G. Introduction. In: G Pastores. ed. *Lysosomal Storage Disorders: Principle and Practice.* Singapore: World Scientific Publishing; 2010:5–22.
24. Jardim LB, Villanueva MM, de Souza CF, et al. Clinical aspects of neuropathic lysosomal storage disorders. *J Inherit Metab Dis.* 2010;33(4):315–329.
25. Stein P, Yu H, Jain D, et al. Hyperferritinemia and iron overload in type 1 Gaucher disease. *Am J Hematol.* 2010;85(7): 472–476.
26. Wraith JE, Baumgartner MR, Bembi B, et al. Recommendations on the diagnosis and management of Niemann–Pick disease type C. *Mol Genet Metab.* 2009;98(1–2):152–165.
27. Stein P, Yang R, Liu J, et al. Evaluation of high density lipoprotein as a circulating biomarker of Gaucher disease activity. *J Inherit Metab Dis.* 2011;34(2):429–437.
28. Weinreb NJ, Aggio MC, Andersson HC, et al. Gaucher disease type 1: Revised recommendations on evaluations and monitoring for adult patients. *Semin Hematol.* 2004;41(4 Suppl 5):15–22.
29. Klein A, Lebreton A, Lemoine J, et al. Identification of urinary oligosaccharides by matrix-assisted laser desorption ionization

time-of-flight mass spectrometry. *Clin Chem.* 1998;44(12): 2422–2428.

30. He M, Xia B, Li X, et al. Comprehensive biochemical and molecular analysis of congenital disorders of glycosylation. American College of Medical Genetics (ACMG) Annual Clinical Genetic Meeting. 3-24-2010.

31. Sewell AC. Urinary oligosaccharide excretion in disorders of glycolipid, glycoprotein and glycogen metabolism. A review of screening for differential diagnosis. *Eur J Pediatr.* 1980; 134(3):183–194.

32. Meikle PJ, Fuller M, Hopwood JJ. Mass spectrometry in the study of lysosomal storage disorders. *Cell Mol Biol (Noisy-le-grand).* 2003;49(5):769–777.

33. Duran M. Miscellaneous analyses. In: N Blau, M Duran, ME Blaskovics. eds. *Physician's Guide to the Laboratory Diagnosis of Metabolic Diseases.* 2nd ed. Germany: Springer; 2003:45–56.

34. Andria GPG. Oligosaccharidoses and related disorders. In: N Blau, M Duran, ME Blaskovics, KM Gibson. eds. *Physician's Guide to the Laboratory Diagnosis of Metabolic Diseases.* 2nd ed. Heidelberg, Germany: Springer; 2005:399–410.

35. Andria G, Parenti G. Oligosaccharidoses and related disorders. In: CR Scriver, AL Beauder, WS Sly. eds. *The Metabolic and Molecular Bases of Inherited Disease.* 8th ed. New York: McGraw-Hill; 2001:399–410.

36. Peltonon L, Hofmann SL. The neuronal ceroid lipofuscinoses. In: D Valle, AL Beaudet, B Volgelstein. eds. *The Online Metabolic and Molecular Bases of Inherited Disease (OMMBID).* Available at www.ommbid.com. 2011. Accessed May 25, 2011.

37. Marie-Therese V. Disorders of sphingolipid metabolism. In: J Fernandes, JM Saudubray, G van den Berghe. eds. *Inborn Metabolic Disease: Diagnosis and Treatment.* 4 ed. Heidelberg, Germany: Springer; 2006:479–494.

38. Wraith JEd. Mucopolysacchridoses and oligosaccharidoses. In: J Fernandes, JM Saudubray, G van den Berghe. eds. *Inborn metabolic Diseases: Diagnosis and Treatment.* 4 ed. Heidelberg, Germany: Springer; 2006:495–508.

39. Thompson JN. The mucopolysacharidoes. In: N Blau, M Duran, ME Blaskovics, KM Gibson. eds. *Physician's Guide to the Laboratory Diagnosis of Metabolic Diseases.* 2nd ed. Heidelberg, Germany: Springer; 2005:377–398.

40. Grabowski GA, Petsko GA, Kolodny EH. Gaucher disease. In: D Valle, AL Beaudet, B Volgelstein. eds. *Metabolic and Molecular Bases of Inherited Disease (OMMBID).* Available at www.ommbid.com. 2011. Accessed May 25, 2011.

41. Mole SE, Willams RE. Neuronal ceroid-lipofuscinoses. Available at www.genereviews.org. 2010. Accessed April 25, 2011.

42. Wang RY, Bodamer OA, Watson MS, et al. Lysosomal storage diseases: Diagnostic confirmation and management of presymptomatic individuals. *Genet Med.* 2011.

43. Beck M. Therapy for lysosomal storage disorders. *IUBMB Life.* 2010;62(1):33–40.

44. Weinreb N, Taylor J, Cox T, et al. A benchmark analysis of the achievement of therapeutic goals for type 1 Gaucher disease patients treated with imiglucerase. *Am J Hematol.* 2008;83(12):890–895.

45. Eckhardt M. Pathology and current treatment of neurodegenerative sphingolipidoses. *Neuromol Med.* 2010;12(4): 362–382.

46. Begley DJ, Pontikis CC, Scarpa M. Lysosomal storage diseases and the blood–brain barrier. *Curr Pharm Des.* 2008;14(16): 1566–1580.

47. Beck M. New therapeutic options for lysosomal storage disorders: Enzyme replacement, small molecules and gene therapy. *Hum Genet.* 2007;121(1):1–22.

48. Staretz-Chacham O, Lang TC, LaMarca ME, et al. Lysosomal storage disorders in the newborn. *Pediatrics.* 2009; 123(4):1191–1207.

49. Munoz-Rojas MV, Horovitz DD, Jardim LB, et al. Intrathecal administration of recombinant human *N*-acetylgalactosamine 4-sulfatase to a MPS VI patient with pachymeningitis cervicalis. *Mol Genet Metab.* 2010;99(4):346–350.

50. Orchard PJ, Blazar BR, Wagner J, et al. Hematopoietic cell therapy for metabolic disease. *J Pediatr.* 2007;151(4): 340–346.

51. Kogler G, Sensken S, Airey JA, et al. A new human somatic stem cell from placental cord blood with intrinsic pluripotent differentiation potential. *J Exp Med.* 2004;200(2):123–135.

52. Schiffmann R. Therapeutic approaches for neuronopathic lysosomal storage disorders. *J Inherit Metab Dis.* 2010;33(4): 373–379.

53. Prasad VK, Kurtzberg J. Transplant outcomes in mucopolysaccharidoses. *Semin Hematol.* 2010;47(1):59–69.

54. Orchard PJ, Tolar J. Transplant outcomes in leukodystrophies. *Semin Hematol.* 2010;47(1):70–78.

55. Escolar ML, Poe MD, Provenzale JM, et al. Transplantation of umbilical-cord blood in babies with infantile Krabbe's disease. *N Engl J Med.* 2005;352(20):2069–2081.

56. Ringden O, Remberger M, Svahn BM, et al. Allogeneic hematopoietic stem cell transplantation for inherited disorders: Experience in a single center. *Transplantation.* 2006;81(5): 718–725.

57. Martins AM, Dualibi AP, Norato D, et al. Guidelines for the management of mucopolysaccharidosis type I. *J Pediatr.* 2009;155(4 Suppl):S32–S46.

58. Grewal SS, Shapiro EG, Krivit W, et al. Effective treatment of alpha-mannosidosis by allogeneic hematopoietic stem cell transplantation. *J Pediatr.* 2004;144(5):569–573.

59. Albert MH, Schuster F, Peters C, et al. T-cell-depleted peripheral blood stem cell transplantation for alpha-mannosidosis. *Bone Marrow Transplant.* 2003;32(4):443–446.

60. Miano M, Lanino E, Gatti R, et al. Four year follow-up of a case of fucosidosis treated with unrelated donor bone marrow transplantation. *Bone Marrow Transplant.* 2001; 27(7):747–751.

61. Yeager AM, Uhas KA, Coles CD, et al. Bone marrow transplantation for infantile ceramidase deficiency (Farber disease). *Bone Marrow Transplant.* 2000;26(3):357–363.

62. Autti T, Santavuori P, Raininko R, et al. Bone-marrow transplantation in aspartylglucosaminuria. *Lancet.* 1997; 349(9062):1366–1367.

63. Arvio M, Sauna-Aho O, Peippo M. Bone marrow transplantation for aspartylglucosaminuria: Follow-up study of transplanted and non-transplanted patients. *J Pediatr.* 2001; 138(2):288–290.

64. Grewal S, Shapiro E, Braunlin E, et al. Continued neurocognitive development and prevention of cardiopulmonary complications after successful BMT for I-cell disease: a long-term follow-up report. *Bone Marrow Transplant.* 2003;32(9): 957–960.

65. Krivit W, Peters C, Dusenbery K, et al. Wolman disease successfully treated by bone marrow transplantation. *Bone Marrow Transplant*. 2000;26(5):567–570.

66. Stein J, Garty BZ, Dror Y, et al. Successful treatment of Wolman disease by unrelated umbilical cord blood transplantation. *Eur J Pediatr*. 2007;166(7):663–666.

67. Cox-Brinkman J, Boelens JJ, Wraith JE, et al. Haematopoietic cell transplantation (HCT) in combination with enzyme replacement therapy (ERT) in patients with Hurler syndrome. *Bone Marrow Transplant*. 2006;38(1):17–21.

68. Wynn RF, Mercer J, Page J, et al. Use of enzyme replacement therapy (Laronidase) before hematopoietic stem cell transplantation for mucopolysaccharidosis I: Experience in 18 patients. *J Pediatr*. 2009;154(1):135–139.

69. Jeyakumar M, Norflus F, Tifft CJ, et al. Enhanced survival in Sandhoff disease mice receiving a combination of substrate deprivation therapy and bone marrow transplantation. *Blood*. 2001;97(1):327–329.

70. Pineda M, Wraith JE, Mengel E, et al. Miglustat in patients with Niemann–Pick disease Type C (NP-C): A multicenter observational retrospective cohort study. *Mol Genet Metab*. 2009;98(3):243–249.

71. Patterson MC, Vecchio D, Prady H, et al. Miglustat for treatment of Niemann–Pick C disease: A randomised controlled study. *Lancet Neurol*. 2007;6(9):765–772.

72. Santos ML, Raskin S, Telles DS, et al. Treatment of a child diagnosed with Niemann–Pick disease type C with miglustat: A case report in Brazil. *J Inherit Metab Dis*. 2008.

73. Arfi A, Richard M, Gandolphe C, et al. Storage correction in cells of patients suffering from mucopolysaccharidoses types IIIA and VII after treatment with genistein and other isoflavones. *J Inherit Metab Dis*. 2010;33(1):61–67.

74. Piotrowska E, Jakobkiewicz-Banecka J, Wegrzyn G. Different amounts of isoflavones in various commercially available soy extracts in the light of gene expression-targeted isoflavone therapy. *Phytother Res*. 2010;24(Suppl 1):S109–S113.

75. Proposal for revised classification of epilepsies and epileptic syndromes. Commission on Classification and Terminology of the International League Against Epilepsy. *Epilepsia*. 1989;30(4):389–399.

76. Federico A, Battistini S, Ciacci G, et al. Cherry-red spot myoclonus syndrome (type I sialidosis). *Dev Neurosci*. 1991;13(4–5):320–326.

77. Sedel F, Gourfinkel-An I, Lyon-Caen O, et al. Epilepsy and inborn errors of metabolism in adults: A diagnostic approach. *J Inherit Metab Dis*. 2007;30(6):846–854.

78. Kuchar L, Ledvinova J, Hrebicek M, et al. Prosaposin deficiency and saposin B deficiency (activator-deficient metachromatic leukodystrophy): Report on two patients detected by analysis of urinary sphingolipids and carrying novel PSAP gene mutations. *Am J Med Genet A*. 2009;149A(4): 613–621.

79. Hoffman GF, Nyhan WL, et al. Storage disorders. In: GF Hoffman, WL Nyhan, J Zschoke, eds. *Inherited Metabolic Diseases*. Philadelphia: Lippincott Williams & Wilkins; 2002:344–356.

80. Gaillard WD, Chiron C, Cross JH, et al. Guidelines for imaging infants and children with recent-onset epilepsy. *Epilepsia*. 2009;50(9):2147–2153.

81. Sevin M, Lesca G, Baumann N, et al. The adult form of Niemann–Pick disease type C. *Brain*. 2007;130(Pt 1):120–133.

82. Sandu S, Jackowski-Dohrmann S, Ladner A, et al. Niemann–Pick disease type C1 presenting with psychosis in an adolescent male. *Eur Child Adolesc Psychiatry*. 2009;18(9):583–585.

83. Vanier MT. Niemann–Pick disease type C. *Orphanet J Rare Dis*. 2010;5:16.

84. Canafoglia L, Bugiani M, Uziel G, et al. Rhythmic cortical myoclonus in Niemann–Pick disease type C. *Mov Disord*. 2006; 21(9):1453–1456.

85. Iturriaga C, Pineda M, Fernandez-Valero EM, et al. Niemann–Pick C disease in Spain: Clinical spectrum and development of a disability scale. *J Neurol Sci*. 2006;249(1):1–6.

86. Uc EY, Wenger DA, Jankovic J. Niemann-Pick disease type C: Two cases and an update. *Mov Disord*. 2000;15(6): 1199–1203.

87. Jalanko A, Braulke T. Neuronal ceroid lipofuscinoses. *Biochim Biophys Acta*. 2009;1793(4):697–709.

88. Fritchie K, Siintola E, Armao D, et al. Novel mutation and the first prenatal screening of cathepsin D deficiency (CLN10). *Acta Neuropathol*. 2009;117(2):201–208.

89. Wolf NI, Bast T, Surtees R. Epilepsy in inborn errors of metabolism. *Epileptic Disord*. 2005;7(2):67–81.

90. Santavuori P, Vanhanen SL, Autti T. Clinical and neuroradiological diagnostic aspects of neuronal ceroid lipofuscinoses disorders. *Eur J Paediatr Neurol*. 2001;5(Suppl A):157–161.

91. Martin JJ. Adult type of neuronal ceroid-lipofuscinosis. *J Inherit Metab Dis*. 1993;16(2):237–240.

92. Nijssen PC, Brusse E, Leyten AC, et al. Autosomal dominant adult neuronal ceroid lipofuscinosis: Parkinsonism due to both striatal and nigral dysfunction. *Mov Disord*. 2002; 17(3):482–487.

93. Haltia M. The neuronal ceroid-lipofuscinoses. *J Neuropathol Exp Neurol*. 2003;62(1):1–13.

94. D'Incerti L. MRI in neuronal ceroid lipofuscinosis. *Neurol Sci*. 2000;21(3 Suppl):S71–S73.

95. Stockler-Ipsiroglu S, Plecko B. Metabolic epilepsies: approaches to a diagnostic challenge. *Can J Neurol Sci*. 2009; 36(Suppl 2):S67–S72.

96. Backman ML, Aberg LE, Aronen ET, et al. New antidepressive and antipsychotic drugs in juvenile neuronal ceroid lipofuscinoses—a pilot study. *Eur J Paediatr Neurol*. 2001; 5(Suppl A):163–166.

97. Aberg LE, Backman M, Kirveskari E, et al. Epilepsy and antiepileptic drug therapy in juvenile neuronal ceroid lipofuscinosis. *Epilepsia*. 2000;41(10):1296–1302.

98. Wong AM, Rahim AA, Waddington SN, et al. Current therapies for the soluble lysosomal forms of neuronal ceroid lipofuscinosis. *Biochem Soc Trans*. 2010;38(6):1484–1488.

99. Macauley S, Roberts Hohms S, Reddy A, et al. Therapeutic approaches for the treatment of infantile neuronal ceroid lipofuscinosis (INCL). 7th World Symposium on Lysosomal Disease, Las Vegas, NV. 2-16-2011.

100. Al SS, Mayatepek E, Hoffmann B. Neurological findings in Hunter disease: pathology and possible therapeutic effects reviewed. *J Inherit Metab Dis*. 2008;31(4):473–480.

101. Matheus MG, Castillo M, Smith JK, et al. Brain MRI findings in patients with mucopolysaccharidosis types I and

II and mild clinical presentation. *Neuroradiology*. 2004;46(8): 666–672.

102. Lai SC, Chen RS, Wu Chou YH, et al. A longitudinal study of Taiwanese sialidosis type 1: an insight into the concept of cherry-red spot myoclonus syndrome. *Eur J Neurol*. 2009; 16(8):912–919.

103. Thomas PK, Abrams JD, Swallow D, et al. Sialidosis type 1: cherry red spot-myoclonus syndrome with sialidase deficiency and altered electrophoretic mobilities of some enzymes known to be glycoproteins. 1. Clinical findings. *J Neurol Neurosurg Psychiatry*. 1979;42(10):873–880.

104. Ramachandran N, Girard JM, Turnbull J, et al. The autosomal recessively inherited progressive myoclonus epilepsies and their genes. *Epilepsia*. 2009;50(Suppl 5):29–36.

105. Lowden JA, O'Brien JS. Sialidosis: a review of human neuraminidase deficiency. *Am J Hum Genet*. 1979;31(1):1–18.

106. Louboutin JP, Nogues B, Caillaud C, et al. Multimodality evoked potentials and EEG in a case of cherry red spot-myoclonus syndrome and alpha-neuraminidase deficiency (sialidosis type 1). *Eur Neurol*. 1995;35(3):175–177.

107. Caciotti A, Di RM, Filocamo M, et al. Type II sialidosis: review of the clinical spectrum and identification of a new splicing defect with chitotriosidase assessment in two patients. *J Neurol*. 2009;256(11):1911–1915.

108. Costello DJ, Eichler AF, Eichler FS. Leukodystrophies: classification, diagnosis, and treatment. *Neurologist*. 2009;15(6): 319–328.

109. Gieselmann V, Krageloh-Mann I. Metachromatic leukodystrophy—an update. *Neuropediatrics*. 2010;41(1):1–6.

110. Sidransky E. Gaucher disease: Complexity in a "simple" disorder. *Mol Genet Metab*. 2004;83(1–2):6–15.

111. Guggenbuhl P, Grosbois B, Chales G. Gaucher disease. *Joint Bone Spine*. 2008;75(2):116–124.

112. Grabowski GA. Recent clinical progress in Gaucher disease. *Curr Opin Pediatr*. 2005;17(4):519–524.

113. Capablo JL, Franco R, de Cabezon AS, et al. Neurologic improvement in a type 3 Gaucher disease patient treated with imiglucerase/miglustat combination. *Epilepsia*. 2007; 48(7):1406–1408.

114. Dobbelaere D, Sukno S, Defoort-Dhellemmes S, et al. Neurological outcome of a patient with Gaucher disease type III treated by enzymatic replacement therapy. *J Inherit Metab Dis*. 1998;21(1):74–76.

115. Grover WD, Tucker SH, Wenger DA. Clinical variation in 2 related children with neuronopathic Gaucher disease. *Ann Neurol*. 1978;3(3):281–283.

116. Neil JF, Glew RH, Peters SP. Familial psychosis and diverse neurologic abnormalities in adult-onset Gaucher's disease. *Arch Neurol*. 1979;36(2):95–99.

117. Conradi N, Kyllerman M, Mansson JE, et al. Late-infantile Gaucher disease in a child with myoclonus and bulbar signs: neuropathological and neurochemical findings. *Acta Neuropathol*. 1991;82(2):152–157.

118. Ledeen RW, Wu G. Nuclear lipids: key signaling effectors in the nervous system and other tissues. *J Lipid Res*. 2004; 45(1):1–8.

119. Brunetti-Pierri N, Scaglia F. GM1 gangliosidosis: review of clinical, molecular, and therapeutic aspects. *Mol Genet Metab*. 2008;94(4):391–396.

120. Suzuki Y, Oshima A, Namba E. Beta-galactosidase deficiency (beta-galactosidosis) GM1 gangliosidosis and Morquio B disease. In: CR Scriver, AL Beauder, WS Sly. eds. *The Metabolic and Molecular Bases of Inherited Disease*. 8th ed. New York: McGraw-Hill; 2001:3775–3809.

121. Kobayashi O, Takashima S. Thalamic hyperdensity on CT in infantile GM1-gangliosidosis. *Brain Dev*. 1994;16(6):472–474.

122. Steenweg ME, Vanderver A, Blaser S, et al. Magnetic resonance imaging pattern recognition in hypomyelinating disorders. *Brain*. 2010;133(10):2971–2982.

123. Tanaka ATN. Gangliosidoses (GM1 gangliosidosis and GM2 gangliosidosis). Diagnosis and treatment based on pathophysiology of pediatric diseases. *Japanese J Ped Med*. 2003; 35:455–460.

124. Pampiglione G, Privett G, Harden A. Tay-Sachs disease: Neurophysiological studies in 20 children. *Dev Med Child Neurol*. 1974;16(2):201–208.

125. Sakuraba H, Itoh K, Shimmoto M, et al. GM2 gangliosidosis AB variant: Clinical and biochemical studies of a Japanese patient. *Neurology*. 1999;52(2):372–377.

126. Shapiro BE, Pastores GM, Gianutsos J, et al. Miglustat in late-onset Tay-Sachs disease: a 12-month, randomized, controlled clinical study with 24 months of extended treatment. *Genet Med*. 2009;11(6):425–433.

127. Maegawa GH, Stockley T, Tropak M, et al. The natural history of juvenile or subacute GM2 gangliosidosis: 21 new cases and literature review of 134 previously reported. *Pediatrics*. 2006;118(5):e1550–e1562.

128. Adams C, Green S. Late-onset hexosaminidase A and hexosaminidase A and B deficiency: family study and review. *Dev Med Child Neurol*. 1986;28(2):236–243.

129. Hendriksz CJ, Corry PC, Wraith JE, et al. Juvenile Sandhoff disease—nine new cases and a review of the literature. *J Inherit Metab Dis*. 2004;27(2):241–249.

130. Shapiro BE, Logigian EL, Kolodny EH, et al. Late-onset Tay-Sachs disease: the spectrum of peripheral neuropathy in 30 affected patients. *Muscle Nerve*. 2008;38(2):1012–1015.

131. Caliskan M, Ozmen M, Beck M, et al. Thalamic hyperdensity—is it a diagnostic marker for Sandhoff disease? *Brain Dev*. 1993;15(5):387–388.

132. Bostantjopoulou S, Katsarou Z, Michelakaki H, et al. Seizures as a presenting feature of late onset metachromatic leukodystrophy. *Acta Neurol Scand*. 2000;102(3):192–195.

133. Fukumizu M, Matsui K, Hanaoka S, et al. Partial seizures in two cases of metachromatic leukodystrophy: electrophysiologic and neuroradiologic findings. *J Child Neurol*. 1992; 7(4):381–386.

134. Fluharty A. Arylsulfatase a deficiency. Available at www.genereviews.org. 2010. Accessed May 20, 2011.

135. d'Azzo A, Andria G, Strisciuglio P, et al. Galactosialidosis. In: D Valle, AL Beaudet, B Volgelstein. eds. *The Online Metabolic and Molecular Bases of Inherited Disease (OMMBID)*. Available at www.ommbid.com. 2011. Accessed May 25, 2011.

136. John J, Hopwood A. Multiple sulfatase deficiency and the nature of the sulfatase family. In: D Valle, AL Beaudet, B Volgelstein. eds. *The Online Metabolic and Molecular Bases of Inherited Disease (OMMBID)*. Available at www. ommbid.com. 2011. Accessed May 25, 2011.

26

Peroxisomal Diseases and Epilepsy

Parastoo Jangouk, Kristin W. Barañano, and Gerald V. Raymond

PEROXISOMAL DISEASES AND EPILEPSY

Peroxisomes represent a class of membrane-bound subcellular organelles present in nearly all eukaryotic cells. Due to this ubiquity, peroxisomal disorders are represented in disorders of multiple organ systems. A significant finding, however, is that nearly all peroxisomal disorders result in neurologic disease, with many affected individuals presenting with recurrent seizures. In Zellweger syndrome (ZS), 92% of patients present with seizures (1). Almost all individuals with D-bifunctional enzyme deficiency (D-BP) have neonatal seizures. Even in X-linked adrenoleukodystrophy (X-ALD), seizures are the first manifestation of disease in 7% of boys. Therefore, it is of key importance to consider peroxisomal disorders, when appropriate, in formulating a differential diagnosis for patients presenting with epilepsy.

PEROXISOMES AND THE NERVOUS SYSTEM

Peroxisomes, which harbor numerous fundamental metabolic enzymes, aid in detoxifying reactive oxygen substrates (ROS) and in various anabolic and catabolic pathways of lipid metabolism. Some of the more notable processes include alpha-oxidation of phytanic acid (a branched-chain fatty acid found predominantly in dairy products) and myelin sphingolipids, and beta-oxidation of the substrates that do not undergo degradation in the mitochondria, such as very-long-chain fatty acids (VLCFAs), bile acid intermediates, and eicosanoids. Peroxisomes also initiate biosynthesis of ether phospholipids, including plasmalogens, which constitute more than 20% of phospholipids in human brain (2–5).

Peroxisomal function is not only essential to the well-being of myelin and neurons (3) but also plays an important role in the developing brain. Peroxisomes are abundant in the developing brain (6), and intact peroxisomes have been shown to play a critical role in neuronal migration during the embryonic period (7).

PEROXISOME BIOGENESIS

The process of peroxisomal biogenesis is highly conserved in all eukaryotic organisms (8). Peroxisomal proteins are encoded by nuclear genes, synthesized on free polyribosomes, and discharged into the cytosol in the mature form. Work in yeast has identified more than 20 genes labeled PEX, whose products are known as peroxins. Peroxins are required for proper importation, and have roles in receptor docking, stability, and translocation across the membrane (8, 9).

The mature polypeptide contains targeting information that directs matrix proteins into the peroxisomes. A majority of proteins destined for the peroxisome use peroxisome targeting sequence 1 (PTS1), which consists of a terminal tripeptide of serine–lysine–leucine (–SKL) that is recognized by the soluble receptor Pex5p (10–13). Other matrix proteins use peroxisomal targeting sequence 2 (PTS2), a nine-residue signal located at the amino terminus. Peroxisomal 3-ketoacyl-coenzyme A (CoA) thiolase and phytanoyl-CoA hydroxylase rely on PTS2, which directs the import of proteins using the soluble receptor Pex7p (14). Both Pex5p and Pex7p receptors bind their targeted proteins in the cytoplasm outside the peroxisome. The present model suggests that the receptor–peptide complex docks at the peroxisome surface by means of membrane-associated complexes that contain other peroxisome assembly proteins. Other peroxins appear to function later in the process of translocation. The importation of proteins to the peroxisome is unique, and the process does not share features with that of the mitochondria or the lysosome.

In a similar fashion, peroxisomal membrane proteins are synthesized on free ribosomes (15, 16); however, they use a distinct trafficking pathway via the endoplasmic reticulum (17–19).

BIOCHEMISTRY OF THE PEROXISOME

Peroxisomes were named for the presence of hydrogen peroxide and catalase, which decomposes the hydrogen peroxide. More than 40 enzymatic functions are found in the peroxisome, and the majority of these are organelle-specific. Examples include oxidation of VLCFAs (fatty acids with carbon length greater than 22), branched-chain fatty acid metabolism, plasmalogen synthesis, pipecolic acid degradation, and the production of DHA. These reactions are abnormal in many peroxisomal disorders, and are often used for diagnostic testing (Table 26.1).

PEROXISOMAL DISORDERS

In humans, disorders of the peroxisome are an expanding group of genetic disorders that can currently be categorized into three groups: peroxisomal biogenesis defects (PBD), single-enzyme disorders (SEDs), and contiguous syndrome (20–22) (Table 26.2).

PBDs are autosomal recessive, heterogeneous disorders based on mutations of different PEX genes that result in alteration of peroxins and disruption of peroxisomal protein importation. Initially classified by complementation studies, 13 different genes have been identified which result in human disorders. Mutations in 12 distinct PEX genes have been identified in the Zellweger syndrome spectrum (PBD, ZSS), and the other complementation group results in rhizomelic chondrodysplasia punctata (RCDP1).

The Zellweger spectrum is a continuum of three phenotypes, including (in order of increasing severity): neonatal adrenoleukodystrophy (NALD), infantile Refsum disease (IRD), and ZS. Phenotypes on the Zellweger spectrum can be identified biochemically by an accumulation of VLCFAs and a deficiency of plasmalogens. There is a direct correlation between the severity of the PEX gene mutation and the number of functional peroxisomes, which in turn determines the spectrum of the clinical disease (2).

The other peroxisome biogenesis disorder consists of the remaining complementation group, and includes all patients with RCDP1. This group of disorders is due to mutations in the PEX7 gene and affects PTS2 only (23, 24).

The SEDs X-ALD, acyl-CoA oxidase deficiency, and D-BP (25) affect beta-oxidation of fatty acids and

TABLE 26.1 Biochemical Markers in Peroxisomal Disorders

Plasma Markers	ZS	NALD	IRD	RCDP1	D-BP
VLCFAs	↑↑	↑	↑	NL	↑
Di- and trihydroxycholestanoic acid	↑	↑	↑		NL- ↑
Phytanic acid	↑	↑	↑	↑	↑
Pristanic acid	↑	↑	↑	NL	↑
Pipecolic acid	↑	↑	↑	NL	↑
Erythrocyte plasmalogens	↓	↓	↓ -NL	↓- ↓↓	NL

D-BP = bifunctional protein deficiency; IRD = infantile Refsum disease; NALD = neonatal adrenoleukodystrophy; NL = normal level; RCDP1 = rhizomelic chondrodysplasia punctata 1; ZS = Zellweger syndrome; ↓ = lower than normal; ↑ = higher than normal. Phytanic and pipecolic acid are age-dependent and may be less useful in establishing diagnosis.

TABLE 26.2 Peroxisomal Disorders

Biogenesis Disorders	Single-Enzyme Disorders	Contiguous Gene Syndrome
Zellweger spectrum disorders (ZSD) – Zellweger syndrome (ZS) – Neonatal adrenoleukodystrophy (NALD) – Infantile Refsum disease (IRD) Rhizomelic chondrodysplasia punctata (RCDP)	X-linked adrenoleukodystrophy (X-ALD) Acyl-coA oxidase deficiency Bifunctional protein deficiency(D-BP) Alkyl-DHAP synthase deficiency DHAP-alkyl transferase deficiency Adult Refsum disease (classic) Glutaric aciduria type III Acatalasemia Hyperoxaluria type I	Contiguous ABCD1 DXS1357E deletion syndrome (CADDS)

are characterized by elevations in VLCFAs. However, while acyl-CoA oxidase deficiency and D-BP result from disruption of their specific enzymes, in X-ALD, the defect is in a gene that codes for a peroxisomal membrane protein responsible for beta-oxidation of VLCFAs (26, 27).

ZELLWEGER SYNDROME

ZS is the most severe phenotype of the PBDs, with characteristic neuronal migration defects, severe neurological impairment early in life, and neonatal seizures. Children affected by this multisystem disorder usually die in the first years of life (20, 21). Individuals with ZS, also known as cerebrohepatorenal syndrome, show numerous congenital anomalies and metabolic problems (28–30). Affected children have distinctive facies, including epicanthal folds, broad nasal bridges, small noses, large fontanelles, hypoplastic supraorbital ridges, and full foreheads. Ocular findings such as cataracts, glaucoma, corneal clouding, and retinal degeneration may occur. Kidney and liver cysts, hepatomegaly, and chondrodysplasia punctata are common.

Patients present in the neonatal period with profound hypotonia, inability to feed, seizures, absence of primitive and deep tendon reflexes, and diminished spontaneous movements (31). Seizures are a common manifestation in patients with ZS, and may be one of the reasons a newborn comes to attention.

Because peroxisomal disorders are generally rare, reports on the nature and pattern of seizures in these disorders is limited. In two studies, between 71% and 92% of patients with ZS developed seizures (1, 32). In a retrospective study by Takahashi et al, five out of seven ZS patients responded to antiepileptic drugs after developing epileptic seizures between 2 days and 1 month of age. The seizures started as partial seizures in the arms, legs, or facial muscles, and very rarely developed into generalized seizures. This might be due to brain immaturity associated with the age of the patients. The site of origin of convulsions alternated in most of the patients during the course of the disease, which suggested bilateral multifocal epileptogenic foci in the frontal motor cortex. Electroencephalogram (EEG) studies were compatible with clinical observations showing multifocal discharges in the central, mid-temporal, or parietal cortex. The authors suggested that the epileptogenic foci in the frontal motor cortex are consistent with the pattern of neuronal migration defect predominately present in the centrosylvian region (32). Agamanolis et al reported one case with twitching of the tongue, arm, and hand, and stiffening of the leg, which could be suggestive of an epileptogenic focus in the frontal motor cortex along with the migration defect pathology (33). However, Gilchricht et al reported two cases of seizures in ZS, with epileptogenic foci from bilateral occipital foci that did not correspond to the typical distribution of the migration defect (34).

NEUROPATHOLOGY OF ZELLWEGER SYNDROME

Pathological investigations in ZS have revealed diverse abnormalities in multiple organs, most notably the brain. In general, nervous system involvement in

PBDs follows one or more of the following patterns: neuronal migration impairment, abnormalities in formation and maintenance of white matter, and selective neuronal degeneration (33).

Unique and specific abnormalities seen in neuronal migration are the most prominent neuropathologies in ZS (34, 35). This impaired migration involves the cerebral hemispheres, large Purkinje cells of the cerebellum, and inferior olive. Failure in migration is most severe in the cerebral cortex, leading to gyral abnormalities around the Sylvian fissure. These abnormalities are characterized by abnormally small and thick gyri (micro- and pachygyria, respectively) and result in neuronal heterotopias in the neocortex and a reduced neuronal population in the outer cortex (1, 36). Interestingly, neuronal migration requires intact peroxisomal function not only in the brain but also in extraneuronal tissues such as the liver. Normal cortical development also depends on peroxisomes in other organs (37, 38). The pathogenesis of the migration defect in ZS is not clearly understood. Some initial studies suggested disordered peroxisomal beta-oxidation (25, 39); however, studies performed on a mouse model of ZS demonstrated that impaired beta-oxidation and biosynthesis of ether lipid cause minor migration defects only (40, 41). It has been suggested that the migration defect is caused partially by dysfunction in *N*-methyl-D-aspartate (NMDA) receptor-mediated calcium mobilization (42).

The white matter abnormality in ZS is not well characterized either. The majority of peroxisomes in white matter are predominantly in oligodendrocytes, particularly during myelination (43, 44). Additionally, among the different cell types in the nervous system, oligodendrocytes have the highest capacity to detoxify ROS (45). Therefore, in the absence of peroxisomes, oligodendrocytes might be more vulnerable to oxidative stress. White matter abnormalities may be both dysmyelinative or demyelinative in nature (33, 46, 47). It is difficult to distinguish abnormal myelination from early demyelination before 2 years of age, and many of the affected children die before substantial myelination has occurred (48). Passarge and McAdams reported severe dysmyelination (49), whereas Volpe and Adams observed a more demyelinative process (35). Agamanolis et al noted longitudinal inclusions along with a demyelinative pattern (50). This pathologic finding is postulated to be identical to the inclusions found in X-ALD that contain VLCFAs (50, 51).

Additional defects, particularly a deficiency in plasmalogen biosynthesis, might contribute to the white matter pathology. Plasmalogens are enriched in myelin, and brain myelin comprises the highest content of plasmalogens in the body (52). The specific role of plasmalogens in the membrane, particularly myelin, has not been well understood. However, evidence suggests that plasmalogens function in multiple roles, including as antioxidants, mediators of membrane fluidity/dynamics, and modulators of signal transduction (53). Recently, it has been shown that plasmalogens have a protective effect against the accumulation of VLCFAs in the brain (54).

Another major CNS lesion in ZS is axonal degeneration, which could be primary or secondary to myelin loss. Primary axonal degeneration is accompanied by an increase in unphosphorylated neurofilament and amyloid precursor protein. Pathological studies have shown that the axonal damage and demyelination were often not colocalized (48). This intriguing finding suggests that peroxisomes have a protective role in axons distinct from the maintenance of myelin (55).

NEONATAL ADRENOLEUKODYSTROPHY, INFANTILE REFSUM DISEASE, AND OTHER VARIANTS

Before the unifying understanding of peroxisome assembly, variants other than ZS on the Zellweger spectrum were identified based on singular biochemical features. It is now recognized that these disorders are part of a spectrum and reflect a less involved genetic and biochemical abnormality than ZS. The clinical presentation of these diseases is also less severe than that of ZS. Affected children have hypotonia, sensorineural hearing loss, retinal disease, liver disease, and delayed development, but longer lifespans that those with ZS. In fact, we are aware of individuals in early adulthood with these variants.

Seizures may occur at any age and do not appear to represent specific neurodegeneration. Migrational defects have been less pronounced in this group, and thus the precise reason for epilepsy is less clear than in ZS. However, epilepsy likely results from a combination of neuronal migration issues, cellular dysfunction, and, in some instances, demyelination.

TREATMENT OF SEIZURES IN ZELLWEGER SPECTRUM DISORDERS

Unlike certain metabolic disorders, any appropriate medication may be used to control seizures in Zellweger spectrum disorders, as there are no medications that are known to have a specific detrimental effect on the peroxisome. Thus, the choice of medication will reflect the age of the patient and the type of seizures. Phenobarbital, topiramate, and levetiracetam have all been used in the neonatal period with reasonable efficacy. In older children, any appropriate agent may be used.

The use of the ketogenic diet deserves special mention. It is known that the ketogenic diet may increase certain fatty acids, including VLCFAs and phytanic acid. This diet has, on occasion, complicated the diagnosis of children with Zellweger spectrum disorders (56). It is not known if these biochemical changes would have a detrimental effect on an affected child. Its use should be reserved for those individuals who have not responded to other therapies and are appropriately monitored.

Some individuals do develop intractable seizures. We have found this symptom to be a poor prognostic feature, but it should not result in therapeutic nihilism. As most physicians who deal with epilepsy are aware, uncontrolled seizures complicate the care and lives of not only the affected individual but also the caretakers. Attempts to minimize hospitalizations for status epilepticus or uncontrolled seizures are warranted.

RHIZOMELIC CHONDRODYSPLASIA PUNCTATA

Classic type RCDP, sometimes referred to as RCDP1, comprises the remaining complementation group of PBD, and involves the mutation of only one PEX gene, PEX7. Clinical features of RCDP1 differ significantly from ZS, and are characterized by proximal shortening of the humerus and femur (rhizomelia) and cartilage calcifications (chondrodysplasia punctata). Bilateral cataracts and spastic tetraplegia are common at birth. Mental deficiency is profound, and the majority of affected children develop seizures. The majority of RCDP1 patients die within the first year or two, but several have survived longer (57). Biochemical defects include abnormal plasmalogen biosynthesis

that is more severe than that of ZS (58), phytanic acid oxidation impairment, and an abnormally processed 3-oxoacyl-coenzyme A. Beta-oxidation of VLCFAs is normal.

Neuropathologic examinations in RCDP are not suggestive of the characteristic neuronal migration defect seen in ZS. In a mouse model of RCDP (PEX7$^{-/-}$), an impairment in neuronal migration has been reported; however, it is less severe than the abnormality seen in the ZS mouse model (59).

White matter abnormalities are common in RCDP, and they may present in the forms of inflammatory demyelination, noninflammatory dysmyelination, or nonspecific reduction in myelin volume (33). A few studies have been conducted on MRIs of affected individuals. MRI studies of a patient with RCDP1 showed a severe delay in myelination and signs of slight demyelination in the occipital area (60). Alkan et al showed abnormally delayed myelination in MR spectroscopy in one case of RCDP (61). In a more recent study on a cohort of 11 patients with RCDP, subjects were categorized in two groups based on MRI findings: those with normal MRIs and those with abnormal MRIs. MRI findings were found to correlate with the phenotype. In the group with normal MRI findings, patients showed milder phenotypes of the disease, including decreased plasmalogen and normal to markedly increased phytanic acid levels. The group with abnormal MRI findings included all of the patients with a severe phenotype. A delay in supratentorial myelination was found before the age of 2 years in five patients. Follow-up imaging in four patients revealed incomplete catch-up in myelination; however, based on MRI findings alone, the dysmyelinative/demyelinative nature of the lesions could not be determined (63). Three patients developed seizures, with two of them on antiepileptic medications. All patients in this group had very low plasmalogen levels with widely varied levels of phytanic acid. As discussed in the ZS section, the role of plasmalogens in myelin abnormalities in PBDs is of increasing interest.

Postdevelopmental degeneration of the cerebellum with loss of Purkinje cells has been seen pathologically in RCDP (62). It has been postulated that phytanic acid accumulation might contribute to the cerebellar atrophy (62, 63). Interestingly, in the same MRI study mentioned above on 11 RCDP cases, cerebellar atrophy was seen in seven patients, and was more profound in the vermis than the hemispheres (63).

However, in this study, the patient with the highest level of phytanic acid showed no cerebellar atrophy, and another case in whom the phytanic acid was normal revealed severe cerebellar atrophy on MRI (64).

Seizures are common in infants with RCDP. In White's study, 27 out of 32 patients (84%) who lived beyond 2 months of age developed seizures (66). According to parents, the average age of the first epileptic presentation was 0.4 ± 2.2 years. Typical presentations have been determined as jerky movements, body stiffening, screaming, and staring episodes. Multiple seizure types have been observed in the same child. The majority of cases (22/27) had unclassified types of seizures. However, 5 out of 27 patients were classified as having typical absence, myoclonic, tonic, and tonic-clonic seizures, and virtually all developed generalized convulsive seizures. Only one patient had partial seizures, and another one developed status epilepticus. EEGs mostly showed nonspecific generalized changes. Twenty out of 27 children received antiepileptic medication, including phenobarbital alone or in combination therapy. In two children with a history of mixed seizures, the ketogenic diet was used in the treatment of intractable seizures (65), and a marked decrease in seizure frequency was reported in both. In one of them, the ketogenic diet was started at age 6, and seizure frequency decreased rapidly. The second one, who had worsening of episodes around age 10, initiated the ketogenic diet at age 11 with continuation of antiepileptic medications. A marked decrease in seizure frequency was observed within 2 weeks. The first patient developed hepatic dysfunction after 5.5 years of being on the ketogenic diet, which resolved with discontinuation of the diet. However, no complications occurred in the second case. Given positive responses to the ketogenic diet, it might be an alternative in the treatment of intractable seizures (66).

BIFUNCTIONAL PROTEIN DEFICIENCY

D-BP, categorized under peroxisomal single-enzyme defects (SEDs), is the deficiency of peroxisomal D-BP, a multifunctional enzyme involved in the second and third steps of certain fatty acid beta-oxidation reactions, as well as the biosynthesis of bile acids (67). The enzyme deficiency is classified into three types, all of which are inherited in an autosomal recessive manner (68). The enzyme has been identified in the

brain and other organs (69, 70). Among the SEDs, D-BP deficiency is relatively common (71), and pathological findings and clinical manifestations resemble what is seen in ZS (67). The clinical phenotype typically includes severe neonatal hypotonia and seizures within the first 2 months of life, resulting in profound developmental delay and, in most cases, death by 2 years of age (72). Biochemical profiles of patients show elevated levels of both VLCFAs and trihydroxycholestanoic acid, with normal values for phytanic acid and pipecolic acid (25).

D-BP deficiency was initially described by Watkins et al (73) in a newborn with severe hypotonia and refractory seizures. Multifocal spikes were reported on his EEG. Visual-evoked responses and brain stem auditory-evoked responses were also abnormal. However, unlike ZS, there was no typical facial dysmorphism or hepatomegaly. The patient died at the age of 5 months, and brain autopsy revealed a polymicrogyric neocortex and focal areas of cortical heterotopia similar to the pattern of neuronal migration defect in ZS. Kaufmann et al. reported a case with severe hypotonia at birth that developed refractory myoclonic seizures on the second day (41). An MRI at 9 months of age revealed delayed myelination and communicating hydrocephalus. He died at the age of 11.5 months. Postmortem neuropathological examination resembled ZS, presenting with centrosylvian pachygyria and microgyria, neocortical heterotopia, decrease in cortical myelin, and Purkinje cell heterotopia. However the neocortical involvement was more limited, white matter heterotopia was diffuse, and the inferior olivary cytoarchitecture was not completely disrupted (41). Itoh et al compared two patients with D-BP with two others with ZS (74). Clinically, they all presented with seizures and severe psychomotor retardation, but, surprisingly, there was not any migrational defect observed in the neuropathology of their D-BP patients (75).

Takahashi et al reviewed two patients with D-BP in their cohort (32). Both patients presented with seizures very early in life. One of the patients presented with seizures at 3 hours after birth. This patient showed diverse ictal manifestations with focal motor seizures and/or tonic convulsions of arms and legs. EEG showed multifocal spikes. In the second case, seizures presented at 2 months of age with tonic-clonic convulsions sometimes accompanied by eye deviation or localized arm and leg convulsing. Seizures developed to a massive myoclonia at 6 months. EEG was initially suggestive of bilateral independent multifocal spikes; however, diffuse high-voltage slow waves replaced this as the disease progressed (32).

In a more recent study, a larger cohort of 126 established D-BP cases was evaluated (75). Virtually all of the patients presented with profound hypotonia (98%) and seizures (93%) within the first month of life. 15% of patients were reported to have experienced infantile spasms. Neurophysiological evaluations showed a high prevalence of impaired vision and hearing and peripheral neuropathy. None of the patients met developmental milestones. Craniofacial abnormalities resembling that of ZS, although less striking, was present in 52% of children. MRI studies revealed neocortical dysplasia and cerebral and cerebellar demyelination similar to that of ZS; however, involvement of the thalamus and globus pallidus was also evident in a number of D-BP deficient patients. Lesions of these areas have not been reported in ZS cases. This neocortical dysplasia found in MRI studies has been confirmed by pathology. In total, 11 brain autopsies were performed, from which polymicrogyria was found in seven patients and heterotopias in three.

Buoni et al reported a case of D-BP deficiency that presented with neonatal intractable seizures from the second day of life (68). They described the seizures as generalized clonic seizures with asymmetric spasms, involving tonic abduction and extension of both arms. EEG revealed the presence of modified hypsarrythmia, with high-voltage slow activity with few multifocal sharp waves and spikes, a consistent focus of abnormal discharge, and the absence of sleep spindles. They suggested that the semiology of the seizure was more compatible with West syndrome showing a modified hypsarrhythmic pattern. The spasms were resistant to valproate, lamotrigine, and clobazam, but showed a partial response to vigabatrin (68).

X-LINKED ADRENOLEUKODYSTROPHY

X-ALD is defined as mutations in the ABCD1 gene, which codes for a peroxisomal membrane protein with homology to the ATP-binding cassette (ABC) transporter super family. X-ALD is the most common peroxisomal disorder, with an approximate frequency of 1:17,000 (76). The disease results in an accumulation of saturated VLCFAs in all tissues, and the measurement of VLCFAs in serum is still the most widely used diagnostic study (79). X-ALD primarily affects the nervous system, adrenal cortex, and testis and shows a wide range of clinical phenotypes that have been described in detail (80,81, Table 26.3). As shown in Table 26.3, the age of clinical presentation varies. One of the most common variants is the childhood cerebral form, with a characteristic clinical presentation of a young male between 6 and 9 years of age with progressive behavioral and cognitive deficits, followed by death within 3 years (2). Initial symptoms are usually subtle and are often misdiagnosed as attention deficit disorder, learning disabilities, or psychiatric disease. Pathologically, there is inflammatory demyelination, seen as a white matter abnormality on MRI, especially in the parieto-occipital regions (77). There is no correlation between phenotype and genotype (78).

It is important to note that the pathology of cerebral forms of X-ALD is significantly different than that of AMN, in which an inflammatory response is virtually absent and the peripheral neuropathy is the dominant manifestation (79). In cerebral X-ALD, the gray matter is often intact. It appears that the cytotoxic effect of accumulation of VLCFAs triggers an inflammatory cascade that leads to a loss of oligodendrocytes and demyelination (80–82). White matter lesions exhibit marked loss of oligodendrocytes and axons along with reactive astrocytosis. The active edges of myelin loss are the sites of profound inflammation characterized by perivascular lipid-laden macrophages and reactive astrocytosis. Chronicity of the lesion determines the type of the inflammatory cells. Diffuse infiltration of macrophages and lymphocytes is highly suggestive of early demyelinating lesions, while perivascular accumulation of periphages typically occurs in older lesions (33, 51). There is increasing evidence that oxidative stress contributes to the pathogenesis of the cerebral inflammatory phenotype (83–86). There is also an increasing understanding of the role of microglia (87).

Despite the fact that the disorder is primarily one of myelin, seizures are a common finding in the course of cerebral X-ALD. In a comprehensive study that reviewed the records of 485 cases of childhood cerebral X-ALD, 45 infants (9.3%) presented acutely at an average age of 5.5 years old, and 44% of those acute cases presented with seizures. The average age of study participants was 5.9 years. Six boys had a

TABLE 26.3   X-ALD Phenotypes in Male

Phenotype	Description	Estimated Relative Frequency (%)
Childhood cerebral (CCER)	Onset at 3–10 y of age. Progressive behavioral, cognitive and neurologic impairments resulting in total disability within 3 y. Inflammatory brain demyelination	31–35
Adolescent	Onset at 11–22 y of age. Resembles CCER, with slower progression	4–7
Adrenomyeloneuropathy (AMN)	Onset 28 ± 9 y and progressive. Mainly involves spinal cord, distal axonopathy, absent/mild inflammatory response, 40% have/develop cerebral involvement, with various degree of inflammatory response and more rapid progression	40–46
Adult cerebral	Dementia, behavioral deficits, some focal deficits without preceding AMN. White matter inflammatory response. Progression parallels that of CCER	2–5
Olivo-ponto-cerebellar	Cerebellar and brainstem involvement in adolescence/adulthood	1–2
Addison only	Onset before 7.5 y. Primary adrenal insufficiency without evident neurologic involvement. Patients mostly develop AMN	Varies with age up to 50% in children
Asymptomatic	Genetic and biochemical disorder without apparent neurologic/adrenal involvement. Detailed evaluations reveal subtle signs of AMN/adrenal hypofunction	Diminishes with age less than 4 y common greater than 40 y rare

focal seizure, with the remainder having generalized seizures. Four boys presented with generalized status epilepticus (77). In another study of six patients with cerebral childhood X-ALD, three developed seizures in the late stage of the disease (88). The seizures were either focal or generalized. EEG studies were either normal or exhibited slowing of the background activity in the posterior regions, compatible with the white matter lesion localization. As demyelinating lesions progressed, slow waves became progressively widespread and accompanied by paroxysmal discharges (88).

Individuals with the "Addison only" phenotype present primarily with adrenocortical insufficiency between age 2 years and adulthood (most commonly by age 7.5 years), without evidence of neurologic abnormality (89, 90). Hypoglycemia is a very common presenting manifestation that may lead to seizures. Recently, a previously healthy 2-year-old boy was reported with generalized tonic-clonic seizures and hypoglycemia. After extensive biochemical and metabolic work-up, the patient was diagnosed with X-ALD (91). It is of utmost importance to consider X-ALD in all male children presenting with idiopathic seizures or seizures in the context of hypoglycemia.

Finally, 20% of men with adrenomyeloneuropathy may develop cerebral disease. While the frequency of incidence has not been established, seizures including status epilepticus have been seen in men with AMN.

CONCLUSIONS

Peroxisomal disorders are an important cause of metabolic encephalopathy. They may be varied in their presentation, but should be considered in the evaluation of both children and adults with epilepsy, especially given that testing for the more common peroxisomal disorders is relatively easy, definitive, and inexpensive. Accurate diagnosis allows the patient to receive appropriate treatment and access to genetic counseling.

KEY POINTS

- Peroxisomal disorders may be divided into two groups.
  - Peroxisome assembly disorders such as Zellweger spectrum or rhizomelicchondrodysplasia punctate.
  - Single enzyme disorders in which X-linked adrenoleukodystrophy and D-bifunctional enzyme deficiency are the most common.
- Seizures are not rare in peroxisomal disorders.
  - Cortical migration defects are common.
  - May be a relatively common cause of neonatal seizures.
  - Leukodystrophies may also be associated with seizures.
- Diagnostic screening may be performed by very long chain fatty acid analysis.
  - Elevation in C26:0, C26/C22, and C24/C22.
  - Other testing may be indicated.
- Treatment is predominantly symptomatic.
  - No group of medications is contraindicated.

REFERENCES

1. Gould SJ, Raymond GV, Valle D. The peroxisome biogenesis disorders. In: CR Scriver, AL Beaudet, WS Sly, D Valle, eds. *The Metabolic and Molecular Basis of Inherited Disease.* New York: McGraw-Hill; 2001:3181–218.
2. Faust PL, Kaye EM, Powers JM. Myelin lesions associated with lysosomal and peroxisomal disorders. *Expert Rev Neurother.* 2010;10(9):1449–1466.
3. Wanders RJ, Ferdinandusse S, Brites P, et al. Peroxisomes, lipid metabolism and lipotoxicity. *Biochim Biophys Acta.* 2010;1801(3):272–280.
4. Schrader M, Fahimi HD. Peroxisomes and oxidative stress. *Biochim Biophys Acta.* 2006;1763(12):1755–1766.
5. Gorgas K, Teigler A, Komljenovic D, et al. The ether lipid-deficient mouse: tracking down plasmalogen functions. *Biochim Biophys Acta.* 2006;1763(12):1511–1526.
6. Ahlemeyer B, Neubert I, Kovacs WJ, et al. Differential expression of peroxisomal matrix and membrane proteins during postnatal development of mouse brain. *J Comp Neurol.* 2007;505(1):1–17.
7. Gressens P. Pathogenesis of migration disorders. *Curr Opin Neurol.* 2006;19(2):135–140.
8. Weller S, Gould SJ, Valle D. Peroxisome biogenesis disorders. *Annu Rev Genomics Hum Genet.* 2003;4:165–211.
9. Ma C, Subramani S. Peroxisome matrix and membrane protein biogenesis. *IUBMB Life.* 2009;61(7):713–722.
10. Gould SJ, Keller GA, Schneider M, et al. Peroxisomal protein import is conserved between yeast, plants, insects and mammals. *EMBO J.* 1990;9(1):85–90.
11. Gould SJ, Keller GA, Subramani S. Identification of peroxisomal targeting signals located at the carboxy terminus of four peroxisomal proteins. *J Cell Biol.* 1988;107(3):897–905.
12. Gould SJ, Krisans S, Keller GA, et al. Antibodies directed against the peroxisomal targeting signal of firefly luciferase recognize multiple mammalian peroxisomal proteins. *J Cell Biol.* 1990;110(1):27–34.
13. Keller GA, Krisans S, Gould SJ, et al. Evolutionary conservation of a microbody targeting signal that targets proteins to peroxisomes, glyoxysomes, and glycosomes. *J Cell Biol.* 1991;114(5):893–904.
14. Swinkels BW, Gould SJ, Bodnar AG, et al. A novel, cleavable peroxisomal targeting signal at the amino-terminus of the rat 3-ketoacyl-CoA thiolase. *EMBO J.* 1991;10(11):3255–3262.
15. Suzuki Y, Orii T, Takiguchi M, et al. Biosynthesis of membrane polypeptides of rat liver peroxisomes. *J Biochem.* 1987;101(2):491–496.
16. Suzuki Y, Shimozawa N, Orii T, et al. Biosynthesis of peroxisomal membrane polypeptides in infants with Zellweger syndrome. *J Inherit Metab Dis.* 1987;10(3):297–300.
17. Hoepfner D, Schildknegt D, Braakman I, et al. Contribution of the endoplasmic reticulum to peroxisome formation. *Cell.* 2005;122(1):85–95.
18. Kim PK, Mullen RT, Schumann U, et al. The origin and maintenance of mammalian peroxisomes involves a de novo PEX16-dependent pathway from the ER. *J Cell Biol.* 2006;173(4):521–532.
19. Van der Zand A, Braakman I, Tabak HF. Peroxisomal membrane proteins insert into the endoplasmic reticulum. *Mol Biol Cell.* 2010;21(12):2057–2065.
20. Raymond GV. Peroxisomal disorders. *Curr Opin Pediatr.* 1999;11(6):572–576.
21. Raymond GV. Peroxisomal disorders. *Curr Opin Neurol.* 2001;14(6):783–787.
22. Shimozawa N. Molecular and clinical aspects of peroxisomal diseases. *J Inherit Metab Dis.* 2007;30(2):193–197.
23. Moser AB, Rasmussen M, Naidu S, et al. Phenotype of patients with peroxisomal disorders subdivided into sixteen complementation groups. *J Pediatr.* 1995;127(1):13–22.
24. Shimozawa N, Tsukamoto T, Nagase T, et al. Identification of a new complementation group of the peroxisome biogenesis disorders and PEX14 as the mutated gene. *Hum Mutat.* 2004;23(6):552–558.
25. Wanders RJA BP, Heymans HSA. Single peroxisomal enzyme deficiencies. In: CR Scriver, AL Beaudet, WS Sly, D Valle, eds. *The Metabolic and Molecular Basis of Inherited Disease.* New York: McGraw-Hill; 2001:3219–3256.
26. Kemp S, Theodoulou FL, Wanders RJ. Mammalian peroxisomal ABC transporters: from endogenous substrates to pathology and clinical significance. *Br J Pharmacol.* 2011;164(7):1753–1766.
27. Kemp S, Wanders R. Biochemical aspects of X-linked adrenoleukodystrophy. *Brain Pathol.* 2010;20(4):831–837.
28. Govaerts L, Monnens L, Tegelaers W, et al. Cerebrohepato-renal syndrome of Zellweger: clinical symptoms and relevant laboratory findings in 16 patients. *Eur J Pediatr.* 1982;139(2):125–128.

29. Kelley RI. Review: the cerebrohepatorenal syndrome of Zellweger, morphologic and metabolic aspects. *Am J Med Genet.* 1983;16(4):503–517.

30. Wilson GN. What is Zellweger syndrome? *J Pediatr.* 1986;109(2):398.

31. Steinberg SJ, Dodt G, Raymond GV, et al. Peroxisome biogenesis disorders. *Biochim Biophys Acta.* 2006;1763(12):1733–1748.

32. Takahashi Y, Suzuki Y, Kumazaki K, et al. Epilepsy in peroxisomal diseases. *Epilepsia.* 1997;38(2):182–188.

33. Powers JM, Moser HW. Peroxisomal disorders: genotype, phenotype, major neuropathologic lesions, and pathogenesis. *Brain Pathol.* 1998;8(1):101–120.

34. Evrard P, Caviness VS, Jr, Prats-Vinas J, et al. The mechanism of arrest of neuronal migration in the Zellweger malformation: an hypothesis based upon cytoarchitectonic analysis. *Acta Neuropathol.* 1978;41(2):109–117.

35. Volpe JJ, Adams RD. Cerebro-hepato-renal syndrome of Zellweger: an inherited disorder of neuronal migration. *Acta Neuropathol.* 1972;20(3):175–198.

36. Faust PL, Banka D, Siriratsivawong R, et al. Peroxisome biogenesis disorders: the role of peroxisomes and metabolic dysfunction in developing brain. *J Inherit Metab Dis.* 2005;28(3):369–383.

37. Janssen A, Gressens P, Grabenbauer M, et al. Neuronal migration depends on intact peroxisomal function in brain and in extraneuronal tissues. *J Neurosci.* 2003;23(30):9732–9741.

38. Krysko O, Hulshagen L, Janssen A, et al. Neocortical and cerebellar developmental abnormalities in conditions of selective elimination of peroxisomes from brain or from liver. *J Neurosci Res.* 2007;85(1):58–72.

39. Kaufmann WE, Theda C, Naidu S, et al. Neuronal migration abnormality in peroxisomal bifunctional enzyme defect. *Ann Neurol.* 1996;39(2):268–271.

40. Baes M, Gressens P, Huyghe S, et al. The neuronal migration defect in mice with Zellweger syndrome (Pex5 knockout) is not caused by the inactivity of peroxisomal beta-oxidation. *J Neuropathol Exp Neurol.* 2002;61(4):368–374.

41. Krysko O, Bottelbergs A, Van Veldhoven P, et al. Combined deficiency of peroxisomal beta-oxidation and ether lipid synthesis in mice causes only minor cortical neuronal migration defects but severe hypotonia. *Mol Genet Metab.* 2010;100(1):71–76.

42. Gressens P. Mechanisms and disturbances of neuronal migration. *Pediatr Res.* 2000;48(6):725–730.

43. Adamo AM, Aloise PA, Pasquini JM. A possible relationship between concentration of microperoxisomes and myelination. *Int J Dev Neurosci.* 1986;4(6):513–517.

44. Kassmann CM, Lappe-Siefke C, Baes M, et al. Axonal loss and neuroinflammation caused by peroxisome-deficient oligodendrocytes. *Nat Genet.* 2007;39(8):969–976.

45. Hirrlinger J, Resch A, Gutterer JM, et al. Oligodendroglial cells in culture effectively dispose of exogenous hydrogen peroxide: comparison with cultured neurones, astroglial and microglial cells. *J Neurochem.* 2002;82(3):635–644.

46. Barkovich AJ, Peck WW. MR of Zellweger syndrome. *AJNR Am J Neuroradiol.* 1997;18(6):1163–1170.

47. Weller S, Rosewich H, Gartner J. Cerebral MRI as a valuable diagnostic tool in Zellweger spectrum patients. *J Inherit Metab Dis.* 2008;31:270–80.

48. Baes M, Aubourg P. Peroxisomes, myelination, and axonal integrity in the CNS. *Neuroscientist.* 2009;15(4):367–379.

49. Passarge E, McAdams AJ. Cerebro-hepato-renal syndrome. A newly recognized hereditary disorder of multiple congenital defects, including sudanophilic leukodystrophy, cirrhosis of the liver, and polycystic kidneys. *J Pediatr.* 1967;71(5):691–702.

50. Agamanolis DP, Robinson HB, Jr, Timmons GD. Cerebrohepato-renal syndrome. Report of a case with histochemical and ultrastructural observations. *J Neuropathol Exp Neurol.* 1976;35(3):226–246.

51. Powers JM, Moser HW, Moser AB, et al. Fetal cerebrohepatorenal (Zellweger) syndrome: dysmorphic, radiologic, biochemical, and pathologic findings in four affected fetuses. *Hum Pathol.* 1985;16(6):610–620.

52. Brites P, Waterham HR, Wanders RJ. Functions and biosynthesis of plasmalogens in health and disease. *Biochim Biophys Acta.* 2004;1636(2–3):219–231.

53. Wanders RJ, Waterham HR. Peroxisomal disorders: the single peroxisomal enzyme deficiencies. *Biochim Biophys Acta.* 2006;1763(12):1707–1720.

54. Brites P, Mooyer PA, El Mrabet L, et al. Plasmalogens participate in very-long-chain fatty acid-induced pathology. *Brain.* 2009;132(Pt 2):482–492.

55. Hulshagen L, Krysko O, Bottelbergs A, et al. Absence of functional peroxisomes from mouse CNS causes dysmyelination and axon degeneration. *J Neurosci.* 2008;28(15):4015–4127.

56. Theda C, Woody RC, Naidu S, et al. Increased very long chain fatty acids in patients on a ketogenic diet: a cause of diagnostic confusion. *J Pediatr.* 1993;122(5 Pt 1):724–726.

57. Oorthuys JW, Loewer-Sieger DH, Schutgens RB, et al. Peroxisomal dysfunction in chondrodysplasia punctata, rhizomelic type. *Ophthalmic Paediatr Genet.* 1987;8(3):183–185.

58. Heymans HS, Oorthuys JW, Nelck G, et al. Rhizomelic chondrodysplasia punctata: another peroxisomal disorder. *N Engl J Med.* 1985;313(3):187–188.

59. Brites P, Motley AM, Gressens P, et al. Impaired neuronal migration and endochondral ossification in Pex7 knockout mice: a model for rhizomelic chondrodysplasia punctata. *Hum Mol Genet.* 2003;12(18):2255–2267.

60. Van der Knaap MS, Breiter SN, Naidu S, et al. Defining and categorizing leukoencephalopathies of unknown origin: MR imaging approach. *Radiology.* 1999;213(1):121–133.

61. Alkan A, Kutlu R, Yakinci C, et al. Delayed myelination in a rhizomelic chondrodysplasia punctata case: MR spectroscopy findings. *Magn Reson Imaging.* 2003;21(1):77–80.

62. Powers JM, Kenjarski TP, Moser AB, et al. Cerebellar atrophy in chronic rhizomelic chondrodysplasia punctata: a potential role for phytanic acid and calcium in the death of its Purkinje cells. *Acta Neuropathol.* 1999;98(2):129–134.

63. Agamanolis DP, Novak RW. Rhizomelic chondrodysplasia punctata: report of a case with review of the literature and correlation with other peroxisomal disorders. *Pediatr Pathol Lab Med.* 1995;15(3):503–513.

64. Bams-Mengerink AM, Majoie CB, Duran M, et al. MRI of the brain and cervical spinal cord in rhizomelic chondrodysplasia punctata. *Neurology.* 2006;66(6):798–803; discussion 789.

65. Woody RC, Brodie M, Hampton DK, et al. Corn oil ketogenic diet for children with intractable seizures. *J Child Neurol.* 1988;3(1):21–24.

66. White AL, Modaff P, Holland-Morris F, et al. Natural history of rhizomelic chondrodysplasia punctata. *Am J Med Genet A.* 2003;118A(4):332–342.

67. Buoni S, Zannolli R, Waterham H, et al. D-Bifunctional protein deficiency associated with drug resistant infantile spasms. *Brain Dev.* 2007;29(1):51–54.

68. Moller G, Van Grunsven EG, Wanders RJ, et al. Molecular basis of D-bifunctional protein deficiency. *Mol Cell Endocrinol.* 2001;171(1–2):61–70.

69. Jiang LL, Kurosawa T, Sato M, et al. Physiological role of D-3-hydroxyacyl-CoA dehydratase/D-3-hydroxyacyl-CoA dehydrogenase bifunctional protein. *J Biochem.* 1997;121(3):506–513.

70. Jiang LL, Miyazawa S, Souri M, et al. Structure of D-3-hydroxyacyl-CoA dehydratase/D-3-hydroxyacyl-CoA dehydrogenase bifunctional protein. *J Biochem.* 1997;121(2):364–369.

71. Paton BC, Pollard AN. Molecular changes in the D-bifunctional protein cDNA sequence in Australasian patients belonging to the bifunctional protein complementation group. *Cell Biochem Biophys.* 2000;32(Spring):247–251.

72. Khan A, Wei XC, Snyder FF, et al. Neurodegeneration in D-bifunctional protein deficiency: diagnostic clues and natural history using serial magnetic resonance imaging. *Neuroradiology.* 2010;52(12):1163–1166.

73. Watkins PA, Chen WW, Harris CJ, et al. Peroxisomal bifunctional enzyme deficiency. *J Clin Invest.* 1989;83(3):771–777.

74. Itoh M, Suzuki Y, Akaboshi S, et al. Developmental and pathological expression of peroxisomal enzymes: their relationship of D-bifunctional protein deficiency and Zellweger syndrome. *Brain Res.* 2000;858(1):40–47.

75. Ferdinandusse S, Denis S, Mooyer PA, et al. Clinical and biochemical spectrum of D-bifunctional protein deficiency. *Ann Neurol.* 2006;59(1):92–104.

76. Bezman L, Moser AB, Raymond GV, et al. Adrenoleukodystrophy: incidence, new mutation rate, and results of extended family screening. *Ann Neurol.* 2001;49(4):512–517.

77. Stephenson DJ, Bezman L, Raymond GV. Acute presentation of childhood adrenoleukodystrophy. *Neuropediatrics.* 2000;31(6):293–297.

78. Smith KD, Kemp S, Braiterman LT, et al. X-linked adrenoleukodystrophy: genes, mutations, and phenotypes. *Neurochem Res.* 1999;24(4):521–535.

79. Powers JM. Adreno-leukodystrophy (adreno-testiculo-leukomyelo-neuropathic-complex). *Clin Neuropathol.* 1985;4(5):181–199.

80. Hein S, Schonfeld P, Kahlert S, et al. Toxic effects of X-linked adrenoleukodystrophy-associated, very long chain fatty acids on glial cells and neurons from rat hippocampus in culture. *Hum Mol Genet.* 2008;17(12):1750–1761.

81. Singh I, Pujol A. Pathomechanisms underlying X-adrenoleukodystrophy: a three-hit hypothesis. *Brain Pathol.* 2010;20(4):838–844.

82. Singh J, Khan M, Singh I. Silencing of Abcd1 and Abcd2 genes sensitizes astrocytes for inflammation: implication for X-adrenoleukodystrophy. *J Lipid Res.* 2009;50(1):135–147.

83. Di Biase A, Di Benedetto R, Fiorentini C, et al. Free radical release in C6 glial cells enriched in hexacosanoic acid: implication for X-linked adrenoleukodystrophy pathogenesis. *Neurochem Int.* 2004;44(4):215–221.

84. Moser HW, Mahmood A, Raymond GV. X-linked adrenoleukodystrophy. *Nat Clin Pract Neurol.* 2007;3(3):140–151.

85. Powers JM, Pei Z, Heinzer AK, et al. Adreno-leukodystrophy: oxidative stress of mice and men. *J Neuropathol Exp Neurol.* 2005;64(12):1067–1079.

86. Vargas CR, Wajner M, Sirtori LR, et al. Evidence that oxidative stress is increased in patients with X-linked adrenoleukodystrophy. *Biochim Biophys Acta.* 2004;1688(1):26–32.

87. Eichler FS, Ren JQ, Cossoy M, et al. Is microglial apoptosis an early pathogenic change in cerebral X-linked adrenoleukodystrophy? *Ann Neurol.* 2008;63(6):729–742.

88. Wang PJ, Hwu WL, Shen YZ. Epileptic seizures and electroencephalographic evolution in genetic leukodystrophies *J Clin Neurophysiol.* 2001;18(1):25–32.

89. Cappa M, Bizzarri C, Giannone G, et al. Is subclinical adrenal failure in Adrenoleukodystrophy/Adrenomyeloneuropathy (ALD/AMN) reversible? *J Endocrinol Invest.* 2011;34:753–756.

90. Cappa M, Bizzarri C, Vollono C, et al. Adrenoleukodystrophy. *Endocr Dev.* 2011;20:149–160.

91. Freedman BD, Hughan K, Garibaldi L. Hypoglycemic seizure. *Clin Pediatr (Phila).* 2010;49:1078–1080.

Leukodystrophies and Epilepsy

Davide Tonduti and Adeline Vanderver

INTRODUCTION

Inherited disorders of the white matter, or genetic leukoencephalopathies, primarily affect the myelinated structures in the brain and in some cases the peripheral nervous system, and are principally recognized based on abnormal white matter on neuroimaging (1). These disorders are classically thought to result in primary motor phenotypes, with lesser encephalopathy and particularly epilepsy than degenerative disorders primarily affecting the central nervous system neurons. However, there are several exceptions to this rule.

The first is that any end-stage leukoencephalopathy can result in secondary symptoms such as epilepsy. These include classic leukodystrophies such as metachromatic leukodystrophy or Krabbe. In general, however, these epilepsies are readily controlled with anticonvulsants and appear later in the disease course.

The second is that some classic leukodystrophies have frequent and significant seizures. The best example of this is Alexander's disease, in which seizures play a significant role in disease manifestations. In many cases, they may even be the presenting symptom.

The third and final exception is the result of the fact that a large number of disorders that are not in fact primary glial cell disorders may have secondary white matter abnormalities. These mimickers represent the largest proportion of patients with white matter abnormalities and epilepsy, in particular early in the disease course.

LEUKODYSTROPHIES WITH EPILEPSY AS A LATE DISEASE MANIFESTATION

Brain white matter is formed by several distinct cellular populations, including astrocytes, oligodendrocytes, and microglia. These glial cells carry out various functions, including guiding development, regulating extracellular concentrations of ions, metabolites, and neurotransmitters, and supporting neuronal and synaptic function (2). The interdependence of neuronal cells and their glial counterparts explains why virtually any primary white matter degeneration may cause secondary neuronal dysfunction and therefore epilepsy. Some specific examples are detailed below, but it is important to know that this list is not exhaustive and if a patient with another leukoencephalopathy manifests seizures, this is likely to be related to their underlying illness.

GLOBOID CELL LEUKODYSTROPHY (OR KRABBE DISEASE)

Globoid cell leukodystrophy (or Krabbe disease) is a leukodystrophy due to defective lysosomal degradation of galactosylceramide, causing an accumulation of psychosine, considered responsible for oligodendrocyte loss (3). The early infantile onset subtype is characterized by hyperirritability, unexplained fevers, hypertonicity, arrest of psychomotor development and after some months rapid motor and mental deterioration, opisthotonus, signs of peripheral nerve involvement, myoclonic jerks, seizures, and optic atrophy. Later onset forms have a more chronic and slowly progressive course with mental deterioration, spasticity, ataxia, dystonia, optic atrophy, seizures, and psychiatric symptoms (3). Epileptic seizures usually begin in the later phases of the disease but exceptionally they have been reported also at symptom onset (4).

METACHROMATIC LEUKODYSTROPHY

Metachromatic leukodystrophy (MLD) is another lysosomal storage disease in which a deficient activity of Arylsulfatase A results in a defect of degradation of sulfatides, which are important components of myelin. Arylsulfatase A deficiency may be the consequence of several different metabolic disorders: (1) a mutation in *ARSA* resulting in a primary Arylsulfatase A deficiency (5); (2) a deficiency of its cofactor, Saposin B, also resulting in Arylsulfatase A deficiency (6); and (3) a mutation in *SUMF1* resulting in a lack of a posttranslational modification that is common to all sulfatases. This Multiple Sulfatase Deficiency leads to a more complex clinical picture which combines features of classic MLD with those of mucopolysaccharidoses (7).

Late infantile and early juvenile MLD variants usually start after a variable symptom free period followed by the onset of ataxia, nystagmus, dysarthria, signs of a progressive polyneuropathy with mental deterioration. Progressively these children develop a spastic tetraplegia with absent deep tendon reflexes with bulbar and pseudobulbar symptoms, seizures, and more rarely dystonia (8). Late juvenile variants are dominated initially by behavioral abnormalities, including learning disabilities. Seizures are usually more frequent in later onset variants and in latest phases of earlier onset variants. More rarely, epileptic seizures at symptom onset have been reported (9).

X-LINKED ADRENOLEUKODYSTROPHY

X-linked adrenoleukodystrophy is a leukodystrophy due to mutations in *ABCD1*, a peroxisomal transporter, leading to an excess of very long-chain fatty acids, which cannot enter the peroxisome for beta oxidation. It is thought that accumulation of this substrate results in oxidative stress and inflammation with myelin destruction (10). The clinical picture is usually initially characterized by psychiatric symptoms, including attention deficit disorder. In some cases adrenocortical insufficiency may be the presenting sign (11). Over time, progressive spastic tetraplegia, visual loss, optic atrophy, hearing impairment and seizures appear as the disease progresses (12).

HEREDITARY DIFFUSE LEUKOENCEPHALOPATHY WITH SPHEROIDS

Hereditary diffuse leukoencephalopathy with spheroids (HDLS) is an adult onset leukodystrophy with an autosomal dominant pattern of inheritance recently attributed to mutations in the colony stimulating factor 1 receptor (*CSF1R*) (13, 14). These patients typically present with psychiatric changes or gait abnormality that progresses to include symptoms such as dementia, gait apraxia, spasticity, ataxia, and urinary incontinence (14). Seizures may be present early in the disease course and may cause significant morbidity (14).

Hypomyelinating leukodystrophies, defined by an unchanged pattern of deficient myelination on two MRIs at least 6 months apart in a child older than 1 y (1), may also have epilepsy in their symptom complex. The prototypic hypomyelinating leukodystrophy is *Pellizaeus–Merzbacher disease*. This x-linked disorder is consequent to mutations on *PLP1*, encoding the Proteolipid Protein, one of the major components of myelin (15). The classical phenotype is characterized by onset in the first year of life of nystagmoid eye movements often with shaking movements of the head. Progressive developmental delay, optic atrophy, spasticity, ataxia, and dystonia become evident (16). As in the other leukodystrophies, epileptic seizures may be part of the clinical picture in the advanced stages of the disease (12).

THE MOST EPILEPTOGENIC LEUKODYSTROPHY: ALEXANDER DISEASE

Alexander disease is an autosomal dominant or sporadic disease due to gain of function mutations in *GFAP*, which encodes an intermediate filament in astrocytes. It leads to an accumulation of mutated GFAP with resulting astrocyte dysfunction and demyelination (17). From a clinical perspective two main forms have been described: one with earlier onset, characterized by progressive downhill course, megalencephaly, psychomotor retardation, spastic tetraplegia (Type 1) and the other with juvenile or adult onset, more frequently characterized by bulbar and pseudobulbar signs and slow mental decline (type 2) (18). Seizures are frequently seen in type I Alexander Disease and often are the first identified symptom, with febrile seizures being a frequent presenting sign (18). The cause of the high frequency of epilepsy in this disorder is poorly understood, but synaptic transmission due to an impairment of astrocytic function has been hypothesized (17). Seizures in this disorder may be more difficult to control than in the above leukodystrophies, but are rarely refractory.

LEUKOENCEPHALOPATHIES WITH SECONDARY WHITE MATTER ABNORMALITIES

White matter abnormalities on neuroimaging may be due not only to a primary degeneration of glial cells but can also be the result of secondary injury in a primary neuronal degenerative disease or in a systemic disease with white matter manifestations (1). The list of these leukodystrophy mimickers is too broad to detail in this chapter (Table 27.1), but include a number of inborn errors of metabolism which can lead to

significant white matter abnormalities. These patients may initially present to the child neurologist as a leukoencephalopathy, later complicated by epilepsy and sometimes diagnostic systemic or biochemical features.

Neuronal disorders with white matter abnormalities on neuroimaging include heritable poliodystrophies such as *Neuronal Ceroid Lipofuscinosis*, a group of diseases caused by mutations in a group of genes *CLN1-8* and *CLN10* which encode a group of proteins expressed in the endosomal–lysosomal system (19). Clinically age of onset differs among the various subtypes and retinal degeneration, motor abnormalities, dementia, and most of all seizures are variably combined (20). White matter abnormalities, mainly in periventricular regions, is almost always present in early-onset subtypes and may initially cause physicians to suspect a primary leukodystrophy (20).

Another family of disorders include *GM1 and GM2 gangliosidoses*, which result from a deficiency of the enzymes beta-galactosidase (in GM1) and beta-hexosaminidase (in the GM2 subtypes including Tay–Sachs disease, AB variant, and Sandhoff disease). The resulting accumulation of gangliosides within central nervous system cells, in particular neurons, leads to a

TABLE 27.1 Inborn Errors of Metabolism With Significant White Matter Involvement

Inborn Errors of Metabolism
- Adenylosuccinatelyase deficiency
- Aspartylglucosaminuria
- Disorders of branched chain amino acids (BCAAS) and other amino acid disorders (including untreated propionic aciduria, methylmalonic aciduria, isovaleric aciduria, maple syrup urine disease (MSUD)) (excluding E3 subunit deficiency)
- Phenylketonuria (PKU)
- Hereditary homocystinurias
- Dihydropterine reductase (DHPR) deficiency
- D-2-Hydroxyglutaric aciduria (D2HGA 1 and 2)
- Defects in N-Glycan synthesis
- Defects in O-Glycan synthesis and other congenital muscular dystrophies
- Disorders of glycoprotein degradation (alpha mannosidosis, beta mannosidosis and sialidosis, excluding fucosidosis)

- Succinic semialdehyde dehydrogenase (SSDH) deficiency (or 4-Hydroxybutyric aciduria)
- Urea cycle disorders (Carbamoylphosphatesynthetase I deficiency, Ornithine trans-carboxylase deficiency, Citrullinemia type I, Argininosuccinicaciduria, Arginase deficiency, NAGS deficiency, HHH syndrome)
- Wilson's disease

Mitochondrial and Energy Metabolism Disorders
- Mitochondrial neurogastrointestinal encephalopathy (MNGIE)
- Mitochondrial myopathy, encephalopathy, lactic acidosis, and stroke (MELAS)
- Pyruvate carboxylase (PC) deficiency
- Pyruvate dehydrogenase deficiency
- Mitochondrial depletion syndromes (*POLG1* and others)

(continued)

TABLE 27.1   Inborn Errors of Metabolism With Significant White Matter Involvement (*continued*)

- Fatty acid hydroxylase-Associated neurodegeneration
- Fumarate hydratase deficiency
- Galactosemia type I
- Glutaric aciduria type I (GA-I)
- Glutaric aciduria type II (GA-II) or Multiple acyl-CoA dehydrogenase deficiency (MADD)
- GM1 and GM2-gangliosidosis, Infantile onset
- HMG-CoA lyase deficiency
- Menkes disease
- Molybdenum cofactor deficiency and isolated sulfite oxidase deficiency
- Mucolipidosis type IV
- Mucopolysaccharidosis including MPS type II (Hunter syndrome)
- Multiple carboxylase deficiency, including biotinidase deficiency and holocarboxylase synthase deficiency
- Neuronal Ceroid Lipofuscinoses (NCL), Infantile onset
- Niemann-Pick C
- Nonketotic hyperglycinemia
- Peroxisomal biogenesis disorders and single enzyme deficiencies
- Serine synthesis defects
- Sialic acid storage disorders

Other

- AGC1-related disorders
- AIMP1-related disorders
- Cockayne syndrome and trichothiodystrophy
- Dentatorubropallidoluysian atrophy (DRPLA)
- Familial Hemophagocytic lymphohistiocytosis
- Fragile X premutation
- Giant axonal neuropathy
- *GPR56* related disorders
- *HSPD1* related disorders (or Mitchap60)
- Hypomelanosis of Ito (HMI) (or incontinentia pigmenti achromians)
- Incontinentia pigmenti
- JAM3 related disorders
- MCT8 (*SLC16A2*) related disorders
- Myotonic dystrophy (DM)
- Neuronopathic form of malignant infantile osteopetrosis
- Oculocerebrorenal syndrome of Lowe (OCRL)
- Polycystic lipomembranous osteodysplasia with sclerosing leukoencephalopathy (PLOSL) or NasuHakola disease
- SPG11 and SPG15
- Spondyloenchondrodysplasia
- Woodhouse Sakatai Syndrome

neurodegenerative condition with dementia, spastic quadreplegia, visual loss and a cherry red spot, and often severe and difficult to control seizures. White matter abnormalities are often diffuse at presentation and may be mistaken for a hypomyelinating disorder. A distinguishing feature is the finding of hyperintense T2 signal abnormalities of the globus pallidus.

SIALIC ACID STORAGE DISORDERS—SALLA DISEASE, INFANTILE SIALIC ACID STORAGE DISEASE (ISSD) AND INTERMEDIATE FORM

Sialic acid storage disorders are another leukoencephalopathy, caused by mutations in *SLC17A5* resulting in a defect of Sialin, the lysosomal membrane-specific carrier for sialic acid and uronic acids. This is leads to an excessive storage of sialic acid in many tissues.

There is diffuse accumulation of storage material in neurons and astrocytes, but also generalized, severe demyelination and gliosis identified both on neuropathology (21) and neuroimaging which is consistent with hypomyelination (22, 23). In both Salla disease, the mildest phenotype and ISSD, the more severe phenotype, patients develop progressive cognitive decline and sometimes severe epilepsy.

A final example are the mitochondrial *POLG1-related disorders* in which early MRI may be dominated by the presence of white matter abnormalities, most of all when clinical onset is dated within the first months of life. Mutations of *POLG1* cause a deficient activity of mitochondrial DNA polymerase gamma (Polγ) leading to an impairment of normal replication and maintenance of mtDNA (24).

POLG1 related disorders may have an extremely variable clinical picture including phenotypes dominated by epilepsy such as in Alpers–Huttenlocher syndrome (AHS), which is characterized by childhood-onset severe drug-resistant seizures and hepatic failure (24).

CONCLUSION

Epilepsy typically occurs in the late stages of primary white matter heritable disease (classic leukodystrophies). However, exceptions to this rule exist, such as Alexander disease. In general, the presence of epileptic seizures early in the clinical course in a patient with white matter abnormalities on MRI should lead to consideration of numerous primary neuronal or systemic inborn errors of metabolism with secondary white matter abnormalities.

CLINICAL PEARLS

- Leukodystrophies classically result in primary motor phenotypes, with lesser degrees of encephalopathy and epilepsy (*although there are exceptions*).
- End stage leukoencephalopathy may result in epilepsy.
- Seizures are a significant manifestation of Alexander's disease and may be the presenting symptom.
- Most patients presenting with epilepsy and white matter abnormalities do not have primary leukodystrophies but instead secondary glial cell dysfunction due to severe neuronal disease.

REFERENCES

1. Schiffmann R and van der Knaap MS. Invited article: an MRI-based approach to the diagnosis of white matter disorders. *Neurology.* 2009;72(8):750–759.
2. Hansson E and Ronnback L. Glial neuronal signaling in the central nervous system. *FASEB J.* 2003;17(3):341–348.
3. Suzuki K. Globoid cell leukodystrophy (Krabbe's disease): Update. *J Child Neurol.* 2003;18(9):595–603.
4. Morse LE and Rosman NP. Myoclonic seizures in Krabbe disease: a unique presentation in late-onset type. *Pediatr Neurol.* 2006;35(2):154–157.
5. Gieselmann V. Metachromatic leukodystrophy: recent research developments. *J Child Neurol.* 2003;18(9):591–594.
6. Kuchar L, et al. Prosaposin deficiency and saposin B deficiency (activator-deficient metachromatic leukodystrophy): report on two patients detected by analysis of urinary sphingolipids and carrying novel PSAP gene mutations. *Am J Med Genet A.* 2009;149A(4):613–621.
7. Annunziata I, et al. Multiple sulfatase deficiency is due to hypomorphic mutations of the SUMF1 gene. *Hum Mutat.* 2007;28(9):928.
8. Gieselmann V and Krageloh-Mann I. Metachromatic leukodystrophy: an update. *Neuropediatrics.* 2010;41(1):1–6.
9. Bostantjopoulou S, et al. Seizures as a presenting feature of late onset metachromatic leukodystrophy. *Acta Neurol Scand.* 2000;102(3):192–195.
10. Singh I and Pujol A. Pathomechanisms underlying X-adrenoleukodystrophy: a three-hit hypothesis. *Brain Pathol.* 2010;20(4):838–844.
11. Moser HW. Therapy of X-linked adrenoleukodystrophy. *NeuroRx.* 2006;3(2):246–253.
12. Wang PJ, Hwu WL and Shen YZ. Epileptic seizures and electroencephalographic evolution in genetic leukodystrophies. *J Clin Neurophysiol.* 2001;18(1):25–32.
13. Rademakers R, et al. Mutations in the colony stimulating factor 1 receptor (CSF1R) gene cause hereditary diffuse leukoencephalopathy with spheroids. *Nat Genet.* 2011;44(2):200–205.
14. Sundal C, et al. Update of the original HDLS kindred: divergent clinical courses. *Acta Neurol Scand.* 2011.
15. Dhaunchak AS and Nave KA. A common mechanism of PLP/DM20 misfolding causes cysteine-mediated endoplasmic reticulum retention in oligodendrocytes and Pelizaeus Merzbacher disease. *Proc Natl Acad Sci.* 2007;104(45):17813–17818.
16. Koeppen AH and Robitaille Y. Pelizaeus–Merzbacher disease. *J Neuropathol Exp Neurol.* 2002;61(9):747–759.
17. Mignot C, et al. Alexander disease: Putative mechanisms of an astrocytic encephalopathy. *Cell Mol Life Sci (CMLS).* 2004;61(3):369–385.
18. Prust M, et al. GFAP mutations, age at onset, and clinical subtypes in Alexander disease. *Neurology.* 2011;77(13):1287–1294.
19. Cooper JD. The neuronal ceroid lipofuscinoses: the same, but different? *Biochem Soc Trans.* 2010;38(6):1448–1452.
20. Haltia M. The neuronal ceroid-lipofuscinoses. *J Neuropathol Exp Neurol.* 2003;62(1):1–13.
21. Lemyre E, et al. Clinical spectrum of infantile free sialic acid storage disease. *Am J Med Genet.* 1999;82(5):385–391.
22. Linnankivi T, Lonnqvist T and Autti T. A case of Salla disease with involvement of the cerebellar white matter. *Neuroradiology.* 2003;45(2):107–109.
23. Parazzini C, et al. Infantile sialic acid storage disease: Serial ultrasound and magnetic resonance imaging features. *AJNR Am J Neuroradiol.* 2003;24(3):398–400.
24. Saneto RP and Naviaux RK. Polymerase gamma disease through the ages. *Dev Disabil Res Rev.* 16(2):163–174.

28

Clinical Approach to Inherited Metabolic Epilepsies

Anna Lecticia Pinto and Phillip L. Pearl

The diagnosis of inherited metabolic epilepsies poses major challenges. Seizures are ominous signs of acquired or inherited brain injury and are a common heralding symptom to a multitude of neurological disorders. The combination of age of onset, seizure semiology, response to treatment and associated clinical features should alert the clinician for a possible underlying metabolic cause for epilepsy. The pathologic features and nature of metabolites accumulated in various elements of the nervous system may provide diagnostic clues. In addition, underlying gene defects for numerous epilepsy syndromes have been mapped to specific chromosomal regions and the causal mutation identified and characterized, although this is a rapidly expanding area of research and discovery.

Inherited metabolic epilepsies tend to have onset during the neonatorum, infancy, or early childhood. The history may provide relevant information regarding other common entities including prenatal or perinatal events, trauma, central nervous system infection, or systemic conditions. A clinical presentation of a newborn with poor feeding, hypotonia, lethargy, respiratory distress, or lactic acidosis associated with myoclonic seizures would be typical of an inherited metabolic disorder. Poor response to traditional antiepileptic drug therapy would merit evaluation for an inborn error of metabolism. Family history is a key point for inherited conditions and

genetically based epilepsies. A detailed physical exam should focus particularly on dysmorphic or neurocutaneous stigmata, micro- or macro-cephaly, and signs of systemic disease. Manifestations such as ocular abnormalities including cataracts, hearing impairment, cardiomyopathy, cholestasis, liver dysfunction, and renal cysts are important clues. The age of onset as well as seizure semiology should guide the clinician during the diagnostic approach. In utero onset seizures in particular are associated with metabolic disorders such as glycine encephalopathy and pyridoxine dependency. The extent of diagnostic investigations should be based on the clinical picture. EEG and MRI are essential components of this evaluation, although a caveat is that MRI abnormalities, especially atrophy, do not rule out metabolic errors and findings "consistent with" hypoxic–ischemic injury without a corroborating sentinel event or clinical history should not be considered a prior proof of hypoxic–ischemic encephalopathy.

The algorithm provided is meant to serve as a guide to enable a logical approach to disease screening and to choose specific diagnostic tests that may be required to identify certain inborn errors. The focus of the algorithm is on metabolic disorders and is not exhaustive. Special emphasis, however, is afforded to identifying treatable disorders that, without timely intervention, have dire prognoses.

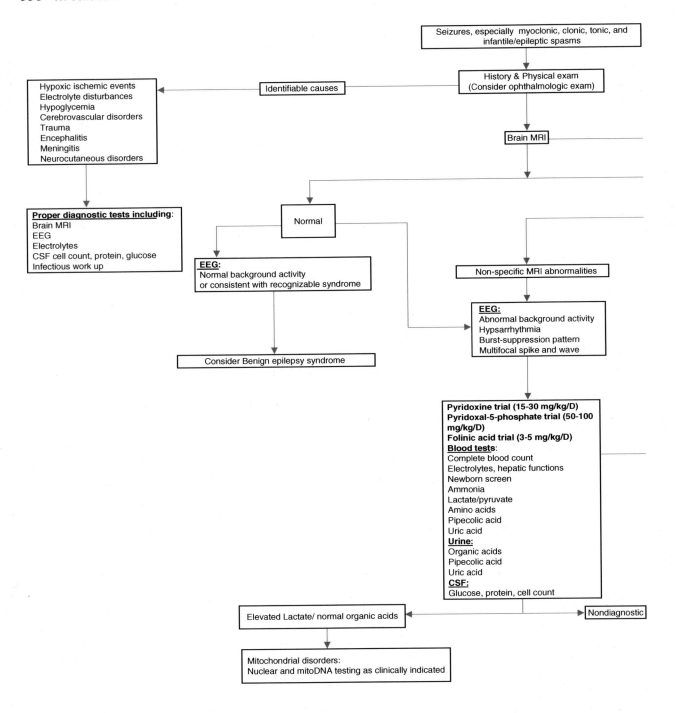

ARX   = Aristaless-related homeobox gene   GABA   = gamma-aminobutyric acid
CDG   = Congenital Disorders of Glycosylation   5-HIAA = 5-hydroxyindoleacetic acid
CDKL5 = cyclin-dependent kinase-like 5   HVA   = homovanilic acid
GAA   = guanidinoacetate   3-OMD   = 3-O-methyldopa

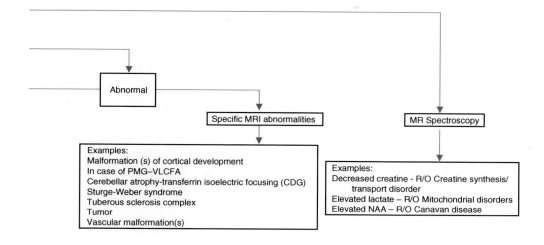

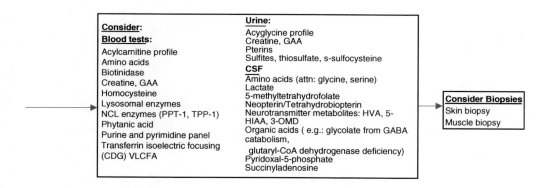

MECP2 = methyl CpG binding protein 2
PMG = Polymicrogyria
PPT1 = palmitoyl-protein thioesterase 1
SCN1A = sodium channel, voltage-gated, type I,
alpha subunit gene

TPP1 = tripeptidyl peptidase 1
UBE3A = ubiquitin protein ligase E3A
VLCFA = Very Long Chain Fatty Acids

Index